Coding for Pediatrics 2023

A Manual for Pediatric Documentation and Payment

For Use With AMA *CPT* 2023

28TH EDITION

Author
Committee on Coding and Nomenclature
American Academy of Pediatrics
Linda D. Parsi, MD, MBA, CPEDC, FAAP, Editor

American Academy of Pediatrics

DEDICATED TO THE HEALTH OF ALL CHILDREN®

American Academy of Pediatrics Publishing Staff

Mary Lou White, *Chief Product and Services Officer/SVP, Membership, Marketing, and Publishing*

Mark Grimes, *Vice President, Publishing*

Mary Kelly, *Senior Editor, Professional/Clinical Publishing*

Laura Underhile, *Editor, Professional/Clinical Publishing*

Leesa Levin-Doroba, *Production Manager, Practice Management*

Amanda Helmholz, *Medical Copy Editor*

Peg Mulcahy, *Manager, Art Direction and Production*

Mary Jo Reynolds, *Marketing Manager, Practice Publications*

Published by the American Academy of Pediatrics
345 Park Blvd
Itasca, IL 60143
Telephone: 630/626-6000
Facsimile: 847/434-8000
www.aap.org

The American Academy of Pediatrics is an organization of 67,000 primary care pediatricians, pediatric medical subspecialists, and pediatric surgical specialists dedicated to the health, safety, and well-being of all infants, children, adolescents, and young adults.

While every effort has been made to ensure the accuracy of this publication, the American Academy of Pediatrics does not guarantee that it is accurate, complete, or without error.

The recommendations in this publication do not indicate an exclusive course of treatment or serve as a standard of medical care. Variations, taking into account individual circumstances, may be appropriate. Vignettes are provided to illustrate correct coding applications and are not intended to offer advice on the practice of medicine.

Any websites, brand names, products, or manufacturers are mentioned for informational and identification purposes only and do not imply an endorsement by the American Academy of Pediatrics (AAP). The AAP is not responsible for the content of external resources. Information was current at the time of publication.

This publication has been developed by the American Academy of Pediatrics. The contributors are expert authorities in the field of pediatrics. No commercial involvement of any kind has been solicited or accepted in the development of the content of this publication. Disclosures: Dr Lago disclosed an employee relationship with Cotiviti, Inc. Dr Parsi disclosed an ownership and consulting relationship with The PEDS MD Company and is part of the Mead Johnson Speaker Bureau.

Please visit www.aap.org/cfp2023 or www.aap.org/errata for an up-to-date list of any applicable errata for this publication.

Special discounts are available for bulk purchases of this publication. Email Special Sales at nationalaccounts@aap.org for more information.

© 2023 American Academy of Pediatrics

All rights reserved. No part of this publication may be reproduced, stored in a retrieval system, or transmitted in any form or by any means—electronic, mechanical, photocopying, recording, or otherwise—without prior written permission from the publisher (locate title at https://publications.aap.org/aapbooks and click on © Get Permissions; you may also fax the permissions editor at 847/434-8780 or email permissions@aap.org). First edition published 1987; 28th, 2023.

CPT copyright 2022 American Medical Association (AMA). All rights reserved.

Fee schedules, relative value units, conversion factors, and/or related components are not assigned by the AMA, are not part of *CPT,* and the AMA is not recommending their use. The AMA does not directly or indirectly practice medicine or dispense medical services. The AMA assumes no liability for data contained or not contained herein.

CPT is a registered trademark of the AMA.

This publication has prior approval of the American Academy of Professional Coders (AAPC) for 4.0 continuing education units. Granting of this approval in no way constitutes endorsement by the AAPC of the publication content or publication sponsor.

Printed in the United States of America

11-35S 1 2 3 4 5 6 7 8 9 10
MA1068
ISBN: 978-1-61002-640-6
eBook: 978-1-61002-641-3
Print ISSN: 1537-324X
Online ISSN: 2833-4361

2022–2023 Committee on Coding and Nomenclature

Eileen D. Brewer, MD, FAAP, Chairperson

Margie C. Andreae, MD, FAAP

Joel F. Bradley, MD, FAAP

Mark Joseph, MD, FAAP

David M. Kanter, MD, MBA, CPC, FAAP, Immediate Past Chairperson

Steven E. Krug, MD, FAAP

Edward A. Liechty, MD, FAAP

Jeffrey F. Linzer Sr, MD, FAAP

Linda D. Parsi, MD, MBA, CPEDC, FAAP

Renee F. Slade, MD, FAAP

Liaisons

Kathleen K. Cain, MD, FAAP

AAP Section on Administration and Practice Management

Kathryn B. Lalor, MD, FAAP

AAP Section on Early Career Physicians

Benjamin Shain, MD, PhD

American Academy of Child and Adolescent Psychiatry

Samuel D. Smith, MD, FAAP

American Pediatric Surgical Association

2022–2023 AAP Coding Publications Editorial Advisory Board

Linda D. Parsi, MD, MBA, CPEDC, FAAP, Editor in Chief

Cheryl Arnold, MHSA, FACMPE

Greg Barabell, MD, CPC, FAAP

Vita Boyar, MD, FAAP

Joel F. Bradley, MD, FAAP

Timothy Ryan Hensley, MD, CPC, CPEDC, FAAP

David M. Kanter, MD, MBA, CPC, FAAP

Steven E. Krug, MD, FAAP

Jamie C. Lago, MD, CPC, FAAP

Edward A. Liechty, MD, FAAP

Jeffrey F. Linzer Sr, MD, FAAP

Richard A. Molteni, MD, FAAP

Karen Nauman, MD, FAAP

Piedade Oliveira-Silva, MD, FAAP

Julia M. Pillsbury, DO, FAAP

Renee F. Slade, MD, FAAP

Karla Nickolas Swatski, MD, FAAP

Sanjeev Y. Tuli, MD, FAAP

AAP Staff

Linda Walsh, MAB

Teri Salus, MPA, CPC, CPEDC

Consulting Editor

Cindy Hughes, CPC, CFPC

Disclaimer

Every effort has been made to include the new and revised 2023 *Current Procedural Terminology* (*CPT*); *International Classification of Diseases, 10th Revision, Clinical Modification* (*ICD-10-CM*); and Healthcare Common Procedure Coding System (HCPCS) codes, their respective guidelines, and other revisions that might have been made. Because of our publishing deadlines and the publication date of the American Medical Association *CPT*, additional revisions and/or additional codes may have been published subsequent to the date of this printing. It is the responsibility of the reader to use this manual as a companion to the *CPT, ICD-10-CM,* and HCPCS publications. Vignettes are provided throughout this publication to illustrate correct coding applications. They are not intended to offer medical advice on the practice of medicine. Further, it is the reader's responsibility to routinely access the American Academy of Pediatrics website (www.aap.org/cfp2023 or www.aap.org/errata) for any errata in the published version. At the time of this publication, final changes for 2023 codes and Medicare payment policies were pending. See www.aap.org/coding for updates.

Copyright Acknowledgment

Current Procedural Terminology (*CPT*) is a listing of descriptive terms and 5-digit numeric identifying codes and modifiers for reporting medical services and procedures performed by physicians. This presentation includes only the *CPT* descriptive terms, numeric identifying codes, and modifiers for reporting medical services and procedures that were selected by the American Academy of Pediatrics (AAP) for inclusion in this publication. The inclusion of a *CPT* service or procedure description and its code number in this publication does not restrict its use to a particular specialty group. Any procedure or service in this publication may be used to report the services provided by any qualified physician or, when appropriate, other qualified health care professional.

The American Medical Association (AMA) and the AAP assume no responsibility for the consequences attributable to or related to any use or interpretation of any information or views contained in or not contained in this publication.

Any 5-digit numeric *CPT* code, service descriptions, instructions, and/or guidelines are copyright 2022 (or such other date of publication of *CPT* as defined in the federal copyright laws) AMA. All rights reserved.

The most current *CPT* is available from the AMA.

No fee schedules, basic unit values, relative value guides, conversion factors or scales, or components thereof are included in *CPT*.

Equity, Diversity, and Inclusion Statement

The American Academy of Pediatrics is committed to principles of equity, diversity, and inclusion in its publishing program. Editorial boards, author selections, and author transitions (publication succession plans) are designed to include diverse voices that reflect society as a whole. Editor and author teams are encouraged to actively seek out diverse authors and reviewers at all stages of the editorial process. Publishing staff are committed to promoting equity, diversity, and inclusion in all aspects of publication writing, review, and production.

Contents

This publication has prior approval of the American Academy of Professional Coders (AAPC) for 4.0 continuing education units (CEUs). Granting of this approval in no way constitutes endorsement by the AAPC of the publication content or publication sponsor. To earn your CEUs, complete the 40-question quiz online (www.aap.org/cfp2023). Click on "2023 AAPC CEU Quiz."

Online Exclusive Content

The following online exclusive content can be accessed at www.aap.org/cfp2023 by following the directions on the inside front cover of this book. (Readers who purchased this product as an eBook have automatic access to the content and do not need to redeem a code.)

- AAP Position on Medicare Consultation Policy
- Asthma, Head Injury, and Laceration: Coding Continuums
- Cardiac Catheterization for Congenital Heart Defect: Code Chart
- Care Management Tracking Worksheet Template
- Care Plan Oversight Billing Worksheet Template
- Centrally Inserted Central Venous Catheter: Codes for Insertion and Replacement
- Coding Education Quiz/Continuing Education Units/Answer Key
- Commonly Administered Pediatric Vaccine Updates
- Emergency Department Procedures
- Evaluation and Management Service Coding in Nursing and Residential Treatment Facilities
- FAQ: Immunization Administration
- General Documentation Checklist
- Global Per Diem Critical Care Codes: Direct Supervision and Reporting Guidelines
- Hospital or Observation Evaluation and Management Services: Code Selection Requirements
- Incident-to Services by Nonphysician Professionals and Clinical Staff: Medicare Requirements
- Medications for Pediatrics: Most Common
- Monthly Care Management and Care Plan Oversight Services: A Comparison
- Office Procedures and Global Days
- Peripherally Inserted Central Venous Catheter: Codes
- Prepare Your Office for a Payer Audit Site Visit
- Preventive Medicine Encounters: What's Included? (Letter Template)
- RUC Times and Values for Pediatric Critical Care/Intensive Care Services
- Screening Laboratory Tests and Codes
- Skin Grafts of Infants and Children: Codes
- Times and Values for Pediatric Critical Care/Intensive Care Services

At www.aap.org/cfp2023, you can also access links to the following American Academy of Pediatrics (AAP) coding resources:

- AAP Coding Hotline
- AAP coding webinars
- *AAP Pediatric Coding Newsletter*™
- AAP Refusal to Vaccinate forms (English and Spanish)
- AAP/Bright Futures "Recommendations for Preventive Pediatric Health Care" (periodicity schedule)
- Coding fact sheets
- Standardized screening/testing coding fact sheet for primary care pediatricians: developmental/emotional/behavioral
- "2022 RBRVS: What Is It and How Does It Affect Pediatrics?"
- "When is it Appropriate to Report an Evaluation & Management Service During Immunization Administration?"

Foreword

The American Academy of Pediatrics (AAP) is pleased to publish the 28th edition of *Coding for Pediatrics,* an instructional manual and reference tool for use by primary care pediatricians, pediatric subspecialists, and others involved in the provision and reporting of care provided to children. This manual supports the delivery of quality care to children by providing the pediatric practitioner with the knowledge to best support appropriate business practices. This edition includes the 2023 *Current Procedural Terminology* (*CPT*) and *International Classification of Diseases, 10th Revision, Clinical Modification* (*ICD-10-CM*) code changes with guidelines for their application.

This edition introduces a wide range of new codes and guidelines, including extensive revisions to many categories of evaluation and management (E/M) services and new codes describing surgical and digital medicine services. In addition, this manual provides pediatric-specific guidance and examples of documentation and code selection using current E/M coding guidelines and other procedural services.

For ease of reference, *Coding for Pediatrics 2023* is divided into the following parts:

- **Part 1. Coding Basics and Business Essentials** includes information on code sets, modifiers, compliance, and business topics such as billing and payment methodologies.
- **Part 2. Primarily for the Office and Other Outpatient Settings** includes information on coding and billing for services such as office visits, outpatient consultations, and preventive services.
- **Part 3. Primarily for Hospital Settings** includes information on coding for facility-based services including emergency department and other hospital E/M services and surgical procedures.
- **Part 4. Digital Medicine Services** includes discussion of the evolving codes for reporting telemedicine services and remote monitoring and interpretation of patient data.
- Quick references to *CPT* and *ICD-10-CM* code changes applicable to pediatrics are provided in **appendixes I and II**. A table of pediatric vaccine product codes can be found in **Appendix III**.
- A **continuing education quiz** to earn 4.0 continuing education units from the American Academy of Professional Coders is included at www.aap.org/cfp2023.
- Supplemental material providing a wealth of information can be found on the *Coding for Pediatrics* website (www.aap.org/cfp2023), including printable quick reference tables for selecting levels of E/M services.

Each chapter includes "Test Your Knowledge!" questions (answers can be located in **Appendix IV**). Additionally, resources for more information on each chapter's contents can be located at the end of chapter.

In 2023, the AAP is also pleased to offer *Coding for Pediatrics 2023* as an eBook on a new, searchable platform.

Coding for Pediatrics 2023 does not replace *CPT, ICD-10-CM,* or the Healthcare Common Procedure Coding System; rather, it supplements those manuals. Every effort has been made to include the 2023 codes and their respective guidelines; however, revised codes and/or guidelines may have been published subsequent to the date of this printing. Errata to this manual will be posted as appropriate on the *Coding for Pediatrics* website (www.aap.org/cfp2023) or www.aap.org/errata.

The AAP actively works with the American Medical Association (AMA) *CPT* Editorial Panel and the AMA/Specialty Society Relative Value Scale Update Committee (RUC) to develop pediatric specialty codes and assign them appropriate relative value units. Since 1995, the AAP has contributed to the process that evaluates and reviews changes to the Medicare Resource-Based Relative Value Scale (RBRVS). Pediatricians have been actively involved in the RUC process to develop work valuation and direct practice expense input recommendations for all existing codes. As importantly, the AAP is represented on the AMA *CPT* Editorial Advisory Panel and on the *ICD-10-CM* Editorial Advisory Board. The AAP continues to be involved in all areas of payment. The AAP Committee on Coding and Nomenclature oversees all areas of coding as related to pediatrics, including *CPT* procedure coding, *ICD-10-CM* diagnosis coding, and the valuation of *CPT* services through the Medicare RBRVS.

The AAP will continue to request new code changes and attempt to expeditiously notify membership of changes through various means. The *AAP Pediatric Coding Newsletter,* a monthly newsletter available in print and online formats, provides up-to-date coding and payment information. The newsletter and other online resources can be accessed through the AAP newsletter website (https://coding.aap.org). Other resources include coding seminars presented at the AAP National Conference & Exhibition; webinars (located at https://coding.aap.org/webinars); instructional materials in *AAP News,* including the Coding Corner; *Pediatric ICD-10-CM: A Manual for Provider-Based Coding; Pediatric Office-Based Evaluation and Management Coding: 2021 Revisions; Pediatric Evaluation and Management Coding Revisions: Facility and Office Services;* and various quick reference cards. Use of these resources should provide pediatricians with the skills needed to report their services appropriately. The AAP Child Health Financing Strategy staff stands ready to assist with coding problems and questions not covered in this manual. The AAP Coding Hotline and Hassle Factor Form can be found at https://form.jotform.com/Subspecialty/aapcodinghotline.

Acknowledgments

Coding for Pediatrics 2023 is the product of the efforts of many dedicated individuals.

Our mission is to make coding easier to understand so pediatric providers can continue to serve children well. We have sought to make this book easier to understand by categorizing care areas and by using many examples (vignettes) of different coding situations. This knowledge is key to helping all pediatric providers stay in compliance and correctly code with confidence. We hope you enjoy reading this book, and we will continue to strive to always serve you with excellence.

This work has been made immeasurably easier and the final edition dramatically improved by the dedicated work of many collaborators. First and foremost, I must thank Cindy Hughes, CPC, CFPC, consulting editor, for her professional input. Additionally, I must thank the Committee on Coding and Nomenclature (COCN) support staff at the American Academy of Pediatrics (AAP), particularly Becky Dolan, MPH, CPC, CPEDC, for her many excellent suggestions and for her review of major portions of the project and Linda Walsh, MAB, for providing and coordinating additional reviews. Thank you also to Teri Salus, MPA, CPC, CPEDC, for her review of new *Current Procedural Terminology* (*CPT*) codes and suggestions for changes to content. I would also like to thank the members of COCN and the AAP Coding Publications Editorial Advisory Board. The members of these groups have each contributed extensive time in reviewing and updating content of the manual. We want to especially thank the following reviewers:

Cheryl Arnold, MHSA, FACMPE
Greg Barabell, MD, CPC, FAAP
Vita Boyar, MD, FAAP
Timothy Ryan Hensley, MD, CPC, CPEDC, FAAP
David M. Kanter, MD, MBA, CPC, FAAP
Jamie C. Lago, MD, CPC, FAAP
Edward A. Liechty, MD, FAAP
Jeffrey F. Linzer Sr, MD, FAAP
Richard A. Molteni, MD, FAAP
Karen Nauman, MD, FAAP
Piedade Oliveira-Silva, MD, FAAP
Julia M. Pillsbury, DO, FAAP
Renee F. Slade, MD, FAAP
Karla Nickolas Swatski, MD, FAAP
Sanjeev Y. Tuli, MD, FAAP

None of this work is possible without the support of the COCN members who work tirelessly to develop and value codes and fight for pediatrics "at the table." The committee strives to keep pediatrics at the forefront of coding and valuation. The excellent teams that follow are truly experts in these areas and are devoted to representing the AAP and its members:

CPT Editorial Panel Advisory Committee Team
Joel F. Bradley, MD, FAAP (*CPT* Advisor)
Renee F. Slade, MD, FAAP (*CPT* Alternate Advisor)
Teri Salus, MPA, CPC, CPEDC (AAP Staff to *CPT*)

American Medical Association/Specialty Society Relative Value Scale Update Committee (RUC) Team
Steven E. Krug, MD, FAAP (RUC Advisor)
Margie C. Andreae, MD, FAAP (RUC Representative)
Eileen D. Brewer, MD, FAAP (RUC Alternate Representative)
Linda Walsh, MAB (AAP Staff to RUC)

International Classification of Diseases (ICD) Team
Jeffrey F. Linzer Sr, MD, FAAP (AAP Representative to *ICD*)
Edward A. Liechty, MD, FAAP (AAP Alternate Representative to *ICD*)
Teri Salus, MPA, CPC, CPEDC (AAP Staff to *ICD*)

I am most grateful to the invaluable input of the following AAP committees and individuals:
- Committee on Medical Liability and Risk Management, specifically, Richard L. Oken, MD, FAAP; Craig H. Gosdin, MD, FAAP; and AAP staff Julie Ake, senior health policy analyst

- Payer Advocacy Advisory Committee, specifically, Sue Kressly, MD, FAAP, and AAP staff Teresa Salaway, senior health policy analyst
- Section on Neonatal-Perinatal Medicine coding trainers

In addition, we reached out to other AAP members for their expertise on specific content areas.

This project would not have been completed were it not for the outstanding work of AAP staff. In Membership, Marketing, and Publishing, Mary Kelly, senior editor, professional/clinical publishing; Laura Underhile, editor, professional/clinical publishing; Leesa Levin-Doroba, production manager, practice management; Amanda Helmholz, medial copy editor; Peg Mulcahy, manager, art direction and production; and Mary Jo Reynolds, marketing manager, practice publications, deserve special recognition for their outstanding skill and dedication to this project. At the AAP, I especially appreciate the support and professional expertise of Linda Walsh, MAB, senior manager, healthy policy and coding, and AAP staff support to the AAP COCN, dedicated advocates for all of us who medically care for children. A special thank-you to our AAP Board of Directors reviewers, Michelle Fiscus, MD, FAAP, and Jeannette Gaggino, MD, FAAP. We are so grateful to have their leadership and review for this manual!

Finally, all of us would like to give a big thank-you to all our readers, billers, coders, medical team, and dedicated pediatric providers who work tirelessly around the clock to best care for all children. Your work inspires us to work very hard behind the scenes to provide you the latest and most accurate coding information. We are always open to ideas to better serve you and welcome your suggestions. By all of us working together, we can accomplish the highest standards of care and be a voice for our children and their future.

Respectfully,
Linda D. Parsi, MD, MBA, CPEDC, FAAP
Editor

How to Use This Manual

Step 1. Use the table of contents or the index to locate information on specific services, codes, or broader subjects.	**Contents** An Introduction to the Official Code Sets............5 Telling the Encounter Story...........................6
Step 2. Use chapter content to review code descriptors and instructions for reporting. Before reporting, verify current codes and complete selection and reporting instructions in the appropriate code set manual or application.	▲**99238** Hospital inpatient or observation discharge day management; 30 minutes or less on the date of the encounter ▲**99239** more than 30 minutes on the date of the encounter Same date admission and discharge services, performed at 2 distinct encounters, are reported with codes **99234–99236**. For admission and discharge services provided at 1 encounter (1 patient visit), report **99221–99223**.

Step 3. Examples are used as guidance on meeting the criteria specified by codes and reporting instructions. However, note that codes must be assigned on the basis of the service provided and supporting documentation.	➤ **A 1-year-old patient presents with a high fever and lethargy.**
	Plan: The patient is admitted to the hospital for diagnostic evaluation to rule out sepsis.
	    Level of problems addressed ⅠⅠ⟹ *High*
	    Teaching Point: The clinical indications of possible sepsis in this patient represent a high-complexity problem.

Step 4. Note highlights and takeaways in each chapter.	● The 4 code sets that are used for reporting professional services are *ICD-10-CM*, HCPCS, *CPT*, and the NDC.
Step 5. Resources for additional information are listed at the end of each chapter and are included at www.aap.org/cfp2023.	CHAPTER 15. EMERGENCY DEPARTMENT SERVICES 373 **Resources** **AAP Coding Assistance and Education** *AAP Pediatric ICD-10-CM 2023: A Manual for Provider-Based Coding* (https://shop.aap.org/pediatric-icd-10-cm-2023-8th-edition-paperback) *ICD-10-CM resources* (www.aap.org/en/practice-management/practice-financing/coding-and-valuation/icd-10-cm-resources) **AAP Pediatric Coding Newsletter™** "Initial Fracture Care: Musculoskeletal or Evaluation and Management," February 2021 (https://doi.org/10.1542/pcco_book202_document005) "You Code It! Integumentary Repair," April 2020 (https://doi.org/10.1542/pcco_book192_document003) **Online Exclusive Content at www.aap.org/cfp2023** "Asthma, Head Injury, and Laceration: Coding Continuums" "Emergency Department Procedures"
Step 6. Although every effort is made to provide accurate and up-to-date coding guidance, changes do happen. Any corrections and code or instruction changes published subsequent to the date of this printing are included at www.aap.org/cfp2023 or www.aap.org/errata.	

Part 1
Coding Basics and Business Essentials

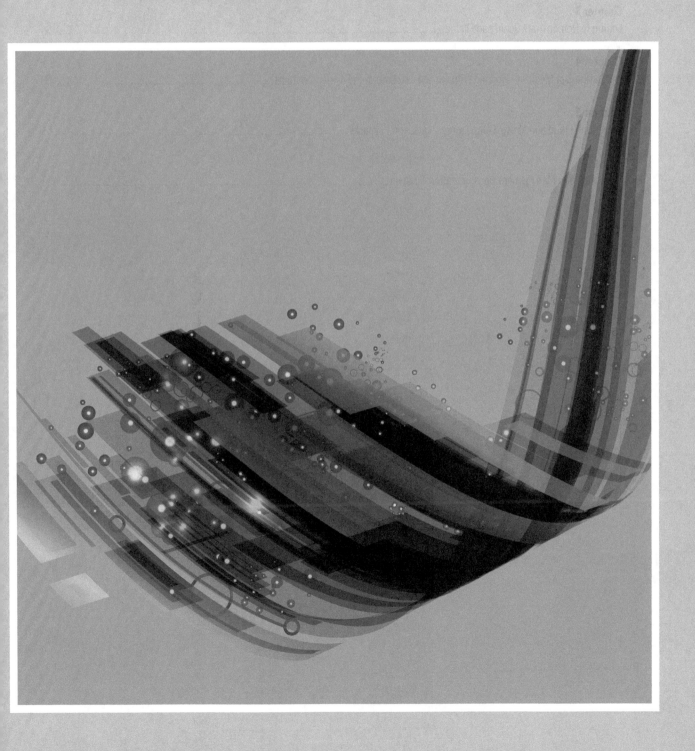

Part 1. Coding Basics and Business Essentials

The Basics of Coding

CPT copyright 2022 American Medical Association. All rights reserved.

Contents

Chapter Highlights

- Identify each of 4 code sets primarily used by physicians and other qualified health care professionals (QHPs) to report professional services.
- Use codes for conveying information to a payer in lieu of submitting actual documentation of an encounter or service.
- Explain the structure and general conventions of each code set.
- Summarize important considerations for selecting and transferring codes to claims.

An Introduction to the Official Code Sets

This chapter introduces the official code sets used for reporting pediatric professional services and briefly discusses the guidelines and conventions of each code set.

In the United States, the Health Insurance Portability and Accountability Act (HIPAA) of 1996 requires the use of 5 specific code sets for the purpose of health care transactions. The 4 code sets primarily used by physicians are listed in **Table 1-1**. The fifth designated code set, *Code on Dental Procedures and Nomenclature* (*CDT*), is primarily used to report dental procedures to dental insurance plans.

The place of service code set, maintained by the Centers for Medicare & Medicaid Services (CMS), is an additional code set that is required on claims. Place of service codes are 2-digit codes that identify the setting (**11**, office) in which a service was provided such that a claims system can differentiate sites of service to apply payer policies and payment differentials (eg, facility or non-facility relative value units). Practice management and billing systems often automatically assign place of service codes based on the site of service selected during charge entry. See **Chapter 4** for more information on place of service codes.

Every HIPAA code set, other than *CDT*, facilitates communication of standardized health information for purposes such as prior authorization of medical care and submission of health care claims in pediatric practice. Understanding the purpose and constructs of the 4 code sets used by physicians is important for successful interactions with health plans and supports accurate health care statistics.

New and revised codes are listed in quick references in **appendixes I** and **II**.

- Quick Reference to 2023 *ICD-10-CM* Pediatric Code Changes (effective with services provided on or after October 1, 2022)
- Quick Reference to 2023 *CPT*® Pediatric Code Changes (effective with services provided on or after January 1, 2023)

This chapter discusses pertinent guidelines and key points for accurately reporting codes. Refer to the American Academy of Pediatrics (AAP) manual, *Pediatric Coding Basics*, for more information on each code set.

Table 1-1. Health Insurance Portability and Accountability Act of 1996 Code Sets

Code Set	Used to Report	Examples
ICD-10-CM	Diagnoses and other reasons for encounters	**Z00.110** Health examination for newborn under 8 days old **Z00.111** Health examination for newborn 8 to 28 days old
CPT[a]	Most professional services, vaccine and immunoglobulin products, and performance measurement tracking	**99291** Critical care, evaluation and management of the critically ill or critically injured patient; first 30–74 minutes
HCPCS[b]	Supplies, medications, and services (when a *CPT* code does not describe the service as covered by health plan benefits)	**S0630** Removal of sutures; by a physician other than the physician who originally closed the wound **J0171** Injection, Adrenalin, epinephrine, 0.1 mg
NDC	Specific prescription drug, vaccine, and insulin products and dosages	**00006-4047-41** RotaTeq 2-mL single-dose tube, package of 10 **60574-4114-01** Synagis 0.5-mL in 1 vial, single dose

Abbreviations: CMS, Centers for Medicare & Medicaid Services; *CPT, Current Procedural Terminology*; HCPCS, Healthcare Common Procedure Coding System; *ICD-10-CM, International Classification of Diseases, 10th Revision, Clinical Modification*; NDC, National Drug Code.

[a] Also known as Level I of the HCPCS code set.
[b] Refers to Level II HCPCS codes assigned by the CMS.

● indicates a new code; ▲, revised; #, re-sequenced; ✚, add-on; ★, audiovisual technology; and ◀, synchronous interactive audio.

Telling the Encounter Story

Because physicians do not submit full documentation, various code sets and other supportive information (eg, procedure code modifiers) tell payers what happened and what is represented by the fees listed on each claim line (**Table 1-2**).

Table 1-2. The Encounter Story Told Through Codes	
Code or Modifier	**Information Provided**
ICD-10-CM	Why were services rendered?
CPT/HCPCS	What services or supplies were provided?
Modifier	Was something about the service altered or unusual?
NDC	What specific medicine or vaccine product and dosage were administered?

Abbreviations: *CPT, Current Procedural Terminology;* HCPCS, Healthcare Common Procedure Coding System; *ICD-10-CM, International Classification of Diseases, 10th Revision, Clinical Modification;* NDC, National Drug Code.

Codes submitted on a claim tell the story of what happened during a patient encounter. However, documentation of an encounter must support the codes assigned for each diagnosis and service and may be requested by a payer to support the accuracy of code assignment. The following 7 general principles of documentation apply to all services:

1. The medical record should be complete and legible.
2. The documentation of each patient encounter should include
   - Reason for the encounter and relevant history, physical examination findings, and prior diagnostic test results
   - Assessment, clinical impression, or diagnosis
   - Plan for care
   - Date and legible identity of the observer
3. If not documented, the rationale for ordering diagnostic and other ancillary services should be easily inferred.
4. Past and present diagnoses should be accessible to the treating and/or consulting physician.
5. Appropriate health risk factors should be identified. Also, social determinants of health should be documented.
6. The patient's progress, response to and changes in treatment, and revision of diagnosis should be documented.
7. The *Current Procedural Terminology* (CPT) and *International Classification of Diseases, 10th Revision, Clinical Modification* (ICD-10-CM) codes reported on the health insurance claim form or billing statement should be supported by the documentation in the medical record.

International Classification of Diseases, 10th Revision, Clinical Modification (ICD-10-CM)

Physicians assign diagnoses and other reasons for encounters to which *ICD-10-CM* codes are assigned for use in payment and public health data.

Although the values assigned to procedure codes are the basis for amounts paid for services, payers are increasingly using *ICD-10-CM* codes when determining the appropriateness of services submitted on a claim (eg, level of evaluation and management [E/M] service). *ICD-10-CM* codes are also used in prior authorization of services. Use of the most specific code for the diagnosis known at the time of an encounter may facilitate both payment and approval of additional health care services.

Updates to *ICD-10-CM* are implemented each April 1 and October 1 following publication a few months before implementation.

Oversight and resolution of coding questions related to *ICD-10-CM* is performed by the American Hospital Association (AHA) Editorial Advisory Board for *Coding Clinic for ICD-10-CM and ICD-10-PCS* and the public-private "cooperating parties": the CMS, National Center for Health Statistics, AHA, and American Health Information Management Association. The increased granularity and specificity in *ICD-10-CM* are also at the specific request of certain medical societies. No clinical diagnosis codes are added for payment purposes.

The AAP holds a seat on the editorial advisory board. Findings are published quarterly by the AHA in *Coding Clinic.* *ICD-10-CM* codes and accompanying guidelines and findings by the editorial advisory board are part of the standard transaction code sets under HIPAA and must be recognized by all payers. For *ICD-10-CM,* the hierarchy of official coding guidelines and instructions is as follows:

1. *ICD-10-CM* alphabetical index and tabular list
2. *Official Guidelines for Coding and Reporting*
3. AHA *Coding Clinic* advice

Pediatricians with suggestions for changes to existing or new *ICD-10-CM* codes related to pediatric care are encouraged to forward their suggestions to coding staff at the AAP headquarters. The AAP staff and advisor who are involved in the process can be of great assistance. To contact the AAP coding staff, complete the form at https://form.jotform.com/Subspecialty/aapcodinghotline.

ICD-10-CM Guidelines

The official conventions found in the *ICD-10-CM Official Guidelines for Coding and Reporting* are outlined in sections that include descriptions of symbols, abbreviations, and other instructional notes. The guidelines are organized into 4 sections. Only sections I and IV pertain to reporting physician services. Sections II and III relate to hospital or facility technical services and are not discussed here. *ICD-10-CM* guidelines can be found in *ICD-10-CM* manuals or at www.cdc.gov/nchs/icd/icd-10-cm.htm.

The following excerpts from the *ICD-10-CM* guidelines provide an overview of the information pertinent to pediatric care as provided in each section of the guidelines:

Section I—Conventions, General Coding Guidelines, and Chapter-Specific Guidelines

A. Conventions

The conventions of *ICD-10-CM* include punctuation, notes, and terminology used throughout the code set.

[ ] Brackets
- Identify manifestation codes in the Alphabetic Index. For instance, otitis externa due to impetigo **L01.00** [**H62.40**] indicates that both impetigo (**L01.00**) and otitis externa in other diseases classified elsewhere (**H62.40**, unspecified ear) are used to report this condition. (Documentation should support the specific site of infection as **H62.41**, right ear; **H62.42**, left ear; or **H62.43**, bilateral ears.)
- Enclose synonyms, alternative wording, or explanatory phrases in the tabular list (eg, **S04.811**, injury of olfactory [1st] nerve, right side).

( ) Parentheses—Enclose supplementary words (ie, nonessential modifiers) that may be included in the medical record but do not affect code selection, for example, sepsis (generalized) (unspecified organism) **A41.9**. If a nonessential modifier is mutually exclusive to a sub-term of the main term, the sub-term is given priority. For instance, the sub-term *candidal* directs to code **B37.7** for candidal sepsis, overriding the nonessential modifier, *unspecified organism.*

- Dash—Indicates that additional characters are required for code completion (eg, **R10.-**). A dash is also used throughout this publication to indicate incomplete codes.

Notes
- Includes: Further defines or gives examples of the content of a category.
- Excludes1: Not coded here—used to indicate codes for conditions that would not occur in conjunction with the code category where the note is found. An exception to the *Excludes1* definition is the circumstance when the 2 conditions are unrelated to each other. If it is not clear whether the 2 conditions involving an *Excludes1* note are related, coders are instructed to query the provider.

Examples

➤ *Excludes1* **notes follow J06.9 (acute upper respiratory infection, unspecified) to prohibit reporting the code in conjunction with less specific acute respiratory infection not otherwise specified (J22) or more specific codes for influenza virus with other respiratory manifestations (J09.X2, J10.1, J11.1) or streptococcal pharyngitis (J02.0).**

> **Excludes1:
> Report only
> if an unrelated
> condition**

    Excludes2: Not included here—used to indicate codes for conditions that are not included in the code category where the note is found but may be additionally reported when both conditions are present.

➤ *Excludes2* **notes apply to code J02.0 (streptococcal pharyngitis).** An *Excludes2* note that applies to all codes in subcategory **J02** (**J02.0–J02.9**) indicates that **J31.2** (chronic pharyngitis) is not included here, and another *Excludes2* note that applies to code **J02.0** indicates that **A38.-** (scarlet fever) is not included here.

Excludes2: Report both codes when present

- Code first: A sequencing rule in the tabular list to report first a code for an underlying cause or origin of a disease (etiology), if known.
- Code also: An instruction that another code may be necessary to fully describe a condition. The sequence of the codes depends on the circumstances of the encounter.
- See: In the alphabetical index, this instructs that another term should be referenced to find the appropriate code.
- See also: In the alphabetical index, this instructs that another term may provide additional entries that may be useful.
- Use an additional code: A sequencing rule often found at the listing of an etiology code; this instruction directs to also report a code for the manifestation.

Terminology
- And: Means and/or when appearing in a title in *ICD-10-CM;* for example, **Q16.1**, congenital absence, atresia and stricture of auditory canal (external), includes absence, atresia, or stricture.
- Combination code: A single code that represents multiple conditions or a single condition with an associated secondary process or complication.
- First-listed diagnosis: For reporting of professional services, the diagnosis, condition, problem, or other reason for the encounter or visit shown in the medical record to be chiefly responsible for the services provided is listed first and followed by other conditions that affected management or treatment.
- NEC: Not elsewhere classifiable. Indicates a code for other specified conditions that is reported when the medical record provides detail that is not captured in a specific code.
- NOS: Not otherwise specified. Indicates a code for an unspecified condition that is reported when the medical record does not provide sufficient detail for assignment of a more specific code.
- Sequela: A late effect of an illness or injury that is no longer in the acute phase. There is no time limit on when a sequela code can be used. The residual may be apparent early, such as that in cerebral infarction, or it may occur months or years later, such as that due to a previous injury.
- With, In: The classification presumes a causal relationship between the 2 conditions linked by the terms *with* or *in.* These conditions should be coded as related even in the absence of provider documentation explicitly linking them, unless the documentation clearly states that the conditions are unrelated or when another guideline exists that specifically requires a documented linkage between 2 conditions (eg, sepsis guideline for "acute organ dysfunction that is not clearly associated with the sepsis").

For conditions not specifically linked by these relational terms in the classification or when a guideline requires that a linkage between 2 conditions be explicitly documented, provider documentation must link the conditions to code them as related.

B. General Coding Guidelines
- Do not report codes for conditions documented as "ruled-out," "suspected," "possible," or "probable." Instead, report codes for signs or symptoms. Exceptions are influenza diagnoses from category **J11** that are assigned for diagnostic statements, such as "possible avian influenza" or "influenzalike illness."
- A confirmatory test is not always required to make a final diagnosis (eg, streptococcal infection may be based on clinical findings in lieu of laboratory findings).
- Do not report additional codes for symptoms or conditions that are integral or routinely associated with a disease process (eg, wheezing in asthma).
- When the same condition is documented as acute and chronic, codes for both conditions are reported if the alphabetical index lists the conditions at the same indentation level. The acute condition is sequenced first.
- When a combination code describes 2 diagnoses, or a diagnosis and its associated manifestation or complication, report only the combination code. If a manifestation or complication is not identified in a combination code, it should be separately reported.
- When reporting a sequela (late effect) of an injury or illness, report first the current condition and then the sequela code.

- If both sides are affected by a condition and the code category does not include a code for the bilateral condition, assign codes for right and left. When a patient has a bilateral condition and each side is treated during separate encounters, assign the bilateral code for each encounter where the condition exists on both sides. Do not assign a bilateral code if the condition no longer exists bilaterally.
- Generally, coders may not assume a complication of care without documentation of the cause-and-effect relationship (eg, infection in a patient with a central venous catheter).
- Unspecified codes are appropriately selected when information to support a more specific code was not available at the time of the encounter (eg, type of pneumonia is not known).

C. Chapter-Specific Guidelines

See guidelines for specific diagnoses and/or conditions found in each chapter of *ICD-10-CM*. Chapter guidelines must be followed for appropriate code selection.

When selecting electronic coding applications, look for inclusion of chapter-specific guidelines when using the code search functionality. *Pediatric ICD-10-CM: A Manual for Provider-Based Coding*, published by the AAP, adds chapter-specific guidance to each chapter for easy reference.

Section IV—Diagnostic Coding and Reporting Guidelines for Outpatient Services

Selecting a Code

- The codes selected must be supported by the physician's or other QHP's documentation of the diagnoses, signs and symptoms, and/or reasons for an encounter as determined after evaluation. Each health care encounter should be coded to the level of certainty known for that encounter.
- Never assign a code for a condition that is unconfirmed (eg, probable or ruled-out obstruction). Instead, assign a code for a confirmed but nonspecific condition (eg, viral pneumonia, unspecified) or sign or symptom (eg, vomiting, abdominal distension).

Examples

➤ **A patient presents with concern of sore throat.** A rapid streptococcal antigen test confirms streptococcal pharyngitis, which is reported with code **J02.0**.

➤ **A patient presents with concern of sore throat.** A specimen is sent to an outside laboratory. Diagnosis at the time of code assignment is pharyngitis, reported with code **J02.9** (acute pharyngitis, unspecified). If a definitive diagnosis is added to the record before claims submission (eg, test results are received later on the same date), the code for the final diagnosis is reported.

- Certain information documented by the patient and/or clinical staff (eg, body mass index) may be used in code selection when the physician or QHP has documented an associated diagnosis (eg, overweight or obesity). See the "Documentation by Other Than a Physician or Other Qualified Health Care Professional" box later in this chapter for more information.
- The coding conventions and guidelines of Section I take precedence over these outpatient guidelines.
- Use codes in categories **Z00–Z99** when circumstances other than a disease or an injury are recorded as the reason for encounter.

Sequencing of Diagnosis Codes

- Physicians and other providers of professional services should list first the condition, symptom, or other reason for encounter that is chiefly responsible for the services provided. List also any coexisting conditions. However, always defer to the manual to determine if sequencing is outlined in the guidelines.

Diagnosis codes must be appropriately linked to a service on a claim to support the medical necessity of that service. See the Reporting Codes for Payment section later in this chapter for more information.

● indicates a new code; ▲, revised; #, re-sequenced; ✚, add-on; ★, audiovisual technology; and ◀, synchronous interactive audio.

Documentation by Other Than a Physician or Other Qualified Health Care Professional

Code assignment is based on documentation by the physician or other qualified health care professional (QHP) legally accountable for establishing the patient's diagnosis, with few exceptions. Documentation by another clinician (eg, nurse, medical assistant, social worker) supports reporting codes for the items on the following list when the associated diagnosis has been documented by the patient's physician or QHP:

- Body mass index with diagnosis of underweight, overweight, or obesity
- Depth of diagnosed nonpressure chronic ulcers or pressure ulcer stage
- Coma scale in acute medical or traumatic brain injury
- National Institutes of Health Stroke Scale
- Social determinants of health
- Laterality of either a condition or an injury
- Blood alcohol level with a condition classifiable to category F10 (alcohol-related disorders)

Patient self-reported documentation may also be used to assign codes for social determinants of health, as long as this documentation is signed off by and incorporated into the medical record by a clinician or a provider.

Reporting Previously Treated Conditions

- Do not code conditions that have been previously treated but no longer exist. Personal history codes **Z85–Z87** may be used to identify a patient's historical conditions. Codes for family history that affects current care are also reported (**Z80–Z84**).
- Report codes for chronic or recurring conditions as many times as the patient receives care for each condition.

Reporting Diagnoses for Diagnostic Examinations

- The condition, symptoms, or other reason for a diagnostic examination or test should be linked to the service. For laboratory or radiology testing in the absence of related conditions, signs, or symptoms, report code **Z01.89**, encounter for other specified special examinations.
- When diagnostic tests have been interpreted by a physician and the final report is available at the time of coding, code any confirmed or definitive diagnosis(es) documented in the interpretation. Do not code related signs and symptoms as additional diagnoses.
- The code that explains the reason for the test (ie, sign or symptom; diagnosis when known at the end of the encounter) should be reported. A screening code is reported only when a test is performed in the absence of signs or symptoms of a condition.

Examples

➤ **A chest radiograph is ordered because of positive purified protein derivative testing.** Code **R76.11** (nonspecific reaction to tuberculin skin test without active tuberculosis) is assigned on the order to indicate the reason for testing.

➤ **A tuberculin purified protein derivative test is performed to screen for tuberculosis in a patient with no symptoms and no known exposure.** Code **Z11.1** (encounter for screening for respiratory tuberculosis) is assigned as the reason for the test.

➤ **A patient presents with symptoms suggestive of urinary tract infection (UTI).** After urinalysis and evaluation, the diagnosis is UTI. Assign a code for UTI (eg, **N39.0**, urinary tract infection, site not specified) and link to codes for the urinalysis and the E/M service.

Reporting Preoperative Evaluations

- When the reason for an encounter is a preoperative evaluation, a code from subcategory **Z01.81-**, encounter for preprocedural examinations, is reported first, followed by codes for the condition that is the reason for surgery and codes for any findings of the preoperative evaluation.

Please see Chapter 8 for discussion of reporting routine health examinations (preventive care).

Chapter 1. The Basics of Coding

The Pathway to *ICD-10-CM* Code Selection

To correctly select codes in *ICD-10-CM*, it is important to recognize and follow instructions found in the alphabetical index and tabular list to locate the most specific code for documented diagnoses. These are the prevailing instructions for reporting that are supplemented by the guidelines and guidance published in AHA *Coding Clinic*.

Indexes

Code selection begins in the alphabetical index, table of drugs and chemicals (eg, to report an adverse effect or poisoning), and/or table of neoplasms. The instructions (eg, instructions to see other terms) in the index will direct to the most specific code in the tabular list. An external cause of injuries index is also useful for locating codes to describe causes such as animal bites, falls, or motor vehicle accidents.

Tabular List

The tabular list is the end point for code selection. It is an alphanumeric list of *ICD-10-CM* codes structured as an indented list of 22 chapters with further divisions, including blocks, categories, subcategories, and codes.

> Look for instructional notes at each division within the tabular list (ie, chapter, block, category, or code), as these give important guidance to correct code selection.

The *ICD-10-CM* tabular list displays codes in an indented format to help users identify complete codes (eg, **P08.21**, post-term newborn) in each category (eg, **P08**, disorders of newborn related to long gestation and high birth weight) or subcategory (eg, **P08.2**, late newborn, not heavy for gestational age) of codes. Only complete codes are reported.

Some code categories include instruction to add a seventh character. The most commonly required seventh characters are **A**, **D**, and **S**. Categories for traumatic fractures have additional seventh character values (eg, **C**, initial encounter for open fracture type IIIA, IIIB, or IIIC).

Assignment of the seventh character **A** (initial encounter) is based on whether the patient is undergoing active treatment (ie, services to establish a pattern of healing) and not on whether the provider is seeing the patient for the first time over the course of treatment of an injury or illness. Encounters during the routine healing phase are reported with seventh character **D** (subsequent encounter) even if the patient is new to the physician or QHP for this condition. Sequelae or late effects are reported with seventh character **S**.

> When selecting a seventh character to indicate the type of encounter, a helpful mnemonic for this character is **A** as active treatment/management, **D** as during healing, and **S** as scars and other sequelae.

Examples

➤ **A (initial encounter):** A physician repairs a facial laceration (active treatment) and reports **S01.81XA** (laceration without foreign body of other part of head, initial encounter). This is active management.

➤ **D (subsequent encounter):** A pediatrician removes facial sutures placed by an emergency department physician and reports **S01.81XD** (laceration without foreign body of other part of head, subsequent encounter). This is care during the healing phase.

➤ **S (sequela or late effect):** A pediatrician evaluates a concern of scar contracture that resulted from repair of a facial laceration. Codes **L90.5** (scar conditions and fibrosis of skin) and **S01.81XS** (laceration without foreign body of other part of head, sequela) are reported. This is care for a scar or other sequelae.

Teaching Point: A sequela (eg, scar) must always be reported first.

Refer to the AAP manuals *Pediatric Coding Basics* and *Pediatric ICD-10-CM* for more information on codes and code selection.

● indicates a new code; ▲, revised; #, re-sequenced; ✚, add-on; ★, audiovisual technology; and ◄, synchronous interactive audio.

Chapter 1. The Basics of Coding

Diagnosis Coding Tips

- Specificity in coding is important in demonstrating the reason for a service or encounter, including the nature or severity of conditions managed. For further discussion of this important topic, see the Appropriate Use of Unspecified Codes section later in this chapter.
- Physicians and other practitioners should become familiar with the documentation elements that are captured in *ICD-10-CM* code categories for conditions commonly seen in their practice. For example, when documenting care for otitis media, key documentation elements include whether the condition
  — Affects the right, the left, or both ears
  — Is acute, acute recurrent, or chronic
  — Is suppurative or nonsuppurative
  — Is with or without spontaneous rupture of the tympanic membrane

  Exposure to or use of tobacco is also reported in conjunction with otitis media.
- Assign codes for social determinants of health (eg, homelessness, food insecurity, or lack of transportation) that increase the complexity and risk of management or treatment (eg, higher risk of nonadherence caused by separation or divorce of parents who do not agree on patient treatment).
- Pay close attention to the terminology for nonspecific diagnoses. For example, the diagnosis "reactive airways disease" is to be coded as asthma per the guidelines.

  In children treated for an asthma-like condition who have not been diagnosed with asthma, it may be more appropriate to report the signs or symptoms as the primary diagnosis.

When a diagnosis is assigned to a child's medical record and reported, the child is then included in the population of any associated quality measure. For example, a child who is 5 years or older and diagnosed with persistent asthma is included in the following measures:

- Receiving a prescription for and continuing to take an asthma-control medication for at least 75% of a treatment period
- Having had a ratio of controller medications to total asthma medications of 0.50 or greater during the measurement year

If asthma is diagnosed but not managed, the physician or qualified health care professional appears to fail to meet the quality measures.

- If, after evaluation and study of a suspected condition, there is no diagnosis or there are no signs or symptoms that are appropriate, report the codes for observation and evaluation for suspected conditions not found (eg, urinary symptoms without diagnosed cause).

  Codes for observation and evaluation for reporting suspected conditions not found in a neonate (*ICD-10-CM* codes **Z05.0–Z05.9**) are distinct from those for reporting suspected conditions not found in older children and adults (*ICD-10-CM* code **Z03.89**).
- Use aftercare codes (**Z42–Z49**, **Z51**) for patients who are receiving care to consolidate treatment or management to address residual conditions.
- Conditions that were previously treated and no longer exist cannot be reported. Therefore, it is correct coding to report care following completed treatment with *ICD-10-CM* code **Z09**, encounter for follow-up examination after completed treatment of conditions other than malignant neoplasm.
  — Personal history codes (**Z86.-**, **Z87.-**) may be used to provide additional information on follow-up care.
  — If a payer does not accept follow-up care codes as primary and requires that the service be reported with the diagnosis code that reflects the condition that had been treated, report the follow-up care codes as secondary. However, get the payer's policy in writing and inquire why it is not following coding guidelines.

Example

➤ **A patient is seen to follow up on otitis media with effusion, which has now resolved.** The physician reports codes **Z09** and **Z86.69** (personal history of other diseases of the nervous system and sense organs) in lieu of the code for otitis media with effusion (no longer applicable).

- Do not select a diagnosis code that is "close to" the diagnosis or condition documented in the medical record. For example, do not report unspecified joint pain (**M25.50**) if the diagnosis is right knee pain (**M25.561**). Modify code selection methods to support correct code assignment.
- Pay attention to age factors within certain code descriptors. For example, report *ICD-10-CM* code **R10.83** for infantile colic and *ICD-10-CM* code **R10.84** for colic in a child older than 12 months.

● indicates a new code; ▲, revised; #, re-sequenced; ✚, add-on; ★, audiovisual technology; and ◀, synchronous interactive audio.

- There is no limit to the number of diagnosis codes that can be documented.
  - Space is only allotted for up to 12 codes on the CMS-1500 paper claim form, and each service line may be connected to 1 to 4 of the included codes. You may submit as many claim forms as necessary to report all current diagnoses.
  - Electronic claims in HIPAA version 5010 may also include up to 12 diagnosis codes.
- "Recurrent" is not defined by *ICD-10-CM*. Therefore, to use a recurrent code, the documentation should reflect that a practitioner believes the condition to be a recurrence.
- "Confirmed" influenza, COVID-19, or other conditions do not require a positive result from a laboratory or other test. What is required is that the practitioner, through training and experience, believes that the patient has the condition, on the basis of clinical assessment, and documents the condition in the medical record.
- Do not report suspected or ruled-out diagnoses for physician services. Code to the nearest clinical certainty, which may be signs or symptoms. Exposure to communicable disease (category **Z20**) may be reported when a patient has known or suspected exposure or when a disease is endemic but ruled out after evaluation.

Appropriate Use of Unspecified Codes

Unspecified codes are valid *ICD-10-CM* codes used to report conditions for which a more specific diagnosis has not yet been determined and/or to report testing to determine that a more specific diagnosis would not be medically necessary. However, misuse of unspecified codes may result in claim denials and unnecessary delays in receiving prior authorizations for testing or procedures.

Do not report the default code (first code listed in the alphabetical index) when more detail about the patient's condition(s) should be documented to support another, more specific code. For example, do not report **J45.909** for unspecified asthma, uncomplicated, for reevaluation of asthma, which includes clinical classification of intermittent, mild-persistent, moderate-persistent, or severe-persistent asthma. The diagnosis code reported should reflect what is known at the end of the current encounter. Unspecified codes are not appropriate when information to support a more specific code would generally be known (eg, laterality, type of attention-deficit/hyperactivity disorder).

Examples of unspecified codes that may be acceptable are as follows:
- Viral intestinal infection, unspecified (**A08.4**)
- Infectious gastroenteritis and colitis, unspecified (**A09**)
- Acute pharyngitis, unspecified (**J02.9**)
- Pneumonia, unspecified organism (**J18.9**)
- Sprain of unspecified site of right knee (**S83.91X-**)

The following examples of unspecified codes indicate inappropriate coding due to failure to document information (eg, location) that would typically be known at the time of the encounter and/or inappropriate code selection:
- Acute suppurative otitis media without spontaneous rupture of eardrum, unspecified ear (**H66.009**)
- Otitis media, unspecified, unspecified ear (**H66.90**)
- Cutaneous abscess of limb, unspecified (**L02.419**)
- Extremely low birth weight newborn, unspecified weight (**P07.00**)

In short, unspecified codes are necessary and should be reported when appropriate. Physicians must document in enough detail to capture what is known at the time of the encounter, and codes selected must reflect the documented diagnosis(es). If, at the time of code selection, documentation does not appear to include information that would be known at the time of the encounter, it is appropriate for coders to query the physician for more information and/or request an addendum to the documentation to more fully describe the conditions addressed at the encounter.

More About *ICD-10-CM*

You can find additional resources from the AAP on *ICD-10-CM* topics at www.aap.org/en/practice-management/practice-financing/coding-and-valuation/icd-10-cm-resources.

The AAP manual, *Pediatric ICD-10-CM* (https://shop.aap.org/pediatric-icd-10-cm-2023-8th-edition-paperback), is a condensed version of the entire *ICD-10-CM* manual and provides only the guidelines and codes that are applicable and of importance to pediatric practitioners. The manual was designed for use in conjunction with the complete *ICD-10-CM* code set. The *ICD-10-CM* codes and guidelines are found at www.cdc.gov/nchs/icd/Comprehensive-Listing-of-*ICD-10-CM*-Files.htm.

AAP Pediatric Coding Newsletter provides timely articles on diagnosis coding for pediatric conditions (https://shop.aap.org/aap-pediatric-coding-newsletter).

Healthcare Common Procedure Coding System

The Healthcare Common Procedure Coding System (HCPCS) includes Level I codes (*CPT*) and Level II codes (CMS national codes). HCPCS Level II codes are the standardized coding system for describing and identifying health care services, equipment, medications, and supplies (eg, **Q4011**, cast supplies, short arm cast, pediatric [0–10 years], plaster) that are not identified by HCPCS Level I (*CPT*) codes. To differentiate discussion of *CPT* and HCPCS Level II codes, the abbreviation HCPCS is typically used in reference to Level II codes unless otherwise stated.

HCPCS procedure codes may be reported when no *CPT* code describes the service provided or when the narrative (code descriptor) differs from and more accurately describes the service provided than a similar *CPT* code. Payer policies, particularly Medicaid plan policies, often drive the decision between reporting with *CPT* and reporting with HCPCS.

Example

➤ **A physician provides critical care services to a pediatric patient via a real-time audiovisual telecommunications system.** *CPT* does not designate codes for critical care services (**99291** and **99292, 99468–99472**) as services reportable with modifier **95** (synchronous telemedicine service rendered via a real-time interactive audio and video telecommunications system). As an alternative, the payer has adopted policy requiring HCPCS codes for critical care provided via telemedicine. The physician reports one of the following codes based on the service provided:

G0508   Telehealth consultation, critical care, initial, physicians typically spend 60 minutes communicating with the patient and providers via telehealth

G0509   Telehealth consultation, critical care, subsequent, physicians typically spend 50 minutes communicating with the patient and providers via telehealth

Reporting Medications Supplied by the Billing Provider

HCPCS **J** codes (eg, **J0696**, injection, ceftriaxone sodium, per 250 mg) represent only the medication and not the administration of the medication.

● The term *injection* is included in the descriptor to specify that the medication code is reported for the medication that is labeled for administration via injection or infusion. This does not limit reporting of these codes when delivered via an alternative route.

Example

➤ **A physician orders and clinical staff deliver an oral administration of 9 mL of injectable dexamethasone sodium phosphate (from a 10-mg/mL single-dose vial) diluted in a flavor solution to a concentration of 2 mg/mL to a patient in the office.** The physician reports **J1100** (injection, dexamethasone sodium phosphate, 1 mg) with 9 units (1 unit per milligram administered). Also, they include a note on the claim (field 19 of a paper claim or the electronic equivalent) that the drug was orally administered. Additional codes are reported for other services (eg, office visit) provided on the same date.

Because 9 mg of the medication administered was a portion of a 10-mg/mL single-dose vial, there is wastage of 1 mL that may be reportable to the health plan by appending modifier **JW** (drug amount discarded/not administered to any patient) to a second listing of code **J1100** on an additional claim line. Payer policies for use of and payment for services reported with modifier **JW** may vary.

● Separate procedure codes, typically *CPT* codes, are used to report each medication administration by injection (**96372**) or infusion.

● HCPCS codes for drugs specify the unit of measure for each unit reported on the claim (eg, 250 mg of ceftriaxone sodium is reported with 1 unit on the claim line reporting provision of the medication). (See the National Drug Code section later in this chapter for information on reporting units of service in conjunction with National Drug Code [NDC] reporting.)

● indicates a new code; ▲, revised; #, re-sequenced; ✚, add-on; ★, audiovisual technology; and ◀, synchronous interactive audio.

Example

➤ **A physician administers 900 mg of ceftriaxone sodium by injection.** Code **J0696** (injection, ceftriaxone sodium, per 250 mg) is reported with 4 units in addition to code **96372** (therapeutic, prophylactic, or diagnostic injection; subcutaneous or intramuscular). Additional codes may be reported for E/M and other services provided at the encounter.

Do not report the number of milligrams (mg) as the unit of service on a claim. Reporting 900 mg of ceftriaxone sodium with 900 units would be incorrect; 900 mg of ceftriaxone sodium is reported per 250 mg with 4 units (rounding up is allowed by Medicare; other payers may require 3.6 units).

New permanent HCPCS codes are released by the CMS each November for implementation on January 1 of each year. However, temporary HCPCS codes may be implemented on a quarterly basis. Temporary codes are added to address the need for a reporting mechanism before the annual update (eg, to meet the requirements of a legislative mandate or to add a new product).

Current Procedural Terminology (CPT®)

CPT is published annually by the American Medical Association (AMA). *CPT* codes are Level I codes of HCPCS but are commonly treated as a separate code set. This is the primary procedural coding system for professional services by physicians and other QHPs. *CPT* codes are commonly included in electronic health record (EHR) systems, but instructions for reporting may not be included. *CPT* manuals and code applications or software provide important instructions for appropriate code selection.

Category I *CPT* codes (commonly performed services and procedures with documented clinical efficacy) are generally updated annually with release of new codes each fall to allow physicians and payers to prepare for implementation on January 1 of each year.

- Exceptions include the vaccine, toxoid, immunoglobulin, serum, and recombinant product codes, which are updated twice annually (January and July) and may be released earlier when specific criteria for rapid release are met. Newly released vaccine codes are posted to www.ama-assn.org/practice-management/cpt/category-i-vaccine-codes.
  — New vaccine codes released July 1 are implemented on January 1, or vice versa.
- New molecular pathology tier 2 codes and codes for multianalyte assays with algorithmic analyses are updated 3 times per year (April 1, October 1, and January 1). Proprietary laboratory analyses codes are released quarterly (July 1, October 1, January 1, and April 1).

Category II *CPT* codes (supplemental tracking used for performance measurement) are released online up to 3 times a year, with an effective date of 3 months after release, at www.ama-assn.org/practice-management/cpt/category-ii-codes.

> **See Chapter 3 for more discussion and illustration of Category II codes.**

Category III *CPT* codes (emerging technology, services, procedures, and service paradigms) are released biannually with an implementation date 6 months after the release date. For instance, a code released on January 1, 2023, is implemented on July 1, 2023, even before it is published in *CPT 2024*. The most recent Category III code listing is found at www.ama-assn.org/practice-management/cpt/category-iii-codes.

> **Category III *Current Procedural Terminology (CPT)* codes are not assigned relative value units, and payment for these services is based strictly on payer policies. If you are performing any procedure or service identified with a Category III *CPT* code, work with your payers to determine their coverage and payment policies.**

The AMA hosts a website devoted to *CPT*, www.ama-assn.org/practice-management/cpt, with information on code development and maintenance, summaries of recent *CPT* Editorial Panel actions, and newly released codes.

CPT Guidelines Applicable to All Services

Correct coding is important in obtaining correct claims payment. Always read the applicable guidelines and instructions before selecting a code.

● indicates a new code; ▲, revised; #, re-sequenced; ✚, add-on; ★, audiovisual technology; and ◀, synchronous interactive audio.

The following general guidelines are applied for selecting and reporting all *CPT* codes:

- *CPT* guidelines do not establish documentation requirements or standards of care.
- Each level of E/M services may be used by all physicians and other QHPs whose license and scope of practice include provision of E/M services.
- In the *CPT* code set, the term *procedure* describes services, including diagnostic tests. The section of the book in which a code is placed does not indicate whether the service is a surgery or not a surgery for insurance or other purposes.
- Select the code for the procedure or service that accurately identifies the service performed.
  - Do not select a code that merely approximates the service provided.
  - If no specific code exists, report the service by using the appropriate unlisted procedure code. Unlisted procedure codes are provided in each section of *CPT* (eg, **99429**, unlisted preventive medicine service). When reporting an unlisted procedure code, medical records need to be submitted to the health plan to identify the service rendered (attach the records to the claim to prevent delay caused by a health plan request for them).
  - In some cases, a modifier may be reported in conjunction with a procedure code to indicate a reduced (**52**), discontinued (**53**), or increased (**22**) procedural service. For more about procedure code modifiers, see **Chapter 2**.
- A code that is reported "per day" or for services "on the same date" is not reported for all services in a 24-hour period but, rather, for all services on a single calendar date.

Examples

99463	Initial hospital or birthing center care, per day, for E/M of normal newborn infant admitted and discharged on the same date
99468	Initial inpatient neonatal critical care, per day, for the E/M of a critically ill neonate, 28 days of age or younger

- A midpoint time rule is applied when codes are selected on the basis of time *and no specific time requirement is provided* in the section guidelines, prefatory instructions, parenthetical instructions, or code descriptor.
  - A unit of time is attained when the midpoint is passed (eg, a code described as 30 minutes may be reported when service time of 16 minutes has elapsed).
  - When codes are ranked in sequential typical times and the actual time is between 2 typical times, the code with the typical time closest to the actual time is used. If the actual time of service falls exactly between the typical times of 2 codes, report the code with the lower typical time (ie, the midpoint must be passed to report the greater service).

Documentation of Time

Documentation of time spent providing services should be evident in the medical record for each service reported on the basis of time (ie, total minutes of service or start and stop times).

- Documentation of time may be automated in an electronic health record (EHR), but physicians should be able to demonstrate that the EHR functionality captures the correct time for code selection as specified by *Current Procedural Terminology*.
- When multiple services are provided on the same date, time spent in time-based services must be clearly distinguished from time spent in provision of other services. For instance, time spent in any separately reportable procedure (eg, 31500, endotracheal intubation) is not included in the time of hourly critical care services (99291, 99292). Documentation should clearly reflect total times and activities of each service.
- In addition to documentation of total times or start and stop times of service, documentation should clearly support the service reported. For example, documentation of counseling should include discussion of diagnosis and treatment options, patient and/or caregiver questions and concerns that were addressed, shared decision-making for management, and any social determinants of health that affect care and were addressed (eg, advice to enroll in a prescription discount program).
- All documentation must be signed or electronically authenticated with the name and credentials of the physician or other provider of care and date of service.

- Time is the physician's or other reporting provider's time unless otherwise stated. Time spent by clinical staff is reported only when specified in *CPT* or allowed under incident-to policy established by a payer.

See Chapter 7 for information on reporting services that are incident to a physician's service.

CPT also includes not only specific guidelines that are located at the beginning of each of 6 sections but also additional prefatory instructions for subsections of codes throughout the *CPT* manual. Code-specific instructions often follow a code in parentheses (referred to as *parenthetical instructions*).

● indicates a new code; ▲, revised; #, re-sequenced; ✚, add-on; ★, audiovisual technology; and ◀, synchronous interactive audio.

Example

> **Codes 99238 and 99239 are to be used by the physician or other QHP who is responsible for discharge services.**
> Services by other physicians or other QHPs that may include instructions to the patient and/or family and coordination of post-discharge services may be reported with **99231**, **99232**, or **99233**.
> ▲**99238**   Hospital inpatient or observation discharge day management; 30 minutes or less on the date of the encounter
> ▲**99239**   more than 30 minutes on the date of the encounter
>   (For hospital inpatient or observation care, including the admission and discharge of the patient on the same date, see **99234–99236**.)
>   (For discharge services provided to newborns admitted and discharged on the same calendar date, use **99463**.)

Additional guidance can be found in *CPT Assistant,* a monthly newsletter published by the AMA that provides additional information about the intended use of codes, the related guidelines, and parenthetical instructions. Although widely considered authoritative, *CPT* instructions, guidelines, and *CPT Assistant* are not part of the HIPAA standard transaction code sets. All payers must accept *CPT* codes but are not required to adhere to the published *CPT* guidelines and instructions. When payer policy differs from *CPT,* payer contracts typically require adherence to payer policy.

Example

> **A health plan policy does not allow separate payment for vision screening in conjunction with a routine child health examination even though *CPT* instructs that the screening be separately reported.** Although the health plan may deny charges associated with a vision screening, the plan must not reject the claim due to inclusion of a vision screening code (eg, **99173**, screening test of visual acuity, quantitative, bilateral).

Provider Terminology

Throughout the *CPT* code set, the use of terms such as *physician, QHP,* or *individual* is not intended to indicate that other entities may not report the service. In select instances, specific instructions may define a service as limited to certain professionals or to other entities (eg, hospital, home health agency).

Of particular importance to correct reporting of services that include clinical staff and other nonphysician providers is identifying the providers included when terms such as *physician or other QHP* and *qualified nonphysician health care professional* are used in *CPT* and/or payer instruction.

CPT defines providers as follows:

- Physician or other QHP: an individual who is qualified by education, training, licensure/regulation (when applicable), and facility privileging (when applicable) who performs a professional service within his or her scope of practice and independently reports that professional service

> Codes in the evaluation and management (E/M) section are reported only by a physician or qualified health care professional (QHP) whose scope of practice includes E/M services (eg, nurse practitioner, physician assistant). In contrast, assessment and management codes are found in the medicine section for reporting services by nonphysician QHPs (eg, physical or occupational therapists and speech pathologists) who may independently provide and report medical services. Coding for services by qualified nonphysician health care professionals whose scope of practice does not include E/M services is discussed in Chapter 13.

- Clinical staff member: a person who works under the supervision of a physician or other QHP and who is allowed by law, regulation, and facility policy to perform or assist in the performance of a specific professional service but does not individually report that professional service

Services performed by clinical staff under the supervision of a physician or QHP are reported by the supervising physician or QHP.

Note: CPT does not include any requirements for licensure but, rather, advises physicians to follow state regulations and the related scopes of practice defined by regulations (eg, regulations defining services that require a nursing license).

CPT Conventions

CPT codes are presented in the 3 categories previously discussed. Additionally, Category I is divided into 6 sections of codes.

1. Evaluation and Management Services (**99202–99499**)
2. Anesthesia (**00100–01999**)
3. Surgery (**10004–66990**)
4. Radiology (**70010–79999**)
5. Pathology and Laboratory (**80047–89398, 0001U–0284U**)
6. Medicine (**90281–99607**)

Symbols are used throughout *CPT* to indicate certain code characteristics.

● A bullet at the beginning of a code indicates a new code for the current year.

▲ A triangle means the code descriptor has been revised.

✚ A plus sign means the code is an add-on code.

Ø A null sign means the code is a "modifier **51** exempt" code and, therefore, does not require modifier **51** (multiple procedures) even when reported with other procedures.

⚡ The lightning bolt identifies codes for vaccines pending US Food and Drug Administration approval.

\# The pound symbol is used to identify re-sequenced codes that are out of numerical sequence. Related codes are placed in an appropriate location, making it easier to locate a procedure or service.

◀ An audio speaker symbol means that the service is included in Appendix T of the *CPT* manual and may be reported with modifier **93** when provided via audio-only telecommunications technology (eg, telephone).

★ A star means the service can be reported as a telemedicine service and is included in Appendix P of the *CPT* manual as a code to which modifier **95** (synchronous telemedicine service) may be appended to indicate that the service was rendered via real-time telemedicine services using audiovisual technology.

Appendixes of the *CPT* manual provide quick references to modifiers; a summary of new, revised, and deleted codes; add-on and modifier-exempt codes; and other procedure code references.

CPT includes an index of procedures used to find codes and code ranges to help guide the user to the correct section(s) of codes.

● Terms in the index cover procedures and services, organs and anatomical sites, conditions, synonyms, eponyms, and abbreviations (eg, *EEG* for *electroencephalography*).

● Codes should not be selected from the index without verification in the main text of the manual.

● Many diagnostic services require both technical and professional components.

— It is important to understand that the technical component (eg, obtaining an electrocardiogram) leads to results or findings.

— The interpretation and creation of a report of the results or findings is a professional service. Some services specifically require a professional's interpretation and report.

— Other services include only a technical component and require only documentation of the results or findings (eg, scoring of a developmental screening instrument).

— Codes and modifiers exist to report the technical or professional component when the complete service is not provided by the same individual or provider (eg, facility provides technical component and physician provides professional component).

> **Never report a code for a global service without a modifier when only the technical or professional component is provided. See Chapter 2 for discussion of appropriate modifiers (eg, 26, TC).**

● Add-on codes (marked with a ✚ before the code) are always performed in addition to a primary service and are never reported as stand-alone services. Add-on codes describe additional intraservice work and are not valued to include pre-service and post-service work like most other codes.

Example

➤ ▲✚★**99417** Prolonged outpatient evaluation and management service(s) time with or without direct patient contact beyond the required time of the primary service when the primary service level has been selected using total time, each 15 minutes of total time (List separately in addition to the code of the outpatient Evaluation and Management services)

● indicates a new code; ▲, revised; #, re-sequenced; ✚, add-on; ★, audiovisual technology; and ◀, synchronous interactive audio.

(Use **99417** in conjunction with **99205**, **99215**, **99245**, **99345**, **99350**, or **99483**.)

(Do not report **99417** on the same date as **90833**, **90836**, **90838**, **99358**, **99359**, **99415**, or **99416**.)

Teaching Point: Code **99417** is never reported without one of the outpatient E/M codes listed in the first parenthetical instruction having been provided and reported on the same date of service. The second parenthetical instruction includes psychotherapy and other prolonged service codes that are not reported on the same date as **99417**.

In *CPT 2023*, the inclusionary parenthetical notes following the add-on codes are not all inclusive but, rather, include the typical base code(s) and not every possible reportable code combination.

National Drug Code

National Drug Codes are universal product identifiers for prescription drugs including vaccines and insulin products. Codes are 10-digit, 3-segment numbers that identify the product, labeler, and trade package size. Medicare, Medicaid, and other government payers (eg, Tricare), as well as some private payers, may require the use of NDCs when reporting medication and vaccine product codes.

- The HIPAA standards for reporting NDCs do not align with the 10-digit format; they require an 11-digit code.
  - Conversion to an 11-digit code in 5-4-2 format is required.
  - Leading zeros are added to the appropriate segment to accomplish the 5-4-2 format, as illustrated in **Table 1-3**.

  It is important to verify each payer's requirements for NDC reporting. A payer may require either
- The NDC that is provided on the outer packaging when a vaccine or another drug is supplied in bulk packages
- The NDC from the vial that was administered

  When reporting NDCs,
- A qualifier (N4) precedes the NDC number on the claim form (eg, N400006404720).
- The correct number of NDC units must also be included on claims.
  - The NDC units are often different from HCPCS or *CPT* units.
  - For most payers, NDC units are reported as grams (GR), milligrams (ME), milliliters (ML), or units (UN).
  - The qualifiers GR, ME, ML, and UN are reported before the number of NDC units on a claim to indicate the measure.

Table 1-3. National Drug Code Format Examples		
Product	**10-Digit NDC Format**	**11-Digit NDC Format (Added 0 [Zero] Underscored)**
Gardasil 9 (human papillomavirus vaccine) carton of ten 0.5-mL single-dose vials	0006-4119-03 (4-4-2)	00006-4119-03 (5-4-2)
Fluarix Quadrivalent (influenza vaccine) prefilled syringe	58160-887-41 (5-3-2)	58160-0887-41 (5-4-2)
Pfizer-BioNTech COVID-19 Vaccine (10-mcg/0.2-mL dosage) single-dose vial	59267-1055-1 (5-4-1)	59267-1055-01 (5-4-2)
Abbreviation: NDC, National Drug Code.		

For examples of how NDC codes and units are reported on a claim, see **Figure 1-1**.

If you are not currently reporting vaccines with NDCs, be sure to coordinate the requirements with your billing software company. For more information on NDCs, visit www.fda.gov/drugs/informationondrugs/ucm142438.htm for updates.

Beyond Code Sets

Who Assigns the Codes?

- Diagnoses should be assigned by the clinician (ie, physician or QHP), indicating a principal (primary) diagnosis that best explains the reason with the highest risk of morbidity or mortality for the patient encounter. Code assignment may take place in conjunction with documentation or at a later date, depending on the workflow processes of the practice.

- All contributing (secondary) diagnoses that help explain the medical necessity for the episode of care should also be listed. However, only those conditions that specifically affect the patient's encounter should be listed.

> Documentation of diagnoses, signs and symptoms, or other reasons for a service is not accomplished through code assignment. Per official guidance from *Coding Clinic*, selection of a code cannot replace a written diagnostic statement. Multiple clinical conditions may be represented by a single diagnosis code, and more than one code may be required to fully describe a condition. Codes should be assigned to the documented diagnostic statement.

- When codes are selected by physicians at the time of EHR documentation, having trained administrative staff verify the levels of service, need for modifiers, and compliance with *ICD-10-CM*, *CPT*, and payer policies is advised before billing. Electronic health records often fail to show complete code descriptors and/or *ICD-10-CM* instructions (eg, exclusion notes).
- Assignment of the specific diagnosis code by clinical or administrative staff should be done under the physician's or reporting provider's supervision.
- The first-listed code on the claim should be the principal reason for the service unless the tabular instructions direct to "code first" another reason (eg, code first routine child health examination [**Z00.121, Z00.129**] when immunizations [**Z23**] are provided at the time of a preventive E/M service).
- For those practices using a printed encounter form, including 50 to 100 of the most commonly used diagnoses *and* their respective codes on the outpatient encounter form allows the physician or other QHP to mark the appropriate code(s), indicating which is primary.
  - If a specific diagnosis code is not included on the form, write it in.
  - Do not select a diagnosis code that is "closest to" the diagnosis.
  - The AAP has developed the *Pediatric Office Superbill*, a convenient card that includes the most-reported *CPT* and *ICD-10-CM* codes (https://shop.aap.org/pediatric-office-superbill-2023).

Reporting Codes for Payment

In addition to establishing standard code sets, HIPAA has established electronic transaction standards for patient benefit inquiries and submission of health claims and related reports.

- Claims for professional services are typically submitted electronically in a format known as 837P (professional claim) as currently configured in version 5010A1.
- Paper claim form submissions using the National Uniform Claim Committee 1500 claim form, version 02/12 (1500 form), are allowed for providers who meet an exception to the HIPAA requirements for electronic claim submission (eg, provider with <10 full-time employees).
  - Paper claim submissions increase the length of time between submission and payment and the chance of error in either completion of the form or claims processing. Because of this, it is advisable to submit electronic claims whenever possible.
  - The 1500 form contains the same information as an electronic claim and is valuable for demonstrating how codes and other information necessary for claims processing must be relayed to payers. An example of a completed 1500 form is found in **Figure 1-1**.

Linking the Diagnosis to the Service

- Every claim line for a physician service must be linked to the appropriate *ICD-10-CM* code that represents the reason for the service.
  - Each *ICD-10-CM* code is placed in a diagnosis field labeled "21A–L."
  - A diagnosis pointer in field 24E indicates which diagnosis codes relate to each service line by indicating the letter(s) of the related diagnosis field. Up to 4 diagnosis fields may be linked to a service line.
- When using an EHR, physicians should list the primary diagnosis in the EHR first and make certain that the software knows it should be reported as the first listed. In addition, the EHR should be able to link diagnosis codes to the appropriate services.
- The diagnosis code may be the same or different for each service performed.

● indicates a new code; ▲, revised; #, re-sequenced; ✚, add-on; ★, audiovisual technology; and ◀, synchronous interactive audio.

Figure 1-1. Example of a Completed 1500 Form

HEALTH INSURANCE CLAIM FORM

APPROVED BY NATIONAL UNIFORM CLAIM COMMITTEE (NUCC) 02/12

ABC Health Plan
123 Money St
Anywhere, AK 00000

CARRIER

| | PICA | | | | | | PICA | | |

1. MEDICARE (Medicare#) MEDICAID [X] (Medicaid#) TRICARE (ID#/DoD#) CHAMPVA (Member ID#) GROUP HEALTH PLAN (ID#) FECA BLK LUNG (ID#) OTHER (ID#)

1a. INSURED'S I.D. NUMBER (For Program in Item 1)
123456789

2. PATIENT'S NAME (Last Name, First Name, Middle Initial)
Smith, Child

3. PATIENT'S BIRTH DATE MM 11 DD 22 YY 2021 SEX M [X] F

4. INSURED'S NAME (Last Name, First Name, Middle Initial)
Smith, Parent A

5. PATIENT'S ADDRESS (No., Street)
123 Main St

6. PATIENT RELATIONSHIP TO INSURED
Self [X] Spouse Child Other

7. INSURED'S ADDRESS (No., Street)

CITY
Anywhere

STATE
KS

8. RESERVED FOR NUCC USE

CITY

STATE

ZIP CODE
12345

TELEPHONE (Include Area Code)
(555) 555-5555

ZIP CODE

TELEPHONE (Include Area Code)
( )

9. OTHER INSURED'S NAME (Last Name, First Name, Middle Initial)
Smith, Parent B

10. IS PATIENT'S CONDITION RELATED TO:

11. INSURED'S POLICY GROUP OR FECA NUMBER
98765432102

a. OTHER INSURED'S POLICY OR GROUP NUMBER
4561237890

a. EMPLOYMENT? (Current or Previous) YES [X] NO

a. INSURED'S DATE OF BIRTH MM 01 DD 01 YY 1992 SEX M F [X]

b. RESERVED FOR NUCC USE

b. AUTO ACCIDENT? YES [X] NO PLACE (State)

b. OTHER CLAIM ID (Designated by NUCC)

c. RESERVED FOR NUCC USE

c. OTHER ACCIDENT? YES [X] NO

c. INSURANCE PLAN NAME OR PROGRAM NAME
Good Health Plan

d. INSURANCE PLAN NAME OR PROGRAM NAME
Another Good Plan

10d. CLAIM CODES (Designated by NUCC)

d. IS THERE ANOTHER HEALTH BENEFIT PLAN?
[X] YES NO If yes, complete items 9, 9a, and 9d.

READ BACK OF FORM BEFORE COMPLETING & SIGNING THIS FORM.

12. PATIENT'S OR AUTHORIZED PERSON'S SIGNATURE I authorize the release of any medical or other information necessary to process this claim. I also request payment of government benefits either to myself or to the party who accepts assignment below.

SIGNED Signature on file DATE 02/22/2022

13. INSURED'S OR AUTHORIZED PERSON'S SIGNATURE I authorize payment of medical benefits to the undersigned physician or supplier for services described below.

SIGNED Signature on file

14. DATE OF CURRENT ILLNESS, INJURY, or PREGNANCY (LMP) MM DD YY QUAL.

15. OTHER DATE QUAL. MM DD YY

16. DATES PATIENT UNABLE TO WORK IN CURRENT OCCUPATION FROM MM DD YY TO MM DD YY

17. NAME OF REFERRING PROVIDER OR OTHER SOURCE
17a.
17b. NPI

18. HOSPITALIZATION DATES RELATED TO CURRENT SERVICES FROM MM DD YY TO MM DD YY

19. ADDITIONAL CLAIM INFORMATION (Designated by NUCC)

20. OUTSIDE LAB? YES NO $ CHARGES

21. DIAGNOSIS OR NATURE OF ILLNESS OR INJURY Relate A-L to service line below (24E) ICD Ind. 0

A. Z00.129 B. Z23 C. D.
E. F. G. H.
I. J. K. L.

22. RESUBMISSION CODE ORIGINAL REF. NO.

23. PRIOR AUTHORIZATION NUMBER

24. A. DATE(S) OF SERVICE From MM DD YY	To MM DD YY	B. PLACE OF SERVICE	C. EMG	D. PROCEDURES, SERVICES, OR SUPPLIES (Explain Unusual Circumstances) CPT/HCPCS	MODIFIER	E. DIAGNOSIS POINTER	F. $ CHARGES	G. DAYS OR UNITS	H. EPSDT Family Plan	I. ID. QUAL.	J. RENDERING PROVIDER ID. #
1	02 22 22		11	99391	25	A	111 00	1		NPI	1234567890
	N44928105105 ML05										
2	02 22 22		11	90698		AB	200 00	1		NPI	1234567890
	N400006404741 ML2										
3	02 22 22		11	90680		AB	200 00	1		NPI	1234567890
	N400005197105 ML05										
4	02 22 22		11	90670		AB	200 00	1		NPI	1234567890
5	02 22 22		11	90460		AB	150 00	3		NPI	1234567890
6	02 22 22		11	90461		AB	100 00	1		NPI	1234567890

25. FEDERAL TAX I.D. NUMBER SSN EIN [X]
12-4567897

26. PATIENT'S ACCOUNT NO.
11111

27. ACCEPT ASSIGNMENT? (For govt. claims, see back)
[X] YES NO

28. TOTAL CHARGE
$ 961 00

29. AMOUNT PAID
$

30. Rsvd for NUCC Use

31. SIGNATURE OF PHYSICIAN OR SUPPLIER INCLUDING DEGREES OR CREDENTIALS (I certify that the statements on the reverse apply to this bill and are made a part thereof.)
Signature on file 02232022
SIGNED DATE

32. SERVICE FACILITY LOCATION INFORMATION
Pediatric Practice
111 Some St
Anywhere, USA 999
a. NPI b.

33. BILLING PROVIDER INFO & PH # (555) 555-5555
Pediatric Practice
111 Some St
Anywhere, USA 999
a. 0123456789 b.

NUCC Instruction Manual available at: www.nucc.org **PLEASE PRINT OR TYPE** APPROVED OMB-0938-1197 FORM 1500 (02-12)

PATIENT AND INSURED INFORMATION

PHYSICIAN OR SUPPLIER INFORMATION

Chapter 1. The Basics of Coding

● indicates a new code; ▲, revised; #, re-sequenced; ✚, add-on; ★, audiovisual technology; and ◀, synchronous interactive audio.

Example

> ➤ If a child is diagnosed with a UTI, the code for UTI (*ICD-10-CM* code N39.0) should be linked to the E/M service (eg, 99213) and to a performed dipstick urinalysis without microscopy (81002).

Other Coding and Billing Information

Correct code assignment and claim completion are important steps in compliant and effective practice management. However, many other processes and policies are required. Please see **Chapter 4** for additional guidance on coding and billing procedures.

To test your knowledge of the information presented in this chapter, complete the quiz found at the end of it, after the resources. Answers to each quiz are found in **Appendix IV**. Add to your knowledge through the information provided in other chapters that discusses codes for specific types of service.

Chapter Takeaways

Readers of this chapter should generally know the code sets used to report professional services. Following are takeaways from this chapter:

- The 4 code sets that are used for reporting professional services are *ICD-10-CM*, HCPCS, *CPT*, and the NDC.
- To correctly select codes in *ICD-10-CM*, it is important to recognize and follow instructions found in the alphabetical index and tabular list to locate the most specific code for documented diagnoses.
- HCPCS procedure codes may be reported when no *CPT* code describes the service provided or when the narrative (code descriptor) differs from and more accurately describes the service provided than a similar *CPT* code.
- Use of *CPT* guidelines and full code descriptors is important in correct coding. Correct coding is important in obtaining correct claims payment.
- Every claim line for a physician service must be linked to the appropriate *ICD-10-CM* code that represents the reason for the service.

Resources

AAP Coding Assistance and Education

AAP Coding Hotline (https://form.jotform.com/Subspecialty/aapcodinghotline)

AAP *ICD-10-CM* resources (www.aap.org/en/practice-management/practice-financing/coding-and-valuation/icd-10-cm-resources)

AAP *Pediatric Office Superbill* (https://shop.aap.org/pediatric-office-superbill-2023)

AAP *Pediatric ICD-10-CM: A Manual for Provider-Based Coding* (https://shop.aap.org/pediatric-icd-10-cm-2023-8th-edition-paperback)

AAP Pediatric Coding Newsletter™

ICD-10-CM article collection (https://publications.aap.org/codingnews/collection/510/ICD-10-CM)

Current Procedural Terminology

AMA *CPT* general information (www.ama-assn.org/practice-management/cpt-current-procedural-terminology)

Category II code descriptors and clinical topics listing (www.ama-assn.org/practice-management/cpt/category-ii-codes)

Category III codes (www.ama-assn.org/practice-management/cpt/category-iii-codes)

Category I vaccine codes (www.ama-assn.org/practice-management/cpt/category-i-vaccine-codes)

ICD-10-CM Code Files and Guidelines

National Center for Health Statistics *ICD-10-CM* (www.cdc.gov/nchs/icd/icd-10-cm.htm)

National Drug Codes

US Food and Drug Administration National Drug Code Directory (www.fda.gov/drugs/informationondrugs/ucm142438.htm)

Test Your Knowledge!

1. **Which of the following code sets is used to convey the reason for services provided to a patient?**
   a. *International Classification of Diseases, 10th Revision, Clinical Modification*
   b. *Current Procedural Terminology*
   c. Healthcare Common Procedure Coding System
   d. National Drug Code

2. **How are the Healthcare Common Procedure Coding System (HCPCS) units determined for a drug administered to a patient?**
   a. Always report the number of milligrams of medication administered.
   b. Always report on the basis of units included in the HCPCS code descriptor.
   c. Only 1 unit is reported per medication administered.
   d. Report either milliliters or units on the basis of the product packaging.

3. **What is indicated by a plus sign (✚) before a *Current Procedural Terminology* code?**
   a. The code has been revised since the previous year.
   b. The code is new.
   c. The code may be reported with modifier **95** for telemedicine services.
   d. The code is reported for a service performed in addition to a primary service and is never reported as a stand-alone service.

4. **What does the first-listed diagnosis code indicate?**
   a. A condition that is most likely to affect the patient's long-term health
   b. The principal reason for the service provided on that date
   c. The patient's past medical history
   d. The condition that is most likely to result in payment for the service provided

5. **Which of the following statements is true of reporting *International Classification of Diseases, 10th Revision, Clinical Modification (ICD-10-CM)* diagnosis codes?**
   a. Only 1 diagnosis code is reported per claim.
   b. The first-listed diagnosis code must be linked to each service reported on a claim.
   c. A diagnosis pointer in field 24E links the appropriate *ICD-10-CM* code(s) to services on each claim line.
   d. *ICD-10-CM* codes do not affect whether a claim for a service is paid or denied.

Chapter 1. The Basics of Coding

Coding Edits and Modifiers

CPT copyright 2022 American Medical Association. All rights reserved.

Contents

Chapter Highlights 29

Coding Edits 29

  National Correct Coding Initiative (NCCI) Edits 29

  Procedure-to-Procedure Edits 29

  Appropriate NCCI Modifiers 30

  Medically Unlikely Edits 30

  Keeping Up to Date With the NCCI 31

  Reviewing and Using These Edits 32

Modifiers 32

  Current Procedural Terminology Modifiers 33

    Modifiers Appended Only to Evaluation and Management (E/M) Codes 33

      24—Unrelated E/M Service by the Same Physician or Other QHP During a Postoperative Period 33

      25—Significant, Separately Identifiable E/M Service by the Same Physician or Other QHP on the
         Same Day of the Procedure or Other Service 34

      57—Decision for Surgery 35

    Modifiers Appended Only to Codes for Procedures, Not to E/M Services 36

      22—Increased Procedural Services 36

      26—Professional Component 36

        Professional, Technical, or Global Services 36

        Reporting Modifier **26** 37

      47—Anesthesia by Surgeon 38

      50—Bilateral Procedure 38

      51—Multiple Procedures 39

      52—Reduced Services 40

      53—Discontinued Procedure 40

      54—Surgical Care Only 41

      55—Postoperative Management Only 41

      56—Preoperative Management Only 41

      58—Staged or Related Procedure or Service by the Same Physician or Other QHP During the
         Postoperative Period 41

      59—Distinct Procedural Service 42

      62—Two Surgeons 42

      63—Procedure Performed on Infants Less Than 4 kg 43

      66—Surgical Team 43

      76—Repeat Procedure or Service by Same Physician or Other QHP 44

      77—Repeat Procedure or Service by Another Physician or Other QHP 44

      78—Unplanned Return to the Operating/Procedure Room by the Same Physician or Other QHP
         Following Initial Procedure for a Related Procedure During the Postoperative Period 45

      79—Unrelated Procedure/Service by the Same Physician or Other QHP During the Postoperative Period 45

      80—Assistant Surgeon 45

      81—Minimum Assistant Surgeon 45

      82—Assistant Surgeon (When Qualified Resident Surgeon Not Available) 45

      90—Reference (Outside) Laboratory 46

      91—Repeat Clinical Diagnostic Laboratory Test 46

      92—Alternative Laboratory Platform Testing 46

    Modifiers Appended to Either E/M or Procedural Services 46

      32—Mandated Services 46

      33—Preventive Services 47

      93—Synchronous Telemedicine Service Rendered via Telephone or Other Real-time Interactive
         Audio-Only Telecommunications System 48

● indicates a new code; ▲, revised; #, re-sequenced; ✚, add-on; ★, audiovisual technology; and ◀, synchronous interactive audio.

Chapter Highlights

- Learn how payers commonly use 2 types of code edits to prevent errors in claims payment, and recognize when modifiers do or do not affect application of code edits.
- Learn about appropriate use of modifiers, including those from *Current Procedural Terminology* (*CPT*®) and the Healthcare Common Procedure Coding System (HCPCS).

Coding Edits

Coding edits and modifiers are important tools for getting paid correctly. Coding edits are used by most payers in electronic claims adjudication to determine which reported services are payable when multiple services are provided on the same date by the same physician, qualified health care professional (QHP), or multiple individuals practicing in the exact same specialty and same group practice. Edits also determine what number of units are allowed on the basis of common utilization (eg, typical medication doses) and payment policies. Correct modifier use can bypass some edits.

Modifiers are used to communicate information to payer systems about the service described by a procedure code.

Modifiers are also used to indicate either a change in the way a service was provided or additional information, such as laterality of a body site or certain circumstances (eg, a significant problem was addressed at an encounter for a routine child health examination).

National Correct Coding Initiative (NCCI) Edits

The National Correct Coding Initiative (NCCI) edits were developed for use by the Centers for Medicare & Medicaid Services (CMS) in adjudicating Medicare claims, and all Medicaid programs use a Medicaid-specific version of the NCCI edits. The NCCI edits may form the basis for proprietary claim editors used by private payers.

The NCCI edits

- Have been developed on the basis of *CPT* code descriptors and instructions, coding guidelines developed by national medical societies (eg, American Academy of Pediatrics [AAP]), Medicare billing history, local and national Medicare carrier policies and edits, and analysis of standard medical and surgical practice
- Are commonly used by payers in the claim processing system for physician services and for promotion of correct coding through publication of the edits and manuals that provide rationales for certain edits
- Include 2 types of edits: procedure-to-procedure edits and Medically Unlikely Edits (MUEs)

Physicians should not inconvenience patients or increase risks to patients by performing services on different dates of service to avoid MUE or NCCI procedure-to-procedure edits.

- This instruction comes from the Medicaid NCCI manual and prohibits practice policies that focus on achieving maximum payment.
- Delaying patient care to avoid code edits could be seen as an abusive billing practice; policies or practices that might be perceived in this way should be avoided.

Procedure-to-Procedure Edits

- Identify code pairs that should not normally be billed by the same physician or physicians of the same group practice and same specialty (*provider* is used in NCCI manuals) for the same patient on the same date of service.
- Include edits based on services that are mutually exclusive on the basis of code descriptor or anatomical considerations (**Table 2-1**), services that are considered to be inherent to each other, and edits based on coding instructions.
  - If 2 codes of an edit are billed by the same provider for the same patient for the same date of service without an appropriate modifier, only the column 1 code is paid.
  - If clinical circumstances justify appending the appropriate modifier to the column 2 code, payment of both codes may be allowed. (The Medicaid NCCI will allow payment when an NCCI modifier is appended to either code in a code pair, provided that the modifier is appropriately reported in conjunction with either code.)

> The Centers for Medicare & Medicaid Services allows physicians to append modifiers 59, XE, XP, XS, and XU to the column 1 or column 2 code when reporting 2 codes paired by the Medicare National Correct Coding Initiative (NCCI) edits. Other payers may adopt this policy or require that the modifier be appended to the code in column 2 of the NCCI edit file.

● indicates a new code; ▲, revised; #, re-sequenced; ✚, add-on; ★, audiovisual technology; and ◀, synchronous interactive audio.

Appropriate NCCI Modifiers

Modifier indicators are assigned to every code pair identified in the NCCI. They dictate whether modifiers are needed or will be accepted to override the edit. These indicators are

0   Under no circumstance may a modifier be used to override the edit.

1   An appropriate modifier may be used to override the edit.

9   This edit was deleted.

Refer to **Table 2-1** for examples.

Table 2-1. Examples of Medicaid National Correct Coding Initiative Edits				
Column 1 Comprehensive Code		**Column 2 Component Code**		**Modifier Indicator**	**Effective Date**
Edits apply to services provided on the same date by 1 physician or QHP or multiple individuals of the same specialty and same group practice.				
99460	Initial hospital or birthing center care, per day, for E/M of normal newborn infant	**99462**	Subsequent hospital care, per day, for E/M of normal newborn	0	10/1/2010
The NCCI edits preclude any payment for the column 2 code because the services are mutually exclusive. Each code represents all normal newborn care on a single date of service.				
10121	Incision and removal of foreign body, subcutaneous tissues; complex	**10120**	Incision and removal of foreign body, subcutaneous tissues; simple	1	10/1/2010
*The component code (**10120**) would be denied unless a modifier indicating a distinct procedural service (eg, **59**) were appended (eg, **10120 59**). Medicaid payment policy allows both services only if the incisions and removals are from separate noncontiguous sites or the procedures occurred at separate encounters.*				
44970	Laparoscopy, surgical, appendectomy	**99221–99223**	Initial hospital inpatient or observation care	0	10/1/2010
*The NCCI edits preclude payment for the component code (ie, a column 2 code **99221–99223**) except when a modifier is appropriately used to override the edit. When a physician makes a decision for surgery on the same date as performing the procedure, modifier **57** (decision for surgery) may be appended to the component code (eg, **99222 57**) to indicate that the E/M service did not occur after the decision for surgery and is not included in the preoperative work of the procedure.*				
10120	Incision and removal of foreign body, subcutaneous tissues; simple	**99212–99215**	Office or other outpatient E/M service	1	10/1/2020
*The component code (**99212–99215**) would be denied if modifier **25** were not appended to it. To report modifier **25**, E/M services must require significant and separate MDM or time beyond that included in the preservice and post-service work of a procedure performed at the same encounter. Be aware that the higher-valued service may be the component code and would be denied without the application of the correct modifier.*				
Abbreviations: E/M, evaluation and management; MDM, medical decision-making; NCCI, National Correct Coding Initiative; QHP, qualified health care professional.				

- Only certain modifiers can be used to override edits when the service or procedure is clinically justified, and they may be used only on the code pairs that are assigned the 1 indicator. See **Box 2-1** for a list of modifiers that override NCCI edits.
- The appropriate modifier is typically appended to the code that appears in column 2 because that is considered the bundled or exclusive procedure.
- To append the appropriate modifier and override an edit, it is imperative that the conditions of that modifier are met (eg, **XE**, separate encounter [different session]).

Medically Unlikely Edits

The *National Correct Coding Initiative Policy Manual for Medicaid Services* describes MUEs as unit of service edits that were established by the CMS to prevent payment for an inappropriate number or quantity of the same service (eg, unintentional reporting of 100 rather than 10 units). An MUE for a HCPCS or *CPT* code is the maximum number of units of service, under most circumstances, allowable by the same provider for the same beneficiary on the same date of service.

Medicaid MUEs

- Are applied separately to each line of a claim. If the unit of service on a line exceeds the MUE value, the entire line is denied

● indicates a new code; ▲, revised; #, re-sequenced; ✚, add-on; ★, audiovisual technology; and ◀, synchronous interactive audio.

Box 2-1. Modifiers That Can Be Used to Override National Correct Coding Initiative Edits

24	Unrelated E/M service by the same physician or other QHP during a postoperative period	F6	Right hand, second digit
25	Significant, separately identifiable E/M service by the same physician or other QHP on the same day of the procedure or other service	F7	Right hand, third digit
		F8	Right hand, fourth digit
		F9	Right hand, fifth digit
57	Decision for surgery	LC	Left circumflex, coronary artery
58	Staged or related procedure or service by the same physician or other QHP during the postoperative period	LD	Left anterior descending coronary artery
		LM	Left main coronary artery
59	Distinct procedural service	LT	Left side
78	Unplanned return to the OR by the same physician or other QHP following initial procedure for a related procedure during the postoperative period	RC	Right coronary artery
		RI	Ramus intermedius coronary artery
		RT	Right side
79	Unrelated procedure/service by the same physician or other QHP during the postoperative period	TA	Left foot, great toe
		T1	Left foot, second digit
91	Repeat clinical diagnostic laboratory test	T2	Left foot, third digit
E1	Upper left, eyelid	T3	Left foot, fourth digit
E2	Lower left, eyelid	T4	Left foot, fifth digit
E3	Upper right, eyelid	T5	Right foot, great toe
E4	Lower right, eyelid	T6	Right foot, second digit
FA	Left hand, thumb	T7	Right foot, third digit
F1	Left hand, second digit	T8	Right foot, fourth digit
F2	Left hand, third digit	T9	Right foot, fifth digit
F3	Left hand, fourth digit	XE	Separate encounter (different session)
F4	Left hand, fifth digit	XP	Separate practitioner
F5	Right hand, thumb	XS	Separate structure (site/organ)
		XU	Unusual nonoverlapping service

Abbreviations: E/M, evaluation and management; OR, operating/procedure room; QHP, qualified health care professional.

- Are coding edits rather than medical necessity edits
- May be established on the basis of claims data
- May limit units of service based on anatomical structures
- May limit the number of units of service based on *CPT* code descriptors or *CPT* coding instructions
- Are published on the CMS Medicaid NCCI website at www.medicaid.gov/medicaid/program-integrity/ncci/index.html
- Are published with an *edit rationale* for each HCPCS and *CPT* code
  - The MUE value assigned for code **96110** (developmental screening, per instrument) is 3 on the basis of CMS NCCI policy. (No further explanation of this rationale is provided in the current Medicaid or Medicare NCCI manuals but may be based on historical claims data.)
  - The MUE value assigned to code **96127** (brief emotional/behavior assessment, per instrument) is 2 on the basis of the nature of the service or procedure (typically determined by the amount of time required to perform a procedure/service or clinical application of a procedure/service).
- Are applied separately to each claim line for a service when modifiers (eg, **59**, **76**, **77**, anatomical) cause the same HCPCS or *CPT* code to appear on separate lines of a claim

It is important to recognize that the use of modifiers to override the MUE must be justified on the basis of correct selection of the procedure code, correct application of the number of units reported, medical necessity and reasonableness of the number of services, and, if applicable, reason the physician's practice pattern differs from national patterns.

Keeping Up to Date With the NCCI

Medicaid and Medicare NCCI edits are updated quarterly. Each Medicare NCCI version ends with .0 (point zero), .1, .2, or .3 indicating its effective dates.

- Versions ending in .0 (point zero) are effective from January 1 through March 31 of that year.
- Versions ending in .1 are effective from April 1 through June 30 of that year.
- Versions ending in .2 are effective from July 1 through September 30 of that year.
- Versions ending in .3 are effective from October 1 through December 31 of that year.

The CMS releases the Medicare NCCI edits free of charge on its website (www.cms.gov/NationalCorrectCodInitEd/NCCIEP/list.asp). Medicaid NCCI files are published separately free of charge at https://data.medicaid.gov/ncci.

- Although many of the Medicaid edits mirror Medicare edits, this is not always the case. The CMS has instructed that use of the appropriate NCCI file is important for correct coding.
- Online NCCI edits are posted in spreadsheet form, which allows users to sort by procedure code and effective date.
- There is a "Find" tool that allows users to look for a specific code. The edit files are indexed by procedure code ranges for simplified navigation.
- Policy manuals that explain the rationale for edits and correct use of NCCI-associated modifiers are published to the web pages listed previously (see "Reference Documents" link on the Medicaid NCCI page).
  — Updated manuals for the year ahead are published annually in late fall.
  — Changes in the manual are shown in red font for easy identification.
  — Be sure to update your NCCI edit files quarterly and review changes to the NCCI manual each year.

Practice management and electronic health record software may also contain tools for identifying codes affected by NCCI edits.

Reviewing and Using These Edits

1. Be aware of all coding edits that are applicable to your specialty; as each update replaces the former edits, it is important to review them quarterly. Always look for new or deleted edits. Updated files can be found at www.aap.org/coding under the "Coding Edits and Modifiers" topic block.
2. Pay close attention to the modifier indicator because it may have changed from the last quarterly update. For example, a code set that would not initially allow override with a modifier may now subsequently allow one, or vice versa.
3. Pay attention to the effective date and deletion date of each code set. The edits are applicable only if they are effective. The effective date is based on the date of service, not the date the claim was submitted. Sometimes an edit is retroactively terminated. If so, you may resubmit claims for payment if the date of service is within the filing time frame of the payer.
4. Use modifiers as appropriate.
   a. Modifiers should be used only when applicable on the basis of coding standards, when medically justified or necessary, and when supported by medical record documentation (progress notes, procedure notes, diagrams, or pictures) or, as previously mentioned, when dictated by payers.
   b. Refer to the CMS written guidelines (because they are very explicit about billing surgical procedures) or to your payer's provider manual.
5. When billing surgical procedures, you may need to look at several different codes for possible edits. Be sure to always use the code that is reflective of the total service performed. When no existing code accurately describes the procedure as performed, report an unlisted procedure code and attach documentation of the procedure to the claim when submitted for payment.
6. Appeal denied payment for services for which there is no edit and the policy manual and/or payment policies do not preclude reporting, for which a reported modifier should have allowed payment, and/or for which the edit is inconsistent with *CPT* guidelines. Having knowledge of how this system works is to your benefit when appealing the denial.
7. Some payers have developed or adopted coding edit programs that are different from and often more comprehensive than the NCCI.
   a. If a payer policy differs from the CMS NCCI policy and is not clearly defined in its provider manual, refer to the payer's website.
   b. Make sure you get policies in writing for the services you commonly perform. Your contracts with health plans should be explicit regarding how you will receive initial and updated policies.
8. Report the services provided correctly on the basis of *CPT* code guidelines (unless a payer has clearly stated otherwise).

Modifiers

CPT defines a *modifier* as an indicator that a service or procedure has been altered by some specific circumstance but not changed in its basic code definition. Modifiers are also used to show compliance with payment policy. Medical record documentation must always support the use of the modifier.

Modifiers from *CPT* and HCPCS are used with codes from either *CPT* or HCPCS. Most state Medicaid programs and many commercial payers recognize HCPCS modifiers and *CPT* modifiers.

When are modifiers needed? In brief, a modifier or combination of modifiers is appended to a procedure code when it is necessary to add context of how or when the service was provided. Context often affects payment, such as when a bilateral procedure is reported with a code that does not indicate unilateral or bilateral. By appending modifier **50** (bilateral procedure), the claim for services provides context allowing claims adjudication systems to process for payment at a higher rate (typically 150% of the allowable amount for the unilateral service). Examples of information provided by modifiers include

- A service provided on the same date or within the global period of a previous service is unrelated, more extensive, performed on a different body area, or performed at separate encounters.
- A face-to-face service was provided via telemedicine by using real-time, interactive communication technology.
- The same service was repeated on the same date.
- An evaluation and management (E/M) service that might otherwise be considered part of another service is significantly beyond the typical preservice and/or post-service components of the other service.
- The units of services provided were medically necessary but exceed the payer's unit of service edits.
- A service that may be provided for diagnostic or preventive purposes was provided for preventive purposes.

Payers use coding edits (ie, paired codes and/or unit of service limitations) to aid in automated claims adjudication. Modifiers play an important role in this process.

- When a modifier is appropriately applied to 1 code in a pair of codes reported by a physician on 1 date of service or to a code for services that exceed the units of service typically allowed by payer edits, the payer may allow charges that would otherwise be denied as bundled or non-covered.

The Health Insurance Portability and Accountability Act of 1996 requires recognition of all *CPT* and HCPCS modifiers, but payers may have their own payment and billing policies for the use of modifiers that can vary from *CPT* guidelines.

- Know and understand their policies. This is important in capturing all payments allowed under your contract.
- If payment is denied inappropriately because of nonrecognition or the incorrect application of a modifier, you should appeal the denied services.
- For additional assistance, contact the AAP Coding Hotline (https://form.jotform.com/Subspecialty/aapcodinghotline).

Current Procedural Terminology Modifiers

Some *CPT* modifiers are used exclusively with E/M services, and others are reported only with surgical or other procedures (eg, medical, laboratory, or radiological testing). Refer to **Table 2-2** to review modifiers used with E/M service codes and those used only for other services. Multiple modifiers can be appended to a single *CPT* or HCPCS code.

Table 2-2. Modifiers and Evaluation and Management Services	
24, 25, 57	E/M-only modifiers
22, 26, 47, 50, 51, 52, 53, 54, 55, 56, 58, 59, 62, 63, 66, 76, 77, 78, 79, 80, 81, 82, 91, 92	Procedure-only modifiers (Do not append to E/M services.)
32, 33, 93ᵃ, 95ᵃ, 96, 97, 99	Either E/M or procedures

Abbreviation: E/M, evaluation and management.

ᵃ See Appendix T in your *Current Procedural Terminology* reference for codes reportable with modifier **93**, and see Appendix P for codes reportable with modifier **95**.

Modifiers Appended Only to Evaluation and Management (E/M) Codes

24—*Unrelated E/M Service by the Same Physician or Other QHP During a Postoperative Period*

> The global period (preoperative, intraoperative, and postoperative periods) for surgical procedures is assigned by the Centers for Medicare & Medicaid Services, private payers, or Medicaid and not by the American Medical Association or *Current Procedural Terminology*. For more information on global surgery guidelines, see chapters 14 and 19.

- Modifier **24** is appended to an E/M code when the physician or other QHP who performed a procedure provides an unrelated E/M service during the postoperative period.
- The CMS has its own system for defining global periods, and many payers will follow those guidelines or assign a specific number of follow-up days for surgical procedures.

● indicates a new code; ▲, revised; #, re-sequenced; ✚, add-on; ★, audiovisual technology; and ◀, synchronous interactive audio.

Link the appropriate *International Classification of Diseases, 10th Revision, Clinical Modification (ICD-10-CM)* code to the E/M visit to support that the service was unrelated to the surgical procedure. Do not report the surgical diagnosis code if it was not the reason for the encounter. However, a different diagnosis is not required, as further treatment of the underlying condition for which surgery was performed is not part of the postoperative work of the procedure and may be separately reported.

Example—Modifier 24

➤ **A physician sees a 10-year-old established patient for follow-up of stable mild persistent asthma and performs a level-3 established patient office or other outpatient E/M service.** The visit occurs within the 90-day global period assigned by the payer to code **25600** (closed treatment of a distal radial fracture) for which the same physician is providing care. Modifier **24** is appended to the E/M code to indicate that the service is unrelated to care of the fracture.

ICD-10-CM	CPT
J45.30 (mild persistent asthma, uncomplicated)	**99213 24** (established office/outpatient E/M)

25—Significant, Separately Identifiable E/M Service by the Same Physician or Other QHP on the Same Day of the Procedure or Other Service

- Modifier **25** is appended only to an E/M service and only when *all the following circumstances are true:*
  - A separate service identified by a separate procedure code is performed by the same physician or other QHP, or by a physician or other QHP of the same specialty and group.
  - The patient's condition requires a significant E/M service (**99202–99499**) above and beyond the other service provided or beyond the usual preoperative and postoperative care associated with the procedure that was performed.
  - The service is separately identifiable in the documentation of the encounter(s).
- Different diagnoses are not required for reporting the E/M service on the same date.
- The performed and documented E/M components must be supportive of the level of service reported and be separately identifiable from the procedure or other service documentation, whether documented in one combined note or separate notes.
- *CPT* procedure codes include evaluative elements routinely performed before the procedure and the routine postoperative care. An assessment of the problem with an explanation of the procedure to be performed is considered inherent to the procedure and should not be reported separately with an E/M service code.
- When appropriate, modifier **25** may be reported on more than one E/M service for a single encounter. See an example below.
- **DO *NOT* USE MODIFIER 25 WHEN**
  - **The medical record does not support both services.**
  - **A problem encountered during a preventive medicine visit is insignificant or incidental (eg, minor diaper rash, renewal of prescription medications without reevaluation) or did not require additional work to perform medical decision-making [MDM] or additional time that is distinct from the time spent providing the preventive E/M service.**
  - **The E/M service is a routine part of the usual preoperative and postoperative care.**
  - **Modifier 57 (decision for surgery) is more appropriate. The ultimate decision on whether to use modifier 25 or 57 requires knowledge of payer policies. (See modifier 57 discussed later in this chapter.)**

Examples—Modifier 25

➤ **A 12-year-old established patient is seen for his preventive medicine visit.** The patient describes increased asthma symptoms. Medical decision-making is moderate for management of moderate persistent asthma with worsening symptoms requiring adjustment to the dose of the control medication, supporting code **99214**. He has not yet received his tetanus, diphtheria, and acellular pertussis (Tdap) or meningococcal (MenACWY-D) intramuscular vaccine. The physician counsels the parents on the risks and protection from each of the diseases. The Centers for Disease Control and Prevention (CDC) Vaccine Information Statements are given to the parents, and the nurse administers the vaccines.

ICD-10-CM	CPT
Z00.121 (well-child check with abnormal findings) **Z23** (encounter for immunization)	**99394 25** (preventive medicine visit, established patient, age 12 through 17 years) **90715** (Tdap, 7 years or older, intramuscular) **90734** (MenACWY-D) **90460** × 2 units **90461** × 2 units
J45.40 (moderate persistent asthma, uncomplicated)	**99214 25** (office/outpatient E/M, established patient)

Teaching Point: Medical record documentation supports that a significant, separately identifiable E/M service was provided and is reported in addition to the preventive medicine service. Modifier **25** is appended to code **99214** to signify that it is significant and separately identifiable from the preventive medicine service. Modifier **25** is also appended to code **99394** to signify that it is significant and separately identifiable from immunization administration (required by payers that have adopted Medicare and Medicaid bundling edits).

> **See Chapter 8 for additional examples and guidelines for reporting a preventive medicine visit and a problem-oriented visit on the same day of service.**

➤ **A patient is scheduled for removal of impacted cerumen of the right ear following use of softening drops as directed at a prior visit.** The physician takes a problem-focused history from the patient, who has no other concerns; examines the affected ear; and determines that manual extraction is necessary, explaining the procedure, risks, and benefits. A combination of irrigation and removal through instrumentation is successful in clearing the ear canal.

ICD-10-CM	CPT
H61.21 (impacted cerumen, right ear)	**69210** (removal impacted cerumen requiring instrumentation, unilateral)

Teaching Point: An E/M service with modifier **25** is *not* reported. A separate charge for an E/M service is reported only when the E/M service is significant and separately identifiable from the preservice work of a procedure reported on the same date.

> **See chapters 14 and 19 for more information on reporting an evaluation and management service on the date of a procedure.**

57—Decision for Surgery

- Modifier **57** is appended to an E/M service that resulted in the initial decision to perform the surgery or procedure. Appending modifier **57** to the E/M service indicates to the payer that the E/M service is not part of the global period.
- An E/M code with modifier **57** is reported only by the physician or a physician of the same specialty and group practice of the physician who performs the procedure. Other physicians providing E/M services on the day before or day of a procedure would not append modifier **57**.
- Many payers will follow the CMS Medicare payment policy that allows reporting of modifier **57** only when the visit on the day before or day of surgery results in a decision to perform a surgical procedure that has a 90-day global period (major procedure).
- Know commercial and state Medicaid policies, maintain a written copy of the policy, and adhere to the policy.

Examples—Modifier 57

➤ **A 10-year-old is seen by the pediatrician for the evaluation of pain in her foot and arm after a fall.** Radiograph reveals a metatarsal fracture, and the decision is made to treat the closed fracture. Arm injuries are limited to bruising and abrasions.

● indicates a new code; ▲, revised; #, re-sequenced; ✚, add-on; ★, audiovisual technology; and ◀, synchronous interactive audio.

Code **28470** (closed treatment, metatarsal fracture; without manipulation) has an assigned global surgery period of 90 days. The appropriate E/M code (**99202–99215 57**), based on the clinically indicated performance and documentation of the required MDM, would be reported in addition to code **28470**.

➤ **A circumcision is performed on the day of discharge on a 2-day-old born in the hospital, delivered vaginally.**

ICD-10-CM	CPT
Z38.00 (single liveborn infant, delivered vaginally) **Z41.2** (encounter for routine male circumcision)	**99238 25** (hospital discharge management) **54150** (circumcision, using clamp/device with dorsal penile or ring block)

Teaching Point: The procedure has a 0-day global period. Per CMS guidelines, modifier **25** would be appended to the E/M service instead of modifier **57**.

Modifiers Appended Only to Codes for Procedures, Not to E/M Services

22—Increased Procedural Services

- Modifier **22** is used to report procedures when the work required to provide a service is substantially greater than typically required.
- Modifier **22** is appended only to anesthesia, surgery, radiology, laboratory, pathology, and medicine codes.
- Documentation must clearly reflect the substantial additional work and the reason for the additional work (eg, increased intensity, time, technical difficulty of procedure, severity of patient's condition, physical and mental effort required).
  - It is important that the documentation is specific. For instance, documentation that a procedure took longer than 1 hour is less supportive than documentation that the procedure took a total of 85 minutes or lasted from 9:15 to 10:40 am.
  - Report additional diagnosis codes to support the increased work, when applicable.
- Most payers will require that a copy of the medical record documentation be sent with the claim when modifier **22** is reported.
- For an electronic claim, indicate "additional documentation available on request" in the claim level loop (2300 NTE) or in the line level loop (2400 NTE) segment. If the payer allows electronic claim attachments, follow the payer's instructions to submit the procedure note and, if necessary, a physician statement about the increased difficulty of the procedure.

Examples—Modifier 22

➤ **The physician required 45 minutes to perform a simple repair of a 1-cm laceration on a 2-year-old because the child was combative and several stops and starts were necessary.**

12011 22 (simple repair superficial wound of face; ≤2.5 cm)

➤ **An appendectomy is performed on a 12-year-old with morbid obesity.** The surgery is complicated and requires additional time because of the obesity.

44950 22 (appendectomy)

26—Professional Component

Professional, Technical, or Global Services

Certain procedures (eg, cardiac tests, radiography, surgical diagnostic tests) are broken down into professional and technical components. *CPT* has a modifier for reporting the professional component (**26**) but does not have a modifier for reporting only the technical component. That falls under the HCPCS modifier set (modifier **TC**).

- Professional component only: The physician who does not supply the equipment but performs the written interpretation and report of a service with professional and technical components should report the service with modifier **26** appended to the appropriate *CPT* code.

> **The professional component includes the physician work (eg, interpretation of the test, written report).**

- Technical component only: Most payers recognize modifier **TC** (technical component only). The facility or provider who owns the equipment and is responsible for the overhead and associated costs would report the same procedure code with modifier **TC** appended.
- Technical and professional components (global): If a service includes both professional and technical components and the physician owns the equipment, employs the staff to perform the service, and interprets the test, the procedure is reported *without a modifier*.

Reporting Modifier 26

- When reporting the professional component of diagnostic tests, interpretation should be documented in a report like that which is typical for the physicians who predominantly provide the service. This report should include *all the following items:*
  — Indication(s) for testing
  — Description of test
  — Findings
  — Limitations (when applicable)
  — Impression or conclusion
- If the report of a physician's interpretation is included in the documentation of another service (eg, office visit), it is important that the report is distinct and complete.
- The professional component is not reported when a physician reviews a test and notes agreement with the interpreting physician or when only a quick read without formal interpretation is provided.
- Some codes were developed to distinguish between technical and professional components (eg, routine electrocardiogram [ECG] codes **93000–93010**). Modifier **26** is not appropriate when reporting codes that distinguish professional and technical components and may result in a denial of the charge.

Examples—Modifier 26

➤ **A pulmonologist interprets the results of exercise testing for bronchospasm and creates a report of the findings. The tests were performed in a facility's pulmonary laboratory, and the facility will bill the technical component of the service.**

94619 26 (exercise test for bronchospasm, including pre- and post-spirometry and pulse oximetry; without electrocardiographic recordings)

The physician reports modifier **26**, indicating professional component only, because the hospital provided the technical component.

➤ **A pediatrician electronically accesses the image of a foot radiograph that was taken at the outpatient department of the hospital and will be interpreted by a radiologist at that facility. The pediatrician notes findings in the patient's records.**

The pediatrician's review of the radiograph is not separately reported when a radiologist will provide a final interpretation and report. However, the physician's review of the image increases the level of data to be reviewed and analyzed when determining the level of MDM in a related E/M service.

➤ **A cardiologist performs transthoracic echocardiography with spectral and color-flow Doppler echocardiography on a patient in the hospital.**

The cardiologist would report code **93306 26** (echocardiography, transthoracic, real-time with image documentation [2D], includes M-mode recording, when performed, complete, with spectral Doppler echocardiography, and with color-flow Doppler echocardiography), and the hospital would report code **93306 TC**.

● indicates a new code; ▲, revised; #, re-sequenced; ✚, add-on; ★, audiovisual technology; and ◄, synchronous interactive audio.

47—Anesthesia by Surgeon

- Modifier **47** is used only when a physician performing a procedure *also personally performs* the regional and/or general anesthesia. The physician performing the procedure may not report codes **00100–01999** for anesthesia services. Instead, modifier **47** is appended to the code for the procedure performed.
- When performed, a code for regional anesthesia (nerve block) may be reported to indicate the site of the block.
- Modifier **47** is considered informational by many payers and does not affect payment.
  - Medicaid considers all anesthesia (other than moderate conscious sedation) provided by the same physician performing a procedure to be included in the procedure.
  - Other payers may restrict use of modifier **47** to specific procedure codes and provide specific reporting instructions. Be sure to verify payer policy before reporting.
- **DO *NOT* USE MODIFIER 47 WHEN**
  - **Administering local anesthesia because it is considered inherent to the procedure**
  - **Performing moderate (conscious) sedation**

> For more information on reporting moderate sedation, see chapter 14 .

Example—Modifier 47

➤ **The surgeon performs a nerve block on the brachial plexus (64415) and removal of a ganglion cyst on the wrist (25111).**
> **25111 47** and **64415**
> The regional anesthesia is separate from the procedure.

50—Bilateral Procedure

- Modifier **50** is used to identify bilateral procedures that are performed at the same session.
- It is used only when the services and/or procedures are performed on identical anatomical sites, aspects, or organs.
- Modifier **50** is not appended to any code with a descriptor that indicates that the procedure includes bilateral, "one or both," or "unilateral or bilateral."
- The Medicare Physician Fee Schedule (MFPS) Relative Value Files (www.cms.gov/Medicare/Medicare-Fee-for-Service-Payment/PhysicianFeeSched/PFS-Relative-Value-Files.html) include a column (Column Z, BILAT SURG) that identifies codes that may be reported with modifier **50**. Procedures with a 1 indicator can be reported with modifier **50**.

> Many private payers also publish lists of codes that may be reported as bilateral procedures.

- When the *CPT* code descriptor indicates a bilateral procedure and only a unilateral procedure is performed, modifier **52** (reduced services) should be appended to the procedure code.
- For Medicaid claims that require use of modifier **50**, only report 1 unit of service on the line item for the bilateral procedure.

Examples—Modifier 50

➤ **A physician performs bilateral tympanostomy with insertion of ventilating tubes under general anesthesia.**
> **69436 50** (tympanostomy [requiring insertion of ventilating tube], general anesthesia)

➤ **A physician performs bilateral nasal endoscopy.**
> Modifier **50** would not be appended to code **31231** (nasal endoscopy, diagnostic, unilateral or bilateral [separate procedure]) because the code descriptor indicates a unilateral or bilateral procedure. (Modifier **52** is also not required for reporting a unilateral service when the code descriptor includes unilateral or bilateral.)

Chapter 2. Coding Edits and Modifiers

Coding Conundrum: Modifier 50

The Medicaid National Correct Coding Initiative edits require that bilateral surgical procedures (for which there is no code specifying a bilateral procedure) be reported with modifier **50** and 1 unit of service.

Example: Report removal of foreign bodies from both ears with code **69200 50** with 1 unit.

Bilateral diagnostic procedures may be reported with any of the following methods:

Example: Report bilateral radiographs of clavicles with one of the following 3 methods:
- 2 units of service on 1 claim line: **73000** (radiologic examination; clavicle, complete) × 2
- 1 unit of service and modifier **50** on 1 claim line: **73000 50** × 1 unit
- 1 unit of service and modifier **RT** on 1 claim line plus 1 unit of service and modifier **LT** on a second claim line: **73000 RT** × 1 unit and **73000 LT** × 1 unit

---

51—*Multiple Procedures*

- Modifier **51** is most often used for surgical procedures that are performed during the same session and through the same incision. This modifier identifies potentially overlapping or duplicative relative value units (RVUs) related to the global surgical package or the technical component of certain services (eg, radiology services).
- Some payers, including Medicare administrative contractors, have advised against reporting this modifier, as their systems automatically assign multiple service reductions to the appropriate services. In these cases, the system ignores modifier **51**. Follow payer guidance for reporting modifier **51**.
- When required, modifier **51** is appended to each additional procedure(s) or service(s) when multiple procedures are performed at the same session by the same individual or individuals in the same group practice. The primary procedure or service is reported first without a modifier.
- Although many claims adjudication systems now automatically identify the primary procedure, it is advisable that the first-reported service is that with the highest relative value, followed by additional services appended with modifier **51**, when applicable.
- Modifier **51** does not override NCCI edits.

For information on multiple surgery indicators and payment adjustments, see Chapter 12, Section 40.6, of the *Medicare Claims Processing Manual* at www.cms.gov/Regulations-and-Guidance/Guidance/Manuals/Downloads/clm104c12.pdf or individual payer policies for multiple procedures performed on the same date.

- **DO *NOT* USE MODIFIER 51 WHEN**
  - **Reporting add-on procedure codes (identified with the ✚ symbol) that are exempt from modifier 51 because the services are always performed in addition to a primary service.**
  - **Reporting *CPT* codes identified with the symbol Ø (exempt from modifier 51) because they have no associated preservice or post-service valuation and are already reduced (see *CPT* Appendix E for a list of these codes).**
  - **Different providers perform the procedures.**
  - **Two or more physicians perform different and unrelated procedures (eg, multiple trauma) on the same patient on the same day (unless one of the physicians performs multiple procedures).**
  - **Reporting E/M services, physical medicine and rehabilitation services, or provision of supplies (eg, vaccines).**

Example—*Modifier* 51

➤ **A child undergoes adenoidectomy and bilateral myringotomy with tube placement at the same surgical session. The surgeon reports**

    69436 50 (tympanostomy [requiring insertion of ventilating tube], general anesthesia)

    42830 51 (adenoidectomy, primary; younger than age 12)

    Teaching Point: Code **69436** is reported first because it carries the highest relative value when reported with modifier **50** (7.17 non-facility total RVUs [4.78 × 150%] vs 6.33 for code **42830**). Modifier **51** is appended to code **42830**. If the myringotomy was a unilateral procedure, code **42830** would be listed first and modifier **51** appended to code **69436** (with no modifier **50**).

● indicates a new code; ▲, revised; #, re-sequenced; ✚, add-on; ★, audiovisual technology; and ◀, synchronous interactive audio.

52—Reduced Services

- Modifier **52** is used when a service or procedure is partially reduced or eliminated (ie, procedure started but discontinued) at the discretion of the physician or other QHP.
- Modifier **52** is not used when a procedure is canceled before the induction of anesthesia and/or surgical preparation in the operating/procedure room (OR).
- The diagnosis code linked to the procedure reported with modifier **52** should reflect why the procedure was reduced.
- When reporting a reduced service or a procedure code with modifier **52**, do not reduce your normal fee. Let the payer reduce the payment on the basis of its policy.

Examples—Modifier 52

➤ **A physician begins a circumcision (54150) on a 3-day-old boy.** The physician elects to perform the circumcision without a dorsal penile or ring block. In this circumstance, modifier **52** would be reported with code **54150** to indicate that the service was reduced from its full descriptor on the basis of the physician's discretion.

➤ **A peripherally inserted central venous catheter (PICC) without a subcutaneous port is inserted with imaging guidance, but tip location is not confirmed by imaging.**

ICD-10-CM	CPT
J13 (pneumonia due to *Streptococcus pneumoniae*)	**36572 52** (PICC insertion without subcutaneous port, with imaging guidance; younger than 5 years of age)

Teaching Point: Code **36572** includes confirmation of the tip location. Therefore, modifier **52** would be appended when performed without confirmation of catheter tip location.

53—Discontinued Procedure

- Modifier **53** signifies that a procedure was terminated (ie, started but discontinued) due to extenuating circumstances or circumstances in which the well-being of the patient was threatened (eg, patient is at risk or has unexpected, serious complications, such as excessive bleeding or hypotension) during a procedure.
- It is not used to report the elective cancellation of a procedure before the patient's anesthesia induction and/or surgical preparation in the operating suite.
- The diagnosis code should reflect the reason for the termination of the procedure.
- Most payers will require that operative or procedure reports be submitted with the claim.

Examples—Modifier 53

➤ **An unsuccessful attempt is made to place a central catheter in the right subclavian vein.** The catheter is successfully placed in the left subclavian vein.
  36555 53 RT (insertion non-tunneled centrally inserted central venous catheter; younger than 5 years)
  36555 LT
  Note: Some payers do not recognize modifiers **RT** and **LT**. For the descriptions and use of these modifiers, see the Healthcare Common Procedure Coding System Modifiers section later in this chapter.

➤ **A physician begins a circumcision (54150) on a 3-day-old boy.** During the procedure, the physician notices that the neonate is showing signs of respiratory distress. Due to the severity of the situation, the physician decides not to continue with the procedure.
  54150 53 (circumcision, using clamp or other device with regional dorsal penile or ring block)
  In this circumstance, the physician would link diagnosis codes **Z41.2** (encounter for routine and ritual male circumcision) and **P22.9** (respiratory distress, newborn) to indicate why the procedure was discontinued. When reporting a procedure with modifier **53**, it is important to indicate why the procedure was discontinued.

Chapter 2. Coding Edits and Modifiers

54—Surgical Care Only

Modifier **54** is appended to the surgery procedure code when the physician does the procedure but another physician or other QHP (not of the same group practice) accepts a transfer of care and provides preoperative and/or postoperative management.

55—Postoperative Management Only

Modifier **55** is appended to the surgical code to report that only postoperative care is performed because another physician or other QHP of another group practice has performed the surgical procedure and transferred the patient for postoperative care.

56—Preoperative Management Only

Modifier **56** is appended to the surgical code when only the preoperative care and evaluation are performed because another physician or other QHP of another group practice has performed the surgical procedure. This modifier is seldom applicable.

Coding Conundrum: Modifiers 54, 55, **and** 56

Modifiers **54, 55,** and **56** are typically used to report surgical procedures that have a global period of 10 to 90 days. They are not reported with procedures that have 0-day global periods. It is important to learn which guidelines are followed by your major payers. When reporting these modifiers, coordination and communication between the physicians and their billing staff is imperative. The physician providing follow-up care must know whether the physician who provided the surgical care reported modifier **54** in order to report modifier **55**. Alternatively, the physician providing follow-up care may be limited to reporting evaluation and management codes for each follow-up encounter that does not include a new procedural service.

For more information on global surgery guidelines, see **chapters 14 and 19**.

Example—Modifiers 54 and 55

➤ **An emergency department (ED) physician provides initial care for a Colles fracture of the right radius and instructs the patient to follow up with a primary care or orthopedic physician for care during the global period.** The ED physician reports an ED E/M service (**99281–99285**) with modifier **57** (decision for surgery) and code **25600 54**.

  25600 54 (closed treatment of distal radial fracture [eg, Colles or Smith type] or epiphyseal separation, includes closed treatment of fracture of ulnar styloid, when performed; without manipulation)

  The primary care or orthopedic physician who assumes management of the patient's fracture care will report code **25600 55**. The 2 physicians must coordinate how the services will be reported so each reports the appropriate modifier.

  Teaching Point: If a physician's initial fracture care is limited to stabilization pending referral for fracture treatment, only the E/M and any splinting or casting and supplies are reported. The physician who will provide fracture treatment will report a fracture care code without a modifier.

58—Staged or Related Procedure or Service by the Same Physician or Other QHP During the Postoperative Period

- Modifier **58** is used to indicate that a procedure or service performed during the postoperative period was planned or anticipated (ie, staged), was more extensive than the original procedure, or was for therapy following a surgical procedure.
- Modifier **58** is a recognized modifier under the NCCI.
- Typically, payers recognize modifier **58** only when there is a global surgical period associated with the procedure code.
- ✖ **DO *NOT* REPORT MODIFIER 58 WHEN**
    - **Treating a problem that requires a return to the OR (eg, unanticipated clinical condition) (See modifier 78 discussed later in this chapter.)**
    - **Reporting procedures that include as part of their *CPT* descriptor "one or more visits" or "one or more sessions"**

● indicates a new code; ▲, revised; #, re-sequenced; ✚, add-on; ★, audiovisual technology; and ◀, synchronous interactive audio.

Chapter 2. Coding Edits and Modifiers

Examples—Modifier 58

➤ **An excision of a malignant lesion (1 cm) on the leg is performed.** The pathology report indicates that the margins were not adequate, and a re-excision is performed 1 week later. The excised diameter is less than 2 cm.

    11602 58 (excision, malignant lesion including margins, leg; excised diameter 1.1–2.0 cm) for the second excision
    Note: The first excision would be reported by using code **11601** (margin diameter 0.6–1.0 cm).

➤ **A physician replaces a cast during the global period of fracture care.** (Only the first cast is included in the code for fracture care. For more on fracture care, see **Chapter 14**.)

    29000–29799 58 (appropriate casting code)

59—Distinct Procedural Service

> **Never use modifier 59 in place of modifier 25 or on an evaluation and management service code.**

- Modifier **59** is used to identify procedures or services, other than E/M services, that are not normally reported together but are appropriate under the circumstances.
- Report modifier **59** only when no other modifier better describes the reason for separately reporting a service that might otherwise be bundled with another procedural service on the same date.
- Never append modifier **59** to bypass payer edits without clinical justification.
- See HCPCS modifiers **XE**, **XP**, **XS**, and **XU** for potential alternatives to modifier **59**.
- Per *CPT*, modifier **59** represents one of the following conditions of a procedure:
  - The procedure was provided at a different session from another procedure.
  - The procedure was a different procedure or surgery.
  - The procedure involved a different site or organ system.
  - The procedure required a separate incision or excision.
  - The procedure was performed on a separate lesion or injury (or area of injury in extensive injuries).

Example—Modifier 59

➤ **Three behavioral health assessment instruments are completed and scored during 1 encounter to assess symptoms of depression, mood and feelings, and anxiety.**

    96127 × 2 (brief emotional/behavioral assessment [eg, depression inventory, attention-deficit/hyperactivity disorder (ADHD) scale], with scoring and documentation, per standardized instrument)
    96127 59 × 1 (third assessment instrument)
    Modifier **59** would be appended to the code for the third assessment instrument to reflect that 3 distinct assessment instruments were scored and documented. Medicaid NCCI MUEs limit units of **96127** to 2 units per claim, but modifier **59** may be appended to units on an additional line to indicate that additional instruments were necessary.

62—Two Surgeons

- Modifier **62** is used when 2 surgeons work together as primary surgeons performing a distinct part(s) of a procedure. Do not use modifier **62** when one surgeon assists another.
- Co-surgeons may be of the same specialty or different specialties, although usually of different specialties. Individual payer policies may vary regarding coverage of co-surgery by 2 physicians of the same specialty.
- Each surgeon should report their distinct operative work by adding modifier **62** to the procedure code and any associated add-on code(s) for that procedure as long as both surgeons continue to work together as primary surgeons.
- Each surgeon should report the co-surgery once by using the same procedure code.
- If an additional procedure(s) (including an add-on procedure[s]) is performed during the same surgical session, a separate code(s) may also be reported without modifier **62** added.
- Simultaneous bilateral services are procedures during which each surgeon performs the same procedure on opposite sides. Each surgeon should report the simultaneous bilateral procedures with modifiers **50** and **62**.

- Column AB (CO SURG) of the MPFS (Resource-Based Relative Value Scale [RBRVS]) identifies procedures that may or may not be performed by co-surgeons. Indicator 1 is assigned to procedures for which co-surgery is allowed under the Medicare program. See www.cms.gov/Medicare/Medicare-Fee-for-Service-Payment/PhysicianFeeSched/PFS-Relative-Value-Files.html.

Example—Modifier 62

> **A neurosurgeon and a general surgeon work together to place a ventriculoperitoneal shunt.**
> Both physicians would report code **62223 62** with the same diagnosis code. The operative note must include the name of each surgeon, specific role of each surgeon, and necessity for 2 surgeons. Each surgeon should dictate their own operative report.
> Most payers will require authorization before the procedure.

63—Procedure Performed on Infants Less Than 4 kg

- Modifier **63** is used to report procedures performed on neonates and infants up to a *present body weight of 4 kg* that involve significantly increased complexity and physician work commonly associated with these patients.
- Unless otherwise designated, this modifier may be appended only to procedures or services listed in the **20100–69990** code series and to codes **92920**, **92928**, **92953**, **92960**, **92986**, **92987**, **92990**, **92997**, **92998**, **93312–93318**, **93452**, **93505**, **93593–93598**, **93563**, **93564**, **93568**, **93569**, **93573–93575**, **93580–93582**, **93590–93592**, **93615**, and **93616**.
- Use of modifier **63** may require submission of an operative note with the claim. The operative note should include the patient's weight. It is also beneficial to report the patient's weight on the claim.
- ✖ **DO *NOT* REPORT MODIFIER 63**
  - **When the code is included in *CPT* Appendix F, as codes in this appendix were valued to include the increased complexity and physician work associated with modifier 63**
  - **With any *CPT* codes listed in the E/M Services, Anesthesia, Radiology, Pathology/Laboratory, or Medicine sections (other than those previously identified from the Medicine/Cardiovascular section)**
  - **When the *CPT* code includes a parenthetical instruction prohibiting reporting modifier 63**

Example—Modifier 63

> **A surgeon performed right- and left-sided heart catheterization through normal native connections on a 4-week-old with a weight of 3.1 kg and positive findings of congenital anomalies.**
> **93596 26 63** (right and left heart catheterization for congenital heart defect[s] including imaging guidance by the proceduralist to advance the catheter to the target zone[s]; normal native connections)
> Because the procedure may be performed on patients weighing more than 4 kg, the complexity and work associated with performing the procedure on an infant weighing up to 4 kg *was not* included in the valuation assigned to code **93596**.

66—Surgical Team

- Modifier **66** is appended to the basic procedure code when highly complex procedures (requiring the concomitant services of several physicians or other QHPs, often of different specialties, plus other highly skilled, specially trained personnel and various types of complex equipment) are carried out under the surgical team concept.
- Each surgeon reports modifier **66**.
- Each surgeon should dictate their own operative report, and it should reflect the medical necessity for team surgery.
- Column AC (TEAM SURG) of the MPFS (RBRVS) identifies procedures that may or may not be performed by a team of surgeons. Indicator 1 is assigned to procedures for which team surgery is allowed under the Medicare program.
- The operative notes are usually required by the payer.
- If a surgeon is assisting another surgeon, modifier **80**, **81**, or **82** would be more applicable.

Example—Modifier 66

> **Multiple surgeons perform different portions of an organ transplant.**
> Each physician would report their services with modifier **66** appended to the procedure code.

• indicates a new code; ▲, revised; #, re-sequenced; ✦, add-on; ★, audiovisual technology; and ◄, synchronous interactive audio.

76—Repeat Procedure or Service by Same Physician or Other QHP

- Modifier **76** is used when a procedure or service is repeated by the same physician or other QHP subsequent to the original procedure or service. Use of this modifier may prevent denial as a duplicate service line.
- When a procedure is repeated on the same date, it may be helpful to include the start times of each procedure in a narrative statement on the claim (eg, field 19 on a paper claim).
- The repeated procedure may be performed on different days. (Payer guidance may vary.)
- This modifier is appended only to non-E/M procedure codes and is not reported when the code definition indicates a repeated procedure.
- Use of this modifier advises the payer that this is not a duplicate service. (See also modifier **91** discussed later in this chapter for a repeated clinical diagnostic laboratory test.)
- The CMS recognizes this modifier only for ECGs and radiographs or for a procedure performed in an OR or another location equipped to perform procedures. Medicaid programs or other commercial payers may follow this guideline. Check with payers to determine their policy on use of the modifier.

Examples—Modifier 76

➤ **You see a patient in your office with severe asthma and give them 3 nebulized albuterol treatments and steroids over the course of the visit. You report**

94640 × 1 (pressurized or nonpressurized inhalation treatment for acute airway obstruction for therapeutic purposes and/or for diagnostic purposes such as sputum induction with an aerosol generator, nebulizer, metered dose inhaler or intermittent positive pressure breathing [IPPB] device)

94640 76 × 1 on 2 separate claims lines to support adjudication of each repeated service

Teaching Point: Only report **94640 76** with 3 units if directed to do so by payer policy because most payers will deny on the basis of the lack of an initial service (ie, code reported without modifier **76**). Note that some payers require you to *report each service on a separate line*, by using a quantity of 1 and appending modifier **76** to the subsequent procedures.

> The Medicare and Medicaid National Correct Coding Initiative manuals contradict *Current Procedural Terminology* (*CPT*) instruction for code **94640**, stating that *CPT* code **94640** be reported once during a single patient encounter regardless of the number of separate inhalation treatments that are administered. Follow individual payer guidance.

➤ **The same physician performs re-reduction (closed treatment with manipulation) of radial and ulnar shaft fractures within the global period of the initial closed treatment of the fractures.**

Re-reduction: **25565 76** (closed treatment of radial and ulnar shaft fractures; with manipulation)

77—Repeat Procedure or Service by Another Physician or Other QHP

- Modifier **77** is used when a procedure or service is repeated by another physician or health care professional subsequent to the original procedure or service. Be sure that the same code(s) is reported by each physician to prevent denials when reporting modifier **77**.
- Payers may require documentation to support the medical necessity of performing the same service or procedure on the same day or during the global surgical period (if applicable).

Example—Modifier 77

➤ **An orthopedic physician performs re-reduction (closed treatment with manipulation) of radial and ulnar shaft fractures. The initial closed treatment of the fractures was reported by a physician of another specialty or another group practice.**

Re-reduction: **25565 77** (closed treatment of radial and ulnar shaft fractures; with manipulation)

● indicates a new code; ▲, revised; #, re-sequenced; ✦, add-on; ★, audiovisual technology; and ◀, synchronous interactive audio.

78—Unplanned Return to the Operating/Procedure Room by the Same Physician or Other QHP Following Initial Procedure for a Related Procedure During the Postoperative Period

- Modifier **78** is used when another procedure is unplanned and related to the initial procedure, requires a return to the OR, and is performed during the postoperative period of the initial procedure by the same physician.
- The related procedure might be performed on the same day or at any time during the postoperative period. (For repeated procedures, see modifier **76** discussed earlier in this chapter.)
- Link the appropriate diagnosis code(s) that best explains the reason for the unplanned procedure.
- ✖ Do not report modifier **78** for treatment of complications that do not require a return to the OR. Payers that use the Medicare description of the global period do not pay separately for additional services caused by complications that do not require a return to the OR.

Example—Modifier 78

➤ **A pediatric surgeon returns to the OR to stop bleeding from an abdominal procedure performed earlier in the day.**

35840 78 (exploration for postoperative hemorrhage, thrombosis, or infection; abdomen)

Teaching Point: The second procedure will usually be paid only for the intraoperative service, not the preoperative or postoperative care already paid in the original procedure.

79—Unrelated Procedure/Service by the Same Physician or Other QHP During the Postoperative Period

- The physician may need to indicate that the performance of a procedure or service during the postoperative period was unrelated to the original procedure. This circumstance may be reported by using modifier **79**.
- The diagnosis must identify the reason for the new procedure within the global period. (For procedures repeated by the same physician on the same day, see modifier **76** discussed earlier in this chapter.)

Example—Modifier 79

➤ **An adolescent patient requires an emergency appendectomy within 90 days of undergoing left-sided inguinal hernia repair.**

44970 79 (laparoscopy, surgical, appendectomy)

80—Assistant Surgeon

- Modifier **80** is used when the assistant surgeon assists the surgeon during the entire operation. *Note:* Modifier **62**, not **80**, is used when 2 surgeons work together as primary surgeons performing a distinct part(s) of a procedure.
- The primary surgeon reports the appropriate *CPT* code for the procedure, and the assistant surgeon reports the same code with modifier **80** appended. Some payers require modifier **AS** (assistant at surgery) in lieu of **80** when any other QHP (ie, physician assistant/associate [PA], nurse practitioner, or clinical nurse specialist) acts as assistant surgeon.
- Payers vary on payment rules. The CMS establishes guidelines for payment of assistant surgery for each procedure code. Most payers, including the CMS, do not pay for nonphysician surgery technicians in this role.
- Many payers require documentation to support the necessity of an assistant surgeon.

81—Minimum Assistant Surgeon

- Modifier **81** is used when an assistant surgeon is required for a short time and minimal assistance is provided.
- The assistant surgeon reports the same procedure code as the surgeon with modifier **81** appended.
- Many payers require documentation to support the use of an assistant surgeon for only a portion of a procedure.

82—Assistant Surgeon (When Qualified Resident Surgeon Not Available)

- Modifier **82** is used in teaching hospitals when a resident surgeon is not available to assist the primary surgeon.
- The unavailability of a qualified resident surgeon is a prerequisite for the use of modifier **82** appended to the usual procedure code number(s).

Chapter 2. Coding Edits and Modifiers

Modifiers 80, 81, and 82

The Medicare Physician Fee Schedule includes in column AA (ASST SURG) indicators identifying procedures that may or may not be billed by an assistant surgeon. Indicator 1 is assigned to procedures for which an assistant surgeon is allowed to bill under the Medicare program. Other payers may adopt the same or different policies.

90—*Reference (Outside) Laboratory*

- Modifier **90** is used to indicate that a laboratory service is being billed by the physician but performed at an outside laboratory.
- Modifier **90** indicates pass-through billing in that the payer will pay the physician for the laboratory service and the laboratory will charge the physician.
- Many payers do not accept modifier **90** and require that the laboratory performing the service bill directly to the health plan for the services. Check with your payers before using modifier **90**.

91—*Repeat Clinical Diagnostic Laboratory Test*

- Modifier **91** is used to indicate that it is necessary to repeat the same laboratory test on the same day to obtain subsequent test results.
- Modifier **91** is reported only when the laboratory test is performed more than once on the same patient on the same day.
- Modifier **91** cannot be reported when tests are repeated to confirm initial results, because of testing problems with the specimen or equipment or for any reason when a normal onetime, reportable result is all that is required.
- Do not substitute modifier **59** (distinct service) for modifier **91**.

Example—Modifier 91

➤ **In the course of treatment of hypoglycemia by administration of oral carbohydrate, a patient underwent 3 blood glucose determinations (82947) on the same day in the same office.**

    82947 91 × 3 units of service

    Some payers will require separate claim lines for each test performed, with modifier **91** appended to the codes for repeated services.

92—*Alternative Laboratory Platform Testing*

- Modifier **92** is used to indicate that laboratory testing was performed by using a kit or transportable instrument that wholly or partially consists of a single-use, disposable analytic chamber.
- This modifier is not required or acknowledged by all payers.
- *CPT* instructs to report this modifier with HIV test codes **86701–86703** and **87389**.

Modifiers Appended to Either E/M or Procedural Services

32—*Mandated Services*

- Modifier **32** is appended to services (eg, a second opinion) mandated by a third-party payer or by governmental, legislative, or regulatory requirements.
- The modifier may be reported with codes for E/M services (eg, for a second opinion required by a payer).
- Modifier **32** would be used when, for example, radiological services are requested from a worker's compensation carrier, when laboratory testing (eg, a drug test) is requested by a court system, or when a physical therapy assessment is requested by an insurer.

Example—Modifier 32

➤ **A Medicaid managed care organization requires modifier 32 to indicate off-schedule provision of a routine child health examination for purposes of clearance to attend child care or preschool.** A pediatrician provides an age- and gender-appropriate preventive E/M service to an established 3½-year-old patient who will be entering the Head Start program.

ICD-10-CM	CPT
Z02.0 (encounter for examination for admission to educational institution)	**99392 32** (established patient preventive service, age 1–4 years)

Teaching Point: Health plan policies vary regarding reporting of preventive E/M services provided more frequently than specified by the periodicity schedule. See **Chapter 8** for further discussion of preparticipation physical evaluations performed for child care, school, or sports clearance.

33—Preventive Services

CPT modifier **33** is used to communicate to payers that a preventive medicine service (as defined by the Patient Protection and Affordable Care Act [PPACA] provisions; the 4 categories follow) was performed on a patient enrolled in a health care plan subject to the preventive service coverage requirements of the PPACA and, therefore, should not be subject to cost sharing.

- Appropriate use of modifier **33** reduces claim adjustments related to preventive services and facilitates correct payments to members.
- Modifier **33** should be appended only to codes represented in one or more of the following 4 categories:
  — Services rated A or B by the US Preventive Services Task Force
  — Immunizations for routine use in children, adolescents, and adults as recommended by the Advisory Committee on Immunization Practices of the CDC
  — Preventive care and screenings for children as recommended by Bright Futures (AAP) and newborn testing (American College of Medical Genetics and Genomics)
  — Preventive care and screenings provided for women supported by the Health Resources and Services Administration
- **DO *NOT* USE MODIFIER 33**
  — **When the *CPT* code(s) is identified as inherently preventive (eg, preventive medicine counseling)**
  — **When the service(s) is not indicated in the categories noted previously**
  — **With an insurance plan that continues to implement the cost-sharing policy on preventive medicine services**
- Check with your payers before reporting modifier **33** to verify any variations in reporting requirements.

Example—Modifier 33

➤ **A 17-year-old established patient is seen for an office visit and requests contraception.** The physician determines that the patient is not pregnant but has been sexually active with multiple partners and would like contraception. The physician then spends approximately 15 minutes discussing contraception and risks of sexually transmitted infection (STI) with the patient. Point-of-care HIV-1 and HIV-2 testing is conducted with negative results. Specimen is collected for chlamydia and gonorrhea screening by an outside laboratory. The patient chooses oral contraception, which is prescribed.

ICD-10-CM	CPT
Z30.09 (encounter for other general counseling and advice on contraception) **Z11.4** (encounter for screening for HIV) **Z11.3** (encounter for screening for STI)	**99401** (preventive counseling, approximately 15 minutes [includes 8–23 minutes]) **86703 33 92** (antibody; HIV-1 and HIV-2; single assay)

Teaching Point: Although recommended as a preventive service, the test reported with **86703** is also used for diagnostic purposes. Modifier **33** indicates that this test was performed as a preventive service. Modifier **92** (alternative laboratory platform testing) is reported to indicate use of the HIV test kit (not all payers recognize modifier **92**). Typically, health plans cover services related to contraception (eg, **99401**) without cost to the patient. When performed, a pregnancy test (eg, **81025,** urine pregnancy test, by visual color comparison methods) may be separately reported with *ICD-10-CM* code **Z32.01** (encounter for pregnancy test, result positive) or **Z32.02** (encounter for pregnancy test, result negative).

Chapter 2. Coding Edits and Modifiers

93—Synchronous Telemedicine Service Rendered via Telephone or Other Real-time Interactive Audio-Only Telecommunications System

Synchronous telemedicine service is defined as a real-time interaction through audio-only technology between a physician or QHP and a patient who is located at a distant site from the physician or QHP. The modifier is not reported for back-and-forth voice messaging.

- *CPT* Appendix T lists codes that may be reported with modifier **93**. Codes eligible for use with modifier **93** are preceded by an audio speaker symbol (◀).
- Verify payer policies for audio-only telemedicine services before provision of services.
- The totality of communication during the course of the audio-only telemedicine service must be of an amount and nature sufficient to meet the requirements of the same service when rendered with face-to-face interaction.
- Note that modifier **93** is different from modifier **FQ** (audio-only service; discussed later in this chapter), which was created for the Medicare program and is reported *only when mental or behavioral health services* are provided via audio-only technology unless otherwise specified by a health plan.

95—Synchronous Telemedicine Service Rendered via a Real-time Interactive Audio and Video Telecommunications System

Modifier **95** is used to indicate that a service was rendered via real-time (synchronous) interactive audio and video telecommunications system. This modifier is not applied if the communication is not real-time interactive audio and video.

Codes to which modifier **95** may be applied are found in Appendix P and are preceded by a star symbol (★) in the *CPT* manual.

> For more information on reporting synchronous telemedicine services, see Chapter 20.

99—Multiple Modifiers

CPT instructs that modifier **99** be reported under certain circumstances when 2 or more modifiers are required to completely describe a service. However, current paper and electronic claims allow listing of up to 4 modifiers per claim line, and payers often instruct to report modifier **99** only when more than 4 modifiers are required on a single code.

Follow individual payer instructions regarding use of modifier **99** and placement of additional modifiers on the claim (eg, in narrative field 19 of the paper claim form).

> For more information on reporting modifiers, see the April 2022 *AAP Pediatric Coding Newsletter* article, "Getting Paid: Correctly Using Modifiers With Correct Coding Edits" (https://doi.org/10.1542/pcco_book216_document003).

Healthcare Common Procedure Coding System Modifiers

The HCPCS modifiers are used to report specific information not conveyed in code descriptors or by *CPT* modifiers, such as

CR	Catastrophe/disaster related
E1	Upper left eyelid
QW	Performance of tests waived by Clinical Laboratory Improvement Amendments (CLIA)
RT	Right side
SL	State-supplied vaccine
TC	Technical component only
XE	Procedural services performed at separate encounters on the same date

Medicaid programs often use a variety of HCPCS modifiers for state-defined purposes. See your Medicaid provider manual for information on HCPCS modifiers and definitions assigned in your state (eg, modifier **SY** [persons who are in close contact with member of high-risk population] may be used with codes for certain immunizations).

Anatomical Modifiers

An anatomical modifier may be reported to identify specific sites, such as right foot, fifth digit (**T9**).

- The anatomical modifiers are designated as appropriate modifiers under NCCI edits.
- The Medicaid NCCI manual indicates that procedures performed on fingers be reported with modifiers **FA** and **F1–F9**, and procedures performed on toes should be reported with modifiers **TA** and **T1–T9**. See also modifiers for eyelids (**E1–E4**) and coronary arteries (**LC, LD, LM, RC, RI**).

Medically Unlikely Edit values for many finger and toe procedures are 1 (one) on the basis of use of these modifiers for clinical scenarios in which the same procedure is performed on more than one finger or toe. (See the Medically Unlikely Edits section earlier in this chapter for more information.)

Example—Anatomical Modifiers

➤ **A physician performs nail avulsion (11730) on the patient's right ring finger and evacuation of blood under the nail (11740) on the patient's right middle finger.**

    11730 F8 (avulsion, nail plate, partial or complete, simple; single—right hand, 4th digit)

    11740 F7 (evacuation of subungual hematoma—right hand, 3rd digit)

    Note: Some payers may require that modifier **59** (distinct procedural service) or **XS** (separate structure) be reported. Verify coding edits and payer policy before reporting.

X {E, P, S, U} Modifiers

Modifiers **XE, XP, XS,** and **XU** more specifically identify reasons for separate reporting of procedures or services that may otherwise be identified by *CPT* modifier **59**.

XE	Separate encounter (different operative session)
XP	Separate practitioner
XS	Separate structure (site/organ)
XU	Unusual nonoverlapping service

- As payer adoption and guidance on use of these modifiers may vary, it is important to verify individual payer policy before reporting. While accepted by most payers, few resources are available to describe appropriate reporting of these modifiers.
- As the **XE, XP, XS,** and **XU** modifiers are more specific, payers may require reporting in lieu of modifier **59**.
- Modifiers **XE, XP, XS,** and **XU** should not be appended to an E/M code.
- Do not append modifier **59** and the **XE, XP, XS,** and **XU** modifiers to the same service line of a claim (ie, single code).

> **Learn more about modifiers XE, XP, XS, and XU in the July 2020** *AAP Pediatric Coding Newsletter* **article, "Modifiers: Do You Use 59 or XE, XP, XS, XU?" (https://doi.org/10.1542/pcco_book195_document003).**

CR—Catastrophe/Disaster Related

Modifier **CR** is used on the basis of payer instruction during a federal- or state-declared disaster or public health emergency to indicate that a service was provided in a manner or under circumstances for which payment may otherwise be prohibited by government statute or payer policies.

Example—Modifier CR

➤ **A well-child examination is conducted via telemedicine on a patient in her home during a public health emergency.** Per payer policy, the service requires a comprehensive, unclothed physical examination. A waiver has been issued allowing billing for the incomplete preventive E/M service with modifier **CR** (eg, **99391 CR**). Payer policy may require an in-person visit within a specified period.

EP—Service Provided as Part of Medicaid Early and Periodic Screening, Diagnostic, and Treatment (EPSDT) Program

Some Medicaid and private payers require the use of modifier **EP** to denote services that are provided to covered patients as part of the Early and Periodic Screening, Diagnostic, and Treatment (EPSDT) program services required in the state.

Modifier **EP** can be appended to the preventive medicine service (eg, **99392**) or screening services, such as developmental screening (**96110**).

● indicates a new code; ▲, revised; #, re-sequenced; ✚, add-on; ★, audiovisual technology; and ◀, synchronous interactive audio.

Modifier **EP** can also be applied to services provided on the basis of a referral prompted by findings of an EPSDT well-child examination (eg, **96112 EP**, developmental test administration [including assessment of fine and/or gross motor, language, cognitive level, social, memory and/or executive functions by standardized developmental instruments when performed], by physician or other qualified health care professional, with interpretation and report; first hour).

Example—Modifier EP

➤ **A 9-month-old established patient presents for her routine preventive medicine service.** As part of her state EPSDT services, she receives an age-appropriate history and physical examination, preventive counseling, and anticipatory guidance. A standardized developmental screening, which is required of EPSDT services, is also completed and scored.

99391 EP (preventive medicine service, established patient <1 year)
96110 EP (developmental screening)

FQ—*The Service Was Furnished Using Audio-Only Communication Technology*

Modifier **FQ** was added specifically for reporting expanded Medicare coverage of telehealth for mental health services furnished to a beneficiary in their home through audio-only communications technology. (See also modifier **93** discussed earlier in this chapter.) Report modifier **FQ** only as instructed by payer policy.

- This modifier and the related payment policy do not apply to services for conditions other than mental health or substance use disorders (SUDs).
- Evaluation and management services addressing diagnosis, evaluation, or treatment of a mental health condition and/or an SUD are reported with modifier **FQ**, when applicable.

FS—*Split or Shared Evaluation and Management (E/M) Visit*

This modifier indicates that a service was provided in a facility setting as a split or shared E/M service by more than one physician or QHP in the same group practice. Medicare requires the reporting individual to append modifier **FS** to an E/M code when the E/M service was performed as a split/shared service. Other payers may adopt Medicare policy for use of modifier **FS**.

FT—*Separate, Unrelated E/M*

The CMS created modifier **FT** for reporting critical care services provided within a 10- or 90-day postoperative period when the services are above and beyond and unrelated to the specific anatomical injury or general surgical procedure performed. See individual health plan guidance before reporting this modifier.

- The Medicare program advises that modifier **25** (significant and separately identifiable E/M service) continue to be reported when 2 E/M services are provided to a patient by the same physician or QHP or another physician or QHP of the same specialty and same group practice on the same date but for different reasons (eg, hospital care before critical care).

GA—*Waiver of Liability Statement Issued as Required by Payer Policy, Individual Case*

GU—*Waiver of Liability Statement Issued as Required by Payer Policy, Routine Notice*

GX—*Notice of Liability Issued, Voluntary Under Payer Policy*

Modifiers **GA**, **GU**, and **GX** may or may not be recognized by Medicaid and private payers when reporting services that are not covered under the patient's benefit plan. Follow individual payer policies regarding provision and reporting of advance notice of noncoverage to patients/responsible parties.

GC—*This Service Has Been Performed in Part by a Resident Under the Direction of a Teaching Physician*

- Modifier **GC** indicates that a teaching physician is certifying that the service was rendered in compliance with the CMS requirements for services reported by teaching physicians.
- Requirements for reporting modifier **GC** may vary among commercial health plans. This modifier is typically *informational*, meaning it does not affect the amount paid for a service.
- If the service was provided solely by the teaching physician, the claim should not be billed with the **GC** modifier.

GE—*This Service Has Been Performed by a Resident Without the Presence of a Teaching Physician Under the Primary Care Exception*

- Modifier **GE** indicates that a teaching physician is certifying that the service was rendered in compliance with the CMS primary care exception rule. Please see **Chapter 6** for discussion of this rule.
- Requirements for reporting modifier **GE** may vary among Medicaid and commercial health plans. This modifier is typically *informational*, which means it does not affect the amount paid for a service.

GT—*Via Interactive Audio and Video Telecommunication Systems*

Modifier **GT** indicates that a face-to-face service was provided via a telecommunication system that included audio and video components. This modifier preceded *CPT* development of modifier **95** (telemedicine via audiovisual technology) and is reported in lieu of **95** when specified in payer policy (eg, appended to a code not included in *CPT* Appendix P).

JW—*Drug Amount Discarded/Not Administered to Any Patient*

- Practice administrators may use as a tool to internally track wasted drugs and vaccines.
- This modifier is reported on claims only when allowed or required by certain payers.
- Medicare requires use of modifier **JW** on codes for the unused portion of a drug or biologic from a single-dose vial or package. Medicaid plans may also require reporting of modifier **JW**.
  - Report only when the full amount of a single-dose vial is not used due to patient indications (eg, patient requires lower dose) and required by a payer.
  - Report only when the amount of drug wasted is equal to at least 1 billing unit (ie, do not report wastage when 7 mg of a 10-mg vial is administered and the billing unit is 10 mg, as the remaining 3 mg is already accounted for in the billing unit).
  - Never report for discarded amounts from a multidose vial.
  - Never report modifier **JW** for overfill wastage (ie, an excess amount placed in the single-dose vial by the manufacturer to ensure that an adequate amount can be drawn into the syringe for use).
- Modifier **JW** is not applicable for reporting the following circumstances. However, some practices use the modifier for internal tracking of drug waste.
  - A parent decided to forego an immunization after the vaccine had been drawn up. Report on a claim only when specifically allowed by payer policy. Practices should keep a log of all wasted vaccines.
  - The vial is dropped, and the medication must be discarded.
  - A vaccine is discarded due to temperature out of range during storage.

> Learn more in the July 2020 *AAP Pediatric Coding Newsletter* article, "Coding for Vaccines Not Administered" (https://doi.org/10.1542/pcco_book195_document007).

KP—*First Drug of a Multiple Drug Unit Dose Formulation*

KQ—*Second or Subsequent Drug of a Multiple Drug Unit Dose Formulation*

Some payers require only the distinct National Drug Code for each vial administered and do not require use of modifiers **KP** and **KQ**. When required by a payer, append modifier **KP** to the procedure code to indicate either of the following reports:
- When reporting the first drug in a multiple drug formulation compounded from drugs supplied in a unit dose form
- When reporting the first dose of a single drug supplied in a unit dose form when the total dose is greater than the amount supplied in a single vial or container

Append modifier **KQ** to the procedure code to indicate either of the following reports:
- When reporting the second drug in a multiple drug formulation compounded from drugs supplied in a unit dose form
- When reporting the second dose of a single drug supplied in a unit dose form when the total dose is greater than the amount supplied in a single vial or container

Example—*Modifier* KP

➤ **An infant requires administration of 150-mg palivizumab to prevent serious lower respiratory tract disease caused by respiratory syncytial virus (RSV). Two single-dose vials (one 100 mg and one 50 mg) are administered.**

90378 KP × 2 units 100-mg single-dose vial (RSV, monoclonal antibody, recombinant, for intramuscular use, 50 mg, each)

90378 KQ × 1 unit 50-mg single-dose vial

QW—*Clinical Laboratory Improvement Amendments–Waived Tests*

- The CLIA-waived tests are those commonly done in a laboratory or an office that are considered simple and low risk.
- One common test in the *CPT* **80000** series that is CLIA waived is the rapid streptococcal antigen test (**87880**).
- Laboratories and physician offices performing waived tests may need to append modifier **QW** to the *CPT* code for CLIA-waived procedures. The use of modifier **QW** is payer specific.
- Some of the CLIA-waived tests are exempt from the use of modifier **QW** (eg, **81002**, **82272**). To determine whether a test is CLIA waived, search the US Food and Drug Administration database at www.accessdata.fda.gov/scripts/cdrh/cfdocs/cfCLIA/search.cfm.

RT, LT—*Right and Left Side*

- Modifiers **RT** and **LT** are used for information only and do not affect payment of a procedure unless otherwise specified by a payer.
- Used to identify procedures performed on the left or right side of the body.
- Some plans allow modifiers **RT** and **LT** in place of modifier **50**, but be sure of payer policy for reporting bilateral diagnostic procedures.

Some payers may require that modifier **59** (distinct procedural service) be reported in addition to or in lieu of the laterality modifiers.

Example—*Modifiers* **RT** *and* **LT**

➤ **Radiographs of the left elbow and wrist are ordered.**
   73110 LT (radiologic examination, wrist; complete, minimum of 3 views)
   73080 LT (radiologic examination, elbow; complete, minimum of 3 views)

SA—*Nurse Practitioner Rendering Service in Collaboration With a Physician*

- Modifier **SA** is typically appended to a procedure code to indicate that a physician is reporting a service provided by a nurse practitioner under incident-to policy. However, some payers require the modifier on all services provided by nurse practitioners.
- Some payers include PAs and other QHPs who can provide E/M services in policies requiring use of modifier **SA**. Other payers may use alternative modifiers for services performed by PAs and other QHPs.
- Not all payers require modifier **SA**, but where required, failure to include the modifier could result in overpayment or coding errors.

Example—*Modifier* **SA**

➤ **A nurse practitioner provides a follow-up visit to reevaluate a patient's type 1 diabetes in continuation of a plan of care developed by the patient's physician.** The physician is in the office suite and available during the visit but does not directly participate in the visit. The service provided is a level-4 established patient office E/M service (**99214**). The physician reports **99214 SA**.

Learn more about incident-to policy in Chapter 7.

To test your knowledge of the information presented in this chapter, complete the quiz found at the end of it, after the resources. Add to your knowledge through the information provided in other chapters that discusses codes for specific types of services.

● indicates a new code; ▲, revised; #, re-sequenced; ✚, add-on; ★, audiovisual technology; and ◄, synchronous interactive audio.

Chapter Takeaways

Readers of this chapter should generally know coding edits and modifiers.

Following are takeaways from this chapter:

- Payers use coding edits to promote correct coding and provide correct payment for services.
- When applicable, use of modifiers to override coding edits must be clinically indicated. Not all edits can be overridden with a modifier.
- The *CPT* and HCPCS include modifiers that may be appended to procedure codes from either code set.
- Some modifiers are limited to use with E/M codes or with other procedure codes. Some modifiers are applicable to either an E/M code or other procedure codes.
- Modifier use may be affected by payer-specific policies requiring knowledge of payer policies for modifier use.

Resources

AAP Coding Assistance and Education

AAP Coding Hotline (https://form.jotform.com/Subspecialty/aapcodinghotline)

AAP Pediatric Coding Newsletter™

"Modifiers: Back to Basics," April 2022 (https://doi.org/10.1542/pcco_book216_document002)

"Modifiers: Do You Use **59** or **XE, XP, XS, XU**?" July 2020 (https://doi.org/10.1542/pcco_book195_document003)

"Coding for Vaccines Not Administered," July 2020 (https://doi.org/10.1542/pcco_book195_document007)

"Getting Paid: Correctly Using Modifiers With Correct Coding Edits," April 2022 (https://doi.org/10.1542/pcco_book216_document003)

"The Surgical Package and Related Services," May 2018 (https://doi.org/10.1542/pcco_book169_document003)

Assistant Surgeon Procedure Identification

MPFS Relative Value Files (www.cms.gov/Medicare/Medicare-Fee-for-Service-Payment/PhysicianFeeSched/PFS-Relative-Value-Files.html; see Column AA [ASST SURG] in the file applicable to the date of service)

Bilateral Procedure Identification

MPFS Relative Value Files (www.cms.gov/Medicare/Medicare-Fee-for-Service-Payment/PhysicianFeeSched/PFS-Relative-Value-Files.html; see Column Z [BILAT SURG] in file applicable to the date of service)

CLIA-Waived Tests

CLIA test category database (www.accessdata.fda.gov/scripts/cdrh/cfdocs/cfCLIA/search.cfm)

Co-surgery and Team Surgery Procedure Identification

MPFS Relative Value Files (www.cms.gov/Medicare/Medicare-Fee-for-Service-Payment/PhysicianFeeSched/PFS-Relative-Value-Files.html; see Column AB [CO SURG] or Column AC [TEAM SURG] in the file applicable to the date of service)

Multiple Surgery Indicators and Adjustments

Medicare Claims Processing Manual, Chapter 12, Section 40.6 (www.cms.gov/Regulations-and-Guidance/Guidance/Manuals/Downloads/clm104c12.pdf)

NCCI Edits

Medicaid NCCI website (https://data.medicaid.gov/ncci)

Medicare NCCI website (www.cms.gov/NationalCorrectCodInitEd/NCCIEP/list.asp)

● indicates a new code; ▲, revised; #, re-sequenced; ✚, add-on; ★, audiovisual technology; and ◀, synchronous interactive audio.

Test Your Knowledge!

1. **Which of the following types of code edits pairs codes that should not normally be billed to the same patient by the same physician or physicians of the same specialty and same group practice on the same date?**
   a. Certain denial edits
   b. Procedure-to-procedure edits
   c. Medically unlikely edits
   d. Abusive billing edits

2. **What does modifier indicator 9 mean in the procedure-to-procedure code edit file?**
   a. A modifier cannot override this edit.
   b. An appropriate modifier may override this edit.
   c. This edit was deleted.
   d. Up to 9 units of service are allowed.

3. **Which of the following modifiers is reported when the physician or qualified health care professional who treated a fracture provides an evaluation and management service for asthma during the postoperative period?**
   a. **25**
   b. **59**
   c. **51**
   d. **24**

4. **Which of the following modifiers indicates that a physician performed a procedure but is not providing postoperative care?**
   a. **52**
   b. **53**
   c. **54**
   d. **55**

5. **True or false? Healthcare Common Procedure Coding System (HCPCS) modifiers can be appended to *Current Procedural Terminology* (*CPT*) codes and *CPT* modifiers can be appended to HCPCS codes.**
   a. True
   b. False

Coding to Demonstrate Quality and Value

CPT copyright 2022 American Medical Association. All rights reserved.

Contents

Chapter 3. Coding to Demonstrate Quality and Value

● indicates a new code; ▲, revised; #, re-sequenced; ✚, add-on; ★, audiovisual technology; and ◀, synchronous interactive audio.

Chapter Highlights

- Learn about the impact of quality and performance measurement on pediatric physicians and patients.
- Learn ways that correct coding supports performance measurement.
- Learn about measure specifications and coding.

Quality and Performance Measurement

Quality and performance measurement are important aspects of the pediatric medical home and the movement from payment by fee for service alone to value-based payment. Performance measures are developed by national organizations, including the National Committee for Quality Assurance (NCQA), and based on quality indicators currently accepted and used in the health care industry. Physicians who have successfully participated in quality measurement may see incentive payments, such as per-member-per-month payments, annual incentives, or a percentage of savings.

For more information on value-based payment and other emerging payment models, see Chapter 4.

Physicians, payers, and accreditation organizations may use codes or claims data as a first line of quality measurement. When diagnosis or procedure codes provide necessary information for reviewing quality performance data, more time-consuming and costly medical record review may be avoided.

In January 2017, the American Academy of Pediatrics (AAP) published a policy statement, "A New Era in Quality Measurement: The Development and Application of Quality Measures" (https://doi.org/10.1542/peds.2016-3442). This policy statement includes the following recommendation to national policy makers:

> "Quality measures, as much as possible, should be reportable by either *International Classification of Diseases, 10th Revision, Clinical Modification,* or *Current Procedural Terminology*® category II codes to reduce burden on pediatric health care providers. However, the inclusion of measures that also capture patient-centered perspectives on care is essential."

Clinical registries and other electronic data may also be used in quality measurement. This chapter discusses 3 ways that correct coding may support performance measurement.
- *Current Procedural Terminology* (*CPT*) Category II codes
- Hierarchical condition categories (HCCs)
- Codes that may support specific performance measures

Also discussed in this chapter are other measures that affect the perceived quality and/or value of care, such as surveys of patient/caregiver perception of care received from physicians and other qualified health care professionals (QHPs), and how practices can affect those perceptions.

Following the public health emergency for COVID-19, use of telemedicine has expanded and performance measures may now include services provided via telemedicine. See guidance from health plans for those measures that may be met during telemedicine services.

CPT® Category II Codes: Performance Measure Codes

When codes are used to collect quality and performance measurement data, one category of *CPT* codes that is useful for conveying this information is *CPT* Category II. Category II codes were developed and are used by physicians and hospitals to report performance measures and certain aspects of care not yet included in performance measures.

Category II codes may or may not be used by payers in pediatric performance measurement. Assignment of Category II codes also allows internal monitoring of performance, patient adherence, and outcomes.

Category II codes
- Are intended for reporting purposes only
- Describe clinical conditions (including complete performance measurements sets) and screening measures
- Have no relative values on the Medicare Physician Fee Schedule (Resource-Based Relative Value Scale)
- Are reported on a voluntary basis

- Are reported in addition to, *not in place of,* Category I *CPT* codes
- Describe the performance of a clinical service typically included in an evaluation and management (E/M) code or the result that is part of a laboratory procedure/test

Category II codes are included after the Category I procedure codes in the *CPT* manual and online at www.ama-assn.org/practice-management/cpt/category-ii-codes. Also available at this link is the alphabetical clinic topics listing, an overview of the performance measures, a listing of *CPT* Category II codes that may be used with each measure, and any applicable reporting instructions. Abbreviations (eg, *PV* for *preventive care and screening*) following code descriptors of Category II codes indicate the performance measure to which the code is associated.

Examples

3008F	Body mass index (BMI), documented (PV) [preventive care and screening]
4056F	Appropriate oral rehydration solution recommended (PAG) [pediatric acute gastroenteritis]

Hierarchical Condition Categories

Hierarchical condition categories are categories of conditions that are assigned weight values and used along with certain demographic and prescription drug claims data in calculating a patient's risk of increased health care use or risk adjustment. **Figure 3-1** shows other components of risk adjustment.

- Health plans offered to individuals under the Patient Protection and Affordable Care Act are subject to revenue adjustment based on the average risk of insured members based in part on HCCs.
- Hierarchical condition categories are also used in shared savings agreements with accountable care organizations (ACOs) and value-based payment to hospitals.
- Even if a physician is not part of an ACO or alternative payment model, health plans and hospitals rely on physicians to document conditions that affect HCC assignment.

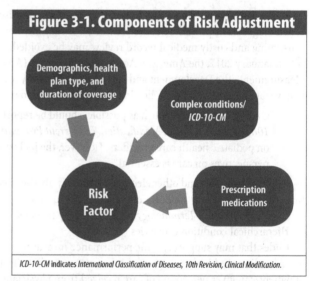

Figure 3-1. Components of Risk Adjustment

Demographics, health plan type, and duration of coverage

Complex conditions/ICD-10-CM

Risk Factor

Prescription medications

ICD-10-CM indicates *International Classification of Diseases, 10th Revision, Clinical Modification.*

International Classification of Diseases, 10th Revision, Clinical Modification (ICD-10-CM) codes are collected from the claims submitted to health plans and used to identify HCCs. Only a small percentage of *ICD-10-CM* codes are assigned to HCCs. Examples of values assigned for certain HCCs can be found in **Table 3-1.**

Most physicians do not need to know the weights assigned to various conditions or how those weights are used to calculate risk adjustment factors. What physicians need to know is how their documentation affects risk adjustment and how risk adjustment may affect physicians and their patients. In addition, choosing a less-specific code than a code supported in the documentation could affect that weight.

- Payment to physicians and QHPs may increasingly be based on quality and cost of care.

Risk adjustment is used to set the expected cost of care for a patient panel. Physicians and QHPs will be affected (especially individuals whose employers may already gain or lose revenue based on risk factor adjustment). Correct and complete diagnosing is necessary to tell the health plan the disease burden of your patients. Showing the true nature of your patient's health status may have not only a short-term effect on rates paid per visit but also long-term implications in contracting with health plans.

- Patient access to care may be affected when conditions are not documented or are documented in insufficient detail.

If risk adjustment results in lower revenue for health plans, health plan coverage and benefits will undoubtedly be affected.

It is also important to know

- Like all health care payments, those based on HCCs are audited for accuracy. Documentation must support the *ICD-10-CM* codes used in assigning HCCs.

Table 3-1. Examples of US Department of Health and Human Services Hierarchical Condition Categories and Weights[a] by Plan Type (2022)					
Diagnosis Category	Health Plan Type				
	Platinum	Gold	Silver	Bronze	Catastrophic
Asthma, Severe	0.807	0.642	0.473	0.284	0.277
Asthma, Except Severe	0.326	0.244	0.155	0.081	0.078
Autistic Disorder	2.668	2.474	2.307	2.135	2.128
Cleft Lip/Cleft Palate	1.185	1.042	0.922	0.789	0.784
Chromosomal Anomalies and Congenital Malformation Syndromes	1.447	1.334	1.245	1.151	1.148
Extremely Immature Severity Level 5 (Highest)	219.854	218.550	217.927	217.743	217.744
Extremely Immature Severity Level 4	142.713	141.194	140.396	140.023	140.018
Immature Severity Level 5 (Highest)	130.150	128.727	128.031	127.783	127.781

Abbreviation: HCC, hierarchical condition category.

[a] Weights attributed to HCCs are one of several factors in the calculation of a risk adjustment factor. Multiple HCCs may be supported for a single patient encounter, but only the highest-valued HCC describing a condition (eg, extremely immature or immature) can be assigned to a patient.

Health plans may request medical records to validate *ICD-10-CM* codes supporting assigned HCCs.

- Pediatric HCC categories apply to children younger than 2 years (ie, before their second birthday) or to patients aged 2 through 20 years (ie, before their 21st birthday).
- Hierarchical condition category values are cumulative, making documentation of all diagnoses that affect management important for accurate calculation of risk.

Learn more in the July 2019 *AAP Pediatric Coding Newsletter* article, "Hierarchical Condition Categories: What They Are and Why They Matter to Pediatricians" (https://doi.org/10.1542/pcco_book183_document006).

Healthcare Effectiveness Data and Information Set (HEDIS)

Most physicians and QHPs should be aware of the Healthcare Effectiveness Data and Information Set (HEDIS). The NCQA describes HEDIS as a tool used by more than 90% of American health plans to measure performance on important dimensions of care and service. It is intended to allow purchasers and consumers to compare quality among health plans. The HEDIS measures are often incorporated in physician quality initiatives.

Altogether, HEDIS consists of more than 90 measures across the following 5 domains of care (not all measures apply to pediatric populations):

1. Effectiveness of Care

Examples of effectiveness of care measures are
- Childhood immunization status
- Immunizations for adolescents
- Appropriate testing for children with pharyngitis
- Follow-up care for children prescribed attention-deficit/hyperactivity disorder (ADHD) medication

2. Access/Availability of Care

Examples of access to and availability of care measures are
- Use of first-line psychosocial care for children and adolescents prescribed antipsychotics
- Annual dental visit

3. Utilization

Examples of utilization measures are
- Child and adolescent well-care visits
- Antibiotic utilization for respiratory conditions

4. Risk-Adjusted Utilization

An example of a risk-adjusted utilization measure is emergency department (ED) utilization.

5. Measures Collected by Using Electronic Clinical Data Systems

- Childhood immunization status
- Immunizations for adolescents
- Follow-up care for children prescribed ADHD medication

To ensure HEDIS stays current, the NCQA has established an annual update to the measurement set.

Each health plan reviews a select set of measures every year. Because so many plans collect HEDIS data and the measures are so specifically defined, it is important to become familiar with the HEDIS system as it relates to quality measures and pay for performance (P4P).

Why HEDIS Matters to Physicians and QHPs

The Centers for Medicare & Medicaid Services (CMS) has directly linked payment for health care services to patient outcomes. Consequently, health plans and providers, including physicians, are being asked to close gaps in care and improve overall quality. This focus on quality outcomes can help patients and members get the most from their benefits, which ultimately means better use of limited resources.

There are large sums of money at stake for health plans. For example, for a health plan with just 100,000 members being evaluated by HEDIS, each quality measure could mean millions in payments from federal or state agencies. When you consider that there are 20 to 25 measures directly tied to payment (depending on the health plan and population served), this is a significant amount of money! Now consider what that might look like for larger managed care organizations that have 1 million or more members enrolled. This is what keeps health care plans running. However, they cannot do it without physicians.

A fundamental concept behind P4P quality initiatives is that the plans will pay the physicians to help them attain these funds from the CMS.

What Is a Physician's or QHP's Role in HEDIS?

You and your office staff can help facilitate HEDIS process improvement by
- Providing appropriate care within the designated time frames.

> **Pay close attention to time frames for providing recommended screenings and services across the patient population.**

Example

➤ **A practice uses a reminder system to track immunizations for children younger than 24 months to prevent failure to provide the recommended immunizations on or before the second birthday.**

Teaching Point: If patients reach 25 months of age without receiving the recommended vaccines, this negatively affects the HEDIS score for the physician until the child turns 3 years old (ie, is no longer included in the patient count for the measure).

- Documenting all care in the patient's medical record.

> **When a measure is met during an inpatient or observation stay (eg, newborn immunization during the birth admission), supporting documentation may be required in the record of the primary care physician even if the care was ordered or provided by another physician or qualified health care professional.**

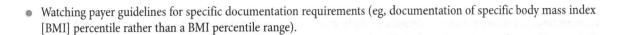

- Watching payer guidelines for specific documentation requirements (eg, documentation of specific body mass index [BMI] percentile rather than a BMI percentile range).

> **Many health plans provide specific information on documentation and codes that do or do not support Healthcare Effectiveness Data and Information Set measurement.**

- Recognizing that not all patients will be included in a physician's patient count for HEDIS purposes, as continuous enrollment in the health plan without a gap of more than a specified number of days may be required for inclusion.

Example

➤ **The measure for appropriate prescribing for pharyngitis includes members continuously enrolled without a gap in coverage from 30 days before the encounter date through 3 days afterward (34 days total).**

> **Many payers will automatically exclude any patient who has had a hospice claim or another indication of ineligibility within the measurement year from the population for Healthcare Effectiveness Data and Information Set measures.**

- Accurately coding all claims. Providing information accurately on a claim may reduce the number of records requested. Use a full spectrum of diagnosis, procedure, and National Drug Codes to show that each measure is met. Health plans typically produce educational resources giving examples of codes that indicate that a measure has been met.
- Responding to a health plan's requests for medical records in a timely fashion (typically within a week). This is required under many health plan contracts.
  Health plans typically include a specific turnaround time for providing records. The time frames are set each year.
  - January to May 15: Medical record requests will come in from the plans. All data must be gathered by the plan by May 15, with no exceptions.
  - June: The plans must report their results to the NCQA.
  - July to October: The NCQA releases the new Quality Compass (a quality comparison tool) nationwide—commercial plans in July, Medicaid and Medicare in September and October.

Medical Record Requests

Some information cannot be captured through claims data, so requests for medical records related to health plan HEDIS surveys are necessary.

- The Health Insurance Portability and Accountability Act of 1996 allows disclosure of protected health information to a health plan for the plan's HEDIS purposes as long as the period for which information is needed overlaps with the period for which the patient is or was enrolled in the health plan.
- Health plans may contract with outside vendors to conduct HEDIS record reviews.
- Providers are notified of record requests.
- The request will include a member list, the measure that is being evaluated, and the minimum necessary medical record information needed.
- Data collection may vary by plan but may include fax, mail, on-site visits for large requests, remote electronic health record access, and electronic data interchange via a secure web portal.

Consumer Assessment of Healthcare Providers and Systems

The Consumer Assessment of Healthcare Providers and Systems (CAHPS) is a program developed by the Agency for Healthcare Research and Quality (AHRQ), part of the US Department of Health and Human Services, that uses surveys to capture patient experience with health care. Different surveys are used to learn about patient experiences in primary care and specialty care settings, in hospitals, and with health plans. The surveys must be conducted by approved survey vendors under a specific framework that is designed to eliminate bias in sample selection and results.

The CAHPS Clinician & Group Survey may be used to measure patient experience in primary and specialty care settings in the following categories. A version of this survey may be used by ACOs to meet a requirement to measure patient experience.

- Getting timely appointments, care, and information

> To provide timely appointments, care, and information, consider offering same-day appointments for sick visits or for sick and well visits and providing patients with written information addressing diagnosed conditions such as attention-deficit/hyperactivity disorder, headaches, and abdominal pain. Telemedicine is also an increasingly covered benefit that may provide patients with easier access to care while maintaining continuity of care in the medical home.

- How well providers communicate with patients

> Accommodations for patients with language barriers, such as assistive technology or use of the free nationwide teletypewriter relay network to call patients/caregivers who are hearing impaired, are ways to improve communication. Use of appropriate language interpreters (eg, clinical staff, translation services) is also an important factor in patient communication. Learn more about meeting patient needs for communication assistance in the December 2021 *AAP Pediatric Coding Newsletter* article, "Coding and Use of Interpretation Services" (https://doi.org/10.1542/pcco_book212_document002).

- Providers' use of information to coordinate patient care

> The use of information to coordinate patient care can be facilitated, at least for initial referrals to other providers, by practice staff assisting patients with scheduling and transfer of relevant clinical and demographic information.

- Helpful, courteous, and respectful office staff

> Physicians and other qualified health care professionals seldom make the first and last impressions on patients/caregivers. Training all office staff to be professional, respectful, and empathic to patient/caregiver concerns is necessary to support a positive image of the practice.

- Patients' rating of the provider

> A rating by a patient/caregiver can be influenced by anything from a clear understanding of a plan of care to the level of customer service received from the practice's billing staff or agency. Each of the previous recommendations along with empathy for patients/caregivers who have concerns with their experience can drive a positive rating.

Health plans use a HEDIS version of CAHPS for gathering, reporting, analyzing, and acting on patient experience (CAHPS) data for Medicaid and commercial health plan members. The surveys are required not only by the CMS but also for health plans to receive or maintain HEDIS accreditation. The health plan surveys are typically a retrospective random sampling of patients from the prior 6 or 12 months.

These surveys measure patient experience based on the following criteria:
- Getting needed care
- Getting care quickly (eg, asking parents how frequently their child was able to receive urgently needed care from the physician [ie, never, sometimes, frequently, always])
- How well doctors communicate
- Health plan customer service
- How people rated their health plan

Health plans must rely on physician practices and other sites of service to participate in quality improvement initiatives focused on patient experiences and may offer incentives to adopt policies and procedures that support an improved patient experience of care (eg, more timely access to care).

> Learn more about the Consumer Assessment of Healthcare Providers and Systems at www.ahrq.gov/cahps/index.html.

Medicaid and Children's Health Insurance Program Quality Measures

Medicaid and the Children's Health Insurance Program (CHIP) plans select and report measures from the Core Set of Children's Health Care Quality Measures for Medicaid and CHIP (Child Core Set). The Child Core Set includes many HEDIS measures and a few measures developed by the CMS or other parties.

Examples

➤ **Percentage of newborns who did not pass hearing screening and have an audiological diagnosis no later than 3 months of age (90 days) (Centers for Disease Control and Prevention).** Specific use of the *ICD-10-CM* code, **P09.6** (abnormal findings on neonatal screening for neonatal hearing loss) can assist in tracking these patients.

➤ **The percentage of children screened for risk of developmental, behavioral, and social delays by using a standardized screening tool in the 12 months preceding or on their first, second, or third birthday (Oregon Health and Science University [formerly an NCQA measure])**

> See the current set of quality measures at www.medicaid.gov/medicaid/quality-of-care/performance-measurement/adult-and-child-health-care-quality-measures/childrens-health-care-quality-measures/index.html.

Coding and Documentation for Performance Measures

Following are documentation and coding tips for some of the pediatric performance measures for 2022 (2023 measures were not finalized at the time of this publication). See guidance from health plans in your area for more specific documentation and coding guidance.

Note that each measure includes a defined patient population (eg, children who turn 2 years of age during the measurement year).

> Healthcare Effectiveness Data and Information Set requires that measures be met within specific time frames (eg, before the second birthday). Catching up after the specified time will not be counted in the number of patients for whom the measure was met.

Physicians and group practices may also report performance measures as part of a pediatric medical home or other quality improvement initiative by using data pulled from internal administrative data (eg, number of preventive medicine service *CPT* codes reported for population of patients 3–21 years old). Pediatric medical home and quality improvement initiatives vary by state or region and may include a combination of HEDIS and other nationally recognized quality measures.

Some measures include criteria that exclude a patient from the population for the measure. For example, adolescents with history of anaphylactic reaction to a vaccine or its components before their 13th birthday may be excluded from the measure for immunizations for adolescents. *ICD-10-CM* codes such as **Z28.04** (immunization not carried out because of patient allergy to vaccine or component), **Z87.892** (personal history of anaphylaxis), and **Z88.7** (allergy status to serum and vaccine status) may be reported to indicate this patient history. Most measures exclude patients receiving hospice care.

Coding Conundrum: Quality Measurement and Vaccine Refusal

Codes for patient or caregiver vaccine refusal do not exclude a patient from the population for immunization measures. This creates a dilemma for physicians whose quality scores and payment may be affected by unimmunized patients within their patient panel. Does the physician continue providing care to patients whose parents refuse immunization despite any effect on quality scores?

The American Academy of Pediatrics policy statement, "Responding to Parental Refusals of Immunization of Children" (https://doi.org/10.1542/peds.2005-0316), provides the following guidance:

"In general, pediatricians should endeavor not to discharge patients from their practices solely because a parent refuses to immunize his or her child. However, when a substantial level of distrust develops, significant differences in the philosophy of care emerge, or poor quality of communication persists, the pediatrician may encourage the family to find another physician or practice. Although pediatricians have the option of terminating the physician-patient relationship, they cannot do so without giving sufficient advance notice to the patient or custodial parent or legal guardian to permit another health care professional to be secured. Such decisions should be unusual and generally made only after attempts have been made to work with the family. Families with doubts about immunization should still have access to good medical care, and maintaining the relationship in the face of disagreement conveys respect and at the same time allows the child access to medical care. Furthermore, a continuing relationship allows additional opportunity to discuss the issue of immunization over time."

Preventive Screening and Utilization Measures

Following are some examples of measures in the categories of preventive screening and utilization with tips for coding and documentation:

Well-Child Visits—First 30 Months of Life

Measurement is based on the age of the patient at 2 distinct points *during the measurement period*.
- Children who turned 15 months—6 or more well-child visits

Health plans may count normal newborn care provided during the birth admission as 1 of 6 well-child visits before 15 months. Inclusion of history from a child's birth admission (eg, date and provider of initial hospital care, hepatitis B immunization) in the patient's medical record may support this and other measures.

- Children who turned 30 months—2 or more well-child visits

This measure can be met by completing each child's recommended well-child visits at 18 and 24 months or, if delayed, before the child reaches 30 months of age.

Annual Child and Adolescent Well-Care Visits

The measure applies to patients aged 3 to 21 years. To meet the measure, one comprehensive well visit must be provided during the calendar year.

Documentation of a comprehensive well visit should include specific information such as the Tanner stage, assessed skills that support the child's developmental milestones, and context of anticipatory counseling (eg, discussed diet, screen time, sleep).

A comprehensive well-care visit provided in conjunction with a preparticipation physical evaluation for school or sports participation may also support this measure.

Developmental Screening in the First 3 Years of Life

This measure applies to children who reached age 1, 2, or 3 years in the measurement year and requires use of a standardized screening instrument for motor, language, cognitive, and social-emotional development (must include all skills). Developmental screening is counted in each measurement year and for the 3-year period (ie, measure counts 4 times).

ICD-10-CM code **Z13.42** (encounter for screening for global developmental delays) and *CPT* code **96110** (developmental screening, with scoring and documentation, per standardized instrument) are typically reported for these services. Code **96110** alone is not sufficient because this code is also reported for screening for specific conditions (eg, autism spectrum disorder [ASD]).

Child/Adolescent Weight Assessment and Counseling for Nutrition and Physical Activity

Percentage of patients aged 3 to 17 years whose BMI was measured and documented as a BMI percentage (eg, 20%) and with documented counseling for nutrition and physical activity (a checklist of counseling topics may be acceptable).

Most health plans require physicians to report a code for the BMI percentile (**Z68.51–Z68.54**). The BMI value is reported as an additional code to counseling for nutrition (**Z71.3**) and codes for any related condition (eg, overweight, obesity).

> *International Classification of Diseases, 10th Revision, Clinical Modification (ICD-10-CM)* **codes for pediatric body mass index (BMI) percentiles (Z68.51–Z68.54) are reported only in conjunction with physician documentation of a related condition (eg, overweight, obesity). If a physician is reporting codes Z68.51–Z68.54 only on the basis of a payer's written guidance for reporting quality measures, it is advisable to keep a copy of the payer's guidance. An alternative method for reporting that the patient's BMI was documented is to report** *Current Procedural Terminology* **Category II code 3008F (BMI, documented) in lieu of** *ICD-10-CM* **codes for BMI.**

Code **Z71.82** (exercise counseling) is used to report counseling for physical activity.

> **When obesity is diagnosed and at least 15 minutes is spent in counseling specific to the obesity, code G0447 (face-to-face behavioral counseling for obesity, 15 minutes) may be separately reportable in addition to a preventive evaluation and management (E/M) service (eg, 99383). Verify individual health plan policies to determine if benefits for counseling for obesity are separately paid on the same date as a preventive E/M service.**

● indicates a new code; ▲, revised; #, re-sequenced; ✚, add-on; ★, audiovisual technology; and ◀, synchronous interactive audio.

Immunization Status

These measures are as follows:

- Child: Patients who received all recommended immunizations on or before their second birthday. This includes administration of 2 doses of influenza vaccine in addition to other recommended immunizations.
- Adolescent: Percentage of patients who are fully immunized by their 13th birthday.

> Documentation of immunizations that require a series of administrations (eg, 3 doses) should be documented as such (dose 2 of 2 or dose 2 of 3). This may be accomplished through use of a chart/template that indicates each vaccine/toxoid product administered, doses required to complete the series, and the date that each dose is administered.

The following *ICD-10-CM* codes (not all inclusive) may indicate a patient's reason for exclusion from 1 or more recommended immunizations:

Z87.892	Personal history of anaphylaxis
Z88.7	Allergy status to serum and vaccine
B20	Human immunodeficiency virus (HIV) disease
Z21	Asymptomatic human immunodeficiency virus (HIV) infection status
D81.9	Combined immunodeficiency, unspecified
D81.31	Severe combined immunodeficiency due to adenosine deaminase deficiency
D84.9	Immunodeficiency, unspecified

Lead Screening

This measure is of the percentage of children who turn 2 years old during the measurement year who had at least 1 capillary or venous blood test for lead poisoning (**83655 QW**).

Example

➤ **A 23-month-old presents as a new patient for clearance to attend child care.** Records from the child's former physician indicate that a preventive E/M service was provided when the child was 18 months old and all immunizations are up to date, including 2 doses of influenza in the prior year. However, the prior preventive service was provided via telemedicine, and immunizations were provided at a separate encounter. The physician identifies that screenings for lead, global development, and ASD were not performed. These are performed (with parental permission) at this encounter in addition to performing the 24-month well-child examination.

ICD-10-CM	CPT	Related HEDIS Measures
Z00.129 (encounter for routine child health examination without abnormal findings)	**99392** (periodic comprehensive preventive medicine reevaluation and management, age 1–4 years)	*Well-Child Visits—First 30 Months of Life* Patients turning 30 months old during measurement year 2 or more comprehensive well-care visits completed between 15 and 30 months after birth
Z13.42 (encounter for screening for global developmental delays [milestones])	**96110** (developmental screening, with scoring and documentation, per standardized instrument)	*Developmental Screening in the First 3 Years of Life* Once within each of the first 3 years after birth
Z13.41 (encounter for autism screening)	**96110 59** (developmental screening, with scoring and documentation, per standardized instrument)	*Not applicable—the measure for developmental screening is limited to screening for global developmental delay.*
Z13.88 (encounter for screening for disorder due to exposure to contaminants)	**36416** (collection capillary blood specimen) **99000** (handling and/or conveyance of specimen)	*Lead Screening* Patients turning 2 years old in the measurement year At least 1 capillary or venous lead blood test completed on or before their second birthday

● indicates a new code; ▲, revised; #, re-sequenced; ✚, add-on; ★, audiovisual technology; and ◀, synchronous interactive audio.

Teaching Point: The physician in this scenario has proactively provided preventive care that is recommended for this patient and, in doing so, is able to report diagnosis and procedure codes demonstrating that quality measures have been met.

Code **Z02.0** (encounter for examination for admission to educational institution) is not reported because an *Excludes1* note prohibits reporting codes in category **Z02** with codes in category **Z00**.

> **See Chapter 8 for more details on coding for preventive medicine services.**

Effectiveness of Care

Certain measures are used to determine the effectiveness of care. Some effectiveness of care measures use a combination of medical and pharmacy claims data to assess overuse or appropriate use of medications. Other measures are of the percentage of patients receiving follow-up care after new diagnoses, ED visits, or hospital stays. Following are examples of these measures:

Pharyngitis and Antibiotic Prescriptions

Percentage of patients 3 years and older diagnosed with pharyngitis who were tested for streptococcal infection and, only if appropriate, prescribed an antibiotic.

Physician, pharmacy, and laboratory claims may be used for this measure. Codes for testing for streptococcal infection (eg, **87880**, infectious agent antigen detection by immunoassay with direct optical [ie, visual] observation; streptococcus, group A) and *ICD-10-CM* codes (eg, **J02.0**, streptococcal pharyngitis) are indicative of meeting this measure.

Depression Screening and Follow-up

Percentage of patients aged 12 years and older who were seen during the measurement year and were screened for depression with a structured instrument and, for positive results, for whom an appropriate follow-up was planned. Code **96127** (brief emotional/behavioral assessment using standardized instrument) may be reported for providing screening, but Healthcare Common Procedure Coding System (HCPCS) codes are used to indicate the screening result and follow-up plan. (Individual payers may or may not require use of HCPCS codes, but reporting appropriate HCPCS codes can provide information that is not conveyed by other codes.)

G8510	Screening for depression is documented as negative, a follow-up plan is not required
G8431	Screening for depression is documented as being positive AND a follow-up plan is documented
G9717	Documentation stating the patient has had a diagnosis of depression or has had a diagnosis of bipolar disorder

Example

> **A physician sees an established patient (aged ≥12 years) for follow-up of major depressive disorder.** The patient is also experiencing a runny nose and sore throat. The caregiver requests an antibiotic but is instructed that the condition is viral so over-the-counter medicine may be used as necessary for the child's comfort. No antibiotic is ordered. The diagnoses are a single episode of moderate major depression, with improvement measured through a standardized rating scale, and acute nasopharyngitis. The plan is for the child to continue antidepressant medication and be reevaluated in 1 month. Home care for acute nasopharyngitis is to gargle with salt water, push fluids, and rest. The patient and caregiver are advised against use of cold and cough medications.

ICD-10-CM	CPT	Related HEDIS Measures
F32.1 (major depressive disorder, single episode, moderate) **J00** (acute nasopharyngitis)	**99214** (office or other outpatient visit for the E/M of an established patient [See full code descriptor in **Chapter 7**.])	*Appropriate Treatment for Children With Upper Respiratory Infection (URI)* Patients 3 mo–18 y with • Diagnosis of URI (includes **J00, J06.0, J06.9**) *and* • Not prescribed an antibiotic within 3 d of URI diagnosis

F32.1 (major depressive disorder, single episode, moderate)	**96127** (brief emotional/behavioral assessment [eg, depression inventory, attention-deficit/hyperactivity disorder (ADHD) scale], with scoring and documentation, per standardized instrument)	*Not applicable—code **96127** is not indicative of depression screening because **96127** is used to report use of a standardized instrument in diagnosis and management of other disorders in addition to depression.*
F32.1 (major depressive disorder, single episode, moderate)	**G9717** (documentation stating the patient has had a diagnosis of depression or has had a diagnosis of bipolar disorder)	*Depression screening and follow-up—code **G9717** indicates that the patient is not included in the population for whom screening is appropriate.*

Teaching Point: Because this patient had no symptoms of a bacterial infection, the physician did not prescribe an antibiotic. This supports the measure for appropriate treatment of URI.

Reporting code **G9717** removes this patient from the population measured for screening for depression and a follow-up plan.

Performance measures change annually. Physician practices should maintain awareness of how health plans collect data for performance measurement and the documentation and coding practices that may reduce burdens associated with associated medical record reviews. An updated Child Core Set is published on www.Medicaid.gov annually. Many plans publish their HEDIS measures and supporting codes, as it is important to payers that physicians achieve optimal HEDIS measurements.

Chapter Takeaways

Readers of this chapter should understand how coding may support quality and performance measurement initiatives.

Following are takeaways from this chapter:

- Physicians, payers, and accreditation organizations may use codes or claims data as a first line of quality measurement.
- Physicians and QHPs need to know how their documentation affects risk adjustment and how risk adjustment may affect their practice and patients.
- A patient's reported experience of care can affect not only quality ratings but also contractual relations between physicians and payers.
- The details of each measure (eg, patient population, exclusions) are important in either providing care within the time frame of a measure or indicating why a patient was excluded from the activity of a measure (eg, not immunized because of patient history or a condition that prevents immunization).

Resources

AAP Coding Assistance and Education

AAP clinical report, "Responding to Parental Refusals of Immunization of Children" (https://doi.org/10.1542/peds.2005-0316)

AAP policy statement, "A New Era in Quality Measurement: The Development and Application of Quality Measures" (https://doi.org/10.1542/peds.2016-3442)

AAP Pediatric Coding Newsletter™

"Coding and Use of Interpretation Services," December 2021 (https://doi.org/10.1542/pcco_book212_document002)

"Hierarchical Condition Categories: What They Are and Why They Matter to Pediatricians," July 2019 (https://doi.org/10.1542/pcco_book183_document006)

● indicates a new code; ▲, revised; #, re-sequenced; ✚, add-on; ★, audiovisual technology; and ◀, synchronous interactive audio.

Consumer Assessment of Healthcare Providers and Systems

AHRQ CAHPS program (www.ahrq.gov/cahps/index.html)

CPT Category II Codes and Alphabetical Clinical Topics Listing

www.ama-assn.org/practice-management/cpt-category-ii-codes

Quality Measures

National Committee for Quality Assurance (www.ncqa.org)

Medicaid Children's Health Care Quality Measures (www.medicaid.gov/medicaid/quality-of-care/performance-measurement/adult-and-child-health-care-quality-measures/childrens-health-care-quality-measures/index.html)

Test Your Knowledge!

1. **Which of the following data are used in calculating a patient's risk of increased health care use or risk adjustment?**
   a. Claims data for physician services
   b. Demographics, health plan type, and duration of coverage
   c. Claims data for prescription drugs
   d. All of the above

2. **Which of the following activities does a physician do that supports Healthcare Effectiveness Data and Information Set (HEDIS) measurement?**
   a. Learning about HEDIS measures applicable to the patient panel and proactively providing related services
   b. Reporting diagnosis codes for all problems in the patient's problem list
   c. Learning everything about all HEDIS measures
   d. Documenting that preventive services are recommended but not scheduled or provided

3. **Which of the following statements is true of the Consumer Assessment of Healthcare Providers and Systems (CAHPS) surveys?**
   a. Each health plan creates its own version of the surveys.
   b. The CAHPS has no impact on physicians and qualified health care professionals.
   c. The patient's experience with office staff can affect survey results.
   d. All physicians must personally survey patients by using a CAHPS survey instrument.

4. **Which of the following statements is true for performance measures related to provision of preventive services?**
   a. Health plans may count normal newborn care provided during the birth admission as 1 of 6 well-child visits before 15 months.
   b. Sports preparticipation physical evaluations that are not comprehensive preventive medicine services count as well-child visits for performance measurement.
   c. When parents refuse immunization, their child is excluded from measures for immunization.
   d. Preventive measures are not affected by the diagnosis codes reported by the physician or qualified health care professional.

Chapter 3. Coding to Demonstrate Quality and Value

The Business of Medicine: Working With Current and Emerging Payment Systems

CPT copyright 2022 American Medical Association. All rights reserved.

Contents

Chapter Highlights

- To maintain a viable practice, physicians and their staff must respond to changing payment systems and continually refine their practice management skills.
- *Fee-for-service and alternative payment models:* Learn how services are currently valued and how assigned values may be used to guide practice management and payer contract negotiations.
- *Contracting and negotiating with payers:* Learn how data are leveraged to negotiate contract terms and payment.
- *Steps to getting paid:* Learn about guidelines and tools that may be used to monitor and manage charge accumulation, claims filing, review of payments, the appeals process, and the use of audits to protect against lost revenue and incorrect billing practices.

Fee-for-Service Payment for Physician Services

Values Assigned to Physician Services

A fee-for-service payment methodology based on both the Medicare Resource-Based Relative Value Scale (RBRVS) and submission of claims reporting physician services is the basis for a large portion of payment for physician services in 2023. Although other payment methodologies are growing, fee-for-service is often part of these methodologies. Before a claim is generated, a physician practice must establish fees for services that are greater than the cost of providing the service. A simple fee schedule methodology involves use of the RBRVS. An understanding of how values are assigned to the codes for services, how the values relate to payment, and how this information contributes to a practice's finances is critical for the practice's financial viability and success.

The 3 components of the RBRVS are as follows:

1. *Physician work:* Physician work represents approximately 50% of the total relative value units (RVUs) assigned to most services. Work RVUs are commonly used in employment contracts as a factor in physician payment.
2. *Practice expense:* This component is an estimate of the following items:
   - Preservice, intraservice, and post-service clinical staff time
   - Medical supplies
   - Procedure-specific and overhead equipment

     Practice expense makes up about 44% of the total RVUs for most services. Practice expense varies by site of service (ie, facility vs non-facility). See the Place of Service Codes section later in this chapter for more information about how place of service affects payment.
3. *Professional liability:* This smallest component (about 4% of the total RVUs) is based on medical malpractice premium data.

Each RVU component may be independently adjusted slightly upward or downward as a function of geographic area. The American Academy of Pediatrics (AAP) RBRVS Conversion Spreadsheet allows you to calculate Medicare payment rates by using your geographic location (https://downloads.aap.org/AAP/Excel/2022%20RBRVS%20Conversion%20Spreadsheet.xls; download required). The Centers for Medicare & Medicaid Services (CMS) calculates Medicare payment for a procedure code by multiplying total RVUs by a dollar conversion factor (CF) that is set annually.

Components of Physician Work

Work is described as time required to perform the service, mental effort and judgment, technical skill, physical effort, and psychological stress associated with concern about iatrogenic risk to the patient.

For most services, physician work is further broken down into *preservice, intraservice,* and *post-service* components. Correct coding requires understanding these components of work, as preservice and post-service components should not be separately reported.

- *Preservice work:* For nonsurgical services, this preparatory non–face-to-face work includes typical review of records and communicating with other professionals. (Prolonged preservice work, such as extensive record review, may be separately reportable.) For surgical services, this includes physician work from the day before the service to the procedure but excludes the encounter that resulted in the decision for surgery or unrelated evaluation and management (E/M) services.

- *Intraservice work:* For most nonsurgical services, this includes time spent by the physician or other qualified health care professional (QHP) in direct patient care activities. Surgical intraservice work begins with incision or introduction of instruments (eg, needle, scope) and ends with closure of the incision or removal of instruments.
  - A physician's intraservice time on the date of an E/M service for which the level of service is selected on the basis of total time or medical decision-making (MDM) includes all time spent on the date of the encounter. Pre-visit planning and post-visit work, such as documenting the service provided, are included in intraservice time when performed on the date of the encounter.
  - Certain services (eg, chronic care management [CCM]) are inclusive only of intraservice time of physicians and/or clinical staff and are not valued to include preservice and post-service work.
- *Post-service work:* Documentation of services provided is included in the post-service work of most services.
  - For nonsurgical services, post-service work includes arranging for further services, reviewing and communicating test results, preparing written reports, and/or communicating by telephone or secure electronic means. Separately reported services, such as CCM or care plan oversight, are not included in post-service work.
  - For surgical services, post-service work includes typical work in the procedure or operating room after the procedure has ended, stabilization of the patient in the recovery area, communications with family or other health care professionals, and visits on the day of surgery. Surgical services are also valued to include typical follow-up care for the presenting problem during a defined global period (eg, 10 or 90 days after the service).

> **For more on the global period for surgery, see chapters 14 and 19.**

Participation in Relative Value Scale Update Committee Surveys

Pediatricians can also play a role in recommending values for services to the CMS by participation in AAP surveys conducted through the American Medical Association/Specialty Society Relative Value Scale Update Committee (RUC). These surveys are conducted to estimate the time and complexity of performing a service in comparison with another service. American Academy of Pediatrics staff sends out requests for participation to AAP section members to allow completion by physicians who most typically perform the service being surveyed. To learn more about participation in RUC surveys, see the "Understanding the RUC Survey Instrument: Physician Services without Global Period" video at www.youtube.com/watch?v=nu5unDX8VIs; for information on code valuation, RBRVS, and payment, see www.aap.org/en/practice-management/practice-financing/coding-and-valuation/code-valuation-and-payment-rbrvs.

Fee Schedules and Calculations

The CMS calculates Medicare payment for a procedure code by multiplying total RVUs by a dollar CF that is set annually.

Example

> **A payer uses the 2022 Medicare Physician Fee Schedule (MPFS) as a basis for physician payment with a CF or contracted fee schedule amount of $40 per RVU.** A physician submits established patient office visit code **99214** to the payer.
>
> The total MPFS non-facility RVUs (3.75) assigned to code **99214** are a combination of RVUs for physician work (1.92), non-facility practice expense (1.71), and professional liability (0.12). The total non-facility RVUs (3.75) are multiplied by the $40 CF to determine the allowed amount for the service.
>
> (Total Medicare RVUs) × (Payer CF) = Allowed amount
>
> (3.75) × ($40) = $150
>
> Actual payment by the payer may vary on the basis of the patient's out-of-pocket obligation.

Medicaid fee schedules vary by state, and although often based on RVUs or the MPFS, state regulations may also designate amounts paid for specific services. Commercial payments for many procedure codes are often linked to a percentage of Medicare payment (eg, 140% of MPFS rate). Alternatively, payers may offer their own fee schedule (eg, a particular year's MPFS) for a practice's most used procedure codes.

> If a health plan contract states that payment is based on the Medicare Physician Fee Schedule (MPFS), it is important to verify the year of the MPFS used by the health plan because the schedule is not always current or may not be updated annually. Resetting payment according to the MPFS for the year of service may result in higher or lower payments.

● indicates a new code; ▲, revised; #, re-sequenced; ✚, add-on; ★, audiovisual technology; and ◀, synchronous interactive audio.

Understanding how health plan rates in your area compare to the current MPFS rates can help inform contract negotiations. For examples of how commercial health plan payments compared to Medicare payments based on amounts paid by 3 large commercial health plans, review the Health Care Cost Institute's "Comparing Commercial and Medicare Professional Service Prices" at https://healthcostinstitute.org/hcci-research/comparing-commercial-and-medicare-professional-service-prices.

- It is important to obtain the payer's fee schedule for all codes used or likely to be used by a practice (including codes for vaccines and administration) and compare these with the current year's MPFS and other published fee schedules. Although Medicare assigns a status of N (noncovered) to *Current Procedural Terminology* (*CPT*®) preventive medicine E/M codes **99381–99385** and **99391–99395** in the MPFS, component RVUs are published in the MPFS allowing calculation of Medicare equivalent payments.

> When reviewing a payer's fee schedule, make sure the payer also fully discloses its policies for paying for services that it considers to be *bundled* (ie, payment for ≥2 codes during the same encounter may be less than the sum of the individual payments) and those whose cost it shifts to the patient/family.

The RBRVS payment methodology may be used with practice- and physician-specific data generated from a practice's accounting and practice management systems to estimate an approximate cost of providing each service. This should result in a list of services that are each assigned a share of the practice's overhead costs as well as the margin and actual cost of providing the service.

- From the accounting system, an administrator may calculate the total practice expenses for a period, subtracting billable services that are not paid on the basis of RVUs such as vaccines and medications.
- From the practice management system, reports may be generated to provide a total of the number of procedures billed by code, RVUs for each service, and total RVUs billed by the practice for the same period.
- By dividing total practice expenses by total RVUs, an administrator can calculate the practice cost per RVU.
- Additional calculations may be used to compare payment per RVU or per service among contracted payers. (Calculations should be viewed in context of other factors, such as history of timely and correct payment.)

> It may be important to consider several years of data to account for seasonal, year-to-year, or public health emergency impacts, which may significantly limit the accuracy of data to predict future service costs and volume.

Such calculations should be used to inform decisions on acceptance of contractual fee schedules, number of services necessary to break even or profit from provision of services, and return on investment potential for new equipment or services.

Keep in mind that some accountable care organizations (ACOs) have financial agreements that require certain services be paid with a single lump payment that is then distributed among all providers of the service. (For discussion of ACOs, see the Organizational Support for Entering Value-Based Payment Contracts section later in this chapter.) To negotiate a fair portion of that lump payment, you need to know the cost of providing the service. More accurate cost estimates may be determined on an actual cost basis. However, RVU calculations are straightforward and typically provide a reasonably reliable result.

Alternative Payment Models

Alternatives to fee-for-service payment have been offered and reimagined many times over the years. However, a fee-for-service component is typically included in alternative payment models.

Capitation is one payment model. In capitation arrangements, the health plan typically pays a specified amount per health plan member assigned to the physician or practice on a per-member-per-month (PMPM) basis. Amounts may vary by patient age, patient sex, and plan design. Under capitation plans, physicians and other QHPs provide sick- and well-child services that are included in the PMPM payment. In addition to PMPM payments, plans may pay separately for provision of vaccine products and other specified services. Capitation arrangements may also include elements of other alternative payment models that are focused on valued-based payment.

Value-based payment models offer physicians and other providers (eg, QHPs and other qualified nonphysician health care professionals [QNHCPs]) incentive payments based on the quality of care, outcomes, and cost containment attributable to their practices. The intent is to promote patient value and efficiency, but some risk is shifted to physician practices and there could be a lack of clarity about how payments are calculated. Value-based payment models are widely variable in regional implementation but are growing in national importance and impact.

Chapter 4. The Business of Medicine: Working With Current and Emerging Payment Systems

Important Considerations in Value-Based Payment Models

In value-based payment programs, it is not always transparent to families how the value is calculated (ie, how much is quality and how much is cost). When discussing such programs with payers, practices should be aware of whether immunizations and preventive care are counted in the total cost of care, or they may find that if they improve well-child visit and immunization rates, the costs of those services are counted against the practice in total cost of care calculations. In addition, some payers prefer to drive patients to high-value practices or have tiered co-payments based on individual physician or practice performance.

Under value-based payment models, practice viability depends on how well quality, cost, and efficiency are managed. Examples of some of these value-based payment models include bundled payments, shared savings/risk, and pay for performance (P4P). Physician payments may be based on a combination of fee for service and alternative payment methodologies.

- *Bundled payments:* These are a type of prospective payment in which health care providers (eg, hospitals, physicians, and other health care professionals) share 1 payment for a specified range of services as opposed to each provider being paid individually. The intent of bundled payments is to foster collaboration and accountability among multiple providers to coordinate services and control costs, thereby reducing unnecessary utilization.
- *Shared savings/risk:* Shared savings/risk models may include upside reward or both upside reward and downside risk. In an upside-reward–only arrangement, the provider shares only in any savings and does not have risk for a loss. Under reward-and-risk arrangements, the practice shares not only a reward if costs are less than budgeted but also the loss should actual total costs exceed budgeted costs.
  - The contractual arrangement among the payer(s) and providers specifies how savings and/or risk is to be calculated and distributed.
  - Shared savings should include an up-front agreement to continue additional payments for ongoing support of infrastructure for future years when the payer may want to cut back on the shared savings margin or reduce as those savings plateau.

The target or expected budgeted amount should be reviewed periodically and renegotiated to account for the current savings opportunity. After implementing many initiatives and achieving significant cost savings early in a contract, providers may then target maintaining cost performance and limiting increases in total cost of care.

  - Quality metrics are typically tied to payment of shared savings, with physicians not receiving a portion of savings when not meeting established quality benchmarks.

See Chapter 3 for more information on coding to support quality and performance measurement.

- *Pay for performance:* In this arrangement, physician payments are based on a prospectively determined comparison of the provider's performance against acknowledged benchmarks. If the provider meets or exceeds those benchmarks, an enhanced payment or bonus is provided.
  - Benchmarks are often like the National Committee for Quality Assurance Healthcare Effectiveness Data and Information Set (HEDIS) quality metrics (some common metrics for pediatrics include rates of immunizations; rates of patient adherence to Early and Periodic Screening, Diagnostic, and Treatment visits; and rates of appropriate prescription of asthma medications). These metrics should be relevant to pediatrics.
  - Benchmarks based on transparent rubrics allow providers to track their performance against the benchmark on an ongoing basis. In contrast, if benchmarks are based on comparison to peers, providers might not know whether they meet the metrics until the period is over.
  - Payers should provide information on how benchmarks are defined and measured. They should also provide quarterly data on provider performance against benchmarks. This way, providers are aware of their performance standing and have an opportunity to improve throughout the measurement incentive year.
  - Providers should be rewarded for achieving incremental improvements and maintaining high levels of quality once achieved.

When considering whether to participate in one of these alternative payment models, practices need to determine expected costs and utilization and assess whether they can deliver services under the projected budget. Using *CPT* codes and their RVUs will aid in this assessment. Projections can be made by using RVUs of the services currently provided and projected to be provided. With these types of data, the practice can assess the effect of new payment methodologies on its bottom line.

● indicates a new code; ▲, revised; #, re-sequenced; ✚, add-on; ★, audiovisual technology; and ◀, synchronous interactive audio.

In some parts of the country, practices can earn additional incentives if the total cost of care for patients compares favorably to that of geographically and specialty matched peers. In addition, some payers are incentivizing around "care efficiency measures." Both of these are often risk adjusted on the basis of claims data about the overall patient population of the practice. Payers should define measures (eg, what constitutes an avoidable emergency department [ED] visit) and data that can be used to improve performance. As with other quality or cost measures, these measures should be relevant to pediatrics.

Participating in Alternative Payment Models

The following payment models are already in place for pediatrics in some areas and may soon be adopted in others. Whether your practice provides primary or specialty care, there are steps you should take to prepare for success. When payment is based on the costs of care and patient experience, practices must take responsibility for keeping costs low and for keeping quality of care and patient experience high. Steps that practices may take include

- Learning more about value-based payment options
- Generating and using reports of your costs, quality measurement, and other data
- Learning who your active patients are and staying up to date through routine data analysis
  - Obtain lists of patients attributed to your practice by payers (patient panels) and reconcile to your active patient list.
  - Identify and agree on a methodology by which patients will be assigned and any disputes over attributed patient panels will be reconciled.

Assignment, Engagement, and Attribution of Patient Panels

Value-based payment may be based on the patients assigned and/or attributed to a practice (patient panel) by a payer. This may be limited to comparison of the cost of care for a physician's patient panel to other patients in a geographic area or to another subset of patients. The cost of care for all attributed patients may lead to additional payment based on shared cost savings or may limit the amount of payments that the practice retains. It is important to understand the distinction between what you view as your practice panel and how the insurer views it.

It is also important to differentiate assignment from engagement and attribution.

- *Assignment:* The patients the insurance company lists on your panel roster.

  For Medicaid managed care, every patient must be assigned to a provider (or provider practice) when patients are enrolled in the health plan. These patients may choose your practice or can be automatically assigned on the basis of insurer algorithms.
- *Engagement:* Patients you have seen and with whom you have a medical home relationship.

  If you have an after-hours clinic and you see patients from other practices, it is essential you communicate to those patients that they are not part of your medical home (ie, they are part of another physician's or practice's panel).
- *Attribution:* Patients who fall into the denominator of a metric in which value (ie, payment) is assigned. Physicians should understand how health plans attribute patients to individual physicians and/or groups for purposes of performance measurement and cost of care.
  - Factors such as time of continuous enrollment with the health plan and number of visits to a provider may affect how patients are attributed.

To ensure you are engaging patients who are assigned to your practice, make sure you receive a panel roster monthly, preferably an Excel file, through the payer's portal. Identify new patients assigned to your practice, and plan for what services they will need on the basis of their age.

- Use the roster at check-in to make sure all patients seen in your medical home are assigned to you. This step is just as important as identifying those you are not seeing on your roster. It will ensure you are getting credit for the quality work your office is providing.

Know the payer's rules for requesting that a patient be removed from your roster. They may require specific documentation, such as number of outreach attempts by phone or mail, to fulfill your request.

- Track the number of patients assigned to your office each month. If there is a large increase, a group of patients from another practice may have been shifted to your practice. Consider including language in your contract that specifies that no panel transfers can be done without prior authorization of your practice.
- If the insurer is nonresponsive in working to ensure that only patients who can be or are engaged are assigned, consider limiting the ages that can be assigned to your practice or closing your practice to auto-assignment altogether.

For HEDIS measures, patients must meet certain age-, utilization-, or encounter-based criteria to fall into your denominator. Knowing when they will be attributed (and show up on your "gaps in care" reports) is essential. For further discussion, see **Chapter 3**. For primary care physicians, the cost of preventive services should not negatively affect the physician's calculated cost of care per patient.

Remember that your revenue comes from encounters with engaged patients regardless of assignment or attribution in a value-based payment model. Your practice will never have a 100% accurate assigned panel. The effort you put in to reaching this perfection must be balanced by what is being measured and how much payment is at risk.

Steps that may increase successful participation in value-based payment include

- Embracing automation and alternatives to paper handling and traditional office-based care.
- Seeking to remove inefficiencies by reviewing routine tasks and patient flow. Provide staff with incentives and an expectation to create consistency and efficiency.
- Learning about the communities of your patients (ie, school and community resources, school schedules, average income and education of caregivers, urgent and emergency care utilization patterns) and using that information in providing care.
- Knowing the costs of the care you provide and order for your patients. Recognize that every provider within and outside your practice must contribute to reducing the cost of care to reduce the practice's risk under new payment models.
  — Remember that care received in the ED and urgent care clinics and from subspecialists or QNHCPs (eg, physical therapists) is included in the cost of care attributed to your cost to care for your patients.
  — Collaborate with other health care professionals to ensure that patients receive evidence-based and cost-effective care, including consideration of formulary and total cost of coordinated care.
- Setting shared goals and shared priorities with the payer. Evaluate your progress against goals and reevaluate targets each year with the payer. Targets might need to be adjusted on the basis of past achievements and future opportunities.
- Considering options for adding nonphysician health care professionals, such as care coordinators, patient educators, and emotional/behavioral health specialists, to your practice. (These clinicians may also add separately reportable services under fee-for-service contracts.)
- Embedding clinical guidelines into care delivery through protocols and reminders.
- Configuring and using your electronic health record (EHR) and other automated systems to promote efficiency (eg, display generic drugs first when a brand name is entered).
- When considering an alternative payment model contract, seeking expert consultation to help identify and, as necessary, negotiate points of concern within the contract.

Other considerations for pediatricians include

- Recognizing that, depending on how the payment model is set up, managing a healthy population of patients may not result in significant cost savings.
- Having the ability to access and monitor patient population and performance metric data, which is important for successful participation in new payment methodologies. Physicians must be aware of not only the patients they are seeing but also those who are not receiving preventive and/or follow-up care.
- For physicians, understanding the links between new payment methodologies and data collection to support quality metrics (eg, failure to report codes for screening services performed may result in negative performance measurement and lost opportunity for enhanced payment).
- Remembering that in states where the Children's Health Insurance Program (CHIP) operates independent of a Medicaid program, children covered by CHIP may or may not be included in new payment methodologies and/or performance measurement.

See the *AAP News* article, "PPAAC: Chapter Pediatric Councils Work With Payers on Medical Home Programs," at https://publications.aap.org/aapnews/news/13007 for examples of how AAP chapters and their pediatric councils advocate for developing adequate financing for pediatric medical homes under value-based payment methodologies.

Contracting and Negotiating With Payers

Participating in a payer's network typically involves entering into a contract with the payer. Physicians should not sign contracts without reading and considering the impact of entering into the contractual agreement. The payer is going to seek terms that are most favorable to its business. Negotiation is important to ensure that your practice is profitable and able to provide quality care without burdensome payer requirements (eg, panel attribution methodology and primary care provider reassignment, dispute process for quality or other P4P programs).

The Importance of Data and Leverage

Successful negotiation requires data and leverage. Negotiating payment with payers can be more successful if a practice is prepared to provide data on the complexity of its patient panel, on its quality performance according to standard quality measures, and on any current initiatives and future opportunities to influence total cost of care. Be prepared to demonstrate the cost savings that may be recognized by the plan as well as the value the practice brings to the plan in quality of care and/or patient satisfaction.

> Refer to Chapter 3 for more information on demonstrating quality and patient satisfaction.

Organizational Support for Entering Value-Based Payment Contracts

Demonstrating that a practice provides care at lower cost and higher value can significantly burden small practices. Entering into a contract to participate in a network or an organization with other physician practices, and sometimes hospitals or health care systems, can offer support on multiple levels. Through these contractual relationships, physicians may achieve objectives such as improved capitation rates, entrance into other risk-sharing contracts, and increased ability to demonstrate quality and cost reductions. There are multiple types of contractual entities that can influence success in value-based payment arrangements.

> Various federal and state regulations (eg, antitrust regulations and price-fixing, physician self-referral, false claims) must be accounted for when entering into a contractual agreement that organizes multiple independent physicians into an organization that will influence health care referrals and health plan fee schedule negotiations.

- *Management services organization:* These organizations focus solely on administrative tasks such as provision of space, equipment, nonclinical staff, billing and compliance, accounts payable, insurance credentialing (not contract negotiation), and human resources.
- *Independent physician or practitioner association:* Joining these organizations of independent physician practices often includes entering into risk-sharing or capitation contracts that place the organization as an intermediary between payers and physician members. These organizations cannot negotiate fee-for-service contracts.
- *Clinically integrated network (CIN):* A group of physicians and providers (eg, hospitals or health systems) who are integrated at the clinical level to be able to jointly contract with and participate in performance incentive programs. The practices continue *independent medical practice* and the CIN members work together to achieve and demonstrate better quality and lower cost. A CIN is much like an ACO (as follows) but is not governed by the Medicare/Medicaid rules for ACOs.
- *Accountable care organizations:* An ACO is an organization of health care professionals that agrees to be accountable for the quality, cost, and overall care of beneficiaries. The ACO is a legal entity with a management structure capable of delivering and reporting on evidence-based and informed care to a defined population, effectively engaging patients, and receiving and distributing shared savings.
  - The Patient Protection and Affordable Care Act of 2010 included provisions that establish ACOs in Medicare, Medicaid, and CHIP. Federal regulations, such as anti-kickback and self-referral prohibitions, continue to be revised to allow more cooperation and technical support among ACO participants.
  - From a practical standpoint, an ACO is a community of physicians and other QHPs who work collaboratively to reduce health care costs and improve the quality of care for their patient population. Accountable care organization members typically focus on data sharing and care coordination to help deliver timely preventive and care management services to generate health care savings that are then shared by the ACO members.
  - Most pediatric ACOs are affiliated with children's hospitals and/or health plans. Commercial health insurers are actively exploring the development of ACOs and may support establishment of an ACO.
- Learn more about establishing and participating in an ACO from the *Pediatrics* article, "Pediatric Accountable Care Organizations: Insight From Early Adopters" (https://doi.org/10.1542/peds.2016-1840).

Preparing for Negotiation

Successful negotiation requires preparation. The following suggestions can help:

- Fully read and ask questions, as necessary, about the terms of the contract.
  - Initial term and any automatic renewal (evergreen) clause
  - Time frame and notice required for termination with/without cause
  - Payment methodology, annual CF, and any automatic increases or updates (eg, whether payment updates align with Medicare updates or are tied to a specific year of the Medicare fee schedule)
  - Time frame for payer recoupment and claim appeals
  - Notice and consent required for amendments and material changes
  - Types of products (eg, HMO, PPO) and health plans included and whether there is a requirement to accept all products
- Verify payer rules about modifier usage, as this may affect payment. For example, when preventive and problem-oriented E/M services are provided on the same date, modifier **25** (significant and separately identifiable E/M service) is appended to the code for the problem-oriented E/M service (eg, **99213 25**). Some payers reduce the payment to 50% of the fee schedule amount for that code.
- Ask whether there is any tiering of network providers based on quality or cost-efficiency rankings and, if so,
  - Whether tiering is done at the provider or practice/group level
  - Whether adding new providers will result in them carrying over their previous ranking
  - How tiering affects provider payment and/or patient cost sharing

Why Health Plan Tiering Matters

Many health plans assign in-network physicians to tiers based on the cost and value of care provided by the individual physician or the group practice.

Tiering is often tied to patient cost sharing (eg, deductible, co-payments, and coinsurance), with patients being responsible for the highest cost sharing if they see providers in the lowest tier. This may affect how and whether a patient receives health care services.

Tiering may also affect both the number of patients who select a particular health plan (eg, a tiered plan in which their current physician is in a high tier) and how the health plan negotiates with a physician or group practice (eg, by offering a lower fee schedule as a larger number of patients enroll in the tiered health plan).

Becoming a contracted network provider might not place you into the highest (preferred) tier, as this depends on how tiering is determined. Language on tiering may or may not be in the contract, so there is value in requesting information about the payer's use of tiering and tier assignment methodology.

- Know a health plan's policies and procedures and their effect on pediatric services. Develop a system to monitor all policy and procedure updates and to receive and review in detail any communications from the payer on changes to the physician contract. The payer may automatically amend the contract if no response is received to a notice of proposed amendment in the specified time frame. Be aware of updates to the provider manual, updates provided via periodic email bulletins, and information posted on a payer website that practices have been instructed to review periodically. Practices must be aware that these alternative ways of disseminating payment information are often considered legal and binding.
- Know a health plan's processes and time frame for adding new *CPT* codes/services and how each plan pays for new services reported before developing and updating their systems with payment policy and fee schedule amounts. This preparation is especially important for new vaccines to make sure you will get paid. (New codes are often paid at a low rate or a percentage of charges, if covered at all.)
- When adding new physicians to your practice, be aware of each payer's fee schedule policies. Do not assume that the same fee schedule will be applied across all physicians in the practice (eg, a payer may assign a reduced fee schedule to new physicians or carry forward a physician's contract from a previous practice).

  Be aware of the potential that patients may incur higher out-of-pocket costs (eg, co-pays) with services by different providers within the practice. When this occurs, discussion with a health plan should include the potential effect of delayed care when the patient/family opts to wait to see a provider for whom the out-of-pocket costs are lower.
- Be aware of any accountability (eg, penalties or other effect on shared savings) that a plan attributes to the practice when patients receive care outside their plan's network without referral by physicians within the practice.
- Know *CPT* codes and modifiers and the guidelines for their use.
- Understand how the National Correct Coding Initiative (NCCI) adopted by some payers (including Medicaid) may relate to your practice.

● indicates a new code; ▲, revised; #, re-sequenced; ✚, add-on; ★, audiovisual technology; and ◀, synchronous interactive audio.

- Understand and be able to describe the scope of services provided and the time requirements for the service.
- Be prepared to demonstrate the cost savings that may be recognized by the plan as well as the value the practice brings to the plan in savings, quality of care, and/or patient satisfaction. *This is your leverage.*
- Monitor and know the use (distribution) of codes by each physician and, if in a group practice, for the practice as a whole.
- Identify your payer mix. Know how many patients you have in each plan and what percentage of your total patients that represents. In addition, know what percentage of RVUs each payer pays for your most frequently used codes and how these percentages compare in payment with each other. Accurate information on payer mix and potential value/ loss to the practice is essential in making participation decisions.
- Know and understand the payment basis and process.
- Have specific codes or issues to discuss, not generalities (agreement with general ideas may not address specific issues).

  In negotiations,

- Try to negotiate for coverage and adequate payment of services. If payers refuse to cover services, ensure there is language in your contract stating that you can bill the patient for non-covered services. If the plan will allow for billing the patient for non-covered services, you must then advise your patients of this policy (a written notification is usually required before rendering the service).
- If the plan does agree to cover a particular service, make certain you understand how the carrier will cover and pay for the service and if there will be any restrictions or limitations.
- Keep notes during the discussion and be certain you understand answers to any of your questions. Any specific agreements should be in writing and signed by both parties with the effective date clearly stated.

  Seek assistance in negotiations.

- Engage parents or employers to work in partnership to help you negotiate with a plan. Encourage parents to work through their human resources department to communicate and appeal with payers. Petitions from parents can be very effective. See the resources for health insurance education from HealthyChildren.org at www.healthychildren.org/ English/family-life/health-management/health-insurance/Pages/default.aspx.

> It is important, too, to recognize that the employers in your area may offer their employees a self-funded health plan and that it is the employer who may be in control of the plan's network, payment rates, and policies for coverage and payment of specific services, although claims are administered by a third party (eg, health insurance company).

- Many AAP chapters have developed pediatric councils, which meet with payers to address pediatric issues. Advise your chapter pediatric council of specific issues you have experienced, and see how it can work with the plan. (The AAP chapter pediatric councils are not forums for negotiating contracts, setting fees, or discussing payments.)
  - If your chapter does not have a pediatric council, this may be the right time to work with your chapter to begin developing one. For more information, visit www.aap.org/en/practice-management/practice-financing/payer-contracting-advocacy-and-other-resources/aap-payer-advocacy/aap-pediatric-councils.

When Negotiations Fail

If the insurance company is not addressing your concerns satisfactorily, you should be willing to provide notice of intent to terminate your contract if unable to reach an agreement after negotiating in good faith. Check your contract for specifications on the days of notice and notification process required for termination of your provider contract with or without cause. Inform the payer, the patients' families, and even the state insurance commission why continued participation is not possible.

- Some reasons for withdrawal might be slow payment, excessive documentation requirements, and substandard payment compared with those of other plans.
- Many times, negotiation begins when you walk away from the table.

Steps to Getting Paid: Clean Claims to Correct Payment

Getting paid for services provided requires a practice-wide team effort. Opportunities for lost revenue can occur anywhere between patient scheduling and posting of health plan payments (or denials). **Figure 4-1** shows steps in the revenue cycle. Even salaried physicians are affected by lost revenue and should take interest in the effectiveness of the practice's billing processes.

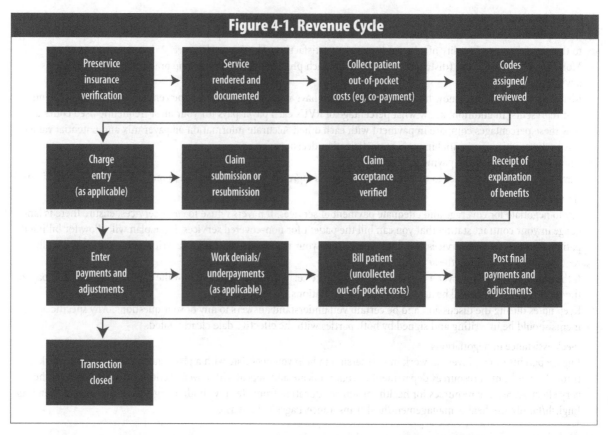

Figure 4-1. Revenue Cycle

An effective charge accumulation system, accurate billing of procedure codes, and an efficient claims filing system are necessary but not sufficient to achieve clean claim submissions. Although the physician is ultimately responsible for the accuracy of codes selected and claims submitted, it typically takes a team effort to create and maintain an effective accounts receivable system, including

- Development and use of management tools.
  - Incorporation of claims processing tools for analysis of your claims processing procedures.
  - Electronic health record and/or billing systems may include automated tools to help identify errors before billing, alert you to payments that do not align with contracted fees, and provide data for monitoring the time lapse from provision of service to payment.
  - Provide access to and create policy for using payer resources such as online code-checking tools that alert to coverage limitations such as bundled services or services covered only in conjunction with specific diagnoses.
- Continuing provider and staff education with constant oversight and communication with staff, payers, and patients.
  - Policies and procedures support continuous monitoring of payer communications and dissemination of information on benefit policy changes that affect coding and payment.
  - Assurance that staff assigned with responsibilities related to correct coding and billing have access to authoritative resources on coding and documentation (eg, health plan provider portals, current Medicaid NCCI edits and manual).

See chapters 2 and 5 for more information on code edits and compliant coding and billing.

- Regularly performing audits to identify potential corrective actions required to remain compliant with billing standards, coding guidelines, and federal rules and regulations (eg, Health Insurance Portability and Accountability Act [HIPAA] of 1996, Anti-Kickback Statute, False Claims Act). Audits benefit the practice by identifying
  - The number of timely and correctly submitted claims, resulting in faster and more appropriate payments and reduced practice cost of obtaining payment
  - The need for physician and staff education on coding and documentation
  - Issues for payer contract negotiations
  - Incorrect coding and related potential risk for charges of fraud or abuse
  - Areas that need written office policies and procedures (eg, pre-authorization and referral processes, claims follow-up processes, control systems)

- Procedures for efficient review of payments and potentially inappropriate denials or reductions. Timely identification of payment errors is necessary to obtain redress because contracts often specify a time limit on appeals.
- Guidance for write-offs and initiation of appeals processes.

Capturing Charges in the Electronic Health Record

Many physicians now capture encounter and billing information in the EHR. The basics of charge capture in the EHR are
- Accurate listing of diagnoses
- Selection of complete codes and access to a complete list of modifiers
- Procedure code selection based on work performed and documented

While integrating charge capture into the encounter documentation should create efficiency, there are pitfalls to be avoided.

> **Compliant documentation and code selection are discussed in Chapter 5.**

When using an EHR, make sure that codes in the system are accurate and updated in accordance with code set updates. It is important to verify with your electronic system vendors how code updates are incorporated into the system. This might happen via scheduled upgrades that may or may not require system downtime, or it could occur via automated upgrades during night or weekend hours. It is important to make sure this information is outlined in your EHR contract.
- Code updates should be based on the effective date of changes (eg, deleted codes may be entered for charges with a date of service before the effective date of deletion even after the update has been made).
- Practice and billing managers must maintain contact with the system vendor's upgrade and support staff and verify what, if any, manual steps are required on the part of the practice in relation to code changes.

> **Any codes saved to favorites lists or included in templates should be reviewed and updated, as indicated, with each release of new and revised codes.**

It is also important that code descriptors displayed in code selection are adequate for accurate code selection. Truncated descriptors may omit key information that differentiates one code from another (eg, attention-deficit hyperactivity disorder [ADHD] should provide options for predominantly hyperactive, predominantly inattentive, or combined ADHD).

Documentation of the diagnoses has been problematic in some EHR systems. As with the paper record, the physician must have the ability to fully describe patient diagnoses for each encounter (ie, not to merely select a diagnosis code).

Example

➤ 1. Neonatal heart murmur; benign versus congenital heart disease (**P29.89**, other cardiovascular disorders originating in the perinatal period)
2. Underachievement in school with grades dropping this semester (**Z55.3**, underachievement in school)
3. Post–COVID-19 loss of taste (**R43.8**, other disturbances of smell and taste; **U09.9**, post-COVID condition, unspecified)

- Systems should not use diagnosis codes for populating the physician's diagnostic statement or assessment. Code descriptors may be generalized and do not capture the physician's differential diagnoses (eg, delayed milestone in childhood—3 years old, late talker in speech therapy; possible autism spectrum disorder—little eye contact and likes to play alone), and many codes do not indicate when a condition is worsening or poorly controlled.
- List first the diagnosis and code most responsible for the encounter, followed by additional diagnoses, in compliance with coding guidelines.

  The EHR should not reorder diagnoses entered by the physician. An EHR that reorders documented diagnoses (eg, alphabetically) results in noncompliance with diagnosis coding guidelines.

> **Sequencing instructions in *International Classification of Diseases, 10th Revision, Clinical Modification* are important for correct coding and for prevention of claim rejections. See Chapter 1 for more on sequencing diagnosis codes.**

● indicates a new code; ▲, revised; #, re-sequenced; ✚, add-on; ★, audiovisual technology; and ◄, synchronous interactive audio.

- The patient problem list should not be pulled forward as the diagnoses for each encounter. Only those conditions addressed or that affected management or treatment of conditions addressed should be reported for that particular encounter.

    Follow payer guidelines for reporting diagnosis codes for chronic conditions that may be reported annually (eg, evaluating problems at preventive service visits) for the purpose of risk stratification (ie, projection of future health care costs for a patient). For example, for an annual well-child visit, a payer may require providers to report all underlying diagnoses for the purpose of risk adjustment, but for non-preventive services, the same payer may want providers to report diagnoses relevant only to the visit performed.

> **Documentation and coding to support risk adjustment are increasingly demanded by payers. Please see Chapter 3 for a discussion of appropriate coding to support risk adjustment.**

Automated code selection is also problematic. An EHR may be designed to determine the level of E/M service provided on the basis of information documented. However, physicians must make the code determination on the basis of the medically necessary services provided and documented and on the basis of code selection criteria (eg, medical decision-making or total time).

- Automatic population of records may result in documentation that overstates the level of work and intensity of the service provided.
- Failure to override suggested codes when appropriate may be considered an abusive practice.

Example

➤ **A child is evaluated for concern of ear pain and mild fever.** The EHR's coding algorithm selects **99214** on the basis of the physician's documented diagnosis of acute otitis media with fever and prescription drug management, but the physician knows that the child was not very ill and that the acute, uncomplicated problem addressed, in combination with the moderate risk of prescription drug management, supports **99213**, not **99214**.

   Teaching Point: The physician overrides the code suggested by the EHR and instead reports **99213**. Consistent failure to override incorrectly assigned codes may lead to audits and/or a request for refund of amounts paid. It may also cause the physician to appear as a high-cost provider of services, which may affect health plan rankings (as discussed in the Preparing for Negotiation section earlier in this chapter).

When encounter data are used to show performance of quality metrics, it is essential that the data are configured to correctly populate reports of the patients to whom the measure applies and whether there is documentation of the outcome or process of care specified in the measure (eg, all patients aged 3–17 years and the percentage of those patients who received counseling for diet and exercise).

> **For more on compliant electronic health record documentation, see Chapter 5. See also Chapter 20 for information specific to documentation and coding for telemedicine services.**

Encounter Forms and Other Coding Tools

Encounter forms are useful supplements to EHR-based code selection. Encounter forms may be electronic or print. They can also be used to convey codes to a billing office/system when systems are not integrated.

Designing and Reviewing the Encounter Form

The encounter form, whether electronic or printed, should be designed to help physicians and clinical staff quickly find all codes for diagnoses and services common to the practice. An encounter form or superbill should prompt recognition of separately reported services and use of diagnosis codes that most accurately describe the patient presentation.

When developing the encounter form,

- Include all levels of service for each category of E/M services (eg, **99211–99215**, **99221–99223**) and ensure that time is listed for coding based on time. List routine health examination codes by age and new or established patient.
- List procedures (eg, laboratory) to fit your practice's workflow. For example, group codes together in the order of your workflow (eg, visit codes followed by immunization, laboratory, respiratory, and other procedures) to maximize efficiency and your workflow.

● indicates a new code; ▲, revised; #, re-sequenced; ✚, add-on; ★, audiovisual technology; and ◀, synchronous interactive audio.

- The printed encounter form should prompt staff for specific details of a procedure when required for code verification. For example,

   Code **120**_____ Simple repair: body site _____ size _____

- Include the most commonly reported diagnosis codes. Consider grouping diagnosis codes by organ system, and then alphabetically, within the system.
- Leave space on the form to allow the reporting of the specific diagnosis and full *International Classification of Diseases, 10th Revision, Clinical Modification (ICD-10-CM)* codes.

Example

> **J45.2_**   Asthma, mild intermittent
> **J45.3_**   mild persistent
> **J45.4_**   moderate persistent
> **J45.5_**   severe persistent
>   Add fifth character: **0**, uncomplicated; **1**, w/ (acute) exacerbation; **2**, w/ status asthmaticus.

- Include the most frequently used modifiers.
- Leave space on forms to write in any services or diagnoses that are not included.
- Include codes for prolonged and special services. For example,
   99358   Prolonged evaluation and management service before and/or after direct patient care; first hour
   99024   Postoperative follow-up visit, normally included in the surgical package, to indicate that an evaluation and management service was performed during a postoperative period for a reason(s) related to the original procedure
- Develop a separate encounter form for services performed in hospital or other facility settings. Make sure it includes all the services most commonly performed in the hospital setting.

   Access to a coding application or pocket-sized reference card with required elements of MDM and/or time of services also helps promote accurate code selection in facility settings.
- When quality initiatives are dependent on codes reported (eg, codes supporting HEDIS measures), be sure that these codes are clearly indicated on the encounter form, prompted by the EHR, or provided in an easily accessible quick reference.

   Encounter forms and other coding tools should be reviewed periodically and updated at the time of each code set update to ensure that most of, if not all, the services and procedures commonly performed in the practice are included and the codes are accurate.

See Chapter 1 for the timing of updates to code sets (eg, January, April, July, October).

Completing the Encounter Form

Every practice should develop a written policy of the requirements needed to complete a form. Some points that should be part of the policy include

- The encounter form is *not* part of the medical record. Information such as the need for follow-up care, diagnostic tests, or referrals must always be documented in the medical record even if written on the encounter form.
- If you are using a printed form, services must be clearly identified (eg, circle procedure, use check mark). Procedures or diagnoses must be written on a form if they are not preprinted.

The person providing the service (eg, physician, laboratory technologist, medical assistant) should enter procedure codes or document that service on the encounter form to ensure that only the procedures performed are reported. This ensures that only work that has been performed is reported.

Example

> **A physician marks a vaccine and its administration on the encounter form when she orders the administration.** However, the child becomes distraught about the injection, and the accompanying grandmother chooses to have the child's father bring her back for the immunization.

● indicates a new code; ▲, revised; #, re-sequenced; ✚, add-on; ★, audiovisual technology; and ◀, synchronous interactive audio.

If the clinical staff (under supervision of the physician) had been responsible for reporting the service when performed, it would not have been reported.

- The physician is ultimately responsible for the services reported and billed.
- Procedure codes must be linked to the diagnosis codes for the condition(s) or reasons the services were provided. Multiple diagnosis codes may link to one procedure code, when applicable.

Example

➤ **A 7-year-old boy is seen for an established patient preventive E/M service (99393), and evaluation and removal of a splinter of the right foot are performed with a small incision (10120).** The physician reports the following codes:

ICD-10-CM: **Z00.121**, encounter for routine child health examination with abnormal findings (field 21A), and **S90.851A**, superficial foreign body, right foot, initial encounter (field 21B)

CPT: **99393 25** with *ICD-10-CM* pointer A (**Z00.121**) and pointer B (**S90.851A**) in field 24E and **10020** with *ICD-10-CM* pointer B in field 24 E

Teaching Point: If **Z00.121** were linked to code **10120**, the claim line might be rejected or denied because the preventive diagnosis does not support the reason for the procedure.

Modifier **25** is appended to **99393** to indicate the significant and separately identifiable E/M service provided in conjunction with the splinter removal.

See **Figure 1-1** for an example of how the linking of diagnoses to procedures appears on a claim form. An electronic claim form contains the same data in segments of loops 2300 and 2400.

- A billing manager or clerk should add or change a service or diagnosis only with the agreement of the provider of service.
- A system should be instituted to monitor and ensure capture of charges for all the day's patient encounters (eg, cross-reference to the patient check-in records).

Reviewing Assigned Codes

A staff member who understands correct coding and reporting guidelines should always review the assigned codes before the claim is submitted to ensure that all procedures and services are captured and accurate.

For example, the reviewer should look to see that

- An administration code is reported with vaccines and/or injections.
- Payer instructions for reporting National Drug Code codes and units are followed.
- A venipuncture or finger stick is reported with a laboratory test, when applicable. The practice's Clinical Laboratory Improvement Amendments (CLIA) certificate number is included on claims for laboratory services, when required.

> To learn more about requirements for in-office laboratory certification, see the August 2019 *AAP Pediatric Coding Newsletter* article, "What Is CLIA?" (https://doi.org/10.1542/pcco_book184_document002).

- A handling fee is reported when a specimen is prepared and sent to an outside laboratory.
- A modifier is appended when appropriate (eg, modifier **25** for significant, separately identifiable E/M services).
- The office visit is reported by using the correct new or established patient category of service.

> See Chapter 6 for more information on new and established patients.

- The diagnoses reported as primary and secondary are appropriate and are linked to the appropriate services or procedures.
- The documentation to support each service has been completed with required dates and signatures.

Place of Service Codes

The place of service is indicated on each claim by a *place of service code* (often integrated into billing systems without need for manual entry with each charge). The place of service may appear evident when reporting codes for services such as inpatient hospital care, but this is not always the case.

- It is important to report the correct place of service because differences in practice expense in a facility versus a non-facility setting affect physician payment.

Example

➤ **A physician may be paid a lower rate for a procedure performed in a surgical center than for the same procedure performed in a physician's clinic (not hospital based) because the fee schedule takes into account the overhead or practice expense of providing services (eg, procedure room, supplies, clinical staff).**

> If services provided in a facility setting are reported as if provided in a physician's clinic, an overpayment may occur.
>
> Physicians in provider-based practices (ie, those practices owned and operated as a part of a hospital) should be aware that the place of service code is especially important in this setting. Physician and practice expense portions of the patient's charges are often billed separately in provider-based practices.

- The same services provided in a facility-based practice are often costlier than those provided in an independent (physician-owned) practice. Facility fees charged by the provider are often significantly higher than the non-facility fees charged in independent practices.
- The Medicare program created place of service code **19** to define an "off-campus" hospital practice to adopt site-neutral payment for many physician services provided at provider-based practices. The rules and payment modifications have not been universally adopted, but it is important to know how your office is classified to ensure proper billing regardless. When considering purchase by a hospital system, it is important to consider the effect of billing with a different place of service code.
- The increased number of high-deductible health plans has raised awareness of the greater costs to patients when services are rendered in provider-based facilities and has prompted Medicare and some states to take action to reduce the added costs. Practices should be aware of any such restrictions that apply to billing in their locality and under payer contracts or policies.

Other place of service codes that may be commonly reported for pediatric services include **02**, telehealth provided other than in patient's home; **03**, school; **10**, telehealth provided in patient's home; **11**, office; **12**, home; **14**, group home; **20**, urgent care facility; **21**, inpatient hospital; **22**, on campus—outpatient hospital; and **23**, emergency room—hospital.

Place of service codes are further discussed for certain E/M services in chapters dedicated to those sites of service. See a full list of place of service codes at www.cms.gov/Medicare/Coding/place-of-service-codes/Place_of_Service_Code_Set.html.

Submitting Clean Claims

Many states have enacted laws that require prompt payment of clean claims. In general, *clean claims* are those that contain sufficient and correct information for processing without further investigation or development by the payer (definitions may vary by state).

Although clean claims must be paid within a specified time, payer contracts also typically include a timely filing period (eg, within 90 days of the date of service). Claims submitted after the timely filing period may be denied and cannot typically be billed to the patient.

- Submitted claims must be accurate and in accordance with the process outlined in the executed carrier or health plan agreement. Knowing a payer's claim requirements will decrease chances of denied claims.
- Make sure the practice understands payer rules, for example, for billing for nonphysician services incident to a physician's or other QHP's service. Rules may vary by health plan.

> See chapters 7 and 13 for more information on billing for services provided by clinical staff and health care professionals such as nutritionists, clinical psychologists, and social workers.

- Be aware of any updates issued by the carrier that affect billing and claims submission.

Generally, a clean claim should have the following information:

- Practice information (name, address, phone, National Provider Identifier [NPI], group tax ID number, and, if any laboratory tests are reported, CLIA certificate number)
- Patient information (patient name, birth date, policyholder, policy number, patient ID number, address)
- Codes (*CPT, ICD-10-CM,* Healthcare Common Procedure Coding System, place of service), modifiers, and service dates
- Carrier information
- Secondary and, when applicable, tertiary insurance information
- Referring physician name and NPI, if applicable
- Facility name and address, as appropriate

If additional information is necessary to support a service or explain an unusual circumstance (eg, unlisted procedure code, unusual procedure, complicated procedure),

- Use the attachments feature of the electronic claims system, clearinghouse, or other claim attachment procedure as directed by the payer (eg, submission of attachments by online portal).

    Health plans may have specific instructions for submission of claims attachments (eg, inclusion of a unique identifier [2–50 characters] or internal control number linking the claim and attachment).

- If it is necessary, send a hard-copy claim with a cover letter and a narrative report or copy of the appropriate part of the medical record (eg, progress note, procedure note) to facilitate claim processing.
    - Any documentation (eg, coordination of benefits information, letter of medical necessity, clinical reports) should include the patient's name, service date, and policy number on each page in case the papers become separated.
    - Keep a copy of the claim and supporting information for follow-up of payment.
- When filing claims for patients with coordination of benefits, make certain that all required information (ie, primary and secondary insurance information) has been obtained from the patient and claims are filed with the supporting information (eg, explanation of benefits [EOBs] or electronic remittance advice information), according to plan requirements.

Claims should be submitted for payment as soon as possible and before the deadline for timely filing specified in the agreement.

- The optimum time for filing outpatient claims is on the day of or the day following the service but no more than 2 to 3 days from the date of service.
- Codes for services to patients with prolonged hospitalizations may be collected for 7 consecutive days before billing; in this case, claims should be filed within 2 to 3 days of the end of the service week. It is not necessary to withhold claims until the patient is discharged. It is important to know whether your EHR and billing systems limit how data are captured and reported for services that extend over consecutive dates.

> Practices should monitor lag time between completion of each service and submission of a claim for the service to identify and correct any cause of delayed submission. Timely finalization of documentation is necessary to make sure that codes are supported by the documentation before claims are submitted. Many practices adopt policies for timely completion of documentation.

Policy should be adopted requiring completion of medical record documentation within a specified period to support prompt billing of services. Physicians must understand that timely completion of documentation is required for appropriate code selection, claim filing, and, ultimately, prompt payment. New entries or corrections to documentation that occur after claim submissions may affect the accuracy of codes reported.

Special Consideration for Medicare Claims

Many health plans receive Medicare claims automatically when they are the secondary payer. In this case, the explanation of Medicare benefits will indicate that the claim has been automatically crossed over for secondary consideration. Physicians and providers should look for this indication on their EOBs and should not submit a paper claim to the secondary payer.

Monitoring Claim Status

An important aspect of billing operations is prompt and routine claim monitoring. A defined process for verifying that submitted claims were received and accepted by claim clearinghouses and/or payers should be included in the practice's or billing service's written billing procedures. Steps may include (see the last item in this list if billing is outsourced or centralized outside the practice)

- Identify each type of report and/or dashboard feature of the practice's billing system for use in verifying claim submission and acceptance for processing, assigning follow-up activities for unpaid claims, and tracking average time from date of service and/or submission to receipt of payment.
- Assign responsibilities for verifying that electronic claim submissions were received and accepted for processing as soon after transmission as possible. Failure to verify claim acceptance by the clearinghouse and payer often leads to unrecoverable revenue because of timely filing limitations.
  - Most clearinghouses will send a report indicating acceptance or rejection of a batch of claims within minutes of transmission and a report with individual claim-level detail within 24 hours of submission.
  - It is also necessary to log in to a payer's website or system to verify receipt of claims and monitor acceptance or rejection. Errors and omissions may occur in transmission.
- Electronic claim submission reports must be promptly reviewed for rejections or denials. All rejected or denied claims must be investigated to determine what corrections or payer contact is necessary to resubmit or return the claim for re-adjudication (eg, when a payer system error is corrected).
- Claims should not be resubmitted without investigation, as
  - Resubmission of a claim containing errors is unlikely to result in payment.
  - Resubmission of the claim with errors may reset the aging of the claim in the billing system and result in late follow-up or denial for lack of timely filing.

> **Prevent potential denial of corrected claims due to duplicate charges.** A claim frequency code, placed in box 22 of a CMS-1500 form or loop 2300 of an electronic 837 format, is used to indicate that a claim is a corrected (code 7) or voided (code 8) claim. Correcting or voiding a previously submitted claim typically results in either a complete replacement of a previously processed claim or voiding of the original claim from the health plan's record. See specific instructions from the health plan when submitting a corrected claim.

- Identify staff responsible for claims follow-up and establish standards for timely follow-up on unpaid claims. System-generated reports are useful in identifying the age of claims.
- Policies and procedures should address communication with patients and responsible parties when a payer requests additional information before claims processing (eg, many payers will request information on other coverage and/or details of where and how an injury was sustained).

  Failure to respond to payer requests for information in a timely manner can result in delayed or denied claims payment.
- If centralized billing or an outsourced billing service is used, maintain oversight of performance by reviewing reports and taking action on any areas where potentially delayed or lost revenue are indicated. Examples of potential areas of concern include
  - Lag time between completion of documentation and submission of claims
  - Aging reports that show that the average number of days since claim submission for unpaid claims is more than 45 days
  - Amounts adjusted or written off

Monitoring Payments

Develop a process to monitor the timeliness of all payments. Tips for monitoring payments include
- Identify payers who do not pay clean claims within the time frame agreed on in your contract and follow up on all late payments with the payer.
  - Check the provisions of your state prompt pay law and know the provisions for clean claims, timely filing, and penalties.
  - Report a payer's practice of late or delinquent payments to the proper agency because your practice may be entitled to payment plus interest.
- One efficiency of many electronic systems is automatic application of payments and adjustments. However, systems may apply incorrect adjustments based on payer remark codes. Staff should monitor all denials and reduced payments as appropriate and appeal incorrect adjustments when applicable.
- Review each EOB and/or remittance advice (electronic or paper) carefully to determine if the payment is correct.
  - Identify any discrepancies, such as changes to codes, payments (specifically reductions), or denials.
  - Familiarity with standard claim adjustment reason codes and remittance advice remark codes is essential in identifying denial reasons, such as a non-covered service, bundled payment, or provision of service not typical for physician specialty (not relevant for taxonomy code), and any patient responsibility for denied charges.

- — Find claim adjustment reason code and remittance advice remark code descriptions online at https://x12.org/codes.
- — Make certain that any denials or reductions in payment are not due to practice billing errors (eg, incorrect modifiers, obsolete codes) or to incorrect applications of an NCCI edit that does not pertain to pediatrics. If so, correct the errors immediately and educate staff members as appropriate to ensure correct future claim submissions.
- Review all payer explanations, particularly reasons for denials or down-coding. If the service provided is not a benefit covered by the plan, the patient should be billed directly (may need a signed waiver form).
  - — Bill patients only for amounts deemed non-covered or patient responsibility by the payer and only in compliance with the health plan contract.
  - — Do not bill patients for bundled services or other reduced payments due to the contract between your practice and the payer. Renegotiate your contract if payment is lower than costs of providing care.

> Billing staff must be aware of unique payment policies for health plans whose claims are processed by third-party administrators. For example, health plans A and B are employer-sponsored plans administered by insurance company A, but each plan has policies that may differ from those of health plans offered directly by insurance company A.

- If your system does not provide a variance report, compare the EOBs and/or remittance advice to a spreadsheet listing your top 40 codes and their allowable payments by carrier to monitor contract compliance. Make certain that the payment is consistent with the fee schedule, write-offs, and discounts agreed to by the practice and payer. Follow up with the payer on any discrepancies.

  Health plans may enter contracted fee schedules for each physician or provider individually, resulting in inaccurate payment for 1 or more providers in a practice.
- Maintain a log of all denials or payment reductions. This can be used as a basis for future negotiations or education of the payer. (Identify 1 individual who has billing and coding expertise to monitor as well as accept or reject denials.)

> See Chapter 5 for discussion of monitoring electronic and print remittances to verify and track that payments comply with health plan contracts, fee schedule, and state-specific clean claims payment timelines.

- Review your fee schedule to see if your practice is paid at 100% of the billed charges. This is an indication that your fees are below the maximum payment amount established by the carrier. Payers often base the amount paid on the lesser of the billed charge or the contracted fee schedule amount for the service. This excludes services that are always patient responsibility (eg, form fees, cosmetic services).
- Review your fees annually and understand the Medicare RBRVS, using it to value the services you provide, as discussed in the Values Assigned to Physician Services section earlier in this chapter.

> Tracking vaccine acquisition cost is very important. Costs may change during the course of the contract. Review the carrier contract for mid-contract vaccine cost changes (eg, some contracts will default to a percentage of billed charges during vaccine price transitions).

Review your payment to ensure that it exceeds your cost of providing that service (eg, total vaccine costs), including time of clinical staff, supplies, tracking systems, and charges for electronic interfaces. When applicable, any non–fee-for-service income based on provision of recommended services (eg, vaccinations provided by ages specified in Centers for Disease Control and Prevention schedules) may be considered in determining the value of services.

- When contracting with payers, be aware of payment options that may be specified (eg, paper checks, electronic fund transfers, virtual credit card payment). It is important to understand the pros and cons of each (eg, credit card processing fees typically apply to card-based payment). Some health plans no longer offer payment by paper check and recommend electronic fund transfer.
- *Health plans must provide payment in compliance with electronic fund transfer standards of HIPAA rather than virtual card or wire transfer when requested by a physician.* Agreements to accept electronic fund transfers should not allow health plans to debit an account without notification and consent. Banks may offer additional protections against unauthorized withdrawals.

Appealing Denials

Do not assume that the carrier's denials or audits are accurate. Be prepared to challenge the carrier and request the specific policy on which the denial is based. If you are coding correctly and in compliance with coding conventions, you should appeal all inappropriately denied claims and carrier misapplication of *CPT* coding principles.

Knowing when to appeal a payer denial is just as important as knowing how to properly appeal. Writing an effective appeal letter to payers requires knowledge of *CPT* guidelines, CMS policy, and payer policy. The AAP Payer Advocacy Advisory Committee has developed resources to effectively respond to inappropriate claim denials, handle requests for refunds, manage private payer contracts and denials, and respond to payer audits. (See *Prepare Your Office for a Payer Audit Site Visit* at https://downloads.aap.org/AAP/PDF/PrepareYourOfficeforaPayerAuditSiteVisit.pdf.)

The AAP works directly with major insurance payers regarding policies that adversely affect pediatrics and pediatricians. If you receive inappropriate denials, we urge you to appeal them through the individual payer's processes and include documentation and any other coding support, such as information taken directly from the *CPT* or *ICD-10-CM* manuals.

You can alert the AAP to issues with payer policies that prohibit payment for correctly reported services by electronically submitting the Hassle Factor Form to the AAP Coding Hotline (https://form.jotform.com/Subspecialty/aapcodinghotline).

Filing Appeals

Develop a system to monitor payer updates and any changes to the provider agreement so you are aware of the current payment policies and coding edits used by the payer.

> Appealing a claim denial requires confidence that the claim was correctly coded and supported in documentation. Ongoing coding education and internal compliance reviews are necessary to support compliant claim submissions. Learn more about coding compliance in Chapter 5.

- By accepting inappropriate claim denials, a practice may be setting itself up to charges of abusive billing practices. If a practice recodes claims as a result of inappropriate claim denials, the resubmitted claim may not actually reflect the treatment the patient received.

  Here is a summary of basic guidelines and tips for appealing payment determinations.
- When in contact with the payer, always document the date, name, and title of the payer representative with whom you have talked and a summary of the details of the conversation.
  - If a payer requests that you submit a claim by using codes or modifiers that are not consistent with clean coding standards, ask for written documentation of the direction (preferably via fax or email).
  - Address issues with the person who has the authority to make decisions to overturn denials or reductions in payment.
  - Keep an updated file with names and contact information of the appropriate personnel with each of your contracted payers.
  - Request an email or letter verifying the information provided, and archive written correspondence containing payer representative advice and payer policies. If the carrier does not provide written documentation, prepare a summary and send it to your contact, stating that this will constitute the documentation of the discussion.
- Submit all appeals in writing.
  - Understand the payer's appeal process and appeal within its timeliness guidelines.
  - Format the letter to include the name of the patient, policy number, claim control number, and date of service(s) in question on each page of the letter.
  - The body of the letter should state the reason for the appeal and why you disagree with the payer's adjudication of the claim. Speak to the payer's rules/regulations regarding the decision and how your documentation supports payment.
  - Specify a date by which you expect the carrier to respond.
  - Support your case by providing medical justification and referencing *CPT* coding guidelines. If necessary, consult with the AAP Coding Hotline (https://form.jotform.com/Subspecialty/aapcodinghotline) for clarification of correct coding. It may be helpful to hire a certified coding expert with knowledge in pediatric coding to review your claims. (If hiring a full-time certified coding expert is not practical for a small practice, part-time employment or periodic consultation may be an option for access to coding and compliance expertise.)
  - Consider sending correspondence to the carrier by certified mail to verify receipt. Document and retain copies of all communications with the carrier about the appeal.

> Note that some payers have multiple levels of appeal, with many initial appeals denied only because of the payer's electronic claim edits. Higher levels of appeal may be necessary for a denied claim to actually be reconsidered according to specific details about the service provided and the payer's contract or written policy.

- Maintain an appeals-pending file.
  - If there is no response from the payer within 4 weeks of the date of the letter, send a copy of the appeal letter stamped "Second Request."
  - If there is no response within 2 weeks of the second request, or if the matter continues to remain unresolved, contact the state department of insurance (or other appropriate agency in your state) to file a complaint or engage its assistance.
  - Contact your AAP chapter and pediatric council, if your chapter has one, to make them aware of the situation with the payer. American Academy of Pediatrics chapter pediatric councils meet with health plans to discuss carrier policies and practices affecting pediatrics and pediatricians.

Documentation and Coding Audits

Medicare, Medicaid programs, and commercial payers will audit claims as well as monitor coding profiles (especially E/M coding). Physician practices should also adopt standards for conducting internal audits or reviews. Internal audits provide important information to inform practice policy and procedures, detect missed revenue, protect against erroneous billing and poor documentation habits, and prevent issues with payers and outside auditors. Some key benefits of internal auditing are
- Identification of negative billing and revenue trends, including
  - Increased lag time between encounter and billing (eg, delays in finalization of documentation, delayed coding or billing functions, technology issues)
  - Denial or underpayment of new services or new or revised procedure codes
  - Significant unexpected increase or decrease in revenue
  - Inappropriate adjustments or write-offs of unpaid or underpaid claims that should be appealed
- Charge verification (eg, number of charges is equal to or greater than number of encounters, with exception of unbilled visits included in a global period)
- Identification of incorrect billing and coding practices
- Identification of payment that does not align with payer contract
- Identification of electronic system or workflow issues
- Identification of areas where new or additional training is necessary

> See Chapter 5 for more detailed information on conducting internal audits and responding to payer audits.

Tools for the Pediatric Practice

Working with third-party payers on coding and payment issues can be a difficult task because there is little uniformity between carriers and, frequently, great inconsistencies within the same umbrella organization of carriers (eg, differing payment policies for commercial, health exchange, and Medicaid plans). The AAP Payer Advocacy Advisory Committee is charged with enhancing systems for members and chapters to identify and respond to issues with carriers.

The AAP has several available resources to assist the pediatric practice.
- American Academy of Pediatrics staff are available to clarify coding issues. The AAP Coding Hotline can be accessed at https://form.jotform.com/Subspecialty/aapcodinghotline.
- The AAP policy statement, "Guiding Principles for Managed Care Arrangements for the Health Care of Newborns, Infants, Children, Adolescents, and Young Adults" (www.aap.org/en/practice-management/practice-financing/payer-contracting-advocacy-and-other-resources/payer-contract-negotiations-and-payment-resources) provides key principles that are necessary for managed care plans to minimize patient underutilization and overutilization of services, as well as to enhance quality of care for children.
- Members of the AAP are encouraged to use the AAP Coding Hotline to report payer issues. The AAP Coding Hotline form (https://form.jotform.com/Subspecialty/aapcodinghotline) may be completed online to report insurance administrative and claim-processing concerns. The information submitted is used to assist the AAP and chapters in identifying issues and facilitating public and private payer advocacy related to health plans, including discussion topics with national carriers and at chapter pediatric council meetings with regional carriers.

● indicates a new code; ▲, revised; #, re-sequenced; ✦, add-on; ★, audiovisual technology; and ◀, synchronous interactive audio.

- American Academy of Pediatrics members and their staff are encouraged to attend AAP coding webinars (https://coding.aap.org/webinars), presented by pediatric coding experts.
- The *AAP Pediatric Coding Newsletter* provides articles on coding and documentation of specific services and supplies (eg, vaccines) with updates on new codes and emerging issues affecting coding and billing practices. Subscribers can access current and archived issues and coding resources at https://coding.aap.org.

The resources that follow provide a valuable point of reference to help address issues that arise in payer contracting and resolve issues that arise in payment. Use the quiz found at the end of this chapter to assess your understanding of the information presented in it.

Chapter Takeaways

This chapter details information on how professional services are valued, how physicians are paid, and how charges can be captured and clean claims for payment can be reported. Following are some takeaways from this chapter:

- The underlying basis for physician payment is the RBRVS, although alternative payment models focus largely on payment for demonstrating higher quality and lower costs of care.
- Physicians and QHPs should not enter into payer contracts without understanding the terms and negotiating for terms that are fair to the practice and the payer.
- Receipt of appropriate payment depends on correctly capturing charges, assigning correct codes, and submitting clean claims. Monitoring for and appealing of underpayments and denials are also an important part of revenue management.

Resources

AAP Coding Assistance and Education

"2023 RBRVS: What Is It and How Does It Affect Pediatrics?" (www.aap.org/en/practice-management/practice-financing/coding-and-valuation/code-valuation-and-payment-rbrvs)

AAP Coding Hotline (https://form.jotform.com/Subspecialty/aapcodinghotline)

AAP coding webinars (https://coding.aap.org/webinars)

AAP payer contract negotiations and payment resources (www.aap.org/en/practice-management/practice-financing/payer-contracting-advocacy-and-other-resources/payer-contract-negotiations-and-payment-resources)

AAP "Payment for Child Health Services" (www.aap.org/en/practice-management/practice-financing)

AAP pediatric councils (www.aap.org/en/practice-management/practice-financing/payer-contracting-advocacy-and-other-resources/aap-payer-advocacy/aap-pediatric-councils)

AAP *Pediatric Office Superbill* (https://shop.aap.org/pediatric-office-superbill-2023)

AAP *Prepare Your Office for a Payer Audit Site Visit* (https://downloads.aap.org/AAP/PDF/PrepareYourOfficeforaPayerAuditSiteVisit.pdf)

AAP "Value-Based and Other Alternative Payment Models" (www.aap.org/en/practice-management/practice-financing/value-based-and-other-alternative-payment-models)

"Accountable Care Organizations (ACOs) and Pediatricians: Evaluation and Engagement," *AAP News* (https://publications.aap.org/aapnews/article/32/1/1/8943)

"PPAAC: Chapter Pediatric Councils Work With Payers on Medical Home Programs," *AAP News* (https://publications.aap.org/aapnews/news/13007)

RBRVS Conversion Spreadsheet (https://downloads.aap.org/AAP/Excel/2022%20RBRVS%20Conversion%20Spreadsheet.xls; download required)

AAP Pediatric Coding Newsletter™

"Codes Assigned by Payers: CARCs and RARCs," July 2019 (https://doi.org/10.1542/pcco_book183_document002)

"Coding Compliance: Conducting Internal Audits"; "Planning Chart Audits"; and "Audit Tools: What You Need to Perform and Document Chart Audits," February 2019 (https://publications.aap.org/codingnews/issue/14/5)

"What Is CLIA?" August 2019 (https://doi.org/10.1542/pcco_book184_document002)

Claims Processing

Remittance advice remark codes (https://x12.org/codes/remittance-advice-remark-codes)

Health Insurance

Health insurance education resources from HealthyChildren.org (www.healthychildren.org/English/family-life/health-management/health-insurance/Pages/default.aspx)

Payment/Relative Value Units

AAP policy statement, "Application of the Resource-Based Relative Value Scale System to Pediatrics" (https://doi.org/10.1542/peds.2014-0866)

AAP policy statement, "Guiding Principles for Managed Care Arrangements for the Health Care of Newborns, Infants, Children, Adolescents, and Young Adults" (https://doi.org/10.1542/peds.2013-2655)

Health Care Cost Institute "Comparing Commercial and Medicare Professional Service Prices" (https://healthcostinstitute.org/hcci-research/comparing-commercial-and-medicare-professional-service-prices)

"Understanding the RUC Survey Instrument: Physician Services without Global Period" video (www.youtube.com/watch?v=nu5unDX8VIs)

Place of Service Codes

Place of service code set (www.cms.gov/Medicare/Coding/place-of-service-codes/Place_of_Service_Code_Set.html)

Value-Based Payment

"Accountable Care Organizations (ACOs): General Information" (https://innovation.cms.gov/innovation-models/aco)
"Pediatric Accountable Care Organizations: Insight From Early Adopters," *Pediatrics* (https://doi.org/10.1542/peds.2016-1840)

● indicates a new code; ▲, revised; #, re-sequenced; ✚, add-on; ★, audiovisual technology; and ◀, synchronous interactive audio.

Test Your Knowledge!

1. **Which of the following statements is true of the Medicare Physician Fee Schedule (MPFS)?**
   a. The MPFS is not connected to most fee schedules applicable to pediatric services.
   b. All commercial payers base payment on the current year's MPFS.
   c. The same payment rate is applied regardless of the location where services are provided.
   d. Each relative value unit component may be independently adjusted slightly upward or downward as a function of geographic area.

2. **Which of the following activities does the American Academy of Pediatrics chapter pediatric councils do?**
   a. Negotiating health plan contracts for individual practices
   b. Developing practice fee schedules
   c. Discussing physician fee schedules
   d. Meeting with payers to discuss pediatric issues

3. **How is the place where a service was provided reported on a claim?**
   a. The procedure code always identifies the place of service.
   b. A 2-digit place of service code is entered on the claim.
   c. A modifier identifies the place of service.
   d. The place of service is not necessary on a claim.

4. **Which of the following benefits results from conducting internal audits or reviews?**
   a. Practice policy and procedures are informed.
   b. Missed revenue is detected.
   c. Issues with payers and outside auditors are prevented through early detection of internal errors.
   d. All of the above.

5. **Which of the following terms refers to the patients a payer includes on your panel roster?**
   a. *Attribution*
   b. *Engagement*
   c. *Assignment*
   d. *Active patient list*

● indicates a new code; ▲, revised; #, re-sequenced; ✚, add-on; ★, audiovisual technology; and ◀, synchronous interactive audio.

Preventing Fraud and Abuse:
Compliance, Audits, and Paybacks

This chapter was contributed by the American Academy of Pediatrics Committee on Medical Liability and Risk Management.

CPT copyright 2022 American Medical Association. All rights reserved.

Contents

● indicates a new code; ▲, revised; #, re-sequenced; ✚, add-on; ★, audiovisual technology; and ◀, synchronous interactive audio.

Chapter Highlights

- Learn the importance of safeguarding the health care system from fraud and abuse.
- Learn how compliance programs can protect medical practices from unintentional billing errors.
- Prepare for responding to overpayment notices and inquiries from auditors.

The Importance of Compliance in Medical Practice

Although most physicians work ethically, provide high-quality care, and submit appropriate claims for payment, unfortunately, there are some providers who exploit the health care system for personal gain. These few have necessitated an array of laws to combat fraud and abuse and protect the integrity of the health care payment system.

Just as patients put enormous trust in physicians, so do payers. Medicare, Medicaid, other federal health care programs, and private payers rely on physicians' medical judgment to treat patients with appropriate services. They depend on physicians to submit accurate and truthful claims for the services provided to their enrollees. And most physicians intend to do just that. However, the process is made more difficult by the complex and dynamic nature of payer coding and billing procedures, which, despite efforts to standardize variations, persist from carrier to carrier, policy to policy, state to state, and month to month.

Defining Medical Fraud and Abuse

The federal government has more than a dozen laws in its anti-fraud and anti-abuse arsenal. The 5 most important laws that apply to physicians are the

- False Claims Act: Prohibits and establishes penalties for submitting claims for payment to Medicare or Medicaid that you know *or should know* are false or fraudulent.
- Anti-Kickback Statute: Prohibits the knowledge and willful payment/acceptance of anything of value (eg, money, trips) intended to induce or reward patient referrals or the generation of business involving any item or service payable by the federal health care program.

Anti-kickback Liability

The Anti-Kickback Statute, by its terms, ascribes criminal liability to all parties to an impermissible kickback transaction (ie, those who solicit or receive prohibited remuneration and those who offer or pay the prohibited remuneration).

- Physician Self-Referral Law (Stark law): Prohibits physicians from referring patients to receive designated health services (DHS) payable by Medicare or Medicaid from entities with which the physician or an immediate family member has a financial relationship, unless an exception applies. The following items or services are DHS:
  - Clinical laboratory services
  - Physical therapy services
  - Occupational therapy services
  - Outpatient speech pathology services
  - Radiology and certain other imaging services
  - Radiation therapy services and supplies
  - Durable medical equipment and supplies
  - Parenteral and enteral nutrients, equipment, and supplies
  - Prosthetics, orthotics, and prosthetic devices and supplies
  - Home health services
  - Outpatient prescription drugs
  - Inpatient and outpatient hospital services
- Exclusion Authorities: Prohibits billing a federal health program (eg, Medicaid, Tricare) for any services furnished, ordered, or prescribed by an excluded individual. Physicians are also responsible for ensuring that they do not employ or contract with excluded individuals or entities who may furnish items or services that may be paid for by a federal health care program.

- Civil Monetary Penalties Law: Authorizes the US Department of Health and Human Services (HHS) to impose civil money penalties and/or exclude from the Medicare and Medicaid programs physicians who commit various forms of fraud and abuse involving Medicare and Medicaid (eg, anti-kickback violations, false claims, or submission of false information on enrollment in a federal health program).

Abiding by these laws is not just the right thing to do; violating them, even (for some) unwittingly, could result in criminal penalties, civil fines, exclusion from federal health care programs, or loss of a medical license from a state medical board. It all begins with understanding the definition of *fraud and abuse* in health care.

Fraud

Fraud is obtaining something of value through intentional misrepresentation or concealment of material facts. Examples of fraud in the physician's office may include

- Requiring that a patient return for a procedure that could have been performed on the same day
- Billing Medicare or Medicaid for services not provided, including no-shows
- Billing one member for services provided to another (non-covered) member
- Billing services under a different National Provider Identifier (NPI) (except as allowed by payer guidance) to receive payment for services that would otherwise be non-covered or paid at a lesser rate
- Taking a kickback in money, in-kind, or other valuable compensation for referrals
- Completing a certificate of medical necessity for a patient who does not need the service or who is not professionally known by the provider

Abuse

Abuse includes any practice that is not consistent with the goals of providing patients with services that

- Are medically necessary
- Meet professionally recognized standards
- Are fairly priced

Examples of actions that will likely be considered abusive are

- Charging in excess for services or supplies
- Billing Medicare or Medicaid on the basis of a higher fee schedule than for other patients
- Providing medically unnecessary services
- Submitting bills to Medicare or Medicaid that are the responsibility of another insurance plan
- Waiving co-payments or deductibles (except as permitted for financial hardship)
- Advertising for free services
- Coding all visits at the same level
- Unbundling claims (ie, billing separately for services that are correctly billed under 1 code)

Kickbacks, Inducements, and Self-referrals

The Centers for Medicare & Medicaid Services (CMS) advises providers to be cautious when investing in health care business ventures. Providers may invest in third parties, such as laboratories, imaging centers, equipment vendors, or physical therapy clinics, to expand patient care access. However, referral patterns to these facilities could implicate a provider in an investigation.

The CMS states that "these business relationships can sometimes improperly influence or distort physician decision-making and result in the improper steering of a patient to a particular therapy or source of services in which a physician has a financial interest" (see the Medicare Learning Network booklet, *Medicare Fraud & Abuse: Prevent, Detect, Report,* at www.cms.gov/Outreach-and-Education/Medicare-Learning-Network-MLN/MLNProducts/Downloads/Fraud-Abuse-MLN4649244.pdf). Many of these investment relationships have serious legal risks under the Anti-Kickback Statute and Stark law, according to the CMS.

To prevent allegations of possible illegal kickback schemes with investment partners, the CMS recommends that providers ask the following questions:

- Is the investment venture promising the provider high rates of return for little or no financial risk?
- Is the investment interest for a nominal capital contribution?
- Is the partner asking the provider to guarantee patient referrals or item orders?
- Does the provider believe they will be more likely to refer patients for services provided by the venture just because they made the investment?
- Will the provider's ownership share be greater than their share of the total capital contributions made to the venture?

● indicates a new code; ▲, revised; #, re-sequenced; ✚, add-on; ★, audiovisual technology; and ◀, synchronous interactive audio.

- Is the investment venture, or any possible business partner, offering to loan the provider money to make their capital contribution?
- Will the venture have enough capital from other sources to fund its operations?

Whenever health care vendors offer free samples, business opportunities, and incentives, providers should ask themselves similar questions.

When considering whether to engage in a particular billing practice, enter into a particular business venture, or pursue an employment, a consulting, or another personal services relationship, it is prudent to evaluate the arrangement for potential compliance problems. Use experienced health care lawyers to analyze the issues and provide a legal evaluation and risk analysis of the proposed venture, relationship, or arrangement.

> The state bar association may have a directory of local attorneys who practice in the health care field. The American Health Law Association is another resource (www.americanhealthlaw.org).

Anti-fraud and Anti-abuse Activities

Physician practices are subject to several levels of scrutiny for possible fraudulent activity, including the federal and state levels of government as well as private payers. Increasingly, these groups are sharing information. This means that a provider under investigation by one government health care program will likely be contacted by another program and possibly by private payers.

- The HHS Office of Inspector General (OIG) has several anti-fraud campaigns underway.
- Many states have enacted anti-fraud and anti-abuse legislation, and Medicaid programs have established Medicaid fraud control units.
- The Medicaid program integrity provisions include activities such as
  - Increased fraud detection methods
  - Terminating providers previously terminated from other government health care programs
  - Suspending future payments on the basis of credible allegations of fraud
  - Adopting the National Correct Coding Initiative (NCCI) edits

> See Chapter 2 for more information on National Correct Coding Initiative edits.

The Medicaid Recovery Audit Contractors (RAC) program allows states to hire private contractors to audit Medicaid payments and keep a percentage of what they collect. Because it is Medicaid, pediatricians may be included in RAC audits. With the increase of Medicaid managed care plans that have their own program integrity systems, some states are now excluded from the requirement to use RAC auditors.

Areas of Specific Concern

Many findings and initiatives put physician practices under high scrutiny for miscoded services, failure to adequately document services, and operating in a manner that conflicts with anti-kickback and self-referral laws. Following are examples of audit and evaluation findings:

- Specific areas of concern that affect physicians include billing for a higher level of service than was provided, appropriate billing for telemedicine and other indirect services, and physician self-referral violations.
- Misuse of modifiers to override NCCI edits when not clinically indicated.
- Several cases in recent years involved inappropriate payments or other incentives paid by laboratory companies to physicians for sending business to their laboratories.
- The HHS OIG has published concerns regarding physicians and other qualified health care professionals who participate in speaker programs that potentially pay for increased prescribing, ordering, or use of a company's products that will be billed to a government payer (https://oig.hhs.gov/documents/special-fraud-alerts/865/SpecialFraudAlertSpeakerPrograms.pdf).
- Analysis of claim data is increasingly combined across payers and care settings to identify physicians and other providers who are outliers in their billing and referral patterns to identify potential fraud and abuse.

The fraud and abuse control units of HHS and the US Department of Justice also continue to cross-reference enrollment information for the physicians and providers when there is history of enrollment in multiple states and/or programs. By cross-referencing enrollment data, conflicting information and/or evidence of prior revocation of eligibility to participate in federal programs may be discovered.

Chapter 5. Preventing Fraud and Abuse: Compliance, Audits, and Paybacks

Compliance Programs

Does your practice have a fraud and abuse prevention compliance program? For many years, compliance programs for small practices were voluntary. This is no longer the case; they are now required, even for small practices, but they can be scalable.

A compliance program establishes strategies to prevent, detect, and resolve conduct that does not conform to

- Federal and state law
- Federal, state, and private payer health care program requirements
- The practice's own ethical and business policies

Pediatric practices benefit from having compliance initiatives because they tighten billing and coding operations and documentation. Practices with written compliance programs report having better control on internal procedures, improved medical record documentation, and streamlined practice operations.

Section 6401(a) of the Patient Protection and Affordable Care Act requires physicians and other providers and suppliers who enroll in Medicare, Medicaid, or the Children's Health Insurance Program to establish a compliance program with certain "core elements."

The 7 Elements of the Office of Inspector General (OIG) Compliance Program

The 7 core elements described in the OIG guidance for compliance programs for small physician practices published in 2000 are

- Conduct internal monitoring and auditing.
- Implement written compliance and practice standards.
- Designate a compliance officer, contact, or committee.
- Conduct appropriate training and education.
- Respond appropriately to detected offenses and develop corrective action.
- Develop open lines of communication.
- Enforce disciplinary standards through well-publicized guidelines.

It is also useful to consult the *United States Sentencing Commission Guidelines Manual,* which makes it clear that an organization under investigation may be given more sympathetic treatment if a good compliance program is in place. Compliance programs not only help prevent fraudulent or erroneous claims but also show that the physician practice is making a good-faith effort to submit claims appropriately. However, that would require the program to be integrated into the daily operations of the practice. It cannot be a set of policies and procedures merely kept in a binder or on a computer unrelated to actual business operations.

Here are some reasons cited by the *United States Sentencing Commission Guidelines Manual* to implement an effective compliance program.

- It may save the practice money if it prevents costly civil suits and criminal investigations.
- It sends an unambiguous message to employees that fraud and abuse will not be tolerated.
- It decreases the risk of employees suing the practice under the False Claims Act because employees will have an internal communication system for reporting questionable activities and resolving problems.
- It helps if an investigation occurs. Investigators may be more inclined to resolve the problem as a civil rather than a criminal matter, or it may lead to an administrative resolution rather than a formal false claim action.
- It may help reduce the range used for imposing fines under federal sentencing guidelines.
- It may influence an OIG decision on whether to exclude a provider from participation in federal health care programs.
- It frequently results in improved medical record documentation.
- It improves coding accuracy, reduces denials, and makes claims and payment processes more effective.
- It educates physicians and employees on their responsibilities for preventing, detecting, and reporting fraud and abuse.
- It should meet governmental requirements for practices to have a formal compliance plan.

Steps to Developing a Compliance Program

The CMS has described the steps to create an effective compliance and ethics program. A key aspect is that the organization exercises due diligence to prevent and detect criminal conduct and promotes a culture that encourages ethical conduct and a commitment to compliance with the law.

The CMS specifies that in creating the compliance program, the practice

1. Develop and distribute written policies, procedures, and standards of conduct to prevent and detect inappropriate behavior.

2. Designate a chief compliance officer and other appropriate bodies (eg, a corporate compliance committee) charged with the responsibility of operating and monitoring the compliance program and who report directly to high-level personnel and the governing body.
3. Use reasonable efforts not to include any individual in the substantial authority personnel whom the organization knew, or should have known, has engaged in illegal activities or other conduct inconsistent with an effective compliance and ethics program.
4. Develop and implement regular, effective education and training programs for the governing body; all employees, including high-level personnel; and, as appropriate, the organization's agents.
5. Maintain a process, such as a hotline, to receive complaints and adopt procedures to protect the anonymity of complainants and protect whistleblowers from retaliation. (In a small practice, a hotline could be replaced with an "anonymous fraud report box.")
6. Develop a system to respond to allegations of improper conduct and enforce appropriate disciplinary action against employees who have violated internal compliance policies, applicable statutes, regulations, or federal health care program requirements.
7. Use audits and/or other evaluation techniques to monitor compliance and assist in the reduction of identified problem areas.
8. Investigate and remediate identified systemic problems, including making any necessary modifications to the organization's compliance and ethics program.

Written Policies and Procedures

A compliance program should have written compliance standards and procedures that the practice follows. They should specifically describe the lines of responsibility for implementing the compliance program.
- Standards and procedures should reduce the likelihood of fraudulent activity while also helping identify any incorrect billing practices.
- Policies and procedures should be updated periodically to address newly identified areas of risk, new regulations, or process changes in the practice.
- All staff should receive periodic education on policies and procedures to maintain up-to-date knowledge.

Coding and Billing

The following billing risk areas have been frequent areas of investigations and audits by the OIG and should be addressed in a good compliance program:
- Billing for items or services not provided or not provided as claimed
- Submitting claims for equipment, medical supplies, and services that are not reasonable and necessary
- Double billing or billing separately for bundled services
- Billing for non-covered services as if covered
- Known misuse of NPIs, which results in improper billing
- Misuse of modifiers
- Consistently under- or over-coding services (eg, using only 1 evaluation and management [E/M] service code within a category of service)

  Other areas that may trigger an audit include
- Profile of services reported differs from payer profiles of physicians of your specialty whose patient population has similar health care comorbidities.
- Repeated inappropriate use of unspecified diagnosis codes or use of codes that are not consistent with the service or your specialty.
- Surgical services not consistent with claims submitted by a facility.
- Number of procedures or services reported exceeds the hours in a day.
- High numbers of denials.

Medical Record Documentation

One of the most important physician practice compliance issues is the appropriate documentation of diagnosis and treatment. Patients and other providers must be able to trust that information within shared records is accurate and actionable for the care of the patient.

  Compliant documentation must encompass not only what should be documented but also what must be safeguarded from inaccuracies and potential noncompliant access to or disclosure of information.

●, indicates a new code; ▲, revised; #, re-sequenced; ✚, add-on; ★, audiovisual technology; and ◀, synchronous interactive audio.

The CMS has published guidance for physicians on detecting and responding to fraud, waste, and abuse associated with the use of electronic health records (EHRs) (www.cms.gov/Medicare-Medicaid-Coordination/Fraud-Prevention/Medicaid-Integrity-Education/documentation-matters.html). The CMS instructs that physicians should apply the compliance program components previously discussed to take preventive action to deter the inappropriate use of EHR system features or inappropriate access to patient information. This includes a written compliance plan.

The written compliance plan should specify that medical record documentation should comply with the following documentation principles and guidelines:

- The medical record should be complete (and legible, when handwritten) and individualized for each patient encounter.
  - Do not allow cut-and-paste functionality in the EHR. Any use of copy and paste, copy forward, macros, or auto-population should be regulated by office policies that address maintenance of record integrity and supplementation via free text, where indicated.
  - Guidance from the CMS includes a decision table for ensuring proper use of EHR features and capabilities.
- Retain all signatures when there are multiple authors or contributors to a document so individual contributions are unambiguously identified. For additional information about documentation by multiple authors, see the "Coding Conundrum: Pitfalls of Electronic Health Record Coding" box later in this chapter.
- All staff should receive initial and periodic education on compliant medical record documentation, including, as applicable, use of EHR functionality, use of individual sign-on, and appropriate access to records. See the March 2019 *AAP Pediatric Coding Newsletter* article, "Coding Compliance Education: Standards and Procedures" (https://doi.org/10.1542/pcco_book179_document002) for more information on developing a compliance education program.
- Documentation should be completed at the time of service or as soon as possible afterward.

Coding Conundrum: Pitfalls of Electronic Health Record Coding

One advantage to using electronic health records (EHRs) is enhanced documentation of services. Documentation of an evaluation and management (E/M) service may be easier because of the use of templates or drop-down options, and legibility is not an issue. However, there are disadvantages to documenting in an EHR. When completing an audit, be aware of the following pitfalls:

- Templates may not accurately describe pertinent patient history or abnormal findings on examination. Some EHRs do not allow free texting, thereby prohibiting more detailed, appropriate documentation. If a system does not allow free texting, work with the vendor to add this capability, or add any and all abnormal findings that might be pertinent in the template so documentation can be complete and accurate.
- Avoid templates and documentation tools that feature predefined text that may include information not relevant to the patient presentation and/or services rendered. Review and edit all defaulted data to ensure that only patient-specific data are recorded for that visit, while removing all other irrelevant data pulled in by the default template.
- Become familiar with the way the EHR constructs a note from the data entered into each field and how the system may be customized to enhance the final note.
- Include only the problems that are evaluated and managed in determining the level of medical decision-making (MDM). However, diagnostic tests and treatment options that are considered but not selected after discussion with the patient/caregiver *do count* toward amount and/or complexity of data to be reviewed and analyzed or the risk of management that contributes to the level of MDM. Therefore, physicians should document those options considered and discussed but not selected.
- The EHR usually captures all documentation, whether performed by ancillary staff or the provider. Make certain it is clear who documented each portion of a service. For example, if history is documented by a nurse or medical assistant, the physician must document agreement and any additional relevant history. (Electronic health record systems include audit trails that may be used to prove who entered specific elements of documentation. It is important to understand how the practice's EHR system creates and produces an audit trail.)
- Scribes are not providers of items or services. When a scribe documents an encounter, the Centers for Medicare & Medicaid Services does not require the scribe to sign/date the documentation. The treating physician's or qualified health care professional's (QHP's) signature on a note indicates that the physician/QHP affirms that the note adequately documents the care provided. Private payers may have different documentation requirements.
- Review any information that is automatically carried forward by an EHR (eg, previous problems, medication lists) to verify it is still accurate, and document the review of the pertinent information.
- List the primary diagnosis first because the EHR should report the diagnoses in the order in which they are documented.
- To support management options, it may be necessary to document the diagnoses being considered. These suspected or ruled-out diagnoses should not be reported by the EHR system in the outpatient setting.
- Make certain that any separately reportable procedure or service has documentation to support that it was performed.
- *Each physician or QHP should document* their total time and the problems and activities that support the necessity of time spent providing an E/M service. (This documentation is especially important in facility settings where split or shared E/M services may be provided.)
- Do not depend on the software vendor to add codes to the system. Review all new, deleted, and revised codes with each code set update. Notify the vendor if codes have not been revised, and educate physicians and staff on the appropriate use of codes.

- The documentation of each patient encounter should include the reason for the encounter; any relevant history; physical examination findings; prior diagnostic test results, when pertinent; assessment, clinical impression, or diagnosis; plan of care; and date and legible identity of the observer.
- If not documented, the rationale for ordering diagnostic and other ancillary services should be easily inferred by an independent reviewer or third party.
- Past and present diagnoses and history should be accessible to the treating and/or consulting physician.
- Appropriate health risk factors should be identified. The patient's progress, their response to and any changes in treatment, and any revision in diagnosis should be documented.
- All pages in the medical record should include the patient's name and an identifying number or birth date.
- Prescription drug management should include the name of the medication, dosage, and instructions.
- A diagnosis code may be assigned for any documented social determinant of health. It should be explicitly documented when a social determinant of health increases the risk of patient treatment of an E/M service.
- Clinically important telephone calls should be documented, including date, time, instructions, patient/parent understanding of and agreement with those instructions, and plan for follow-up.
- Anticipatory guidance, patient education, and counseling are best documented when performed.
- Any addenda should be identifiable with the author's signature and labeled with the date the addendum was made. The compliance plan should address what circumstances justify making changes to the EHR and identify who can make changes, requirements for amendments and corrections to an EHR, and what information cannot be changed (ie, author, date, and time of original note).
- Consent forms should be dated; the procedure, documented; and the form, signed by the patient or their legal representative. Documentation should include a summary of the discussion of the procedure and risks.
- All abbreviations used should be explicit.
- Patient nonadherence, including immunization refusal, should be documented, as well as discussion of the risks and adverse consequences of nonadherence.

> **The American Academy of Pediatrics offers templates in English and Spanish for creating a form to document refusal to vaccinate at https://downloads.aap.org/DOPCSP/SOID_RTV_form_01-2019_English.pdf and https://downloads.aap.org/DOPCSP/SOID_RTV_form_01-2019_Spanish.pdf.**

- Allergies and adverse reactions should be prominently displayed.
- Immunization and growth charts must be maintained and current.
- Problem and medication lists should be completed and current, including over-the-counter medications.
- The EHR audit log should always be enabled to ensure it creates an accurate chronological history of changes to the EHR. Practice procedures should describe any exceptions, including who can disable the log and under what circumstances this may be appropriate.

Retention of Records

Policies and procedures should be written to include the creation, distribution, retention, and destruction of documents. In designing a record-retention system, privacy concerns and federal and state regulatory requirements should be taken into consideration. In addition to maintaining appropriate and thorough medical records on each patient, the OIG recommends that the system include the following types of documents:

- All records and documentation (eg, billing and claims documentation) required for participation in federal, state, and private-payer health care programs
- All records necessary to demonstrate the integrity of the physician practice's compliance process and to confirm the effectiveness of the program

The following record-retention guidelines should be used:

- The length of time that a physician's medical record documentation is to be retained should be specified. Federal and state statutes should be consulted for specific time frames. In the event of a disparity between federal and state statutes, it is advisable to select the longer retention period.
- Consulting with an attorney or risk management department of a medical liability insurer is prudent to determine the appropriate retention period.
  - At a minimum, pediatricians may want to retain records until patients obtain the age of majority plus the statute of limitations in their jurisdiction.
  - Longer retention periods may be prudent, depending on the circumstances.

Chapter 5. Preventing Fraud and Abuse: Compliance, Audits, and Paybacks

- Medical records, including electronic correspondence, should be secured against loss, destruction, unauthorized access, unauthorized reproduction, corruption, and damage.
- Policies and procedures should stipulate the disposition of medical records in the event the practice is sold or closed.

Document Advice From Payers

A physician practice should document its efforts to comply with applicable federal, state, and private health care program requirements. For example,

- When requesting advice from a government agency charged with administering a federal or state health care program or from a private payer, document and retain a record of the request and of all written or oral responses.
- Maintain a log of oral inquiries between the practice and third parties.
- Keep copies of all provider manuals, provider bulletins, and communications from payers about coding and submission of claims.

Designate a Compliance Officer

To administer the compliance program, the practice should designate an individual responsible for overseeing the program. More than one employee may be designated with the responsibility of compliance monitoring, or a practice may outsource all or part of the functions of a compliance officer to a third party. Attributes and qualifications of a compliance officer include

- Independent position to protect against any conflicts of interest from "regular" position responsibilities and compliance officer duties
- Attention to detail
- Experience in billing and coding
- Effective communication skills (oral and written) with employees, physicians, and carriers

The primary responsibilities of a compliance officer include

- Overseeing and monitoring the implementation of the compliance program.
- Establishing methods, such as periodic audits, to improve the practice's efficiency and quality of services and reduce the practice's vulnerability to fraud and abuse.
- Revising the compliance program in response to changes in the needs of the practice or changes in the law and in the policies and procedures of government and private payer health plans.
- Developing, coordinating, and participating in a training program that focuses on the elements of the compliance program and seeks to ensure that training materials are appropriate.
- Checking the HHS OIG Excluded Individuals and Entities List (https://exclusions.oig.hhs.gov) and the federal System for Award Management (https://sam.gov/content/exclusions) to ascertain that any potential new hires, current employees, medical staff, or independent contractors are not listed; advising management of findings; and seeing that appropriate action is taken as described in the compliance program.
- Informing employees and physicians of pertinent federal and state statutes, regulations, and standards and monitoring their compliance.
- Investigating any report or allegation concerning suspected unethical or improper business practices and monitoring subsequent corrective action, compliance, or both.
- Assessing the practice's situation and determining what best suits the practice in terms of compliance oversight.
- Maintaining records of compliance-related activities, including meetings, educational activities, and internal audits. Particular attention should be given to documenting violations found by the compliance program and documenting the remedial actions.

Coding Compliance Information Sources

A compliance program should train all employees to seek an authoritative source (eg, *Current Procedural Terminology* instructions, Medicaid National Correct Coding Initiative manual) for coding guidance. Information obtained from coding discussion forums, webinars, conferences, and, especially, medical product vendors should be verified against authoritative sources.

Additionally, payment policies established by health plans vary, and one plan's policy does not necessarily apply to charges billed to other plans.

The Audit/Review Process

1. Obtain and review a productivity report from your billing system.
2. Calculate the percentage distribution of E/M codes within each category of service (new and established office or outpatient visits, initial inpatient or observation services, use of modifier **25**) for each physician in the practice. (Most billing software provides these calculations.)
3. Use data from a 12-month period to include seasonal trends and better reflect practice patterns.
4. Perform a comparative analysis of the distribution with each physician in the practice. Remember that data only reflect the billing patterns and not if one is more correct than another. More frequent oversight and monitoring is necessary for services provided by physicians who are new to the practice and may use documentation or coding guidance that conflicts with practice policy.
5. Review the report to ensure that all procedures performed are being captured and reported appropriately. For example, are discharge visits (**99238** and **99239**) being billed and is the number proportionate to the number of newborn and other hospital admissions performed?
6. Review the practice encounter form or code selection application to ensure that *Current Procedural Terminology* (*CPT*®), Healthcare Common Procedure Coding System (HCPCS), and *International Classification of Diseases, 10th Revision, Clinical Modification* (*ICD-10-CM*) codes are correct and match the corresponding description.
7. Review the actual encounter and claim form with the medical record to ensure that the claim is submitted with the appropriate codes and/or modifiers. (See the Documentation and Coding Audits section later in this chapter.)
8. Review each medical record and encounter form (as applicable) with the following questions in mind:
   - Are the patient's name, identification number, and/or date of birth on every page in the medical record?
   - Does the medical record contain updated demographic information?
   - Are allergies noted and prominently displayed?
   - Is the date of service documented?
   - Was the service medically necessary?
   - Are all the services and/or procedures documented/captured on the encounter form?
   - Does the documentation support the procedure billed (eg, level and type of E/M service, administration of injection, catheterization, impacted cerumen removal)?
   - Does the documentation for the preventive medicine visit meet the requirements of the Medicaid Early and Periodic Screening, Diagnostic, and Treatment program when applicable?
   - Does the documentation support the diagnosis code(s) billed? Were diagnosis codes assigned for all conditions that required or affected management or treatment?
   - If using an EHR, does the documentation support physician review and personal documentation? For example, if the EHR always brings up the patient's history, is there a notation that the physician reviewed and, when indicated, updated the information? If not, it should not be counted as part of the service.
   - Is there a completed growth chart and immunization record?
   - Is handwritten documentation legible?
   - Does any order for medication include the specific dosage and use?
   - Is there documentation of a follow-up plan?
   - Are diagnostic reports (eg, laboratory tests, radiograph) signed and dated to reflect review?
   - Does documentation include the name and credentials of each contributing author in a manner that reflects each author's individual contributions?
   - Was an appropriate modifier reported with sufficient documentation?
   - Is the documentation in compliance with Physicians at Teaching Hospitals guidelines and/or incident-to provisions as appropriate?

Documentation and Coding Audits

Medicare, Medicaid programs, and commercial payers will audit claims as well as monitor E/M coding profiles. While the specialty-specific E/M profiles published by the CMS provide helpful information, keep in mind that these distributions reflect only code use and not code accuracy. An atypical code distribution may be the result of care for a more complex patient population than average (eg, patients with chronic diseases or with social and economic challenges). Correct coding appropriately identifies the risk stratification for your patients and may directly affect your payments.

Also, just because you got paid does not mean that payers will not retrospectively audit and demand repayment or withhold future payments, particularly if claims were processed incorrectly or in error according to your contract. Practices are advised to become familiar with state laws addressing retrospective audits and repayments and with payer procedures for repayment. Your American Academy of Pediatrics (AAP) chapter or state medical society may be able to help you understand your state-specific laws.

Chapter 5. Preventing Fraud and Abuse: Compliance, Audits, and Paybacks

Preparing for the Audit

Before using documentation and coding audits to reduce the practice's vulnerability to fraud and abuse, it is important to consider how your practice can best conduct and use findings of an internal audit. Individual practices must consider how to conduct audits in a manner that offers the most benefit and least disruption to the practice. **Figure 5-1** offers steps to consider when developing a medical record audit process.

Performing the Audit

Make certain that the reviewer has all appropriate and necessary tools, which may include

- Current *CPT, ICD-10-CM,* and HCPCS manuals.
- Access to or copies of all payer newsletters or information bulletins that outline coding and/or payment policies (may require access to a payer's provider portal).
- An audit worksheet. This may be one designed by your practice or one of many published templates. Be certain the audit form includes appropriate requirements for E/M code selection. The CMS does not endorse a specific audit form or coding template.

> Electronic audit programs may be purchased and offer automated report- and record-keeping functions. However, compliance managers should carefully review the program's accuracy periodically (eg, when codes or coding instructions are revised).

- A general documentation checklist of elements of documentation applicable to all records (eg, having patient identification, date, and page numbers on each page of a record), which can help with identification of missing nonclinical documentation and record authentication (an example can be found online at www.aap.org/cfp2023).
- A log to document findings for each provider (**Table 5-1**). This log should include a summary detail of findings for each encounter reviewed. The log and E/M audit worksheets can be used as teaching tools at the conclusion of the audit.
- Audit summary reporting forms—results by individual provider with encounter details (eg, levels of medical decision-making assigned vs audit finding); results by individual with codes and variances (eg, level of service and/or relative value unit variances); and report of key findings (eg, practice accuracy rates; strengths; areas of concern, including historical comparisons; recommendations for correction/improvement).

Following the Audit

- Discuss audit findings with each provider.
- Educate providers and staff as necessary.
- If a problem is encountered (eg, inappropriate use of modifiers, miscoding), a more focused retrospective review should be conducted to determine how long the error has been occurring and its effect. This is especially important when reviewing claims for physicians new to the practice or when a particular coding guideline or code has changed.

Table 5-1. Sample Audit Log				
Physician:	**Date:**		**Auditor:**	
Patient ID	**Date of Service**	**Reported Code**	**Audited Code**	**Comments**
4494	2/3/23	**99239**	**99238**	Total physician time not documented; **99239** is reported only when >30 min is documented.
4494	2/3/23	**J45.901**	**J45.31**	Documentation supports exacerbation of mild persistent asthma (**J45.31**), not unspecified asthma.
2973	6/4/22	**69209**	**None**	Impaction of cerumen not documented
43221	6/4/22	**99222**	**99235**	Patient admitted and discharged on the same date

- If overpayments have occurred because of miscoding or billing errors, the errors should be corrected and education of appropriate staff performed. Requirements (eg, contractual, regulatory) for refunding overpayments and disclosure of errors must be understood and included in practice procedures.

● indicates a new code; ▲, revised; #, re-sequenced; ✚, add-on; ★, audiovisual technology; and ◀, synchronous interactive audio.

Figure 5-1. Preparing and Planning Medical Record Audits

Focus
- Focus audits on documentation and coding of the most commonly performed services, adherence to medical record standards, appropriate reporting of diagnosis codes, use of modifiers, and adherence to coding and federal guidelines (eg, PATH guidelines, Physician Self-Referral Law).

Agree
- Make certain that all physicians in the practice are in agreement with how any audit will be conducted and how results will be used.

Auditor
- The auditor (eg, physician, physician extender, coder or other administrative employee, outside consultant, a combination thereof) must be proficient at coding, understand payer guidelines and requirements, and know medical terminology. Consider a team approach (eg, nurse and coder). If a physician is not actually performing record reviews, one should be available to assist as necessary.

Legal
- Determine whether audits should be performed under the direction of a health care attorney who may offer assistance with developing an audit process and provide guidance on any internal compliance concerns discovered in the process.
- Attorney-client privilege may apply when audits are directed by an attorney.

Timing
- Determine if your audit will be retrospective (ie, performed on paid claims and services) or prospective (ie, performed on services and claims that have not yet been billed).
- Prospective reviews are recommended because any necessary corrections can be made before a claim is filed. Although a prospective review will delay claims submission and introduce additional practice expense, this practice may have a net positive financial effect.

Services
- Select the types of services to be included in the audit. For example, if the review will include only office or outpatient services, include services most frequently reported (eg, a sampling of new and established patient problem-oriented and preventive medicine visits, documentation of nebulizer treatments).
- Include newborn care, critical care, and initial and subsequent inpatient or observation services when performing an audit of facility-based services.

Number
- Determine how many records or encounters will be included in the audit. Most coding consultants recommend at least 10 records per physician or provider per baseline or subsequent review (may be fewer for part-time providers). If a more focused review is required, the sample size may need to be increased. Medical records should be randomly selected for each E/M level of service and from different dates of service.

Schedule
- Determine the frequency of audits. Large practices might consider conducting audits on a rotating schedule of one physician or provider per week or one physician or provider per month throughout the year.

E/M indicates evaluation and management; PATH, Physicians at Teaching Hospitals.

● indicates a new code; ▲, revised; #, re-sequenced; ✚, add-on; ★, audiovisual technology; and ◀, synchronous interactive audio.

Chapter 5. Preventing Fraud and Abuse: Compliance, Audits, and Paybacks

Chapter 5. Preventing Fraud and Abuse: Compliance, Audits, and Paybacks

> The Patient Protection and Affordable Care Act requires any person who has received an overpayment from certain defined government health programs (including Medicaid plans) to report and return the overpayment within 60 days of the date the overpayment is identified. Always seek advice from the practice's attorney before disclosure or repayment.

- If necessary, document a corrective action plan with deadlines for completion (eg, completion of education, attainment of a specified accuracy rate) and administrative sign-off verifying completion.
- Schedule follow-up audits, if indicated, to determine if problems have been resolved (eg, improved documentation, capturing procedures, correct use of modifiers).
- Determine if audits need to be performed on a quarterly or annual basis and follow through with audits on a routine basis.
- If changes need to be made to the EHR system, contact the vendor and discuss how these might be accomplished. Educate physicians and providers on the changes made or the need for additional physician documentation.
- Establish or update written policies and procedures.
- Maintain records of your compliance efforts and training.

As illustrated in **Figure 5-2**, audits are not onetime events. Depending on your practice's resources for conducting audits and education, your practice may choose to conduct small audits monthly (eg, 5 medical records per provider), larger audits quarterly (eg, 10 medical records per provider), or continuous prospective audit of a small number of medical records weekly. There may be a period of trial and error to find what works best for your practice.

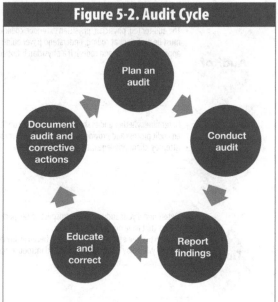

Figure 5-2. Audit Cycle

Do Not Get Caught Without a Plan

Most practices will never have to deal with demands for paybacks or fraud audits. Nevertheless, all practices should have a plan just in case they occur. Because time is of the essence in responding to these communications, it would be a calamity to have a letter sit on someone's desk while precious days tick away. Often, a response must be received within 30 days of the date of the request, and the paperwork demanded is not insignificant.

The first communication may be a request for repayment based on payer software analysis of claims history to detect claims paid in conflict with payment policies. It is important for all staff to be trained to recognize these requests and know to get them to the compliance officer immediately. Then, qualified staff tasked with receiving all requests for paybacks can determine the veracity of the request and, if inaccurate, act in accordance with the payer's rebuttal and appeal processes in a timely manner. Likewise, requests for records must be handled carefully and expeditiously.

Responding to Repayment Demands

In an effort to control costs and stamp out fraud, carrier claims processing and special investigative units use sophisticated software programs to identify providers with atypical coding patterns that could indicate erroneous coding and potential overpayments. For example, some carriers may flag those providers considered outliers in frequently reporting high-level E/M codes or frequent use of modifiers. They then extrapolate the alleged overpayments over several years and demand across-the-board repayments. Worse, carriers will reduce payments on future claims to correct alleged overpayments on past claims. These requests require a swift and skilled response. Usually, several thousand dollars are involved. Given the compressed timeline and dollars at stake, seeking legal advice is invaluable in these situations.

Here is some general guidance for your consideration.

- If it is truly due to a billing error by the practice, take action to correct the problem and demonstrate to the carrier how it has or will be corrected and the measures implemented to prevent the problem in the future.
- Reply in writing to inform the carrier you are willing to work with it and ask that it identify each of the claims in question as well as the specific criteria or standards it is applying to the audit.

- Make sure the practice and the carrier consistently apply current *CPT* guidelines. Reference *CPT* coding guidelines and have appropriate documentation for support. The AAP Coding Hotline can be a resource to you as well (https://form.jotform.com/Subspecialty/aapcodinghotline).
- Review your carrier contract's clauses on audits and dispute resolution as well as applicable state laws on audits and repayments with your attorney.
- Focus any overpayment recovery efforts on a case-by-case basis. Prevent unilateral take-backs by not allowing the carrier to extrapolate repayments on any or all future claims.
- Have the carrier provide documentation as proof of overpayment for each contested claim.
- Obtain and secure written documentation of all contacts with the carrier on this issue. Should a carrier payment policy require reporting that varies from *CPT* guidelines, obtain written, dated documentation from the carrier to verify that is the case. Keep this documentation permanently.
- Use legal counsel skilled in carrier contracting when negotiating contracts and confronted with repayment demands.

What If Your Practice Is Audited?

- Contact legal counsel as soon as possible. Make sure the attorney or legal practice has experience with audits. If it is a Medicaid audit, it is preferable to have an attorney with Medicaid audit experience. An audit is a complex legal process with significant consequences. It is unwise to attempt to maneuver through this process without sound legal advice.
- Designate 1 physician or staff member to serve as the primary contact with the attorney and auditors. However, keep in mind that all physicians and staff members may need to work with auditors to some extent.
- Request that the auditor provide you with an opening and closing conference. At the initial meeting, ask for the individual's credentials and job title and ask them to summarize the purpose of the review or audit.
- Know how far back auditors may conduct reviews, the number of records a contractor may request, the amount of time allowed to respond to each request, any rebuttal process in place, and steps necessary to appeal adverse findings.
- If the time requirements for producing copies or gathering medical records are unmanageable, contact the auditing entity and request an extension in writing. Provide a clear justification for the extension request.
- Keep copies of all written communication (eg, letters, directives, memos, emails). Keep the postmarked envelopes of all letters, including the original notice.
- Fully document all verbal communication, including time, date, persons involved, substance of the discussion, and conclusions and agreements.
- In response to requests for information, provide only the information requested and maintain copies of what you provide auditors. Before providing files, remove any information unrelated to the audit. For example, in a Medicaid audit, you could exclude information related to services provided when the patient was covered under a commercial plan or was uninsured.
- Do not alter any documents or medical records.
- Respond only to questions from the auditors; do not try to engage them in any conversations. If the auditors are conducting the review in your office, try to place them in a separate office away from patients, staff, and business operations.
- Be prepared to respond promptly to each request received. Keep a log of requests received by date, response due date, requesting party, any communication with the requester, date of response, and outcome.
- Know Health Insurance Portability and Accountability Act (HIPAA) privacy regulations, documentation principles, coding guidelines, and payment policies, and verify that all supporting documentation is included in each response.
- If legibility of the record is questionable, include a transcribed copy with attestation by the author of the original document stating that the transcription is accurate and provided to ensure legibility. Any unsigned entry should also be accompanied by a separate attestation by its author.
- Copied or scanned medical records should be carefully reviewed to be sure that all pages were legibly copied (front and back, if applicable) and are straight and within the margins on the page.
- Any questions about the sufficiency of medical record documentation should be addressed with the physician or provider who ordered or documented the service before responding to the request for records.
  - Any corrections to an entry should be performed in a manner that maintains legibility of the original content (eg, single-line strike-through) and should be signed and dated.
  - A summary of the service provided may be included to provide more information but should be distinctly labeled as such and not as part of the original record.
- Include any policy or correspondence from the payer that was used to guide your billing and coding practices related to the service. (Archived payer manuals supportive of claims from previous years may be available on Medicaid websites.) Clinical practice guidelines, policy statements, textbooks, and manuals may also be supportive of medical necessity.

Chapter 5. Preventing Fraud and Abuse: Compliance, Audits, and Paybacks

- Send records in a manner that allows for confirmation of receipt.
- Secure a copy of auditors' contact information in case you need to follow up.
- Obtain, in writing, the expected date of a written summary of findings.

Can This Really Happen?

Conventional wisdom says that auditors will probably go after big organizations when it comes to investigating fraud and abuse, but the OIG has said repeatedly that it has zero tolerance for fraud, so, technically, everyone is at risk. Because most of the software programs used to detect unusual coding and billing patterns are based on adult services, pediatricians may be identified as outliers. As a result, valid pediatric coding may be tagged as improper and honest providers may have to respond to inappropriate recoupment requests or audits. The AAP works hard to minimize these problems and help chapters respond when payers target pediatric coding as inappropriate. This is an ongoing challenge.

Unfortunately, there are instances of fraud involving pediatricians. A review of past OIG reports to Congress and press releases revealed the following cases:

- A whistleblower lawsuit filed under the qui tam provisions of the False Claims Act resulted in a Wisconsin pediatric practice agreeing to pay greater than $700,000 to resolve allegations that the practice submitted false claims to Medicaid for unnecessary treatment and visits. The defendant settled but did not admit liability.
- A Florida pediatrician was sentenced to 63 months in prison after pleading guilty to one count of wire fraud in connection with a clinical research study of an asthma medication for children. The pediatrician and employees falsified medical records to make it appear as though pediatric participants made scheduled visits to the practice, took study drugs as required, and received checks as payment.
- A nonpracticing physician, acting as a chief executive officer of a large group practice, agreed to pay $3,000,000 to settle charges of violating the Anti-Kickback Statute. The physician not only had employed physicians order unnecessary toxicological and genetic testing on patients (including children) but also required physicians to perform unnecessary procedures that used a specific medical device. The physician is also facing criminal charges for filing fraudulent health insurance claims for services that were not medically necessary. This case was brought by an employee who will share in the settlement of the qui tam case.
- A Connecticut pediatrician pleaded guilty to charges of health care fraud for billing Medicaid and other insurance programs for childhood vaccines received free of charge from the joint federal/state Vaccines for Children program.
- A New Jersey pediatrician was accused by 2 former employees of filing fraudulent claims. Although ultimately found not guilty, the pediatrician experienced both professional and personal losses during the investigation and trial. Records of a strong compliance program may have offered a quicker resolution of the charges.

Explore the Need for Additional Insurance

Many medical liability insurers and insurance brokers offer products to provide additional coverage for the consequences of billing errors and omissions. Pediatric practices may want to contact their insurers to see whether their current medical liability policies cover any of the following problems. If they do not, it might be worthwhile to explore insurance options for obtaining that additional protection.

- Defense coverage for a Medicaid audit
- Qui tam action (False Claims Act)
- Unintentional billing errors and omissions
- Physician Self-Referral Law (Stark law) violations
- Unintentional release of medical or financial data
- Breach of computers or network security
- Data recovery
- HIPAA fines or investigation costs

Health care fraud and abuse regulations will likely change as the health care system evolves to new care delivery and claims payment standards, such as value-based payment and accountable care organizations. Providers need to stay abreast of and comply with new regulations to prevent triggering fraud investigations.

● indicates a new code; ▲, revised; #, re-sequenced; ✚, add-on; ★, audiovisual technology; and ◀, synchronous interactive audio.

Chapter Takeaways

Protecting your practice from accusations of fraud or abuse requires thoughtful preparation and ongoing attention. Taking steps such as the ones discussed in this chapter show that your practice has an intent to comply. Following are some takeaways for protecting your practice from loss caused by lack of compliance planning:

- Learn about the fraud and abuse enforcement climate in your state.
- Implement an effective compliance program and follow it.
- Be sure your staff knows what a demand for repayment or audit notice looks like and what they need to do with it just on the off chance that something should happen.
- Have a response plan in place should an auditor knock on your door or a recoupment letter arrive in the mail.
- Consult with an attorney when needed.
- Think about the need for insurance for billing errors and omissions.
- Keep current with coding and billing updates.

Resources

AAP Coding Assistance and Education

AAP payer contract negotiations and payment resources (www.aap.org/en/practice-management/practice-financing/payer-contracting-advocacy-and-other-resources/payer-contract-negotiations-and-payment-resources)

AAP Refusal to Vaccinate forms (English and Spanish) (https://downloads.aap.org/DOPCSP/SOID_RTV_form_01-2019_English.pdf and https://downloads.aap.org/DOPCSP/SOID_RTV_form_01-2019_Spanish.pdf)

AAP Pediatric Coding Newsletter™

"Coding Compliance Education: Standards and Procedures," March 2019 (https://doi.org/10.1542/pcco_book179_document002)

"What Does Your EHR Documentation Say?" March 2017 (https://doi.org/10.1542/pcco_book155_document001)

CMS Medicare Fraud and Abuse Booklet

Medicare Fraud & Abuse: Prevent, Detect, Report (www.cms.gov/Outreach-and-Education/Medicare-Learning-Network-MLN/MLNProducts/Downloads/Fraud-Abuse-MLN4649244.pdf)

Documentation

Program integrity: *Documentation Matters Toolkit* (www.cms.gov/Medicare-Medicaid-Coordination/Fraud-Prevention/Medicaid-Integrity-Education/documentation-matters.html)

HHS OIG Excluded Individuals and Entities List

HHS OIG Excluded Individuals and Entities List (https://exclusions.oig.hhs.gov) and the federal System for Award Management (https://sam.gov/content/exclusions)

HHS OIG Special Fraud Alert: Speaker Programs

https://oig.hhs.gov/documents/special-fraud-alerts/865/SpecialFraudAlertSpeakerPrograms.pdf

Legal Advice

American Health Law Association (www.americanhealthlaw.org)

Online Exclusive Content at www.aap.org/cfp2023

"General Documentation Checklist"

Payer Audits

Medicaid RAC program (www.medicaid.gov)

Test Your Knowledge!

1. **Which of the following laws applies to claims submitted to Medicaid that you know *or should know* are false or fraudulent?**
   a. False Claims Act
   b. Anti-Kickback Statute
   c. Physician Self-Referral Law (Stark law)
   d. Civil Monetary Penalties Law

2. **When should a physician practice seek legal counsel familiar with anti-kickback and self-referral laws?**
   a. When a health plan advises of a claims audit
   b. When hiring a new physician or qualified health care professional
   c. When the practice disagrees with a health plan's denial of charges
   d. When intending to enter a business arrangement that involves making referrals

3. **True or false? Compliance programs for small practices are voluntary.**
   a. True
   b. False

4. **Which of the following components must compliant documentation encompass?**
   a. What should be documented
   b. Safeguards from inaccuracies
   c. Safeguards from potential noncompliant access to or disclosure of information
   d. All of the above

5. **Which of the following responses is recommended when a payer demands repayment based on atypical coding patterns?**
   a. Send the payer the amount demanded without question.
   b. Ignore the demand and do not pay anything.
   c. Seek legal advice.
   d. File bankruptcy and start a new practice.

Evaluation and Management Documentation Guidelines

CPT copyright 2022 American Medical Association. All rights reserved.

Contents

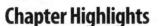

Chapter Highlights

- Recognize the services to which general and specific evaluation and management (E/M) guidelines apply.
- Understand the concepts of new versus established patient and initial versus subsequent encounter.
- Learn the *Current Procedural Terminology* (*CPT®*) terms and definitions used in determining a level of E/M services based on a physician's or other qualified health care professional's (QHP's) total time on the date of an encounter (regardless of the percentage spent in counseling and/or coordination of care) or on medical decision-making (MDM).
- Apply the Centers for Medicare & Medicaid Services (CMS) guidelines for reporting services provided as a teaching physician, when applicable.

This chapter outlines the *CPT* E/M guidelines used in selecting codes for encounters to evaluate and manage a patient's health problems. The content of this chapter provides the basis for learning category-specific instructions for code selection discussed in later chapters.

How Guidelines Have Changed Since 2022

In 2023, the division between guidelines for office and other outpatient evaluation and management (E/M) services and guidelines for other E/M services for which codes are selected on the basis of key components or typical time is unnecessary. The basic format of codes with levels of E/M services based on medical decision-making (MDM) or time is now the same. Revisions to codes throughout the E/M section have resulted in a single set of guidelines that apply to the following services:

- Office or other outpatient services
- Hospital inpatient and observation care services
- Consultations
- Emergency department services
- Nursing facility services
- Home or residence services
- Prolonged service with or without direct contact on the date of an E/M service

Additionally, definitions of initial and subsequent services are added to assist with selecting code categories for services to patients in facility settings. Certain other definitions are added or revised to guide in selecting a level of MDM.

The MDM table in *Current Procedural Terminology* previously used only for office and other outpatient E/M services is revised for use for all the services listed.

General Guidelines

The E/M guidelines in *CPT* are used to guide code selection and are neither documentation guidelines nor standards of care. The E/M guidelines section of *CPT* mostly applies to codes selected on the basis of the physician's or the QHP's total time on the date of an encounter (total time) or on the basis of the level of MDM required for the problems addressed. However, the following portions of the E/M guidelines apply to many E/M services, including those not selected on the basis of total time or MDM:

- Definitions of new versus established patients and initial versus subsequent encounters
- Other services provided on the same date as an E/M service

Additional service-specific guidelines are found preceding categories of E/M service (eg, home and residence E/M services) and subcategories (eg, initial hospital inpatient or observation care services, **99221–99223**) and, in parenthetical instructions, following E/M codes.

Please refer to other chapters of this manual and your *CPT* coding reference for more detailed guidelines for reporting services such as normal newborn care in the hospital, hourly or daily critical care services, intensive care services, care plan oversight, care management services, and preventive medicine E/M services.

● indicates a new code; ▲, revised; #, re-sequenced; ✛, add-on; ★, audiovisual technology; and ◀, synchronous interactive audio.

Chapter 6. Evaluation and Management Documentation Guidelines

---

About Documentation

Although *Current Procedural Terminology* guidelines are not documentation guidelines, the information documented in the medical record must support the reported procedure codes.

When selecting a code based on total time, *the total time* and a summary of activities during that time (eg, history and examination findings, counseling topics) must be documented.

When selecting a code based on the level of medical decision-making, the documentation should demonstrate the basis for the level selected. For instance, the record should include the signs, symptoms, and diagnoses that were addressed, including any conditions that were considered plausible but ruled out. It is also important to demonstrate review of external records or prior test results. The physician or other qualified health care professional might sign the external record or report of test results to indicate review or might document a brief notation of findings in the encounter note. Conversations with external physicians and other health care professionals or sources (eg, social workers) should also be summarized in the documentation (eg, "Spoke with Dr X regarding management options for this patient").

Another clinician or coding auditor should be able to readily determine your basis for the code reported.

New Versus Established Patients

New and established patients are defined in the *CPT* E/M guidelines. The categorization of patients influences coding for the following services:

- Office or other outpatient E/M services (new patient, **99202–99205**; established patient, **99211–99215**)
- Home or residence services (new patient, **99341** and **99342**, **99344** and **99345**; established patient, **99347–99350**)
- Preventive medicine services (new patient, **99381–99385**; established patient, **99391–99395**)

No distinction is made between new and established patients for emergency department (ED) services, for consultations, or for observation, inpatient, or nursing facility care. Evaluation and management services in these categories may be reported for any new or established patient. For E/M services provided to patients in observation or inpatient status or in a nursing facility, services are distinguished as initial or subsequent encounters during the same admission, as discussed in the Initial and Subsequent Services section later in this chapter.

Following are the criteria for distinguishing between new and established patients:

- *New patients* have not received a face-to-face professional service from the physician or other QHP, or any physician or QHP of the same group practice and same exact specialty and subspecialty (eg, primary care, allergist), in the prior 3 years.
- *Established patients* have received, and charged for, a face-to-face professional service from a physician or QHP of the same group practice and same exact specialty and subspecialty within the past 3 years.
- Per *CPT*, a QHP working with a physician(s) and who may report E/M services is considered to be working in the exact same specialty and subspecialty as the physician(s). (Medicare assigns different specialty designations to QHPs and does not consider the specialty of the physician providing supervision when determining whether a patient is new. Medicaid and private plans may follow either *CPT* or Medicare practices.)
- When a physician is covering for another physician of the same specialty, the patient's encounter is reported as it would have been by the physician who is not available. However, a physician covering for another physician of a different specialty determines new or established on the basis of the rules listed earlier in this list for new and established patients (see the first 2 bulleted items).
- If the physician has moved to a different location or changed their tax identification number, patients would still be considered established if they were established patients before these changes took place.
  - When a new physician joins a group practice, patients who follow the physician to the new practice are considered to be established patients to any physician of the same specialty in the new practice because the patients were seen by a physician of the same specialty in the group within the past 3 years.

Examples

➤ **A physician provides an office visit to an infant who received newborn hospital care from a physician of the same group and same exact specialty.** The patient is considered established at the office visit.

➤ **A physician provided an outpatient consultation to a patient within the past 3 years.** Another physician in the same group but *different specialty* is asked to provide an office or other outpatient E/M service to the patient. The patient is new for this encounter.

● indicates a new code; ▲, revised; #, re-sequenced; ✚, add-on; ★, audiovisual technology; and ◀, synchronous interactive audio.

When a physician is covering for another physician of the same specialty, the patient's encounter is reported as it would have been by the physician who is unavailable. When QHPs are working with physicians, they are considered to be working in the exact same specialty and subspecialty as the physician.

Initial and Subsequent Services

The following services are described as initial or subsequent services as opposed to services provided to a new or established patient:

- Hospital inpatient and observation care services (initial, **99221–99223**; subsequent, **99231–99233**)
- Nursing facility services (initial, **99304–99306**; subsequent, **99307–99310**)

> **Intensive and Critical Care Services**
>
> Please see the prefatory guidelines for critical care (99291, 99292), inpatient neonatal and pediatric critical care (99468–99472; 99475, 99476), and neonatal intensive care services (99477–99480) for distinct instructions on reporting initial and continuing services.

As with new and established patients, differentiating between initial and subsequent encounters is based on the timing of the professional (face-to-face) services provided by a physician or other QHP to the patient during an admission/stay.

- Admission/stay: The duration of time from admission to discharge from a facility. For the purpose of determining initial versus subsequent encounters, an admission/stay that includes a transition in levels of care from observation to inpatient or between skilled nursing facility and nursing facility is one admission/stay.
- Initial service: During the inpatient or observation or nursing facility admission/stay, the patient has not received any professional services from the physician or QHP or another physician or QHP of the exact same specialty and subspecialty who belongs to the same group practice.
- Subsequent service: During the admission/stay, the patient has received professional service(s) from the physician or QHP or another physician or QHP of the exact same specialty and subspecialty who belongs to the same group practice.

> For the purpose of selecting between initial and subsequent evaluation and management services provided in a facility setting, a single admission/stay includes any transfers from one level of care to another (eg, observation to inpatient). A transfer in the level of care is not a new admission/stay.

Examples

➤ **A physician provides hospital care to a patient who has received no prior care from the physician or any physician or QHP of the same group practice and same specialty during this admission/stay.** Initial hospital care is reported.

➤ **A physician provides hospital care to a patient who received observation care from a physician of the same group and same exact specialty on a prior date during this admission/stay.** The encounter is reported as subsequent hospital care.

➤ **A physician who is covering for a patient's attending physician who is unavailable sees the patient for the first time during an inpatient stay.** The encounter is subsequent hospital care.

Separately Reported Services

Procedures and services described by *CPT* codes distinct from those of an E/M service provided on the same date may be separately reported except where specifically noted as included/bundled in *CPT*. For example, critical care E/M services include services such as electrocardiographic collection and interpretation and vascular access procedures that are reported in addition to most other E/M services.

> When an evaluation and management service is caused or prompted by the symptoms or condition for which another diagnostic or therapeutic service (eg, electrocardiography, injection of medication, surgery) is provided on the same date, different diagnoses are not required for reporting the 2 services on the same date.

Example

➤ **A physician provides an office E/M service to a patient who describes limited hearing and fullness in their right ear.** Examination of the right ear reveals impacted cerumen that requires removal with instrumentation (performed by the physician on the same date). The physician reports *International Classification of Diseases, 10th Revision, Clinical Modification* code **H61.21** (impacted cerumen, right ear) linked to a code for the E/M service (eg, **99213 25**) and to **69210** (removal of impacted cerumen requiring instrumentation, unilateral).

Modifier **25** (significant, separately identifiable E/M service) is appended to an E/M code when an E/M service provided on the same date as a procedural service is significantly beyond the preservice work of the procedural service.

For more information on modifier **25**, please see **Chapter 2**.

E/M Guidelines for Use of Total Time or MDM

Applicability of E/M Guidelines for Use of Total Time or MDM

Evaluation and management guidelines used for selecting codes from the following categories are further discussed in this chapter:

- Office or other outpatient services (new patient, **99202–99205**; established patient, **99211–99215**)
- Hospital inpatient or observation care services (initial, **99221–99223**; subsequent, **99231–99233**; same date admission and discharge, **99234–99236**; discharge day management, **99238–99239**)
- Outpatient and inpatient consultations (outpatient, **99242–99245**; inpatient, **99252–99255**)
- Emergency department services (**99281–99285**)
- Nursing facility services (initial, **99304–99306**; subsequent, **99307–99310**; discharge day management, **99315** and **99316**)
- Home or residence services (new patient, **99341** and **99342**, **99344** and **99345**; established patient, **99347–99350**)
- Prolonged service with or without direct contact on the date of an evaluation and management service (**99417, 99418**)

Each of the listed code categories involves selecting a code based on the location where a face-to-face service is provided and a physician's or a QHP's total time on the date of the encounter or the level of MDM associated with the encounter. All other E/M services are reported on the basis of guidelines specific to the code category. The guidelines for these other E/M services are addressed in other chapters of this manual (eg, **Chapter 8**, **Chapter 18**). See also **Chapter 1** for general guidelines for *CPT* code selection.

> Telemedicine evaluation and management services (delivered via real-time audiovisual technology) are face-to-face services even though the physician is present only by audiovisual technology. Learn more about coding for services provided via telemedicine in Chapter 20.

Each of the categories and subcategories of E/M service to which these general guidelines apply may also have additional guidelines presented before the list of codes and/or as parenthetical instructions after the codes in *CPT 2023*. For instance, unique prefatory guidelines for hospital inpatient and observation care provide important guidance for reporting the correct subcategory of service: initial care, subsequent care, discharge day management, or same date admission and discharge. These additional guidelines, specific to each category of E/M code, are discussed in other chapters devoted to reporting these services (eg, **Chapter 15**).

History and Examination

History and examination are included components of all evaluation and management (E/M) services addressed by the E/M guidelines. However, the extent of history and examination, while lending support for the amount of time spent or the level of MDM, are not directly used in code selection. A medically appropriate history and examination, as determined by the reporting physician or qualified health care professional (QHP), should be documented for each E/M service.

History and examination are important elements of documentation to support that medical services provided were clinically indicated and to support quality initiatives (eg, verification of timely immunization and review of current medications and supplements). History documented by a patient, caregiver, or clinical staff member should be reviewed, expanded (when indicated), and authenticated by the reporting physician or QHP.

Code Selection Options

Once you have determined the correct code category (eg, outpatient consultation) or subcategory (eg, initial hospital inpatient or observation care), there are 2 options for selecting the appropriate codes based on these guidelines. An exception is services provided in the ED (**99281–99285**) that are selected on MDM alone, with no option for selection based on time.

- Select the code based on the reporting physician's or QHP's *documented total time* directed to care of the individual patient *on the date of the encounter.*
- Select a code based on meeting 2 of 3 elements of MDM.

> **Time and Emergency Department Services**
>
> Per *Current Procedural Terminology,* time is not a descriptive component for the emergency department (ED) levels of evaluation and management services because ED services are typically provided on a variable-intensity basis, often involving multiple encounters with several patients over an extended period.

Box 6-1 provides an overview of code selection based on total time or MDM. For each method of code selection, the documentation should support the clinical indication for the level of service reported.

Box 6-1. Evaluation and Management Code Selection Based on Total Time or Medical Decision-making

Select a code based on the pediatrician's or the QHP's total time on the date of the encounter or the level of MDM.

Time: May be used to select a code level whether or not counseling and/or coordination of care dominates the service.
- Time includes the total time on the date of the encounter (face-to-face and non–face-to-face) personally spent by the physician and/or QHP focused on the care of 1 patient.
  - Do not include time in activities performed or normally performed by clinical staff (eg, rooming the patient).
  - Time does not need to be continuous. Total all time on 1 date.
- Include the time of the following activities when performed by the reporting pediatrician/QHP:
  - Preparing to see the patient (eg, reviewing previous test results)
  - Obtaining and/or reviewing separately obtained history
  - Performing a medically appropriate examination and/or evaluation
  - Counseling and educating the patient, family, or caregiver
  - Ordering medications, tests, or procedures
  - Referring/communicating with other QHPs (when not separately reported)
  - Documenting clinical information in the electronic or other health record
  - Independently interpreting results (when not separately reported) and communicating results to the patient, family, or caregiver
  - Coordinating care (when not separately reported)

MDM: Four types of MDM are recognized: straightforward, low, moderate, and high.
Determine the level of MDM based on the highest 2 of 3 elements of MDM.
1. Number and complexity of problems addressed. Include problems addressed or managed by the reporting pediatrician/QHP as part of the encounter.
2. Amount and/or complexity of data reviewed and analyzed. Data include
   - Tests, documents, orders, or independent historian(s)
   - Independent interpretation of tests (not separately reported)
   - Discussion of management/test interpretation with an external physician, QHP, or appropriate source (not separately reported)
3. Risk of complications, morbidity, and/or mortality of patient management decisions made during the encounter, including decisions against a considered management option.

Abbreviations: MDM, medical decision-making; QHP, qualified health care professional.

Time Guidelines and Application

Time may be used to select a code level in the E/M services to which these guidelines apply *whether or not* counseling and/or coordination of care dominates the service.

- Time is the physician's and/or QHP's total time on the date of service, not their time in a 24-hour period.

> The total time should be documented in the medical record when used as the basis for code selection. No specific verbiage is required by *Current Procedural Terminology*. Remember, when not documented, time is not an option for code selection.

- Only time spent in activities directed to care of the individual patient is counted in the total time on the date of an encounter.
- Both face-to-face and non–face-to-face time or time on or off the unit/floor spent on the date of service are included in the time of the encounter. **Figure 6-1** illustrates the time included in the physician's or QHP's total time.

Code Descriptors and Total Time

It is important to identify the time required in each code's descriptor to accurately assign codes based on total time. There are differences in how time is described across various categories of service.

Office and other outpatient evaluation and management services are described by ranges of time spent on the date of the encounter (eg, code 99202 includes 15–29 minutes).

For most other codes that may be selected on the basis of a physician's or qualified health care professional's total time on the date of the encounter, a specific time must be met or exceeded.

Other codes, such as hourly critical care codes 99291 and 99292, have different guidelines and code descriptors that include only the time spent providing critical care services (ie, not the total time spent on the date of the encounter).

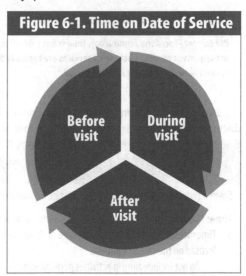

Figure 6-1. Time on Date of Service

Before visit | During visit | After visit

Examples

➤ **A physician spends 10 minutes reviewing laboratory results and consultation reports before an E/M encounter with an established patient on the same date.** Later that day, a face-to-face visit with the patient and caregivers lasts 20 minutes. After the visit but on the same date, the physician spends 10 minutes in discussion with a consulting sub-specialist and another 10 minutes in follow-up with the caregivers and in documentation. The physician's total time on the date of service is 50 minutes.

    Teaching Point: The physician reports code **99215** (40–54 minutes). All the physician's time spent in activities directed to the care of the single patient is counted.

> *Current Procedural Terminology* does not require documentation of each segment of time spent on the date of service or documentation in any specific format. The physician must, however, document the total amount of time spent on the date of the encounter and be able to account for the time spent.

➤ **A physician spends 10 minutes reviewing laboratory results and medical records before an outpatient consultation on the same date.** Later that day, a face-to-face visit with the patient and caregivers lasts 20 minutes, and another 10 minutes is spent documenting the encounter and preparing a report to the QHP who requested the consultation. The physician's total time on the date of the face-to-face E/M service is 40 minutes. On the next day, the physician spends 10 minutes in discussion with the QHP who requested the consultation and another 10 minutes in follow-up with the caregivers and in documentation.

    Code **99244** (40 minutes must be met or exceeded) is reported for the time on the date of the face-to-face visit.

    Teaching Point: The time spent on the next date is not included in the total time on the date of the encounter. However, when a physician or QHP spends at least 30 minutes in patient care and coordination on a date when no other E/M service is provided, code **99358** (prolonged E/M service before and/or after direct patient care; first hour) is reported.

● indicates a new code; ▲, revised; #, re-sequenced; ✚, add-on; ★, audiovisual technology; and ◀, synchronous interactive audio.

➤ **A physician spends 25 minutes on the unit/floor reviewing consultation reports and test results, reevaluating the patient, and discussing care with the patient and the patient's mother.** Another 10 minutes is spent entering orders and documenting the encounter. Later, when not on the patient's unit, the physician also spends 10 minutes on the phone with the patient's father explaining current findings and the plan for further E/M. Total time on the date of the encounter is 45 minutes.

   Teaching Point: Total time on the date of the encounter includes time regardless of the location of the physician (eg, whether on or off the inpatient unit or in or out of the outpatient office). However, the time must be directed to the care of that single patient and must require the skills of a physician or QHP.

● No time spent by clinical staff or time spent by a physician or QHP in activities typically performed by clinical staff is included.
● When the physician and a QHP meet with a patient and caregiver at the same time (incident-to or split or shared encounter), only the reporting individual's time is counted. *Each minute of time is counted only once.*

> Per Medicare policy, a split or shared encounter is an evaluation and management service provided in a facility setting in which a physician and qualified health care professional (QHP) jointly provide the face-to-face and non–face-to-face work. For more information on split/shared encounters, see Chapter 17. Medicare's policy for split/shared encounters does not apply in non-facility settings (eg, office) where incident-to policy applies. Incident-to services are non-facility services provided by a QHP under a physician's direct supervision and in continuation of a physician's plan of care. See Chapter 7 for more information on incident-to services.

Example

➤ **A nurse practitioner provides initial observation care to a patient.** After initially evaluating the patient, the nurse practitioner spends 5 minutes discussing the patient with a physician in her same group practice and specialty and documents a total time of 25 minutes, including the time of the phone call with the physician. Later, on the same date, the physician of the same group practice and specialty reviews the patient's progress notes and test results since admission to observation and, after reevaluating the patient, agrees with continuing the current management overnight. The physician's total time is 20 minutes *not including the time of the phone conversation with the nurse practitioner.*

   Code **99221** (initial hospital inpatient or observation care; 40 minutes must be met or exceeded) is reported for the 45-minute service. The 5-minute conversation between the physician and nurse practitioner is counted by only 1 of the providers.

   Teaching Point: Whether the physician or nurse practitioner reports the service may depend on policy established by the individual payer. In an office or other non-facility setting, a payer may limit physician reporting of split/shared encounters to when incident-to guidelines are met, as discussed in **Chapter 7**.

> Pediatric clinical vignettes are presented throughout this manual. These are only examples, and the associated *Current Procedural Terminology* codes should not be used for every patient with the same diagnosis.

MDM: Guidelines for Selecting a Level

Medical decision-making is the work of establishing diagnoses, assessing the status of a condition, and/or selecting a management option. Medical decision-making is determined by assessing the level at which 2 of 3 elements of MDM are supported in the documentation of an encounter. The 3 elements of MDM are

1. The number and complexity of problem(s) addressed during the encounter
2. The amount and/or complexity of data to be reviewed and analyzed
3. The risk of complications, morbidity, and/or mortality of patient management decisions made at the visit, associated with the patient's problem(s), diagnostic procedure(s), and treatment(s)

   Four types of MDM are recognized, as follows:

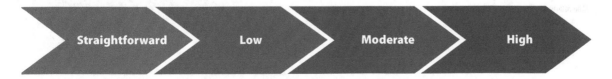

Straightforward   Low   Moderate   High

● indicates a new code; ▲, revised; #, re-sequenced; ✚, add-on; ★, audiovisual technology; and ◀, synchronous interactive audio.

Each level of MDM is based on the same criteria whether the patient is new or established or the encounter is initial or subsequent. (Time and other factors considered in valuing codes further differentiate these E/M services.)

Number and Complexity of Problems Addressed

The first step in determining the level of MDM for an encounter is identification of the number and complexity of problems addressed. A problem is a disease, a condition, an illness, an injury, a symptom, a sign, a finding, a concern, or another matter addressed at the encounter, with or without a diagnosis being established at the time of the encounter.

- Include all problems addressed at an encounter in the number and complexity of problems.
- Complexity is determined by the types of problems addressed. *CPT* instructs that
  - The final diagnosis for a condition does not, in and of itself, determine the complexity or risk of the problem, as extensive evaluation may be required to reach the conclusion that the signs or symptoms do not represent a highly morbid condition.
  - Manifesting symptoms that are likely to represent a highly morbid condition may drive MDM even when the ultimate diagnosis is not highly morbid.

CPT does not provide examples of types of problems included in each level of MDM but does leave the determination to the reporting individual's clinical judgment. Examples included in this manual may not apply to all patient encounters.

Defining Problems Addressed for Inpatient and Observation Services

For hospital inpatient and observation care services, select the complexity of the problem addressed on the basis of the problem status on the date of the encounter, which may significantly differ from that on admission. For example, an encounter with a patient who was admitted in respiratory distress but who presents with no distress at the current encounter may include a lower number and complexity of problems addressed than that of prior encounters in the same admission. Likewise, a patient's condition may deteriorate such that problems at subsequent encounters are of higher complexity than at admission.

Problem(s) managed or comanaged by a reporting physician or qualified health care professional may not be the cause of admission or continued stay (eg, addressing a comorbid condition).

See **Table 6-1** for the levels of problems in MDM. Expanded discussion of each type of problem follows the table.

Table 6-1. Levels of Problems in Medical Decision-making	
Level	**Type of Problem**
NA	Minimal (See **99211, 99281**.)
SF	1 self-limited or minor problem
Low	≥2 self-limited or minor problems
	Acute, uncomplicated illness or injury
	Stable chronic illness
	1 stable acute illness
	1 acute, uncomplicated illness or injury requiring hospital inpatient or observation level of care
Moderate	2 stable chronic illnesses
	Chronic illness with exacerbation, progression, or side effects of treatment
	Acute, complicated injury
	Acute illness with systemic symptoms
	Undiagnosed new problem with uncertain prognosis
High	Chronic illness with severe exacerbation, progression, or side effects of treatment
	Acute/chronic illness or injury posing a threat to life or bodily function
Abbreviations: NA, not applicable; QHP, qualified health care professional; SF, straightforward.	

The guidelines for office E/M services define the types of problems typically addressed at these encounters. See the following "Coding Conundrum: Addressed or Not Addressed" box for guidance on problems considered to have been addressed:

Coding Conundrum: Addressed or Not Addressed

A problem is addressed or managed when evaluated or treated at the encounter by the physician or other qualified health care professional (QHP) reporting the service.

- This includes consideration of further testing or treatment that may not be elected by virtue of risk to benefit analysis or patient, parent, guardian, or surrogate choice.
- Notation in the patient's medical record that another professional is managing the problem without additional assessment or care coordination documented does not qualify as being addressed or managed by the physician or QHP reporting the service.
- Referral without evaluation (by history, examination, or ≥1 diagnostic studies) or consideration of treatment does not qualify a problem as being addressed or managed by the physician or QHP reporting the service.
- Do not include problems simply listed in the medical record when determining code level if those problems were not addressed.

Determination of the type of problem addressed may require a pediatrician's clinical judgment. Coding staff should query the pediatrician when unsure of the appropriate types of problems addressed at an encounter (eg, self-limited vs acute, uncomplicated illness).

Following are definitions for the types of problems identified in each level of MDM from *CPT 2023:*

Minimal: Presence of the physician or QHP is not required, but the service is provided under the physician's or QHP's supervision (see codes **99211**, **99281**).

Self-limited or minor: A problem that runs a definite and prescribed course, is transient in nature, and is not likely to permanently alter health status.

Low

- Two or more self-limited or minor problems.
- Acute, uncomplicated illness or injury. A recent or new short-term problem with low risk of morbidity for which treatment *is considered.*
  - Little to no risk of mortality with treatment and full recovery without functional impairment are expected.
  - May be a self-limited or minor problem that is not resolving consistently with a definite and prescribed course.
  - Examples may include cystitis, allergic rhinitis, or a simple sprain.
- Acute, uncomplicated illness or injury requiring hospital inpatient or observation-level care. A recent or new short-term problem with low risk of morbidity for which treatment *is required.*
  - Little to no risk of mortality with treatment and full recovery without functional impairment are expected.
  - The treatment required is delivered in a hospital inpatient or observation-level setting.
- Stable acute illness. A problem that is new or recent for which treatment has been initiated. The patient is improved and, while resolution may not be complete, is stable with respect to this condition.
- Stable chronic illness. A problem *with an expected duration of at least 1 year* or until the death of the patient *where the risk of morbidity is significant without treatment.*
  - *Stable* is defined by the individual patient's specific treatment goals. A patient who is not at their treatment goal is not stable, even if the condition has not changed and there is no short-term threat to life or function.
  - Examples of stable chronic illness may include well-controlled attention-deficit/hyperactivity disorder (ADHD), asthma, cystic fibrosis, depression, or diabetes.

Conditions are treated as chronic whether or not stage or severity changes (eg, uncontrolled diabetes and controlled diabetes are a single chronic condition).

Moderate

- Two stable chronic illnesses.
- Chronic illness with exacerbation, progression, or side effects of treatment. Acutely worsening, poorly controlled, or progressing with an intent to control progression, *requiring additional supportive care or requiring attention to treatment of side effects.*
  - Examples include non-severe exacerbation of asthma, generalized anxiety disorder now with school avoidance, and ADHD with tics secondary to treatment.

● indicates a new code; ▲, revised; #, re-sequenced; ✦, add-on; ★, audiovisual technology; and ◀, synchronous interactive audio.

- Acute, complicated injury. Requires evaluation of body systems that are not directly part of the injured organ, extensive injury, multiple treatment options, and/or association with risk of morbidity (eg, head injury with brief loss of consciousness).
- Acute illness with systemic symptoms. An illness causing systemic symptoms and *with high risk of morbidity without treatment.*
  - For systemic general symptoms (eg, fever, body aches, fatigue) in a minor illness that may be treated to alleviate symptoms, see *self-limited or minor* or *acute, uncomplicated illness.*
  - Systemic symptoms may not be general but may be single system (eg, juvenile oligoarticular arthritis with only musculoskeletal symptoms).
  - Examples may include pyelonephritis or bacterial gastroenteritis.

> **Although the risk of morbidity without treatment is a consideration in determining the nature of the problem addressed, this does not equate to the risk of mortality or morbidity of management (ie, problem risk is distinct from patient management risk).**

- Undiagnosed new problem with uncertain prognosis. A problem in the differential diagnosis that represents a condition *likely to result in a high risk of morbidity without treatment.* Examples may include unexplained bruising, anterior neck mass, unexpected weight loss, and school failure.

  High
- Chronic illness with severe exacerbation, progression, or side effects of treatment. Severe exacerbation or progression of chronic illness or severe side effects of treatment with significant risk of morbidity and may require escalation in the level of care.
- Acute or chronic illness or injury posing a threat to life or bodily function. Acute illness with systemic symptoms or an acute, complicated injury, or a chronic illness or injury with exacerbation and/or progression or side effects of treatment, that poses a threat to life or bodily function in the near term without treatment.
  - Some symptoms may represent a condition that is significantly probable and poses a potential threat to life or bodily function. These may be included in this category when the evaluation and treatment is consistent with this degree of potential severity.
  - Examples may include severe respiratory distress, psychiatric illness with potential threat to self or others, acute renal failure, or an abrupt change in neurological status.

The following examples focus only on identification of the type of problem addressed. Can you identify the type of problem(s) addressed in each example?

Examples

➤ **A patient presents with a small area of uncomplicated heat rash.** The patient's parents are advised on home care.
   Level of problems addressed ⦙⦙➡ *Minimal*

➤ **A patient presents for follow-up evaluation of a sprained ankle (not within a global period of a procedure).** The sprain is healing well. The patient and caregiver are instructed that a brace is no longer necessary but the patient should continue functional therapy.
   Level of problems addressed ⦙⦙➡ *Low*

➤ **A patient who was seen and admitted with moderate dehydration caused by acute gastroenteritis is reevaluated on the day after admission.** The patient is stable but continues to have some vomiting and diarrhea. The patient will continue to receive intravenous fluids until symptoms resolve.
   Level of problems addressed ⦙⦙➡ *Moderate*
   Teaching Point: The patient is recovering from an acute illness with systemic symptoms.

➤ **A 1-year-old patient presents with a high fever and lethargy.**
   Plan: The patient is admitted to the hospital for diagnostic evaluation to rule out sepsis.
   Level of problems addressed ⦙⦙➡ *High*
   Teaching Point: The clinical indications of possible sepsis in this patient represent a high-complexity problem.

● indicates a new code; ▲, revised; #, re-sequenced; ✚, add-on; ★, audiovisual technology; and ◀, synchronous interactive audio.

➤ **A 16-year-old patient presents to a hospital by ambulance after being hit by a car.** The patient has multiple trauma with potential injury to internal organs.
Plan: Stabilization and admission with decisions for consultations and surgery as indicated.

    Level of problems addressed ⅢⅢ➡ *High*

    Teaching Point: The patient's injuries pose a threat to life or bodily function.

Amount and/or Complexity of Data to Be Reviewed and Analyzed

Data are divided into the following 3 categories:

1. Tests, documents, orders, or independent historian(s) (Each unique test, order, or document is counted to meet a threshold number.)
2. Independent interpretation of tests not separately reported
3. Discussion of management or test interpretation with external physician or other QHP or appropriate source when not separately reported

> **Minimal or no data are required for straightforward medical decision-making.**

When data are used in support of low, moderate, or high MDM, the requirements for either 1 or 2 categories of data must be met. Instructions are provided for each level of data. **Table 6-2** shows the data requirements for limited, moderate, and extensive amounts and/or complexity of data.

Note that Category 1 includes multiple types of data that may be combined to meet a limited, moderate, or high amount and/or complexity of data. Each of the following data would support a limited level of data:

- Review of external notes from 2 unique sources
- Order or review of results of 2 unique tests (represented by separate *CPT* codes)
- Review of external notes from 1 unique source and order or review results of 1 unique test

The following examples illustrate different levels of data to be reviewed and analyzed. Can you identify the amount and/or complexity of data to be reviewed in each example?

Examples

➤ **A 12-year-old boy presents with right ear pain.** On the basis of history and examination, swimmers ear of the right ear is diagnosed.

    Level of data reviewed and analyzed ⅢⅢ➡ *Minimal or none*

➤ **A 16-year-old established patient presents for follow-up of upper respiratory tract (URTI) symptoms.** The patient was evaluated at an urgent care practice 2 days ago, but symptoms have increased. The physician reviews records of the urgent care visit that include a diagnosis of an URTI. An influenza test is ordered and its results positive.

    Level of data reviewed and analyzed ⅢⅢ➡ *Limited*

    Teaching Point: The combination of a review of external records from 1 source and an order for 1 test supports a limited amount and complexity of data to be reviewed and analyzed. If an independent historian were required in addition to the external records reviewed and test ordered, the level of data would be moderate.

> **External records, communications, and/or test results are those from an external physician, qualified health care professional, facility, or health care organization.** *Review of all materials from any unique source counts once toward medical decision-making.*

➤ **A 6-year-old patient presents with a laceration of the thumb.** The patient's mother notes concern that the wound bled until pressure was held for several minutes. After evaluating the laceration, a pediatric nurse practitioner cleanses and bandages the wound.

    Level of data reviewed and analyzed ⅢⅢ➡ *Limited*

    Teaching Point: Data are limited on the basis of assessment requiring an independent historian.

● indicates a new code; ▲, revised; #, re-sequenced; ✚, add-on; ★, audiovisual technology; and ◀, synchronous interactive audio.

Table 6-2. Defining Data Required by Level of Medical Decision-making

Limited *(Must meet the requirements of 1 of the 2 categories)*	**Category 1: Tests and documents** Any combination of 2 from the following data: Review of prior external note(s) from each unique source[a] Review of the result(s) of each unique test[a] Ordering of each unique test[a]
	Category 2: Assessment requiring an independent historian(s)
Moderate *(Must meet the requirements of 1 out of 3 categories)*	**Category 1: Tests, documents, or independent historian(s)** Any combination of 3 from the following data: Review of prior external note(s) from each unique source[a] Review of the result(s) of each unique test[a] Ordering of each unique test[a] Assessment requiring an independent historian(s)
	Category 2: Independent interpretation of tests performed by another physician/other QHP (not separately reported)
	Category 3: Discussion of management or test interpretation with external physician/other QHP/ appropriate source (not separately reported)
Extensive *(Must meet the requirements of at least 2 out of 3 categories)*	**Category 1: Tests, documents, or independent historian(s)** Any combination of 3 from the following data: Review of prior external note(s) from each unique source[a] Review of the result(s) of each unique test[a] Ordering of each unique test[a] Assessment requiring an independent historian(s)
	Category 2: Independent interpretation of tests performed by another physician/other QHP (not separately reported)
	Category 3: Discussion of management or test interpretation with external physician/other QHP/ appropriate source (not separately reported)

Abbreviation: QHP, qualified health care professional.

[a] Each unique test, order, or document is counted.

An independent historian is an individual (eg, parent, guardian, surrogate, witness) who provides a history in addition to one provided by a patient who is unable to provide it completely or reliably (eg, because of developmental stage or loss of consciousness) or because a confirmatory history is judged to be necessary.

If there may be conflict or poor communication between multiple historians and more than one historian is needed, the independent historian(s) requirement is met.

➤ **An established patient presents for follow-up of persistent headaches and fatigue.** Results of tests ordered at the previous visit were reviewed between visits, and 2 additional tests were ordered and completed before this visit. The physician reviews the results of the additional tests and discusses the findings and treatment recommendation with the patient and parents.

  Level of data reviewed and analyzed ⫸ *Limited*

  Teaching Point: The review of 2 unique test results supports a limited level of data to be reviewed and analyzed. The level of MDM for this encounter may be low, moderate, or complex depending on the nature of the problem addressed (eg, undiagnosed new problem with uncertain prognosis) and the risk of morbidity from additional diagnostic testing or treatment.

● indicates a new code; ▲, revised; #, re-sequenced; ✚, add-on; ★, audiovisual technology; and ◄, synchronous interactive audio.

When tests are ordered *between encounters,* the new test results are counted toward the level of data reviewed and analyzed. Review of results of tests ordered at a prior evaluation and management service are included in the order and not counted again at the next encounter.

➤ **A 5-month-old boy presents with suspected viral bronchiolitis.** Parents provide the patient's medical, family, and social history. Respiratory viral panel, basic metabolic panel, complete blood cell count, and chest radiography are ordered.

    Level of data reviewed and analyzed ᵢᵢᵢ➡ *Moderate*

    Teaching Point: A moderate level of data may be supported by any combination of 3 of the following data: review of prior external note(s) from each unique source, order or review of the result(s) of each unique test, or assessment requiring an independent historian(s). In this example, the patient's parents are independent historians and the physician orders 4 unique tests.

Tests include imaging, laboratory, psychometric, or physiological data. A clinical laboratory panel (eg, basic metabolic panel [80047]) is a single test because it is reported with one *Current Procedural Terminology* (*CPT*) code. The differentiation between single or multiple unique tests is defined in accordance with the *CPT* code assignment. *Pulse oximetry is not counted as a test ordered or reviewed for the purpose of medical decision-making.*

Tests considered but not ordered or performed after shared decision-making with the patient/caregivers may be counted toward the amount and complexity of data. Shared decision-making includes soliciting preferences, providing education, and explaining risks and benefits associated with testing.

➤ **A patient is seen by her attending physician for subsequent observation care following an observation admission the previous evening for a head injury.** She was admitted to observation because of recurrent vomiting and confusion and a working diagnosis of postconcussion syndrome. She is now also experiencing a severe headache with nausea. The attending physician discusses the case with a consultant and orders computed tomography and additional nonnarcotic pain medications.

    Level of data reviewed and analyzed ᵢᵢᵢ➡ *Moderate*

    Teaching Point: A moderate level of data may be supported by discussion of management or test interpretation with an external physician, other QHP, or other appropriate source when the discussion is not separately reported (eg, not reported as an interprofessional consultation).

External physicians or other qualified health care professionals (QHPs) are individuals who are not in the same group practice or are of a different specialty or subspecialty, including licensed professionals who are practicing independently. A facility or organizational provider such as a hospital, nursing facility, or home health care agency may also be an independent source.

Professionals who are not in health care but may be involved in the treatment of the patient are appropriate sources. Examples include lawyers, case managers, nonclinical social workers, or teachers. *Family or informal caregivers are inappropriate sources,* although they may be independent historians.

Discussion requires all the following components: is an interactive and direct exchange between the reporting individual and external physician, QHP, or other appropriate source; may be asynchronous but completed within a short period; and is used in medical decision-making for the encounter. Sending medical record notes or a written exchange within medical record notes is not an interactive exchange.

➤ **A 15-year-old established patient presents for follow-up of type 1 diabetes with history of poor control.** The physician reviews results of 2 tests performed on the basis of a recurring order from a prior visit (eg, testing repeated 1 week before each visit). Parents provide the patient's medical, family, and social history since the previous visit.

    Level of data reviewed and analyzed ᵢᵢᵢ➡ *Moderate (3 items in Category 1)*

    Teaching Point: The review of 2 unique test results and use of an independent historian support a moderate amount and complexity of data. With a recurring order, each new result, after the initial result that is included in the order, may be counted toward the level of data reviewed and analyzed in the visit in which it is analyzed. For example, an order for a blood glucose test to be performed every 2 months includes review of the initial test result, but results of future blood glucose tests would count in the encounter at which the result is used in patient management.

● indicates a new code; ▲, revised; #, re-sequenced; ✚, add-on; ★, audiovisual technology; and ◀, synchronous interactive audio.

> **Comparison of multiple results of the same unique test (eg, a new blood glucose test result is compared with previous results) is counted as review of 1 unique test result.**

➤ **A 6-year-old new patient presents with fever, cough, and vomiting for 2 days.** The parents provide history of fever that was as high as 102°F (39°C) and vomiting that may be associated with coughing. Chest radiography and an influenza test are ordered. The physician independently reviews the chest radiograph (pending receipt of the radiologist's report).

    Level of data reviewed and analyzed ⫸ *Extensive*

    Teaching Point: An extensive level of data is based on meeting the requirements of categories 1 and 2. Category 1 is met with orders for 2 unique tests and an assessment requiring an independent historian. Category 2 is met by independent interpretation of a test reported by another physician or QHP.

> **Independent interpretation is the interpretation of a test for which there is a *Current Procedural Terminology* code and an interpretation or report is customary. This does not apply when the same physician or qualified health care professional (QHP) (or physician or QHP of the same group practice and same specialty) is providing or has previously provided an interpretation and report for the test.**
>
> **An interpretation should be documented but need not conform to the usual standards of a complete report for the test (ie, notation of pertinent findings from review of an image or a tracing is sufficient, rather than the typical documentation completed when providing and billing for an interpretation and report).**

Both independent interpretation of a test and discussion of the test result with the interpreting physician can be counted when both are performed for the same encounter.

➤ **A 6-year-old new patient presents with fever, cough, and vomiting for 2 days.** The patient is accompanied by her grandmother, who asks that the child's mother provide history by telephone. The mother speaks with the physician providing history of fever that was as high as 102°F (39°C) and vomiting that is associated with coughing. Chest radiography and combined respiratory virus multiplex testing are ordered. Later that day, the physician independently reviews the chest radiograph via electronic health exchange (pending receipt of the radiologist's report) and calls the parents by telephone with the results.

    Level of data reviewed and analyzed ⫸ *Extensive*

    Teaching Point: The extensive level of data reviewed and analyzed is based on 2 unique tests ordered, assessment requiring an independent historian, and independent interpretation of a test by a physician not reporting a code for the interpretation and report of the findings.

> **The independent history does not need to be obtained in person but does need to be obtained directly from the historian providing the independent information.**

Risk of Complications and/or Morbidity or Mortality of Patient Management

Risk is the probability and/or consequences of an event. For the purpose of code selection, the level of risk considers the risk of morbidity from additional diagnostic testing or treatment. Risk also includes MDM related to the need to initiate or forego further testing, treatment, and/or hospitalization.

> **Morbidity is a state of illness or functional impairment that is expected to be of substantial duration during which function is limited, quality of life is impaired, or organ damage may not be transient despite treatment.**

The risk of patient management criteria applies to the reporting physician's or QHP's patient management decisions associated with the diagnostic procedure(s) and treatment(s) during the reported encounter. *Although condition risk and management risk may often correlate, the risk from the condition is distinct from the risk of the management.*

● Definitions of risk are based on the usual behavior and thought processes of a physician or QHP in the same specialty.

- Trained clinicians apply common meanings to terms such as *high, medium, low,* or *minimal risk* and do not require quantification for these definitions (quantification may be provided when evidence-based medicine has established probabilities).

> *Current Procedural Terminology* does not include examples of minimal or low risk. Coders should seek guidance from a physician or qualified health care professional if unsure of the risk associated with a treatment or management option. For example, a decision to use an over-the-counter medication for a patient who is younger than the age indicated on the product label may carry higher risk than a decision to use it in a patient who is within the indicated age range.

- Assessment of the level of risk is affected by the nature of the event under consideration. For example, a low probability of death may be high risk, whereas a high chance of a minor, self-limited adverse effect of treatment may be low risk. *Social determinants of health may also influence the risk of morbidity.*

> Social determinants of health are economic and social conditions that influence the health of people and communities. Examples may include food or housing insecurity.

- Risk includes the possible management options selected, and those considered but not selected, after shared decision-making with the patient and/or family. For example, a decision about hospitalization includes consideration of alternative levels of care.

> Shared decision-making is soliciting patient and/or family preferences and patient and/or family education and explaining risks and benefits of management options.

Risk levels are minimal, low, moderate, and high. **Table 6-3** exemplifies each level of risk.

Risk of Surgery

> In determining risk associated with a decision about surgery, the surgical package classification does not determine whether the procedure is minor or major. *Current Procedural Terminology* states that the classification of surgery into minor or major is based on the common meaning of such terms when used by trained clinicians. Risk factors are those relevant to the patient and the procedure.

Table 6-3. Examples of Levels of Risk[a]	
Minimal	Rest and plenty of fluids Diaper ointment Superficial wound dressing
Low	Over-the-counter medication(s) following directions as labeled Removal of sutures Physical, language, or occupational therapy
Moderate	Prescription drug management or recommendation for off-label use of an over-the-counter medication Decision about minor surgery with identified patient or procedure risk factors Decision about elective major surgery without identified patient or procedure risk factors Diagnosis or treatment significantly limited by social determinants of health
High	Drug therapy requiring intensive monitoring for toxicity (monitoring for a cytopenia in the use of an antineoplastic agent between dose cycles) Decision about hospitalization or escalation of hospital-level care Decision about emergency major surgery (immediately performed or minimally delayed to allow for patient stabilization) Decision not to resuscitate or to de-escalate care because of poor prognosis Parenteral controlled substances

[a] Examples are subject to clinical judgment for each individual patient and encounter.

The following examples provide information to identify a level of risk of management or treatment decisions made at an encounter. Can you identify the level of risk for each example?

Examples

➤ **A patient presents for follow-up after treatment of impetigo.** The patient appears well and the parents have no concerns but need clearance to return to child care. Clearance to return to child care is provided. The patient is to return as needed or at the next scheduled preventive visit.
   Risk ||||➤ *Minimal to none*

➤ **A 6-year-old boy presents with several days of increasing sneezing, itchy eyes, and fatigue.** After examination, a pediatrician recommends daily use of a nonprescription allergy medication.
   Risk ||||➤ *Low*

➤ **A physician sees a 6-year-old patient who presents with an injury to their left leg.** A fracture is diagnosed, and repair under general anesthesia is recommended. The parents agree to proceed with the procedure.
   Risk ||||➤ *Moderate*
   Teaching Point: Decision for major surgery supports moderate risk.

➤ **A 14-year-old presents for follow-up of asthma.** The patient's asthma is well controlled, and a refill of control medication is prescribed.
   Risk ||||➤ *Moderate*
   Teaching Point: The prescription medication presents a moderate risk.

➤ **A 6-year-old patient is observed for ongoing management of influenzalike illness.** After examination, the pediatrician recommends inpatient hospitalization for management of increasing symptoms.
   Risk ||||➤ *High*
   Teaching Point: The risk associated with the decision to hospitalize the ill child is high. A decision for aggressive outpatient follow-up may also support high risk.

Selection of Codes Based on MDM

To select a code for E/M services based on MDM, you must determine which code is supported by 2 of 3 elements of MDM or the physician's or QHP's total time on the date of service. Refer to **Table 6-4** for an at-a-glance reminder of the levels of MDM.

	Table 6-4. Medical Decision-making Requirements		
	Medical Decision-making (2 of 3 Required: Data,[a] Problems, Risk)		
Level of MDM	**Problems Addressed**	**Data Reviewed and Analyzed[b]**	**Risk**
Straightforward	1 self-limited or minor	Minimal or none	Minimal *Examples* • Rest and plenty of fluids • Diaper ointment • Superficial wound dressing

	Table 6-4 (*continued*)		
	Medical Decision-making (2 of 3 Required: Data,[a] Problems, Risk)		
Level of MDM	**Problems Addressed**	**Data Reviewed and Analyzed[b]**	**Risk**
Low	Low—*Any 1 of* ≥2 self-limited or minor 1 stable chronic illness 1 acute, uncomplicated illness or injury 1 stable acute illness 1 acute, uncomplicated illness or injury requiring hospital inpatient or observation level of care	Limited (*Meet 1 of 2 categories*) Category 1: Tests and documents (*Any 2*) • Review of prior external note(s)—each unique source • Review of the result(s) of each unique test • Ordering of each unique test Category 2: Assessment requiring an independent historian(s)	Low *Examples* • Over-the-counter medication(s) • Removal of sutures • Physical, language, or occupational therapy
Moderate	Moderate—*Any 1 of* ≥1 chronic illness with exacerbation, progression, or side effects of treatment ≥2 stable chronic illnesses 1 undiagnosed new problem with uncertain prognosis 1 acute illness with systemic symptoms 1 acute, complicated injury	Moderate (*Meet 1 out of 3 categories*) Category 1 (*Meet any 3*) • Review of prior external note(s)—each unique source • Review of the result(s) of each unique test • Ordering each unique test • Assessment requiring an independent historian(s) Category 2: Independent interpretation of a test performed by another physician/other QHP[b] Category 3: Discussion of management or test interpretation with external physician/other QHP/appropriate source[b]	Moderate *Examples* • Prescription drug management or off-label use of over-the-counter medication • Decision about minor surgery with identified patient or procedure risk factors • Decision about elective major surgery without identified patient or procedure risk factors • Diagnosis or treatment significantly limited by social determinants of health
High	High—*1 of* ≥1 chronic illness with severe exacerbation, progression, or side effects of treatment 1 acute or chronic illness or injury that poses a threat to life or bodily function	Extensive (*Meet 2 out of 3 categories*) Category 1: (*Meet any 3*) • Review of prior external note(s) from each unique source • Review of the result(s) of each unique test • Ordering of each unique test • Assessment requiring an independent historian(s) Category 2: Independent interpretation of a test performed by another physician/other QHP[b] Category 3: Discussion of management or test interpretation with external physician/other QHP/appropriate source[b]	High *Examples* • Drug therapy requiring intensive monitoring for toxicity • Decision about hospitalization or escalation of hospital level of care • Decision about elective major surgery with identified patient or procedure risk factors • Decision about emergency major surgery • Decision not to resuscitate or to de-escalate care because of poor prognosis • Parenteral controlled substance

Abbreviation: QHP, qualified health care professional.

[a] Each unique test, order, or document contributes to the combination of 2 or combination of 3 in Category 1.

[b] Do not count data review or communications reported with other codes (eg, test interpretation, interprofessional consultation).

Following are key points to remember in code selection:

- Examples given are not clinical recommendations, and levels of service supported may vary on the basis of documentation and patient age and presentation (eg, patient's immunization status).
- Select a code *based on either* total physician/QHP time on the date of service or MDM.
- Use of new versus established patient codes is based on whether the patient has received any face-to-face professional service from the same physician or a physician in the same group practice of the same exact specialty and subspecialty in the 3 years before the date of service.

Chapter 6. Evaluation and Management Documentation Guidelines

- Use of initial versus subsequent care codes is based on whether the patient has received any professional services from the physician or QHP or another physician or QHP of the exact same specialty and subspecialty who belongs to the same group practice during the current inpatient or observation or nursing facility admission/stay.
- When selecting a code level based on MDM as described by *CPT*, the documentation should include the medically appropriate history and examination findings and all problems, diagnoses, management, and treatment options considered.

The following examples provide information sufficient to select a level of service based on the level of MDM. The actual code assigned will vary on the basis of the site of service. Can you identify the level of MDM in each example?

Examples

➤ **A patient encounter includes instruction to keep an uninfected bug bite clean and use an over-the-counter product as labeled to reduce itching.** No tests are ordered, and no results are reviewed. History is obtained from the patient's mother because of the patient's developmental status.

    Problem(s) addressed ⟶ *Minimal—self-limited problem*

    Data reviewed and/or analyzed ⟶ *Limited—independent historian*

    Risk of patient management ⟶ *Minimal—use of over-the-counter medication as labeled*

    Teaching Point: The level of MDM is straightforward. Although the amount and/or complexity of data to be reviewed and analyzed could support a low level of MDM, 2 of 3 elements must be met to support a level of MDM. The problems and risk at this encounter limit the level of MDM to straightforward.

➤ **A patient encounter includes addressing stable type 1 diabetes with history from parents, orders for and review of results for 2 unique tests (eg, hemoglobin A₁c test and urinalysis), and renewal of prescription of insulin.**

    Problem(s) addressed ⟶ *Low—single stable chronic illness*

    Data reviewed and/or analyzed ⟶ *Moderate—independent historian and order/review of 2 tests*

    Risk of patient management ⟶ *Moderate—prescription drug management*

    Teaching Point: The level of MDM is moderate because both data reviewed and risk support this level of service.

➤ **A patient who was admitted for observation of bronchiolitis and dehydration is reevaluated and found to be hypoxic despite treatment. The physician consults a subspecialist for advice on management and transfers the patient to inpatient status.**

    Problem(s) addressed ⟶ *High—1 acute or chronic illness or injury that poses a threat to life or bodily function*

    Data reviewed and/or analyzed ⟶ *Moderate—discussion of management or test interpretation with external physician/other QHP/appropriate source*

    Risk of patient management ⟶ *High—decision regarding hospitalization or escalation of hospital-level care*

    Teaching Point: The level of MDM is high on the basis of the problem addressed and the risk. (The data to be reviewed and/or analyzed could also be high in this example, but 2 of 3 elements are sufficient to support the level of MDM.)

Please see other chapters discussing specific types of E/M services for more examples. For a quick reference to E/M coding, see the American Academy of Pediatrics (AAP) *Pediatric Evaluation and Management: Coding Quick Reference Card 2023* (https://shop.aap.org/pediatric-evaluation-and-management-coding-quick-reference-card-2023).

Teaching Physician Guidelines for Reporting E/M Services

Refer to Chapter 19 for the teaching physician guidelines for billing surgical, high-risk, or other complex procedures.

- Payment is made when a teaching physician involves a resident in providing care only if the teaching physician is present for the key or critical portions of the service, including the portion that is used to select the level of service reported.

● indicates a new code; ▲, revised; #, re-sequenced; ✚, add-on; ★, audiovisual technology; and ◄, synchronous interactive audio.

For residency training sites of a teaching setting that are rural (outside a metropolitan statistical area), the Centers for Medicare & Medicaid Services expanded the teaching physician regulations to allow a teaching physician to use real-time audiovisual communication to interact with the resident to meet the requirement of being present for the key portion of the service, including telehealth services. This provision does not allow use of audio-only (eg, telephone) communication, and the communication must be real-time to allow the teaching physician to observe the resident providing the service.

- The level of service billed will be dependent on the level of work performed and documented by the resident and the teaching physician in combination or by the teaching physician if seen independent of the resident.
- The teaching physician, resident, or nurse must document that they were physically present (ie, in the same room as the patient) during the key or critical portions of the service performed by the resident and participated in the management of the patient. The selected key or critical portion of the visit is at the discretion of the physician.
  - Medicare requires that modifier **GC** (service performed in part by a resident under the direction of a teaching physician) be reported for each service, unless the service is furnished under the primary care exception (reported with modifier **GE**). Other payers may or may not require a modifier.
- Only the teaching physician's total time is counted when total time is used to determine the E/M visit level, not including the time spent by the resident furnishing care without the presence of the teaching physician.
  - Only time spent by the teaching physician performing qualifying activities listed by *CPT* (with or without direct patient contact on the date of the encounter), including time the teaching physician is present when the resident is performing those activities, may be counted in selecting a level of service. This excludes teaching time that is general and not limited to discussion required for the treatment of a specific patient.
- The teaching physician must document the key or critical part of the service personally performed, link their documentation back to the resident's note, and document that the care plan was reviewed and approved. It is not necessary to repeat the resident's documentation.

When a resident admits a patient to the hospital without the teaching physician present and the teaching physician sees the patient later, including on the next day, the teaching physician's date of service is the day they saw the patient. The code reported is based on their personal work of obtaining a history, performing a physical examination, and participating in medical decision-making regardless of whether the combination of the teaching physician's and resident's documentation satisfies criteria for a higher level of service. For payment, the composite of the teaching physician's entry and the resident's entry must support the medical necessity of the billed service and the level of the service billed by the teaching physician.

- The teaching physician documentation must be linked to the resident's note and all exceptions to the resident's findings must be documented. A signature alone is not acceptable documentation.
- Medicare guidelines stipulate that when documenting in an EHR, the teaching physician may use a macro (eg, predetermined text) as the required personal documentation if it is personally entered by the teaching physician. The resident or teaching physician must enter customized information to support medical necessity. If the resident and teaching physician use only macros, the documentation is not sufficient. See **Table 6-5** for minimal documentation required.

Table 6-5. Unacceptable and Minimal Acceptable Documentation Required by a Teaching Physician

Unacceptable	**Minimal Acceptable Documentation Required** *Substitute the resident's name for Dr Resident.*
Countersignature	"I performed a history and physical exam of the patient. Findings are consistent with Dr Resident's note. Discussed patient's management with Dr Resident and agree with the documented findings and plan of care." Signature
"Agree with above." Signature **"Rounded, reviewed, agree." Signature**	"I saw and evaluated the patient. I agree with the findings and plan of care as documented in Dr Resident's note." Signature
"Patient seen with resident and evaluated." Signature **"Seen and agree." Signature**	"I saw the patient with Dr Resident and agree with Dr Resident's findings and plans as written." Signature
"Discussed with resident." Signature	"I was present with Dr Resident during the history and exam. I discussed the case with Dr Resident and agree with the findings and plan as documented in Dr Resident's note." Signature

● indicates a new code; ▲, revised; #, re-sequenced; ✚, add-on; ★, audiovisual technology; and ◀, synchronous interactive audio.

Examples

➤ **A resident admits a patient at 11:30 pm.** The teaching physician's initial visit is performed the following morning at 8:00 am. The teaching physician documents, "I saw and evaluated the patient. Discussed with resident and agree with the findings and plan as documented in Dr Resident's note except as per my addendum and edits within Dr Resident's note." *Note:* Edits should be distinguishable in the note.

  The teaching physician reports an initial hospital care service based on the work personally performed that morning.

➤ **The teaching physician sees the same patient for follow-up inpatient care subsequent to the resident's visit.** The teaching physician documents, "I saw and evaluated the patient. Discussed with Dr Resident and agree with Dr Resident's findings and plan as documented in the resident's note."

➤ **The teaching physician and resident jointly admit on the same patient.** The teaching physician documents, "I was present with Dr Resident during the history and exam. I discussed the case with Dr Resident and agree with the findings and plan as documented in Dr Resident's note."

➤ **The teaching physician and resident jointly provide a subsequent hospital visit.** The teaching physician documents, "I saw the patient with the resident and agree with Dr Resident's findings and plan."

Medical Student Documentation

- Any contribution and participation of a student to the performance of a billable service (other than obtaining history, which is not separately billable but is taken as part of an E/M service) must be performed in the physical presence of a teaching physician or a resident in a service meeting the requirements set forth in this section for teaching physician billing.
- Students may document services in the medical record. However
  - The teaching physician must verify in the medical record all student documentation or findings, including history, physical examination, and/or MDM.
  - The teaching physician must personally perform (or re-perform) the physical examination and MDM activities of the E/M service being billed but may verify any student documentation in the medical record, rather than re-documenting this work.

Primary Care Exception Rule

The primary care exception rule (PCER) in the teaching physician guidelines allows teaching physicians to bill for services provided by residents under their supervision who have completed at least 6 months of approved graduate medical education (GME).

- To qualify for this exception, services must be provided in a teaching hospital or ambulatory care entity. If the services are provided outside a hospital, there must be a written agreement with the teaching hospital that includes a contract outlining the payment for the teaching services or written documentation that the services will be "donated." In general, this exception cannot be applied in a private physician's office or patient's home.
- Preventive medicine visit codes are not included in the Medicare exception at this time. Some Medicaid programs have granted the exemption for preventive medicine services to established patients.
- No more than 4 residents can be supervised at a time by a teaching physician. This may include residents with less than 6 months in a GME-approved residency program in the mix of 4 residents under the teaching physician's supervision. However, the teaching physician must be physically present for the critical or key portions of services furnished by the resident with less than 6 months in a GME-approved residency program. That is, the primary care exception does not apply in the case of the resident with less than 6 months in a GME-approved residency program.
- Patients seen should consider this practice as their primary location for health care.
- The teaching physician
  - Must be physically present in the clinic or office and immediately available to the residents and may not have other responsibilities (including supervising other personnel or seeing patients).

— Must review the care provided (ie, history, findings on physical examination, assessment, and treatment plan) during or immediately after each visit. The documentation must reflect the teaching physician's participation in the review and direction of the services performed.

Example

➤ **The teaching physician is supervising a second-year resident in the clinic under the PCER.** An established patient is diagnosed with acute otitis media.

Unacceptable	Acceptable
Countersignature	"I reviewed Dr Resident's note and agree with Dr Resident's findings and plans as written." Signature "I reviewed Dr Resident's note and agree but will refer to ENT for consultation." Signature

● May only report codes **99202** and **99203** for new patient visits or **99211–99213** for established patient visits. If a higher-level E/M service is necessary and performed, the teaching physician must personally participate in the care of the patient as outlined in the guidelines.

> Evaluation and management code selection is based only on medical decision-making and not on total time when the service is provided under the primary care exception rule.

● Modifier **GE** (service performed by a resident without the presence of a teaching physician under the primary care exception) may be required by a payer that follows Medicare guidelines for teaching physician services.

The AAP continues to advocate for the preventive medicine service codes (99381–99385 and 99391–99395) to be included under the PCER. In some instances, Medicaid plans already consider preventive medicine service codes as part of their primary care exception, so be sure to check with your payers. Look for updates in the AAP Pediatric Coding Newsletter™.

You can access the updated guidelines addressing the PCER at www.aap.org/cfp2023 or Chapter 12, Section 100.1.1c, of the Medicare Claims Processing Manual *(www.cms.gov/Regulations-and-Guidance/Guidance/Manuals/Downloads/clm104c12.pdf).*

To test your knowledge of the information presented in this chapter, complete the quiz found at the end of it, after the resources. Add to your knowledge through the information provided in other chapters that discuss specific categories of E/M service.

Chapter Takeaways

Readers of this chapter should generally understand the *CPT* E/M guidelines and the CMS teaching physician rules. Following are takeaways from this chapter:

● *CPT* provides general and specific E/M guidelines for many codes and code categories. It is important to recognize the guidelines that apply to each E/M service.
● When selecting a code based on time, time must be documented. It is important to note the time required in a code descriptor (eg, time range, required minimum time for reporting).
● *CPT* includes definitions of many terms used in selecting a level of MDM as well as key instructions regarding what activities are counted toward MDM versus what ones are reported separately.
● When selecting a code based on MDM, the documentation must support that at least 2 of 3 elements of MDM were met or exceeded.
● Teaching physicians should maintain awareness of guidelines and PCERs published by the CMS.

● indicates a new code; ▲, revised; #, re-sequenced; ✚, add-on; ★, audiovisual technology; and ◄, synchronous interactive audio.

Resources

AAP Coding Assistance and Education

AAP *Pediatric Evaluation and Management: Coding Quick Reference Card 2023* (https://shop.aap.org/pediatric-evaluation-and-management-coding-quick-reference-card-2023)

Teaching Physician and Primary Care Exception

Medicare Claims Processing Manual, Chapter 12, Section 100.1.1c (www.cms.gov/Regulations-and-Guidance/Guidance/Manuals/Downloads/clm104c12.pdf)

Test Your Knowledge!

1. **Which of the following code categories is not selected on the basis of either medical decision-making or total time on the date of the encounter?**
   a. Office and other outpatient evaluation and management
   b. Initial hospital inpatient or observation care
   c. Inpatient consultation
   d. Critical care (hourly)

2. **Which of the following categories of evaluation and management (E/M) codes is selected solely on the basis of medical decision-making (ie, time is not a factor in code selection)?**
   a. Office and other outpatient E/M
   b. Initial hospital inpatient or observation care
   c. Emergency department services
   d. Inpatient or observation consultation

3. **Which of the following times is not included in a physician's or other qualified health care professional's total time on the date of an encounter?**
   a. Face-to-face time spent obtaining history and performing an examination
   b. Time spent in communication with other health care professionals regarding the patient's care
   c. Time spent documenting the evaluation and management service provided
   d. Time of clinical staff who obtained history and vital signs

4. **Which of the following elements would support a moderate level of medical decision-making?**
   a. Low number and complexity of problems, limited data, and high risk
   b. Low number and complexity of problems, moderate data, and moderate risk
   c. Moderate number and complexity of problems, moderate data, and moderate risk
   d. b and c

5. **Which of the following circumstances meets the requirements for a teaching physician's observation of the key portion of an evaluation and management service provided by a resident in a rural location?**
   a. Presence via real-time audiovisual technology
   b. Presence via audio-only communication technology
   c. Presence via interactive exchange of messages
   d. Presence during medical record review

● indicates a new code; ▲, revised; #, re-sequenced; ✚, add-on; ★, audiovisual technology; and ◀, synchronous interactive audio.

Part 2
Primarily for the Office and Other Outpatient Settings

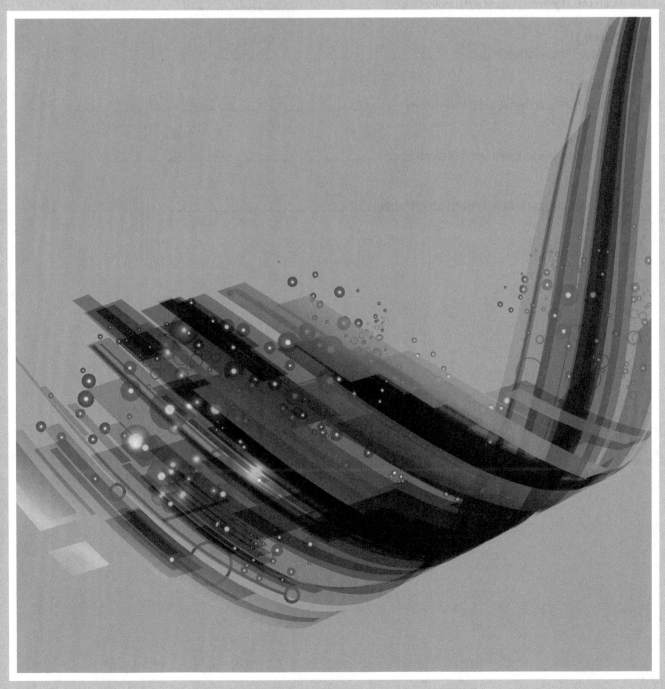

Part 2. Primarily for the Office and Other Outpatient Settings

CHAPTER 7

‖‖‖‖‖

Non-preventive Evaluation and Management Services in Outpatient Settings

‖‖‖‖‖

CPT copyright 2022 American Medical Association. All rights reserved.

Contents

● indicates a new code; ▲, revised; #, re-sequenced; ✚, add-on; ★, audiovisual technology; and ◀, synchronous interactive audio.

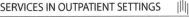

Chapter Highlights

- Select the appropriate codes on the basis of outpatient site of service.
- Distinguish new and established patients, when applicable.
- Use time in code selection for outpatient evaluation and management (E/M) services.
- Select codes based on medical decision-making (MDM).

Outpatient Evaluation and Management (E/M) Codes

This chapter provides information on reporting problem-oriented E/M services when provided in outpatient settings. These codes are reported for most non-preventive E/M services in pediatric outpatient settings and urgent care facilities.

For information on non–face-to-face or indirect E/M services (eg, telephone, online digital, care management services), see **chapters 9 and 10**.

> For services provided in a nursing facility, psychiatric residential treatment facility, or intermediate care facility for individuals with intellectual disabilities, see "Evaluation and Management Service Coding in Nursing and Residential Treatment Facilities" at www.aap.org/cfp2023.

This chapter provides important details and examples of how MDM and total time on the date of the encounter are used in code selection for the following services:

- Office or other outpatient E/M services (**99202–99205, 99211–99215**)
- Office or other outpatient consultations (**99242–99245**)
- Home or residence services (**99341, 99342; 99344, 99345; 99347–99350**)

Sites of Service and Codes for Outpatient Services

The 2023 edition of *Current Procedural Terminology* (*CPT*®) includes simplified guidelines for outpatient consultations and E/M services provided in a patient's home or domiciliary, as with guidelines previously introduced for office and other outpatient services (**99202–99215**).

Outpatient sites of service for codes discussed in this chapter include the following sites:

- Physician office or clinic, including urgent care clinics
- Private residence
- Temporary lodging or short-term accommodation (eg, hotel, campground, hostel, or cruise ship)
- Assisted living facility
- Group home (that is not licensed as an intermediate care facility for individuals with intellectual disabilities)
- Custodial care facility
- Residential substance abuse treatment facility

E/M Services in Urgent Care Facilities

CPT does not include codes specific to E/M services provided at an urgent care facility. Office E/M codes (**99202–99215**) are typically reported.

The Centers for Medicare & Medicaid Services (CMS) describes an *urgent care facility* as a location, distinct from a hospital emergency department (ED), an office, or a clinic, the purpose of which is to diagnose and treat illness or injury for unscheduled, ambulatory patients seeking immediate medical attention.

- Emergency department codes **99281–99285** are not reported for urgent care E/M services.
- The site of service is differentiated by the place of service code (eg, **20** for urgent care facility; **11** for office).
- Other E/M codes that may be applicable to services in an urgent care facility include
  - After-hours service codes, discussed in the After-hours Services section later in this chapter
  - Healthcare Common Procedure Coding System code **S9088** (services provided in an urgent care center) that may be listed in addition to the codes for other services provided
  - Code **S9083** (global fee urgent care centers) when an urgent care clinic contracts to bill all services under a global fee

Some physician practices operate as a primary care pediatric practice and an urgent care center in the same location but with different tax identification numbers and insurance contracts for each. Physicians should consult a health care attorney for assistance in establishing an urgent care practice and contracting with payers to cover the additional overhead costs often applicable to urgent care (eg, extended staffing, radiology, procedural services).

> It is imperative to know your contractual agreements for coding and billing as an urgent care facility or clinic versus a primary care practice, as rates of payment are typically higher for urgent care facilities and so, too, are patient co-payments. Billing and payment also vary for those urgent care facilities owned by hospitals, and guidance on billing and coding for these locations should be obtained from the compliance officer or other administrative personnel.

Office E/M Guidelines

Please see **Chapter 6** for full guidelines that apply to all E/M services reported on the basis of the level of MDM or total time on the date of the encounter.

New Versus Established Patients

Codes for office and other outpatient E/M services (**99202–99215**) and home or residence services (**99341–99350**) designate new or established patient. Following are the criteria:

- *New patients* have not received a face-to-face professional service from the physician or qualified health care professional (QHP), or any physician or QHP of the same group practice and same exact specialty and subspecialty (eg, primary care, allergist), in the prior 3 years.
- *Established patients* have received, and a claim has been submitted for, any face-to-face professional service (eg, hospital care, immunization with physician counseling) from a physician or QHP of the same group practice and same exact specialty within the past 3 years.

> Telemedicine services (delivered via real-time audiovisual technology) are face-to-face services, even though the physician is present only by audiovisual technology.

Codes for outpatient consultations (**99242–99245**) apply to services provided to a new or an established patient.
- Per *CPT*, a QHP working with a physician(s) and who may report E/M services is considered to be working in the exact same specialty and subspecialty as the physician(s). (Medicare assigns different specialty designations to QHPs and does not consider the specialty of the physician providing supervision when determining whether a patient is new. Medicaid and private plans may follow either *CPT* or Medicare practices.)

Examples

➤ **If a physician of a different specialty is covering for another physician (eg, pediatrician covering for a family physician) and has the first face-to-face contact with the other physician's established patient, the encounter is considered new.**

If a physician is covering for another physician of the same specialty, the patient's encounter is coded as it would have been by the physician who is not available. For example, an established patient for a pediatrician is seen by the on-call pediatrician. The on-call pediatrician should report that patient's service as established.

> Per *Current Procedural Terminology*, if a physician is covering for another physician of the same specialty, the patient's encounter is reported as it would have been by the physician who is not available.

➤ **If the physician has moved to a different location or changed their tax identification number, patients would still be considered established if they were established patients before these changes took place.**

When a new physician joins a group of other pediatricians, patients who follow the physician to the new practice are considered to be established patients to any of the pediatricians in the new practice because the patients were seen by a physician of the same specialty in the group within the past 3 years.

● indicates a new code; ▲, revised; #, re-sequenced; ✦, add-on; ★, audiovisual technology; and ◀, synchronous interactive audio.

➤ When a newborn or child is examined in the hospital (eg, nursery or ED care) and is subsequently examined in the office by the same physician or member of the same group and same specialty, the newborn or child is considered an established patient.

Visits Not Requiring a Physician's or Qualified Health Care Professional's Presence

▲99211   Office or other outpatient visit for the evaluation and management of an established patient that may not require the presence of a physician or other qualified health care professional

Services by clinical staff, such as **99211** visits, are considered incidental to a physician's or QHP's services and are reported under the supervising physician's or QHP's name and National Provider Identifier (NPI). Generally, clinical staff, such as nurses and medical assistants (MAs), are not credentialed with payers and cannot independently provide and report these services.

> Per *Current Procedural Terminology*, a *clinical staff member* is a person working under the supervision of a physician or other qualified health care professional and who is allowed by law, regulation, and facility policy to perform or assist in the performance of a specified professional service but who does not individually report that professional service.

Code **99211**
- Is reported only for established patients
- Is not reported on the same date as an office E/M service by a physician or QHP of the same group practice
- Services are provided on the basis of a physician's or QHP's order
- Is reported for clinical staff assessments and other follow-up care not included in services described by other procedure codes (eg, face-to-face patient education not included in time billed as chronic care management services)
- Does not require the presence of a physician or QHP
- Does not require MDM by a physician or QHP
- Is not a time-based service

Do not report **99211** for non-E/M services such as venipuncture (**36415**, **36416**) or injections (**96372**) or for demonstrating or teaching use of an inhalation device (**94664**). Do not report **99211** in conjunction with administration of immunizations (**90471–90474**) without separate and distinct nursing assessment and management.

> Code 99211 is not typically reported for an encounter solely for clinical staff to obtain a sample for laboratory testing. However, exceptions may have allowed physicians to report 99211 for the work of clinical staff who obtained specimens to test for COVID-19 during the public health emergency. Report 99211 only for specimen collection when a payer has expressly provided guidance to report the code for this purpose.

Examples

➤ **An established patient presents for blood pressure and weight check.**
History: The patient is here per a physician's order for follow-up on weight loss plan for obesity and hypertension. The patient is following the recommended diet and began an exercise program at the local recreation center. The mother states she feels more positive about changing the family's diet and routines now.
Physical assessment: Blood pressure is 118/70 mm Hg, weight is 120 lb (down 7 lb since most recent visit), and body mass index is now at the 88th percentile.
Plan: The patient is encouraged to continue diet and exercise. She is already scheduled to follow up with her physician in 1 month. The patient and parent are instructed to call if there are any concerns before the follow-up visit.
Codes reported are **99211** linked to **I10** (hypertension) and **E66.9** (obesity, unspecified).

➤ **An established patient is provided education on use of self-injectable epinephrine by a nurse.** The supervising physician reports **99211**.

● indicates a new code; ▲, revised; #, re-sequenced; ✚, add-on; ★, audiovisual technology; and ◀, synchronous interactive audio.

➤ **An established patient is seen for evaluation of reaction to a tuberculin test.** An MA assesses the site of the injection and finds no signs of reaction. The supervising physician reports **99211**. Note that code **86580** (skin test; tuberculosis, intradermal) includes the work of administering the purified protein derivative but not the work of evaluating for potential reaction on a later date.

Incident-to Requirements: Services Provided Under Physician Supervision

> Incident-to provisions apply only in the office or other outpatient setting where the reporting physician or qualified health care professional is responsible for the practice expense of providing services (eg, labor costs for clinical and support staff, supplies, and other overhead expenses).

Incident-to policy is used by some payers to allow a physician or QHP to report services in 2 different circumstances.
1. Services that do not include direct care by the ordering physician or QHP (eg, nurse-only visit).
2. Services that include significant work by both a physician and a QHP who might otherwise provide and report the service individually. In a facility setting, this would be a split or shared service, but the Medicare split/shared service policy applies only to services provided in a facility setting (eg, hospital).

It is important to know whether a patient's health plan or other payer has adopted an incident-to policy, as this may affect billing and payment.

For payers who align with Medicare policy, see detailed requirements at www.aap.org/cfp2023 ("Incident-to Services by Nonphysician Professionals and Clinical Staff: Medicare Requirements"). See also Chapter 12, Section 30.6, of the *Medicare Claims Processing Manual,* and Chapter 15, Section 60, of the *Medicare Benefit Policy Manual,* at http://cms.gov/manuals (select "Internet-Only Manuals [IOMs]").

Billing for Services Performed Under Supervision

Under incident-to policy, a physician and QHP may bill under their NPI for services performed by a clinical staff member or a qualified nonphysician health care professional (QNHCP) such as a clinical social worker or pharmacist.

The CMS defines *incident to* as "services incident to the service of a physician or other professional permitted by statute to bill for services incident to their services when those services meet all of the requirements applicable to the benefit."
- Incident-to services are always provided as a continuation of a physician's or QHP's services and do not address new problems (eg, a nursing visit performed at patient or caregiver request and not based on a physician's recommendation is not an incident-to service).
  - A treatment plan or order must be documented by a physician or QHP before provision of services billed incident to a physician or QHP.
- A supervising physician or QHP must be present *in the office suite* and available to assist, as needed, at the time of service.

> Medicare makes an exception by not requiring the physician's presence in the office suite for certain activities of principal or chronic care management and behavioral health integration performed by clinical staff. Private payers may also allow inclusion of time spent by clinical staff without direct supervision when reporting these services.

- The individual providing the incident-to service must be an employee (direct or leased) or contracted to work with the physician practice (ie, paid as a practice expense).

Examples

➤ **A patient returns as directed by a pediatrician for evaluation of a tuberculin test result.** The physician is in the office suite at the time of service. An MA evaluates the site of the injection (placed 48 hours earlier) and notes no reaction (0 mm). The MA instructs the patient to notify the practice if any reaction occurs within the next 24 hours.

Code **99211** (established patient E/M, minimal level, not requiring a physician's presence) is reported for this encounter.

➤ **An MA, as allowed under state scope of practice laws, administers an intranasal influenza vaccine that was ordered and directly supervised by the physician who documented counseling provided to the patient and/or caregivers.** Codes for the vaccine and administration (**90460**, **90672**) are reported under the physician's NPI. If a pediatric nurse practitioner had ordered and supervised the treatment, the service would have been reported under that practitioner's NPI.

Incident-to policy may also allow a physician to report services provided by QHPs and QNHCPs who may otherwise bill for their services under their own NPI when they provide medically necessary services (within their state's scope of practice). The incident-to provision allows for reporting under the name and NPI of a supervising physician when the requirements of incident-to billing are met.

- Nonphysician providers (NPPs) without their own NPIs must report services incident to a physician and must meet all incident-to requirements, including physician presence in the office suite and continuation of a physician's previously established plan of care.
- Payment for QHPs and QNHCPs billing under the incident-to provision may be 100% of the physician payment versus 85% when reporting under the QHP's and QNHCP's individual NPIs.

> Although Medicare and many other payers reduce payment to 85% of the Physician Fee Schedule amount when a qualified health care professional provides a service outside the incident-to requirements (eg, new patient visit), this is not the case for all payers.

- Payers may not allow reporting of a certain service as incident to a physician's service (eg, nutrition therapy) when the service is not included under the contract between the payer and physician.

Example

➤ **A patient returns for follow-up of attention-deficit/hyperactivity disorder (ADHD).** The physician is in the office suite at the time of service, but the appointment was scheduled with a QHP in the same group practice. The QHP evaluates the patient and has concerns about the patient's report of side effects of medication. The QHP consults the patient's physician, who obtains additional history from the patient and decides to change the patient's medication. The QHP and physician each individually document the portion of the E/M service that they independently provided.

The code for the established patient office E/M is selected on the basis of the combined MDM or total time of service spent by the physician and QHP. No time is counted twice; any time that was spent simultaneously by the QHP and physician is counted only once. (Examples discussed in the Application of Time Guidelines section later in this chapter illustrate counting time when a physician and QHP each care for the same patient on the same date.)

Documentation Requirements and Tips When Reporting Incident-to Services

- Physicians and QHPs must document their order for a service or treatment (eg, an injection) that will be performed as incident to or document their plan for a follow-up visit in the treatment plan (eg, follow-up visit within 1 week for a weight check).
- To demonstrate compliant incident-to billing, clinical staff providing services in continuation of a physician's plan of care *should, ideally, reference the date of the physician order for the service.* This may be documented in the chief complaint (primary concern) for the encounter (eg, "Patient is seen today per Dr Green's 1/2/2022 order for dressing change to left arm wound in 3 days").
- Documentation of incident-to services should fully describe the services provided, including date of service, assessment, concerns noted and addressed, details of care provided (eg, wound cleansed and new bandage applied), and education and/or instructions for home care and follow-up.
  - Inclusion of the supervising physician's name also supports that incident-to requirements were met.
  - Medical record documentation must reflect the identity, including credentials and legible or digital signature, of the person providing the service.

For Medicare purposes, the physician or QHP billing the service is not required to sign documentation prepared by the clinical staff. Other payer and state regulations may require authentication by the supervising physician or QHP. Documentation might be as simple as "Service performed/provided under the direct supervision of Dr X." When applicable, the signature must be legible.

● indicates a new code; ▲, revised; #, re-sequenced; ✚, add-on; ★, audiovisual technology; and ◀, synchronous interactive audio.

Code Selection Guidelines for Outpatient E/M Services

For all the outpatient visits discussed in this chapter except **99211**, the level of service is determined by either

- The level of MDM alone
- The total amount of time (face-to-face and non–face-to-face) spent by a pediatrician or other QHP on the date of service directed to care of the patient

See **Box 7-1** for an overview of the key guidelines for code selection.

Box 7-1. Key Office Evaluation and Management Coding Guidelines

History and examination: Code selection is not based on the extent of history and examination. Each service includes a medically appropriate history and/or physical examination, when performed. Information supplied directly by the patient/caregiver or obtained by the care team may be reviewed and expanded on (as necessary) rather than re-documented.

Code selection: Select a code based on either MDM or the pediatrician's or QHP's total time on the date of the visit.

MDM: Four types of MDM are recognized: straightforward, low, moderate, and high.

Determine the level of MDM based on the highest 2 of 3 elements of MDM.

1. Number and complexity of problems addressed. Include problems addressed or managed by the reporting pediatrician/QHP as part of the encounter.
2. Amount and/or complexity of data reviewed and analyzed. Data include
   - Tests, documents, orders, or independent historian(s)
   - Independent interpretation of tests
   - Discussion of management/test interpretation with external physician, QHP, or appropriate source
3. Risk of complications, morbidity, and/or mortality of patient management decisions made at the visit, associated with the patient's problem(s), and the diagnostic procedure(s) or treatment(s), including possible management options selected and those considered but not selected.

Time: May be used to select a code level whether or not counseling and/or coordination of care dominates the service.

- Time includes the total time on the date of the encounter (face-to-face and non–face-to-face) personally spent by the physician and/or QHP focused on the care of 1 patient.
  - Do not include time in activities performed or normally performed by clinical staff (eg, rooming the patient).
  - Do not include travel time (eg, travel to a patient's home or residence).
  - Do not count the same minute/period toward >1 service.
  - When >1 physician or QHP meet with or discuss a patient's care, only 1 individual counts that time toward an E/M service.
  - Time does not need to be continuous. Total all time on 1 date.

- Include the time of the following activities when performed by the reporting physician/QHP:
  - Preparing to see the patient (eg, medical record review)
  - Obtaining and/or reviewing separately obtained history
  - Performing a medically appropriate examination and/or evaluation
  - Counseling and educating the patient, family, or caregiver
  - Ordering medications, tests, or procedures
  - Referring to/communicating with other QHPs (when not separately reported)
  - Documenting clinical information in the medical record
  - Independently interpreting results (when not separately reported) and communicating results to the patient, family, or caregiver
  - Coordinating care (when not separately reported)

Abbreviations: E/M, evaluation and management; MDM, medical decision-making; QHP, qualified health care professional.

● indicates a new code; ▲, revised; #, re-sequenced; ✚, add-on; ★, audiovisual technology; and ◀, synchronous interactive audio.

Application of Time Guidelines

- Time is the physician's and/or QHP's total time on the date of service, not the time in a 24-hour period, directed to the care of the individual patient.
- Both face-to-face and non–face-to-face time spent on the date of service are included in the time of the encounter. **Figure 7-1** illustrates the time included in the physician's or QHP's total time.
- The total time should be documented in the medical record when it is used as the basis for code selection. No specific verbiage is required by *CPT*.

> *Current Procedural Terminology* does not require documentation of each segment of time spent on the date of service or any specific format of documentation. The physician must, however, document the total amount of time spent on the date of the encounter and be able to account for the time spent.

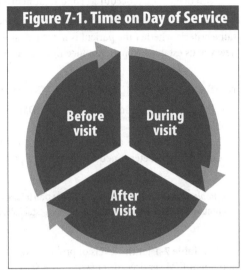

Figure 7-1. Time on Day of Service

Before visit | During visit | After visit

- When selecting a code based on time, it is important to verify the time required for the code selected. Office E/M codes **99202–99215** include a range of time in the descriptor for each code. Codes for outpatient consultations (**99242–99245**) and for home or residence services (**99341–99342**; **99344**, **99345**; **99347–99350**) include a specific time *that must be met or exceeded.* Time for all services discussed in this chapter are provided in **Table 7-1**.

Examples

➤ **A nurse practitioner sees an established patient for a follow-up visit due to parent concerns about the child returning to sports after sustaining a concussion.** Five minutes is spent reviewing the patient medical record and accessing records from the emergency physician's initial management of the injury. History is obtained about the injury and ongoing signs and symptoms that may be related to the injury but have also occurred previously in relation to migraine headaches (10 minutes). The nurse practitioner consults the pediatrician, who joins the practitioner in answering questions and counseling the parents for another 15 minutes. The patient and parents agree to neurological testing before a decision on clearance for sports. The nurse practitioner spends another 10 minutes arranging the testing and documenting the encounter. Total time on the date of the visit is 40 minutes (5 + 10 + 15 + 10).

Code **99215** (40–54 minutes) is reported. Only 15 minutes is counted by 1 individual for the time spent jointly by the pediatrician and the nurse practitioner.

➤ **A physician spends 10 minutes reviewing laboratory results and hospital records before a consultation on the same date.** Later that day, a face-to-face visit with the patient and caregivers lasts 20 minutes. After the visit but on the same date, the physician spends 10 minutes in discussion with the physician who requested the consultation and another 10 minutes in coordination of further treatment and in documentation. The total time on the date of service is 50 minutes.

The physician chooses to report the service based on total time on the date of the consultation service and reports code **99244** (40 minutes must be met or exceeded). If the time on the date of service had met or exceeded 55 minutes, code **99245** would have been reported.

Guidelines for Medical Decision-making

Medical decision-making is the work of establishing diagnoses, assessing the status of a condition, and/or selecting a management option. The level of MDM is determined by assessing the level at which 2 of 3 elements of MDM are supported in the documentation of an encounter. The 3 elements of MDM are

1. The number and complexity of problem(s) that are addressed during the encounter
2. The amount and/or complexity of data to be reviewed and analyzed

3. The risk of complications, morbidity, and/or mortality of patient management decisions made at the visit, associated with diagnostic procedure(s) and treatment(s)

Four types of MDM are recognized: straightforward, low, moderate, and high. Each level of MDM is based on the same criteria whether the patient is new or established. (Time and other factors considered in valuing codes differentiate new versus established patient office E/M services.)

Number and Complexity of Problems Addressed

The first step in determining the level of MDM for an encounter is identification of the number and complexity of problems addressed.

- Include all problems addressed at an encounter in the number and complexity of problems.
- Complexity is determined by the types of problems addressed.

A *problem* is a disease, a condition, an illness, an injury, a symptom, a sign, a finding, a concern, or another matter addressed at the encounter, with or without a diagnosis being established at the time of the encounter.

See **Table 7-1** for the levels of problems in MDM. Expanded discussion of problem types is included in examples of outpatient E/M services, discussed in the Selection of Office and Outpatient E/M Codes section later in this chapter. Use this table to identify the number and complexity of problems in the examples.

The guidelines for office E/M services provide definitions of the types of problems that are typically addressed at these encounters. See the "Coding Conundrum: Addressed or Not Addressed" box in **Chapter 6**.

Amount and/or Complexity of Data to Be Reviewed and Analyzed

Data are divided into the following 3 categories:

1. Tests, documents, orders, or independent historian(s) (Each unique test, order, or document is counted to meet a threshold number.)
2. Independent interpretation of tests that are not separately reported
3. Discussion of management or test interpretation with external physician or other QHP or appropriate source

When data are used in support of low, moderate, or high MDM, the requirements for either 1 or 2 categories of data must be met. For example, Category 1 at the limited level of data is met when a physician orders 2 tests represented by separate *CPT* codes or reviews 1 test result and notes from 1 unique source (eg, hospital records from a recent admission). Instructions are provided for each level of data. Minimal or no data are required for straightforward MDM. **Table 7-1** shows the data requirements for limited, moderate, and extensive data.

A decision to not order a test that was considered is counted as a test ordered when the consideration and reason for not ordering the test are documented. For example, documentation may show that a test was discussed but determined to be unnecessary or that a test that is typically performed is not indicated due to patient risk.

Risk of Complications and/or Morbidity or Mortality of Patient Management

Risk is the probability and/or consequences of an event. For the purpose of code selection, the level of risk takes into consideration the risk of morbidity from additional diagnostic testing or treatment. Risk also includes MDM related to the need to initiate or forego further testing, treatment, and/or hospitalization.

The risk of patient management criteria applies to the patient management decisions made by the reporting physician or other QHP as part of the reported encounter.

Risk levels are minimal, low, moderate, and high. **Table 7-1** provides examples for minimal and low risk that are not included in *CPT* and may vary on the basis of the individual patient presentation.

Table 7-1. Code Selection Requirements for Outpatient Evaluation and Management Service (Excluding 99211)

Level/Codes/Total Time (min)[a]	Medical Decision-making (2 of 3 Required: Data,[b] Problems, Risk)		
	Problems Addressed	**Data Reviewed and Analyzed[c]**	**Risk**
Straightforward *Office* NP **99202** (15–29) EP **99212** (10–19) *Consultation* **99242** (≥20) *Home/residence* NP **99341** (≥15) EP **99347** (≥20)	1 self-limited or minor *Examples* • Mild diaper rash • Cold or mild URTI	Minimal or none	Minimal *Examples* • Rest and plenty of fluids • Diaper ointment • Superficial wound dressing
Low NP **99203** (30–44) EP **99213** (20–29) *Consultation* **99243** (≥30) *Home/residence* NP **99342** (≥30) EP **99348** (≥30)	Low—*Any 1 of* ≥2 self-limited or minor 1 stable chronic illness 1 acute, uncomplicated illness or injury 1 stable acute illness 1 acute, uncomplicated illness or injury requiring hospital inpatient or observation level of care *Examples* • Acute gastroenteritis • Follow-up of stable ADHD • Uncomplicated hand-foot-and-mouth disease • Recheck of wound repaired by other physician/QHP • Resolution of URTI with continued cough	Limited (*Meet 1 of 2 categories*) Category 1: Tests and documents (*Any 2*) • Review of prior external note(s)—each unique source • Review of the result(s) of each unique test • Ordering of each unique test Category 2: Assessment requiring an independent historian(s)	Low *Examples* • Over-the-counter medication(s) • Removal of sutures • Physical, language, or occupational therapy
Moderate NP **99204** (45–59) EP **99214** (30–39) *Consultation* **99244** (≥40) *Home/residence* NP **99344** (≥60) EP **99349** (≥40)	Moderate—*Any 1 of* ≥1 chronic illness with exacerbation, progression, or side effects of treatment ≥2 stable chronic illnesses 1 undiagnosed new problem with uncertain prognosis 1 acute illness with systemic symptoms 1 acute, complicated injury *Examples* • Asthma with respiratory distress but not hypoxia • Stable asthma and stable anxiety disorder • Unexplained bruising • Acute gastroenteritis with dehydration • Intermittent headaches and confusion following concussion	Moderate (*Meet 1 out of 3 categories*) Category 1: Tests and documents (*Meet any 3*) • Review of prior external note(s)—each unique source • Review of the result(s) of each unique test • Ordering each unique test • Assessment requiring an independent historian(s) Category 2: Independent interpretation of a test performed by another physician/other QHP[c] Category 3: Discussion of management or test interpretation with external physician/other QHP/appropriate source	Moderate *Examples* • Prescription drug management or off-label use of over-the-counter medication • Decision about minor surgery with identified patient or procedure risk factors • Decision about elective major surgery without identified patient or procedure risk factors • Diagnosis or treatment significantly limited by social determinants of health

Continued on next page

• indicates a new code; ▲, revised; #, re-sequenced; ✚, add-on; ★, audiovisual technology; and ◀, synchronous interactive audio.

Table 7-1 (*continued*)			
Level/Codes/Total Time (min)ª	**Medical Decision-making (2 of 3 Required: Data,ᵇ Problems, Risk)**		
	Problems Addressed	**Data Reviewed and Analyzedᶜ**	**Risk**
High *NP* **99205** (60–74) *EP* **99215** (40–54) *Consultation* **99245** (≥55) *Home/residence* *NP* **99345** (≥75) *EP* **99350** (≥60)	High—*1 of* ≥1 chronic illness with severe exacerbation, progression, or side effects of treatment 1 acute or chronic illness or injury that poses a threat to life or bodily function *Examples* • Asthma with respiratory distress with hypoxia • Infant with fever, tachycardia, lethargy, and dehydration	Extensive (*Meet 2 out of 3 categories*) Category 1: Tests and documents (*Meet any 3*) • Review of prior external note(s) from each unique source • Review of the result(s) of each unique test • Ordering of each unique test • Assessment requiring an independent historian(s) Category 2: Independent interpretation of a test performed by another physician/other QHP Category 3: Discussion of management or test interpretation with external physician/other QHP/appropriate sourceᶜ	High *Examples* • Drug therapy requiring intensive monitoring for toxicity • Decision about hospitalization or escalation of hospital level of care • Decision about emergency major surgery • Decision not to resuscitate or to de-escalate care because of poor prognosis • Parenteral controlled substance

Abbreviation: ADHD, attention-deficit/hyperactivity disorder; EP, established patient; NP, new patient; QHP, qualified health care professional; URTI, upper respiratory tract infection.

ª Does not include time of clinical staff. Include only time spent by the physician or QHP directed to the individual patient's care on the date of the encounter.

ᵇ Each unique test, order, or document contributes to the combination of 2 or combination of 3 in Category 1.

ᶜ Do not count data review or communications reported with other codes (eg, test interpretation, interprofessional consultation).

Selection of Office and Outpatient E/M Codes

To select a code for an outpatient E/M service, you must determine which code is supported by 2 of 3 elements of MDM or the physician's or QHP's total time on the date of service. Refer to **Table 7-1** for an at-a-glance guide to the levels of MDM or time required for each level of outpatient E/M service.

The following pages provide an overview of a level of office E/M service with time and MDM reporting criteria and examples of each level of service. Following are key points to remember in code selection:

● Examples given are not clinical recommendations and levels of service supported may vary on the basis of documentation and patient age and presentation (eg, ill appearance beyond what is typical for concern).

● Select a code based on either total physician/QHP time on the date of service or MDM.

● The use of new versus established patient codes is based on whether the patient has received any face-to-face professional service from the same physician or a physician in the same group practice of the same exact specialty and subspecialty in the 3 years before the date of service.

● When selecting a code based on time, the total physician and/or QHP time spent devoted to the single patient's care must be documented in addition to the context of the care provided (eg, remarkable findings, counseling, care coordination, shared decision-making).

● When selecting a code level based on MDM, as described by *CPT,* the documentation should include the medically appropriate history and examination findings and all problems, diagnoses, management, and treatment options considered.

The American Academy of Pediatrics *Pediatric Evaluation and Management Coding: Quick Reference Card 2023* **(https://shop.aap.org/ pediatric-evaluation-and-management-coding-quick-reference-card-2023) provides a quick reference for use in selecting evaluation and management codes.**

● indicates a new code; ▲, revised; #, re-sequenced; ✚, add-on; ★, audiovisual technology; and ◀, synchronous interactive audio.

Examples of Code Selection for Office and Other Outpatient E/M Services

Office E/M (99202, 99212)

★**99202**   Office or other outpatient visit for the evaluation and management of a new patient, which requires a medically appropriate history and/or examination and straightforward medical decision making
> When using time for code selection, 15–29 minutes of total time is spent on the date of the encounter.

★**99212**   Office or other outpatient visit for the evaluation and management of an established patient, which requires a medically appropriate history and/or examination and straightforward medical decision making
> When using time for code selection, 10–19 minutes of total time is spent on the date of the encounter.

Example

➤ **A 17-year-old male established patient presents with need for clearance to attend a sports camp.** The patient received a preventive medicine service 3 months before this visit and reports no health concerns at this time. History is unremarkable. After brief examination, a pediatrician clears the patient for participation.

> *Level of problem addressed* ⟫ *Straightforward (request for clearance for participation with no identified problems)*
> *Level of data reviewed and analyzed* ⟫ *Minimal or none*
> *Level of risk of morbidity* ⟫ *Low (decision to clear for participation)*

Teaching Point: Medical decision-making is straightforward because of the number and complexity of problems addressed and because there are minimal or no data to be reviewed and analyzed. Low risk of morbidity, by itself, is insufficient to support a higher level of service.

Had the patient not recently received a recommended preventive medicine service or required additional preventive evaluation, the physician would have likely performed a preventive service in lieu of the sports preparticipation physical evaluation. A sports preparticipation physical evaluation may also represent a higher level of service when the patient has known or newly identified health conditions that must be evaluated before clearance.

> If an evaluation and management service includes history from an independent historian and more than a single self-limited or minor problem, documentation should typically support at least low medical decision-making.

Office E/M (99203, 99213)

★**99203**   Office or other outpatient visit for the evaluation and management of a new patient, which requires a medically appropriate history and/or examination and low level of medical decision making
> When using time for code selection, 30–44 minutes of total time is spent on the date of the encounter.

★**99213**   Office or other outpatient visit for the evaluation and management of an established patient, which requires a medically appropriate history and/or examination and low level of medical decision making
> When using time for code selection, 20–29 minutes of total time is spent on the date of the encounter.

Examples

➤ **An established patient presents for follow-up of mild congenital pulmonary valve stenosis.** The patient and parents have no concerns. The examination and electrocardiogram (ECG; with interpretation and report by the same physician) indicate that the condition remains stable. The child will return for follow-up in 1 year.

> *Level of problem addressed* ⟫ *Low (1 stable chronic illness)*
> *Level of data reviewed and analyzed* ⟫ *Limited (independent historian)*
> *Level of risk of morbidity* ⟫ *Low (return for follow-up in 1 year)*

ICD-10-CM: **Q22.1** (congenital pulmonary valve stenosis)

CPT: **99213** and **93000** (electrocardiogram, routine ECG with at least 12 leads; with interpretation and report) for the separately reportable ECG with interpretation and report by the ordering physician

Teaching Point: Medical decision-making is low because of 1 stable chronic condition addressed, limited data (independent historian), and low risk (return for follow-up in 1 year). The ECG is not counted as a test ordered or reviewed because the physician separately reports the service.

● indicates a new code; ▲, revised; #, re-sequenced; ✚, add-on; ★, audiovisual technology; and ◀, synchronous interactive audio.

➤ **A 5-year-old new patient presents with parental request for antibiotics for an upper respiratory tract infection (URTI).** Extended history is obtained from the child's parents, who state that the child has often required an antibiotic for respiratory infections in the past. The child is in kindergarten, and the parents feel that missing school is not an option. The parents are counseled regarding un-indicated use of antibiotic or over-the counter medication and appropriate home care and infection control precautions for their child. The pediatrician documents a total time of 35 minutes, which includes time spent completing documentation after the visit.

Level of problem addressed ➡ ***Minimal (1 self-limited problem)***
Level of data reviewed and analyzed ➡ ***Limited (independent historians)***
Level of risk of morbidity ➡ ***Moderate (decision against prescription drug management)***
ICD-10-CM: **J06.9** (acute upper respiratory infection, unspecified)
CPT: **99203**

Teaching Point: The total time on the date of the encounter supports code **99203** (30–44 minutes), as does the low level of MDM.

Office E/M (99204, 99214)

★99204 Office or other outpatient visit for the evaluation and management of a new patient, which requires a medically appropriate history and/or examination and moderate level of medical decision making

When using time for code selection, 45–59 minutes of total time is spent on the date of the encounter.

★99214 Office or other outpatient visit for the evaluation and management of an established patient, which requires a medically appropriate history and/or examination and moderate level of medical decision making

When using time for code selection, 30–39 minutes of total time is spent on the date of the encounter.

Examples

➤ **A new patient presents with increasingly symptomatic generalized anxiety disorder.** The patient's father notes that his daughter had previously undergone counseling but has had few symptoms until recently. The patient's mother, who has a long history of illicit drug use, left her home and has not been in contact with her daughter for 6 weeks. The child is not sleeping well and stays with her father rather than plays with friends or visits other relatives. The physician advises that psychiatric counseling be resumed. Although the father agrees, he says that the girl's prior provider has closed her office and the only other psychology practice that accepts the child's health plan is not accepting new patients. The child's father also notes that he does not want the child to be taking anxiety medication. The physician instructs a staff member to contact other providers, seeking an earlier appointment. A rural health care facility that can provide counseling services based on ability to pay has an appointment available in 1 week. The physician provides interim counseling and schedules a follow-up visit in 2 weeks. The physician's total time on the date of the encounter is 40 minutes.

Level of problem addressed ➡ ***Moderate (1 chronic illness that is not stable)***
Level of data reviewed and analyzed ➡ ***Limited (independent historian)***
Level of risk of morbidity ➡ ***Moderate (treatment limited by social determinants of health)***
ICD-10-CM: **F41.9** (anxiety disorder, unspecified), **Z63.32** (other absence of family member), **Z75.3** (unavailability and inaccessibility of health-care facilities)
CPT: **99204**

Teaching Point: Medical decision-making is moderate because of the problem addressed and risk associated with managing the patient's care that is limited by social determinants of health.

➤ **An established patient presents with an itchy rash.** The parents note that the patient developed the rash following a day of playing at a campground. The pediatrician examines the patient and then determines that the rash is poison ivy and provides instruction on home care. However, the child is under-immunized due to the parents' fear of harmful effects of immunization. The pediatrician takes the opportunity to counsel the parents regarding immunization. Twenty minutes are spent in counseling the parents on risks associated with not immunizing their child and how vaccines are produced, tested, and approved. After the parents still refuse immunization at this encounter, the pediatrician requests that the parents sign and date a vaccine refusal form. The pediatrician's total time on the date of service, including documentation after the visit, is 35 minutes.

Level of problem addressed ⟫➡ *Straightforward (self-limited or minor problem)*
Level of data reviewed and analyzed ⟫➡ *Limited (independent historian)*
Level of risk of morbidity ⟫➡ *Low (home care)*
ICD-10-CM: **L23.7** (allergic contact dermatitis due to plants, except food), **Z28.3** (under-immunization), and **Z28.82** (immunization not carried out because of caregiver refusal)

CPT: **99214** is supported by the physician's total time of 35 minutes.

Teaching Point: All the physician's time spent in care of the 1 patient on the date of the encounter is included in the time used to select the level of service for the office visit. There is no requirement that more than 50% of that time be spent in counseling and/or coordination of care.

Office E/M (99205, 99215)

★**99205** Office or other outpatient visit for the evaluation and management of a new patient, which requires a medically appropriate history and/or examination and high level of medical decision making
    When using time for code selection, 60–74 minutes of total time is spent on the date of the encounter.

(For services ≥75 minutes, see prolonged services code **99417**, discussed in the Prolonged Outpatient E/M Service, Physician or Other Qualified Health Care Professional, section later in this chapter.)

★**99215** Office or other outpatient visit for the evaluation and management of an established patient, which requires a medically appropriate history and/or examination and high level of medical decision making
    When using time for code selection, 40–54 minutes of total time is spent on the date of the encounter.

(For services ≥55 minutes, see prolonged services code **99417** discussed in the Prolonged Outpatient E/M Service, Physician or Other Qualified Health Care Professional, section later in this chapter.)

Examples

➤ **A 3-month-old established patient presents to a rural pediatric practice with tachypnea and retraction and is found to have hypoxia.** The diagnosis is bronchiolitis, positive for respiratory syncytial virus (RSV). The infant responds well to administration of oxygen. Because there is no need for a workup to rule out sepsis and the infant is not dehydrated, a decision is made to not refer the patient to the regional medical center but, rather, to provide home oxygen with close monitoring by the physician, including daily visits for reevaluation involving weight and pulse oxygen checks until the infant is weaned off oxygen. The parents are instructed to call the physician directly by phone with any new concerns. Diagnosis is documented as acute RSV bronchiolitis with hypoxemia.

Level of problem addressed ⟫➡ *High (1 acute or chronic illness or injury that poses a threat to life or bodily function)*
Level of data reviewed and analyzed ⟫➡ *Limited (independent historian)*
Level of risk of morbidity ⟫➡ *High (decision regarding hospitalization)*
ICD-10-CM: **J21.0** (acute bronchiolitis due to respiratory syncytial virus), **R09.02** (hypoxemia)

CPT: **99215** is supported by the acute illness that poses a threat to life or bodily function and decision to not hospitalize.

Teaching Point: A decision to hospitalize and a decision to not hospitalize but to closely monitor would each support high risk in this scenario. A limited availability of health care resources may affect MDM by increasing the risk of management.

For the purpose of data reviewed and analyzed, do not count pulse oximetry as a test. Although payers often bundle pulse oximetry to office evaluation and management (E/M) services, in the absence of payer policy that prohibits separate reporting, it is appropriate to report the appropriate pulse oximetry code for single (**94760**) or multiple (**94761**) determinations, when performed. National Correct Coding Initiative edits bundle E/M codes to pulse oximetry, requiring that modifier 25 (significant, separately identifiable E/M service) be appended to the E/M code (eg, **99215 25**).

➤ **A pediatrician reviews records from 3 unique sources for a new patient with complex medical history and later that day sees the patient to develop a plan of care and assists the parents with establishing subspecialty care.**
Prescriptions are reviewed and prescribed, as needed. The physician's total time on the date of the visit is 60 minutes.
Level of problem addressed ▯▯▯➡ *Moderate (assumption of ≥2 chronic illnesses)*
Level of data reviewed and analyzed ▯▯▯➡ *Moderate (review of records from 3 unique sources)*
Level of risk of morbidity ▯▯▯➡ *Moderate (prescription drug management)*
ICD-10-CM: Appropriate codes for the diagnoses addressed at the encounter are reported.
CPT: **99205** is reported on the basis of the physician's total time on the date of the encounter.

Outpatient Consultations (99242–99245)

> Code **99241** has been deleted. To report an outpatient consultation with straightforward medical decision-making, see code **99242**.

CPT defines a consultation as a type of E/M service that is provided at the request of another physician, QHP, or appropriate source to recommend care for a specific condition or problem. Two major factors distinguish consultations from other E/M services.

1. The service is requested by another physician, QHP (eg, nurse practitioner, clinical social worker, or psychologist), or appropriate source (eg, nonclinical social worker, educator, lawyer, insurance company) *to recommend care* for a specific condition or problem. *An E/M service requested by a patient or family member is not a consultation.*
2. The consultant's opinion and any services that were ordered or performed must also be *communicated by written report* to the requesting physician, QHP, or other appropriate source.

The consultant may initiate other services at the time of the consultation or at a subsequent encounter. Follow-up E/M services initiated by the consultant or patient/family are reported as established patient visits on the basis of the site of service (eg, established patient office visit).

Services that constitute transfer of care (ie, that are provided for the management of the patient's entire care or for the care of a specific condition or problem) are reported with the appropriate new or established patient codes for office or other outpatient visits or for home or residence services.

> Services reported with codes **99242–99245** may be provided in an office or other outpatient site, including the home or residence or an emergency department.

When a Payer Does Not Accept Consultation Codes

Not all payers provide payment for services reported with consultation codes. Some payers have implemented policies that require reporting another E/M service code in lieu of consultation codes. The American Academy of Pediatrics (AAP) supports payment for consultation codes as described in its position on Medicare consultation policy (www.aap.org/cfp2023; "AAP Position on Medicare Consultation Policy").

When consultation codes are not accepted, another E/M code reported is based on the site of service and whether the patient is new or established, as shown in **Table 7-2**.

Table 7-2. Coding Consultations Under Medicare Rules	
New Patient	**Established Patient**
99202–99205 (office, outpatient hospital)	99212–99215 (office, outpatient hospital)
99341–99345 (home or residence visit)	99347–99350 (home or residence visit)

When a payer does not accept consultation codes, select the alternative E/M code based on the required level of MDM or the total time on the date of the encounter.

● indicates a new code; ▲, revised; #, re-sequenced; ✚, add-on; ★, audiovisual technology; and ◀, synchronous interactive audio.

Selecting Codes for Outpatient Consultation Services

The following examples are intended to demonstrate how MDM or total time may be used to select each level of service for outpatient consultations. Refer to **Table 7-1** for an at-a-glance guide to the levels of MDM or time required for each level of outpatient E/M service. Each outpatient consultation code is followed by 1 or more examples.

★▲**99242**   Office or other outpatient consultation for a new or established patient, which requires a medically appropriate history and/or examination and straightforward medical decision making.

When using total time on the date of the encounter for code selection, 20 minutes must be met or exceeded.

Example

➤ **An adolescent male patient is referred for evaluation for left inguinal hernia and opinion on necessity of repair.** The referring physician's encounter note is reviewed by the physician who provided the consultation. On examination, no hernia is found and the patient reports no current symptoms. Diagnosis is suspected right inguinal hernia not found, likely a muscle strain that has resolved. The patient is to follow up with his primary care physician as needed.

Level of problem addressed ⟶ *Straightforward (1 self-limited condition, resolved)*

Level of data reviewed and analyzed ⟶ *Straightforward (review of prior external notes from 1 unique source)*

Level of risk of morbidity ⟶ *Moderate (decision regarding elective major surgery without identified risk factors)*

ICD-10-CM: **Z03.89** (encounter for observation for other suspected diseases and conditions ruled out)

CPT: **99242** is supported.

Teaching Point: Although the risk is moderate, the problem addressed and the data to be reviewed and analyzed are straightforward. Because the patient had no current concern, a code for observation for suspected condition that was ruled out was appropriate.

> If an evaluation and management service includes history from an independent historian and more than a single self-limited or minor problem, documentation should typically support low medical decision-making.

★▲**99243**   Office or other outpatient consultation for a new or established patient, which requires a medically appropriate history and/or examination and low level of medical decision making.

When using total time on the date of the encounter for code selection, 30 minutes must be met or exceeded.

Example

➤ **An adolescent ballet dancer is referred for evaluation and recommendation of treatment for pain and swelling to the posterior aspect of the ankle.** The physician reviews an encounter note provided by the physician who requested the consultation and independently interprets magnetic resonance imaging of the ankle. Diagnosis is posterior ankle tenosynovitis caused by os trigonum syndrome. Conservative treatment with rest and physical therapy is recommended, and an order for physical therapy is provided. A report of the encounter is sent to the requesting physician.

Level of problem addressed ⟶ *Low (1 acute, uncomplicated illness or injury)*

Level of data reviewed and analyzed ⟶ *Moderate (independent interpretation of tests)*

Level of risk of morbidity ⟶ *Low (decision for physical therapy)*

ICD-10-CM: **M65.871** (other synovitis and tenosynovitis, right ankle and foot), **Q68.8** (os trigonum syndrome)

CPT: **99243** is supported.

Teaching Point: The problem addressed and the risks of management support low MDM.

★▲**99244**   Office or other outpatient consultation for a new or established patient, which requires a medically appropriate history and/or examination and moderate level of medical decision making.

When using total time on the date of the encounter for code selection, 40 minutes must be met or exceeded.

● indicates a new code; ▲, revised; #, re-sequenced; ✚, add-on; ★, audiovisual technology; and ◀, synchronous interactive audio.

Examples

➤ **A primary care pediatrician consults an otolaryngologist for opinion on tympanostomy with tubes for treatment of chronic otitis media.** The patient is new to the otolaryngologist, who reviews and summarizes records provided by the primary care pediatrician. History is obtained from the patient's parents, who note that the patient finished a course of antibiotics 2 weeks ago and is increasingly missing school and community events because of ear infections. Examination reveals enlarged adenoids and bilateral otitis media with effusion.

Assessment/plan: Diagnosis is bilateral chronic serous otitis media with chronic hypertrophy of adenoids. The otolaryngologist discusses treatment options with the parents, including tympanostomy with tube placement and adenoidectomy, and the parents agree to the surgery. The otolaryngologist sends a report to the primary care pediatrician advising that surgery is recommended.

Level of problem addressed ⟹ *Moderate (≥1 chronic conditions with progression)*
Level of data reviewed and analyzed ⟹ *Limited (independent historians and review of records from 1 source)*
Level of risk of morbidity ⟹ *Moderate (decision for elective major surgery without known risk factors)*
ICD-10-CM: **H65.23** (chronic serous otitis media, bilateral), **J35.2** (hypertrophy of adenoids)
CPT: **99244** is supported.
Teaching Point: The problem addressed and the risks of management support moderate MDM.

➤ **An adolescent patient is seen in consultation for increasingly symptomatic mental health problems.** The patient's psychologist has requested evaluation and recommendation for treatment, as the patient has not adequately responded to current treatment. The physician reviews the patient's current medications and results of psychological tests. History is obtained mainly from the patient's mother, who is present. After extensive discussion, new medication is prescribed and a follow-up visit is scheduled in 1 week. The physician sends the psychologist a report with findings and recommendations. The physician's total time spent in medical management (not psychotherapy, which would be reported separately, when provided) is 50 minutes.

ICD-10-CM: appropriate codes for problems addressed
CPT: **99244** is supported by the time exceeding 40 minutes but not reaching the 55 minutes required for code **99245**.

★▲**99245** Office or other outpatient consultation for a new or established patient, which requires a medically appropriate history and/or examination and high level of medical decision making.

When using total time on the date of the encounter for code selection, 55 minutes must be met or exceeded.

(For services ≥70 minutes, use prolonged services code **99417**, discussed in the Prolonged Outpatient E/M Service, Physician or Other Qualified Health Care Professional, section later in this chapter.)

Example

➤ **A neurologist is consulted by a primary care pediatrician to evaluate a patient who has Down syndrome and possible symptoms of atlantoaxial instability and is requesting clearance to participate in Special Olympics.** The neurologist reviews the patient's history provided by the referring physician. Additional history is provided by the patient's parents, who state that the patient sometimes describes her hands as "tingling" after sleeping or playing a game on a tablet. Following examination of the patient, the neurologist orders radiography of the patient's cervical spine. Later that day, after receiving the radiologist's interpretation of the cervical spine radiographs, the neurologist views the images and then contacts the primary care pediatrician to discuss that there is no evidence of atlantoaxial instability on radiography and, after discussion, recommends clearing the child for participation. The neurologist's total time on the date of the encounter is 65 minutes.

Level of problem addressed ⟹ *Moderate (1 undiagnosed new problem with uncertain prognosis)*
Level of data reviewed and analyzed ⟹ *High (independent interpretation of tests and discussion of management)*
Level of risk of morbidity ⟹ *Low to moderate (decision for participation)*
ICD-10-CM: **Z03.89** (encounter for observation for other suspected diseases and conditions ruled out), **R20.2** (paresthesia of skin), **Q90.2** (trisomy 21, translocation)

CPT: **99245** is supported.

Teaching Point: The physician's total time supports code **99245**, although the MDM for the encounter is moderate.

Home or Residence Services (99341–99350)

In 2023, code **99343** is deleted because both **99343** and **99344** required moderate medical decision-making and were differentiated by levels of history and examination under the prior code structure.

For the purpose of reporting home or residence services, a home or residence may include the following sites. Each site is followed by the applicable place of service code in parentheses.

- Private residence (**12**)
- Temporary lodging or short-term accommodation (**16** [eg, hotel, campground, hostel, cruise ship])
- Assisted living facility (**13**)
- Group home that is not licensed as an intermediate care facility for individuals with intellectual disabilities (**14**)
- Custodial care facility (**33**)
- Residential substance abuse treatment facility (**55**)

To report services provided in an intermediate care facility for individuals with intellectual disabilities and services provided in a psychiatric residential treatment center, see "Evaluation and Management Service Coding in Nursing and Residential Treatment Facilities" at www.aap.org/cfp2023.

Medicaid plans may vary in sites of service reported as home visits. Verify payer policies for E/M services provided in a patient's home or residence before provision of services.

Evaluation and management services provided in a patient's home by an NPP who does not have their own NPI may not be billable unless the physician provides direct supervision. Refer to **Chapter 13** for information on reporting services by professionals such as therapists, clinical social workers, and nutritionists.

Any procedures performed by the physician may be separately reported.

Home or Residence E/M Service Examples

Refer to **Table 7-1** for an at-a-glance guide to the levels of MDM or time required for each level of outpatient E/M service.

▲**99341**   Home or residence visit for the evaluation and management of a new patient, which requires a medically appropriate history and/or examination and straightforward medical decision making.

        When using total time on the date of the encounter for code selection, 15 minutes must be met or exceeded.

▲**99347**   Home or residence visit for the evaluation and management of an established patient, which requires a medically appropriate history and/or examination and straightforward medical decision making.

        When using total time on the date of the encounter for code selection, 20 minutes must be met or exceeded.

Example

➤ **A physician or QHP visits the home of a newborn whose parents are concerned that the newborn is not breathing normally.** On examination, the newborn is breathing normally and is free of any signs or symptoms of illness. The parents are reassured. The total time directed to care of this patient on this date is 10 minutes.

    Level of problem addressed ⇒ *Minimal (1 self-limited problem)*

    Level of data reviewed and analyzed ⇒ *Limited (independent historians)*

    Level of risk of morbidity ⇒ *Minimal (home care)*

    ICD-10-CM: **Z05.3** (observation and evaluation of newborn for suspected respiratory condition ruled out)

    CPT: **99341** if the patient is new or **99347** if the patient is established

    Teaching Point: In this example, the physician's or QHP's total time did not meet the minimum required for code selection. However, straightforward MDM is the highest level supported by 2 of the 3 elements of MDM.

If an evaluation and management service includes history from an independent historian and more than a single self-limited or minor problem, documentation should typically support low medical decision-making.

▲**99342** Home or residence visit for the evaluation and management of a new patient, which requires a medically appropriate history and/or examination and low level of medical decision making.

> When using total time on the date of the encounter for code selection, 30 minutes must be met or exceeded.

▲**99348** Home or residence visit for the evaluation and management of an established patient, which requires a medically appropriate history and/or examination and low level of medical decision making.

> When using total time on the date of the encounter for code selection, 30 minutes must be met or exceeded.

Examples

➤ **A physician or QHP visits the home of an autistic 5-year-old whose parents fear he has an ear infection.** The parents note that the child has been holding his right ear frequently for the past week. They have not seen him pulling at or trying to insert anything into his ear. The physician's examination of the patient takes 15 minutes because of extensive coaching to gain the child's cooperation. The child's ears are free of signs of infection and foreign bodies. The parents are counseled that this may be a self-comfort mechanism or habit and they are not to use cotton swabs to clean the ear canals and to try to dry the ear canals after showers. The option of trying 2 drops of distilled vinegar and alcohol solution in the ear canal once daily is offered, although infection is not suspected. The physician's total time on the date of the encounter is 30 minutes. Diagnosis is suspected ear infection, ruled out; the behavior is likely a self-comfort measure, but the patient does not respond to questions about his ears. *Plan:* If the parents see any indication of itching or discomfort, they will try drops of distilled vinegar solution; otherwise, they will call if any fever or other concerns develop.

> *Level of problem addressed* ⫸ *Minimal (1 self-limited problem)*
> *Level of data reviewed and analyzed* ⫸ *Limited (independent historians)*
> *Level of risk of morbidity* ⫸ *Minimal (home care)*
> *ICD-10-CM:* **Z03.89** (encounter for observation for other suspected diseases and conditions ruled out), **F84.0** (autistic disorder)
> *CPT:* **99342** if the patient is new or **99348** if the patient is established (based on total time of 30 minutes)
> **Teaching Point:** In this example, the physician's or QHP's total time on the date of the encounter supports a higher level of service than the straightforward MDM.
>
> Payers may require documentation of medical necessity for provision of services in the home rather than the office. Inclusion of codes that limit the patient's ability to be seen in the office or outpatient clinic may help demonstrate medical necessity.

> Travel time is not included in the time of service. However, if escorting a patient to a medical facility becomes necessary, code **99082** (unusual travel) may be appropriate.

➤ **A physician visits the home of a 3-year-old who is having infrequent, very hard stools.** Per the patient's mother, the child's stepbrother also has this problem. The physician reviews the patient's diet and level of activity with the mother. After examining the patient, the physician recommends a diet higher in fiber, lower in processed foods, and lower in milk and other dairy products. The total time on the date of the encounter is 20 minutes, including time spent documenting the encounter.

> *Level of problem addressed* ⫸ *Low (1 acute, uncomplicated illness)*
> *Level of data reviewed and analyzed* ⫸ *Limited (independent historian)*
> *Level of risk of morbidity* ⫸ *Minimal (dietary recommendations)*
> *ICD-10-CM:* **K59.00** (constipation, unspecified)
> *CPT:* **99342** if the patient is new or **99348** if the patient is established
> **Teaching Point:** The problem addressed and level of data to be reviewed support low MDM.

▲**99344** Home or residence visit for the evaluation and management of a new patient, which requires a medically appropriate history and/or examination and moderate level of medical decision making.

> When using total time on the date of the encounter for code selection, 60 minutes must be met or exceeded.

● indicates a new code; ▲, revised; #, re-sequenced; ✚, add-on; ★, audiovisual technology; and ◀, synchronous interactive audio.

▲99349   Home or residence visit for the evaluation and management of an established patient, which requires a medically appropriate history and/or examination and moderate level of medical decision making.

              When using total time on the date of the encounter for code selection, 40 minutes must be met or exceeded.

Example

➤ **A pediatrician agrees to provide medically necessary services at the infirmary of a youth ranch where an established patient lives.** The patient presents with concern of increased asthma symptoms. The patient-provided history and an examination are documented in addition to a decision to change the patient's control medication and update the patient's asthma control plan. Diagnosis is moderate persistent asthma with exacerbation.

     Level of problem addressed ⅢⅢ➡ *Moderate (1 chronic condition with exacerbation)*
     Level of data reviewed and analyzed ⅢⅢ➡ *Minimal*
     Level of risk of morbidity ⅢⅢ➡ *Moderate (prescription drug management)*
     ICD-10-CM: **J45.41** (moderate persistent asthma with [acute] exacerbation)
     CPT: **99349** (established patient)
     Teaching Point: The problem addressed and risk associated with management support moderate MDM. If the patient were new, code **99344** would be reported.

▲99345   Home or residence visit for the evaluation and management of a new patient, which requires a medically appropriate history and/or examination and high level of medical decision making.

              When using total time on the date of the encounter for code selection, 75 minutes must be met or exceeded.

▲99350   Home or residence visit for the evaluation and management of an established patient, which requires a medically appropriate history and/or examination and high level of medical decision making.

              When using total time on the date of the encounter for code selection, 60 minutes must be met or exceeded.

Example

➤ **A physician visits the home of an established patient who has cystic fibrosis.** The patient's mother notes that she requested the appointment because the patient is experiencing diarrhea and progressive, cramping abdominal pain in the right left quadrant. The physician recommends admission to the hospital for further E/M of possible intestinal blockage. The physician arranges for the patient to be admitted to the local hospital through the ED (as required by the facility).

     Level of problem addressed ⅢⅢ➡ *High (1 chronic illness with severe exacerbation)*
     Level of data reviewed and analyzed ⅢⅢ➡ *Limited (independent historian)*
     Level of risk of morbidity ⅢⅢ➡ *High (decision regarding hospitalization)*
     ICD-10-CM: **E84.0** (cystic fibrosis with other intestinal manifestations)
     CPT: **99350**
     Teaching Point: The MDM is high because of an illness that poses a threat to life or bodily function and decision to hospitalize. A decision to hospitalize and a decision to not hospitalize but to closely monitor would each support high risk in this scenario.

Prolonged Office E/M Service

Prolonged Outpatient E/M Service, Physician or Other Qualified Health Care Professional

★✚▲99417   Prolonged outpatient evaluation and management service(s) time with or without direct patient contact beyond the required time of the primary service when the primary service level has been selected using total time, each 15 minutes of total time

---

● indicates a new code; ▲, revised; #, re-sequenced; ✚, add-on; ★, audiovisual technology; and ◄, synchronous interactive audio.

> **Code 99417** is reported only when the code for the primary service was selected on the basis of time. The time requirement for the highest-level code for the primary service must be met and exceeded by at least 15 minutes.

Code **99417** is used to report prolonged total time (ie, combined time with and without direct patient contact) provided by the physician or QHP on the same date as one of the following outpatient E/M services. Prolonged total time is time that is 15 minutes beyond the time required to report the highest-level primary service (eg, level-5 office E/M service).

- Office or other outpatient services reported with code **99205** or **99215**
- Office or other outpatient consultation reported with **99245**
- Home or residence service reported with **99345** or **99350**
- Assessment of and care planning for a patient with cognitive impairment reported with **99483** (not typically a pediatric service)

For prolonged services on a date other than the date of a face-to-face E/M encounter with the patient and/or family/caregiver, report **99358** or **99359**. For E/M services that require prolonged clinical staff time and may include face-to-face services by the physician or QHP, report **99415** or **99416**. Do not report **99417** in conjunction with other codes for prolonged service (eg, **99358, 99359; 99415, 99416; 99418**).

There is no limitation on the number of units of **99417** reported per encounter. However, each unit must represent a full 15-minute period beyond the time included in the initial service or the time included in a previous unit of time reported with **99417**.

Do not report **99417**

✖ For prolonged service of less than 15 minutes on the date of the office E/M service
✖ For any additional increment of time that is less than 15 minutes from the most recent
✖ For time spent performing separately reported services other than the E/M service
✖ In addition to codes for less than the highest-level service in a code category (eg, do not report with **99211–99214**)

Payer policies for prolonged service may vary. See the "Coding Conundrum: **G2212** Versus **99417**" box later in this chapter for an example of a payer policy that may deny payment when code **99417** is reported.

Table 7-3 provides the required times for reporting units of **99417** in addition to the appropriate highest-level primary E/M service.

Table 7-3. Time Requirements for Prolonged Service Reported With Code 99417

Only time spent by a physician or QHP in providing care directed to the individual patient is included in the total time on the date of the encounter.

Type of Service and Code	Assigned Time (min)	Minimum Time (min) Required for Reporting 99417	Minimum Time (min) Required for Reporting Additional Units of 99417[a]
Office E/M NP 99205	60–74	75–89 **99205** × 1 and **99417** × 1	90–104 **99205** × 1 and **99417** × 2
Office E/M EP 99215	40–54	55–69 **99215** × 1 and **99417** × 1	70–84 **99215** × 1 and **99417** × 2
Outpatient consultation 99245	≥55	70–84 **99245** × 1 and **99417** × 1	85–99 **99245** × 1 and **99417** × 2
Home or residence NP 99345	≥75	90–104 **99345** × 1 and **99417** × 1	105–119 **99345** × 1 and **99417** × 2
Home or residence EP 99350	≥60	75–89 **99350** × 1 and **99417** × 1	90–104 **99350** × 1 and **99417** × 2

Abbreviations: E/M, evaluation and management; EP, established patient; NP, new patient; QHP, qualified health care professional.

[a] Each unit of service for **99417** is reported only for a *full 15-minute* period beyond the most recent unit reported. Although times for up to only 2 units are shown in this table, there is no limitation on the number of units reported.

● indicates a new code; ▲, revised; #, re-sequenced; ✚, add-on; ★, audiovisual technology; and ◀, synchronous interactive audio.

Examples

➤ **A new patient is referred following discharge from observation care for asthma.** The patient has no usual source of care and has been seen in 3 EDs for a total of 4 visits in the past year. The pediatrician spends 20 minutes before the face-to-face visit, on the same date, reviewing observation and ED records for the child. At the visit, the pediatrician spends 45 minutes evaluating the patient, who also has behavioral issues in school; developing a plan of care; and counseling the patient and caregiver on the plan. After the visit, the pediatrician spends 20 minutes on the same date providing instructions to the school nurse about the patient's use of a rescue inhaler and arranging for teachers to complete rating scales for ADHD. Another 10 minutes is spent in documentation. The pediatrician reports codes **99205** and **99417** × 2 for the 95 minutes devoted to the patient's care on the date of the encounter.

➤ **An adolescent patient and her parents are scheduled for an outpatient consultation to evaluate the patient's treatment options for newly diagnosed Crohn disease.** The physician documentation of the consultation supports moderate-level MDM. Total time is not documented. Later, on that same date, the physician receives a call from the patient's parents with additional questions and concerns and spends 30 minutes communicating on the call and completing the documentation. The outpatient consultation is reported with code **99244**.

 Teaching Point: The total time on the date of the encounter might have supported code **99245** and possibly prolonged service, but the total time was not documented and the consultation code was selected on the basis of MDM.

Coding Conundrum: G2212 Versus 99417

Some payers may not accept code **99417** for prolonged office evaluation and management (E/M) services. The Centers for Medicare & Medicaid Services developed an alternative code **G2212** (described below) in 2021 to require that the time of prolonged office E/M services begins when time exceeds *the higher time in the range of total time* assigned to either code **99205** or **99215** in lieu of the lower time in the range of total time as required for code **99417**.

G2212	Prolonged office or other outpatient evaluation and management service(s) beyond the maximum required time of the primary procedure which has been selected using total time on the date of the primary service; each additional 15 minutes by the physician or qualified health care professional, with or without direct patient contact

G2212 is reported only in conjunction with **99205** (add **G2212** for total time ≥89 minutes) or **99215** (add **G2212** for total time ≥69 minutes) and only when the time requirement is met.

In the absence of a contractual requirement to follow a payer's policy to report **G2212** in lieu of **99417**, physicians should assign code **99417** and follow *Current Procedural Terminology* guidelines. An additional G code for reporting a prolonged home or residence E/M service is anticipated for 2023.

Prolonged Service Without Direct Patient Contact (99358, 99359)

99358	Prolonged evaluation and management service before and/or after direct patient care; first hour
✛99359	each additional 30 minutes (Use in conjunction with code **99358**.)

 Prolonged service without direct patient contact (ie, non–face-to-face) is reported when a physician provides prolonged service *on a date when no face-to-face E/M service has been or will be provided.* The prolonged service must relate to a service during and patient for which direct (face-to-face) patient care has occurred or will occur and to ongoing patient management.

 See codes **99417** and **99418** for prolonged service on the date of a face-to-face E/M service.

 Only time spent by a physician or other QHP may be counted toward the time of prolonged service. Prolonged service of less than 30 minutes on a given date is not separately reported. Report code **99359** for 15 or more minutes beyond the first hour or the last full 30-minute period of prolonged service.

 Codes **99358** and **99359** are not limited to specific sites of service.

Example

➤ **A physician provides an office or other outpatient consultation to a patient to evaluate whether surgery is indicated.** After the consultation, the physician requests records from a prior surgery. The following day, the physician spends 30 minutes reviewing the old records, plans a surgical approach, and speaks with the referring physician about

Chapter 7. Non-preventive Evaluation and Management Services in Outpatient Settings

perioperative management. The total time of service is 45 minutes. The physician reports code **99358** for the first hour of prolonged service (reported for services of ≥30 minutes).

Teaching Point: Payers may or may not allow payment for codes **99358** and **99359**. Code **99359** may be reported for the first and each additional 30 minutes of service time, including a period of 15 minutes or more beyond the first hour or beyond the last 30-minute period.

Prolonged Clinical Staff Service (99415, 99416)

+99415 Prolonged clinical staff service (the service beyond the typical service time) during an evaluation and management service in the office or outpatient setting, direct patient contact with physician supervision; first hour (List separately in addition to code for outpatient Evaluation and Management service)

+99416 each additional 30 minutes

Codes **99415** and **99416** are used to report 30 minutes or more of prolonged clinical staff time spent face-to-face providing care to a patient and/or parent or caregiver under the direct supervision of a physician or other QHP who has provided an office or other outpatient E/M service at the same session.

- Report prolonged clinical staff service **99415** and **99416** only in addition to office or other outpatient E/M codes **99202–99205** or **99211–99215**.
- The starting point for **99415** is 30 minutes beyond the typical clinical staff time that is included in the value assigned to the office or other outpatient E/M code reported for the encounter. This time is not included in the code descriptors in *CPT* but, rather, in a table like **Table 7-4**.

Table 7-4. Time Requirements for Prolonged Clinical Staff Service (99415, 99416)

Only time spent by a physician or QHP in providing care directed to the individual patient is included in the total time on the date of the encounter.

Office E/M Code	Typical Clinical Staff Time (min)	Time Range (min) for +99415	Time Range (min) for +99416 (1st Unit)[a]
99202	29	59–103	104–133
99203	34	64–108	109–138
99204	41	71–115	116–145
99205	46	76–120	121–150
99211	16	46–90	91–120
99212	24	54–98	99–128
99213	27	57–101	102–131
99214	40	70–114	115–144
99215	45	75–119	120–149

Abbreviations: E/M, evaluation and management; QHP, qualified health care professional.

[a] Each unit of service for **99416** is reported only when the time included in **99415** or the prior unit of **99416** is exceeded *by at least 15 minutes*. There is no limitation on the number of units reported, but documentation must support the time spent and the clinical indication for prolonged clinical staff service.

Example

➤ **A physician documents total time on the date of an office E/M service as 30 minutes.** Clinical staff spent a total of 75 minutes monitoring the patient (face-to-face) under the physician's supervision. The physician reports a code for the office E/M service (eg, **99214**) and code **99415** because the clinical staff time exceeded the typical clinical staff time of code **99214** (40 minutes) by at least 30 minutes.

Teaching Point: Because the typical clinical staff time associated with the E/M code reported by the physician was exceeded by at least 30 minutes, code **99415** is reported in addition to the office E/M code.

Documentation should support the clinical indication(s) for the prolonged service and the specific amount of time spent by clinical staff providing face-to-face services to the individual patient. If face-to-face time is discontinuous, each segment of time should be added together to support **99415** and, when applicable, **99416**.

✖ *Never report both* prolonged office E/M service by a physician or other QHP (**99417**) and prolonged clinical staff services together.
✖ Do not include time spent providing separately reported services, such as intravenous medication administration or inhalation treatment, in the time of prolonged service.
✖ Do not include any time that is not face-to-face with the patient and/or family/caregiver.
✖ Do not report more than one unit of **99415** for service to the same patient on the same date. Report **99415** and **99416** for a cumulative time of 75 minutes or more beyond the typical clinical staff time.
● Codes **99415** and **99416** may be reported for *no more than 2 simultaneous patients,* and the time reported is the time devoted only to a single patient.
● Codes **99415** and **99416** were assigned relative value units based only on clinical staff's intraservice time, as the preservice and post-service times were considered to be included in the value of the related E/M service. Relative value units for 2023 services were unavailable at the time of this publication.

The following guidelines apply to reporting of prolonged clinical staff services:
● A physician or other QHP must supervise the duration of prolonged clinical staff service.
● The total clinical staff time (whether continuous or segmented) and clinical indication(s) for the services must be documented.
● When not continuous, document and include the face-to-face time of each episode of clinical staff time.
● Report code **99416** for each additional 30 minutes of clinical staff time beyond the first hour and for the last 15 to 30 minutes of prolonged clinical staff service. Do not report **99416** for a period of less than 15 minutes.

Outpatient Critical Care (99291, 99292)

Regardless of the patient's age, critical care services provided in outpatient settings are reported with hourly critical care codes (**99291, 99292**).

99291	Critical care, evaluation and management of the critically ill or critically injured patient; first 30–74 minutes
✚99292	each additional 30 minutes

> **See Chapter 18 for further discussion of guidelines for critical care services.**

If the same patient requires outpatient and inpatient critical care services on the same day, the physician or a physician of the same group and specialty would report their services on the basis of where the services were provided and the patient's age. Refer to **Figure 7-2** for information on coding when critical care occurs in the outpatient setting.

Examples

➤ **A patient presents to an urgent care clinic with a respiratory illness and has become increasingly short of breath following coughing spells.** During the examination, the patient goes into respiratory failure with hypoxia, and her vital signs deteriorate. The physician provides critical care. An ambulance is called, and the physician continues critical care services until the transport team accepts care of the patient. The total time for critical care services provided by the physician is 40 minutes. The physician provides no further care to the patient and reports outpatient critical care services with a diagnosis of acute respiratory failure with hypoxia. Documentation includes the critical nature of the patient's condition, the care provided, and the total time spent in critical care dedicated to this patient.

ICD-10-CM	CPT
J96.01 (acute respiratory failure with hypoxia)	**99291** (critical care, first 30–74 minutes)

Teaching Point: If the same physician or physician of the same specialty and group practice provided outpatient and inpatient critical care services on the same calendar date and the total critical care time was 75 minutes or more, code **99292** would be reported with 1 unit for each block of time, of up to 30 minutes beyond the first 74 minutes.

● indicates a new code; ▲, revised; #, re-sequenced; ✚, add-on; ★, audiovisual technology; and ◀, synchronous interactive audio.

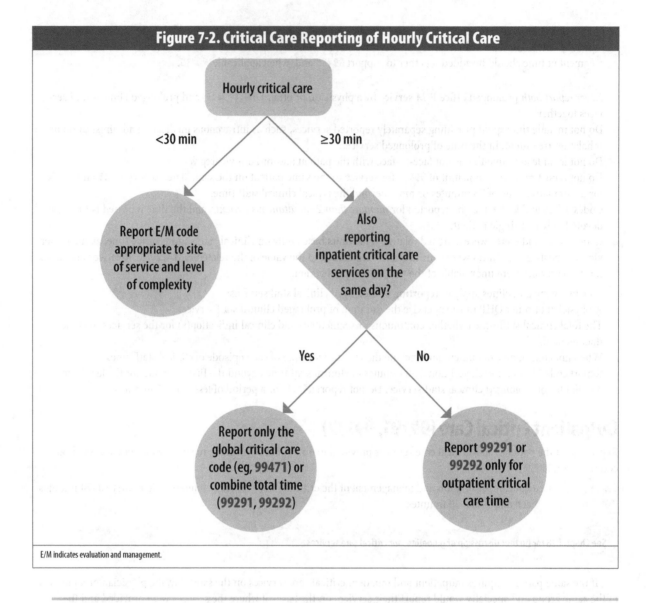

Figure 7-2. Critical Care Reporting of Hourly Critical Care

Hourly critical care

<30 min

Report E/M code appropriate to site of service and level of complexity

≥30 min

Also reporting inpatient critical care services on the same day?

Yes

Report only the global critical care code (eg, 99471) or combine total time (99291, 99292)

No

Report 99291 or 99292 only for outpatient critical care time

E/M indicates evaluation and management.

➤ **An established patient presents with fever and severe cough.** Clinical staff summon the physician to the examination room, where the physician notes that the patient is in respiratory failure. The physician provides critical care to the child for 20 minutes before an ambulance team assumes management. The physician documents a diagnosis of respiratory failure.

Level of problem addressed ⬛➡ *High (1 acute or chronic illness or injury that poses a threat to life or bodily function)*

Level of data reviewed and analyzed ⬛➡ *Limited (assumption of independent historian)*

Level of risk of morbidity ⬛➡ *High (decision regarding hospitalization)*

ICD-10-CM: **J96.00** (acute respiratory failure, unspecified whether with hypoxia or hypercapnia) or code for more specific diagnosis, when known, and **R50.9** (fever unspecified)

CPT: **99205** is supported by the problems addressed (ie, illness with threat to life or bodily function) and risk (ie, hospitalization).

Teaching Point: Although the physician provided outpatient critical care services, the 30-minute minimum time for reporting code **99291** (critical care, first 30–74 minutes) was not met. The office encounter is separately reported in addition to initial hospital care when a physician or QHP of the same specialty and same group practice provides both services on the same date. Modifier **25** is appended to the code for the office E/M service.

● indicates a new code; ▲, revised; #, re-sequenced; ✚, add-on; ★, audiovisual technology; and ◀, synchronous interactive audio.

Codes for Reporting Special Circumstances

The codes discussed in this section are reported in addition to the code(s) for an E/M service when there are special circumstances such as a service provided after the practice's normal business hours to allow care in the practice as opposed to an urgent care clinic or ED.

After-hours Services (99050–99058)

After-hours codes are used to report services that are provided after hours or on an emergency basis and are always reported in addition to the primary service (eg, E/M service).

After-hours service codes **99050–99058** are used by physicians or other QHPs (under their state scope of practice when billing with their own NPI) to identify the services that are adjunct to the basic services rendered. These codes

- Describe the special circumstances under which a basic service is provided
- Are reported only in addition to an associated basic service (eg, E/M, fracture care)
- Are reported without a modifier appended to the basic service because they only further describe the services provided

  Third-party payers will have specific policies for coverage and payment.
- Some carriers pay practices for extended hours because they recognize the cost benefit realized from decreased urgent care and ED visits.
  - Communicate with individual payers to understand their definition or interpretation of the service and their coverage and payment policies.
  - As part of this negotiation and education process, it is important to demonstrate the cost savings recognized by the payer for these adjunct services.
- If appropriate, more than one adjunct code may be reported on the same day of service (eg, **99058** and **99051** for services provided on an emergency basis during regularly scheduled evening or weekend hours).

  Many payers will pay only for the use of a single special services code per encounter and may manually review, question, or deny payment for a claim with multiple after-hours codes.

  Follow individual payer policy when reporting after-hours codes in conjunction with a service provided via telemedicine. Codes **99050** and **99051** are neither preceded by the telemedicine symbol (★) nor included in *CPT* Appendix P.

Services Provided When the Office Is Normally Closed

99050   Service(s) provided in office at times other than regularly scheduled office hours, or days when the office is normally closed (eg, holidays, Saturday, Sunday), in addition to basic service

- Office hours must be posted. *CPT* does not define a holiday or posted office hours. While most commonly applied to evening, weekend, or holiday hours, code **99050** could be applied to services provided at the patient request on a weekday if the office is typically closed on that day.
- Code **99050** is *not* reported when a physician or other QHP is behind schedule and sees patients after posted office hours.
- The service must be requested by the patient, and the physician or other QHP must agree to see the patient.
- Documentation must indicate the time and date of the encounter and the request to be seen outside of normal posted hours.

Services Provided During Regularly Scheduled Evening, Weekend, or Holiday Hours

99051   Service(s) provided in the office during regularly scheduled evening, weekend, or holiday office hours, in addition to basic service

- Regularly scheduled office hours must be posted.
- Documentation must include the time and date of the encounter.
- Evenings and holidays are not defined by *CPT,* but holidays can generally refer to national and/or state holidays, and evenings are generally 6:00 pm and later. Check with payers for coverage and/or ability to bill patients these charges under the health plan contract.

Example

➤ **A pediatric clinic offers urgent care appointments 3 evenings a week with staffing by QHPs (ie, nurse practitioners, physician assistants/associates) working under general supervision.** A patient who has been seen at the clinic by Dr A within the past year is seen in the evening clinic by a nurse practitioner who documents a clinically indicated history and examination with low-level MDM with diagnosis of URTI.

    ICD-10-CM: **J06.9** (acute upper respiratory infection, unspecified)

    CPT: **99213** (established office E/M) and **99051** (service provided in office during regularly scheduled weekend hours)

        Teaching Point: Because the office offers regularly scheduled evening hours, code **99051** is reported. The patient is established because *CPT* instructs that QHPs are to be considered of the same specialty as the physicians with whom they work in a group practice.

Services Provided on an Emergency Basis in the Office

99058   Service(s) provided on an emergency basis in the office, which disrupts other scheduled office services, in addition to basic service

- Report when an office patient's condition, in the clinical judgment of the physician, warrants the physician interrupting care of another patient to deal with the emergency.
- Code **99058** may not be reported when patients are simply fit into the schedule or for walk-ins.
- Document that the patient was seen immediately and the reason for the emergent care.

Example

➤ **A pediatric practice offers scheduled appointments on Saturday mornings from 8:00 am to noon.** A child is scheduled for evaluation of increased symptoms of moderate persistent asthma on a Saturday at 9:00 am. The child arrives 30 minutes before the scheduled time with severe exacerbation and is immediately taken to an examination room by the triage nurse, and the physician disrupts his schedule to see the child urgently.

    ICD-10-CM: **J45.42** (moderate persistent asthma with status asthmaticus)

    CPT: **99202–99215** (new or established office E/M), **99058** (service provided on an emergency basis in office, disrupting other scheduled services), and **99051** (service provided in office during regularly scheduled weekend hours)

        Teaching Point: If the Saturday hours were for walk-in visits only (ie, no scheduled appointments), code **99058** would *not* be reported. If a physician or QHP of the same specialty and same group practice provides inpatient or observation care to the patient on the same date, modifier **25** (significant, separately identifiable service) is appended to the office E/M code. Check individual payer policy for reporting 2 E/M services on the same date.

Out-of-Office Service (99056–99060)

Codes **99056–99060** are used to report services provided after hours or on an emergency basis and are an adjunct to the basic E/M service provided.

Third-party payers have specific policies for coverage and payment. Communicate with individual payers to understand their definition or interpretation of the service and their coverage and payment policies. As part of this negotiation and education process, it is important to demonstrate the cost savings recognized by the payer for these adjunct services. After-hours service codes are used by physicians or other QHPs (under their state scope of practice when billing with their own NPI) to identify the services that are adjunct to the basic services rendered. These codes

- Describe the special circumstances under which a basic procedure is performed
- Are reported only in addition to an associated basic service (eg, home visit)
- Are reported without a modifier appended to the basic service because they only further describe the services provided

99056   Service(s) typically provided in the office, provided out of the office at request of patient, in addition to basic service

        Documentation should include the patient's request to be seen outside the office.

99060   Service(s) provided on an emergency basis, out of the office, which disrupts other scheduled office services, in addition to basic service

        Documentation should indicate that the physician was called away during scheduled office hours to attend to a patient in another location (eg, a nursing facility).

Example

➤ **A physician is seeing patients in the office when a parent calls by phone and asks the physician to provide a house call for her autistic child who has a fever and appears quite ill.** The physician agrees and, later that day, arrives at the patient's home to find that the patient is more withdrawn than typical. The physician spends a total of 40 minutes providing the home visit, which includes examining the child, diagnosing streptococcal sore throat on the basis of clinical signs and symptoms, and prescribing an antibiotic.

ICD-10-CM	CPT
J02.0 (streptococcal pharyngitis) **F84.0** (autistic disorder)	**99349** (established home or residence E/M requiring moderate MDM or total time of 40 minutes or more) **99056** (service[s] typically provided in the office, provided out of the office at request of patient, in addition to basic service)

Teaching Point: Payers may or may not allow payment for code **99056** when services are rendered in a patient's home or residence or when a physician meets a patient in the ED. However, it is appropriate to report **99056** when a service is provided at an alternative location because of a request from the patient and/or caregiver. It is inappropriate to report **99056** when a physician instructs a patient to meet at a location other than the office.

Learn more about coding for special services in the May 2018 *AAP Pediatric Coding Newsletter* article, "Coding for Special Services In and Out of the Office" (https://doi.org/10.1542/pcco_book169_document002).

To test your knowledge of the information presented in this chapter, complete the quiz found at the end of it, after the resources.

Asthma, Attention-Deficit/Hyperactivity Disorder, and Otitis Media: Coding Continuums

Continuum Model for Asthma			
Code selection at any level above **99211** *may be based on the level of MDM or the total time spent on the date of service by the reporting physician or other QHP.* *The extent of history and examination documented does not affect code selection.*			
***CPT* Code and Vignette**	**Medical Decision-making (2 of 3 Elements Required)**		
99211 Nurse visit for a well 10-year-old established patient	*Time and MDM do not apply. Must indicate continuation of physician's plan of care, medical necessity, assessment, and/or education provided.* CC: Review asthma care plan. Current medications documented, peak expiratory flow measured, education topics reviewed, and questions answered		
***CPT* Code With Total Physician Time and Vignette**	**No. and Complexity of Problems Addressed**	**Amount and/or Complexity of Data Reviewed and Analyzed**	**Risk of Complications and/or Morbidity or Mortality of Patient Management**
99212 (10–19 minutes) An 8-year-old with stable asthma presents with a single patch of poison ivy rash on her forearm.	**SF:** 1 self-limited or minor problem	**SF:** None	**SF:** Minimal risk of morbidity from treatment
99213 (20–29 minutes) A 7-year-old with stable persistent asthma who is using a metered-dose steroid inhaler with β-agonist as needed returns for follow-up.	**Low:** 1 stable chronic illness	**Limited:** Assessment requiring an independent historian(s)—Mother provides history of asthma symptoms and medication adherence since most recent visit.	**Moderate:** Prescription drug management
99214 (30–39 minutes) An 8-year-old with unstable asthma is examined because of an acute exacerbation of the disease.	**Moderate:** ≥1 chronic illnesses with exacerbation, progression, or side effects of treatment	**Limited:** Assessment requiring an independent historian(s)—Mother provides history. *Note:* Spirometry and pulse oximetry provided are separately reported and not counted toward data reviewed and analyzed.	**Moderate:** Prescription drug management
99215 (40–54 minutes) A 3-year-old presents with persistent cough that is more frequent at night and during play.	40 minutes are spent on the date of the encounter obtaining patient, family, and social history; examining the patient; ordering tests and reviewing results; educating the family; using shared decision-making to develop a plan of care; prescribing medication and durable medical equipment; and documenting the service. Total time on the date of the encounter is included in the documentation.		
Abbreviations: CC, chief complaint (primary concern); *CPT, Current Procedural Terminology;* MDM, medical decision-making; SF, straightforward; QHP, qualified health care professional.			

●, indicates a new code; ▲, revised; #, re-sequenced; ✚, add-on; ★, audiovisual technology; and ◀, synchronous interactive audio.

Continuum Model for Attention-Deficit/Hyperactivity Disorder

Code selection at any level above **99211** *may be based on the level of MDM or the total time spent by the physician or other QHP on the date of the encounter.*

CPT Code With Total Physician Time and Vignette	Medical Decision-making (2 of 3 Elements Required)		
	No. and Complexity of Problems Addressed	**Amount and/or Complexity of Data Reviewed and Analyzed**	**Risk of Complications and/or Morbidity or Mortality of Patient Management**
99211 Nurse visit to check growth or blood pressure before renewing prescription for psychoactive drugs	*Time and MDM do not apply. Must indicate continuation of physician's plan of care, medical necessity, assessment, and/or education provided.* CC: Check growth or blood pressure. Documentation: Height, weight, and blood pressure. Existing medications and desired/undesired effects. Assessment: Doing well. Obtained physician approval for prescription refill. Advised to keep appointment with physician in 1 month.		
99212 (10–19 minutes) 4-year-old whose parents are concerned about ADHD symptoms (ADHD is not diagnosed; parents are reassured.)	**Minimal:** 1 self-limited problem	**Limited:** Assessment requiring an independent historian	**Minimal:** Parent education
99213 (20–29 minutes) Initial follow-up after initiation of medication, patient responding well	**Low:** 1 stable chronic illness	**Limited:** Assessment requiring an independent historian	**Moderate:** Prescription drug management
99214 (30–39 minutes) Follow-up for recent weight loss in patient with established ADHD otherwise stable on stimulant medication	**Moderate:** 1 chronic illness with side effects of treatment	**Limited:** Assessment requiring an independent historian	**Moderate:** Prescription drug management
99215 (40–54 minutes) Initial evaluation of a patient with ADHD and new onset of suicidal ideation. The patient and mother decide on no hospitalization because of cost. *Tip:* Add **99417** if time on the date of service is ≥55 minutes. Add **99058** if service(s) are provided on an emergency basis in the office, which disrupts other scheduled office services.	**High:** 1 acute or chronic illness or injury that poses a threat to life or bodily function	**Moderate:** Assessment requiring an independent historian; discussion with behavioral health specialist; psychiatric testing	**High:** Decision regarding hospitalization

Abbreviations: ADHD, attention-deficit/hyperactivity disorder; CC, chief complaint (primary concern); *CPT, Current Procedural Terminology;* MDM, medical decision-making; QHP, qualified health care professional.

● indicates a new code; ▲, revised; #, re-sequenced; ✚, add-on; ★, audiovisual technology; and ◀, synchronous interactive audio.

	Continuum Model for Otitis Media		
Code selection at any level above **99211** may be based on the level of MDM or the total time spent by the physician or other QHP on the date of the encounter. (Code **99211** is not included because of lack of indication for follow-up by clinical staff.)			
CPT **Code With Total Physician Time and Vignette**	**Medical Decision-making (2 of 3 Elements Required)**		
	No. and Complexity of Problems Addressed	**Amount and/or Complexity of Data Reviewed and Analyzed**	**Risk of Complications and/or Morbidity or Mortality of Patient Management**
99212 (10–19 minutes) Follow-up for otitis media, uncomplicated	**Minimal:** Follow-up for otitis media, evaluation of effusion and hearing	**Limited:** Tympanometry, audiometry, and/or assessment requiring an independent historian	**Minimal:** Risk associated with diagnostic testing and treatment
99213 (20–29 minutes) 2-year-old presents with tugging at her right ear. Afebrile. Mild otitis media.	**Low:** 1 acute, uncomplicated illness or injury	**Limited:** Assessment requiring an independent historian	**Moderate:** Prescription drug management, delayed prescribing
99214 (30–39 minutes) Infant presents with fever, lethargy, and cough and suspected third episode of otitis media within 3 months.	**Moderate:** 1 acute illness with systemic symptoms	**Limited:** Assessment requiring an independent historian	**Moderate:** Prescription drug management
99215 (40–54 minutes) 6-month-old presents with high fever, vomiting, and irritability. After tests, antipyretics, and fluid, infant's condition is stable.	**High:** 1 acute illness that poses a threat to life or bodily function	**Moderate:** Orders and/or review of laboratory tests, chest radiography, and possible lumbar puncture. Assessment requiring an independent historian.	**High:** Decision about hospitalization (hospitalization discussed with parents and decision made for care at home with strict instructions and close follow-up)

Abbreviations: *CPT, Current Procedural Terminology*; MDM, medical decision-making; QHP, qualified health care professional.

Chapter Takeaways

This chapter focuses on outpatient services that are reported on the basis of either MDM or the total time by a physician or QHP on the date of the encounter. Readers of this chapter should generally understand outpatient code categories and code selection. Following are takeaways from this chapter:

- Codes for outpatient E/M services are selected on the basis of the site of service as directed by *CPT* guidelines.
- To be considered a new patient, the patient must not have received a professional service from a physician or QHP of the same exact specialty and same group practice within the past 3 years.
- Office E/M services provided solely by clinical staff may be reported with code **99211**. Payer policy may limit reporting to services that meet an incident-to policy.
- Prolonged service may be reported when the time requirements are met.
- Critical care provided in outpatient settings is reported with time-based codes **99291** and **99292**.

● indicates a new code; ▲, revised; #, re-sequenced; ✚, add-on; ★, audiovisual technology; and ◀, synchronous interactive audio.

Resources

AAP Coding Assistance and Education

AAP *Pediatric Evaluation and Management Coding: Quick Reference Card 2023* (https://shop.aap.org/pediatric-evaluation-and-management-coding-quick-reference-card-2023)

AAP Initial History Questionnaire Documentation Form for office or outpatient visits (https://shop.aap.org/initial-history-questionnaire-documentation-form)

AAP Pediatric Coding Newsletter™

"Coding for Special Services In and Out of the Office," May 2018 (https://doi.org/10.1542/pcco_book169_document002)

"Is This a Consultation or Other Evaluation and Management Service?" May 2021 (https://doi.org/10.1542/pcco_book205_document005)

Online Exclusive Content at www.aap.org/cfp2023

"AAP Position on Medicare Consultation Policy"

"Evaluation and Management Service Coding in Nursing and Residential Treatment Facilities"

"Incident-to Services by Nonphysician Professionals and Clinical Staff: Medicare Requirements"

Test Your Knowledge!

1. **Which of the following patients is a new patient per evaluation and management coding guidelines?**
   a. A patient who was recently cared for by a pediatrician has a follow-up visit with a qualified health care professional in the same practice.
   b. A patient who was seen most recently by a physician of the same specialty in the same group practice 2 years ago
   c. A patient who has received hospital care from the same physician but is receiving care in the office for the first time
   d. A patient of a primary care pediatrician who is evaluated by an otolaryngologist in the same group practice for the first time (ie, first otolaryngology appointment)

2. **Which of the following data are included in determining the amount and/or complexity of data to be reviewed and analyzed?**
   a. An in-office test for which the physician reports a code for interpretation and report
   b. Review of the result of a test that was ordered between visits
   c. Review of the result of the first test performed under a recurring order
   d. Pulse oximetry

3. **Which of the following services is reported for a follow-up evaluation and management (E/M) service that the providing physician planned at an outpatient consultation on an earlier date?**
   a. Prolonged outpatient E/M service.
   b. Outpatient E/M service based on the site of service (eg, office).
   c. Another outpatient consultation.
   d. The service is not reportable.

4. **At which of the following locations are E/M services reported as home or residence services?**
   a. A hotel or other short-stay accommodation
   b. A psychiatric residential treatment facility
   c. An intermediate care facility for individuals with intellectual disabilities
   d. A nursing facility

5. **Which of the following circumstances supports reporting a prolonged office evaluation and management service (99417)?**
   a. The physician's total time on the date of the encounter met and exceeded the minimum time requirement for the highest level of the primary service by 15 minutes.
   b. The time requirement for any level of primary service must be met and exceeded by at least 15 minutes.
   c. The combined physician and clinical staff time exceeds the minimum time required for the highest level of the primary service by at least 15 minutes.
   d. A physician's total time on the date of an encounter supports code **99215**, and a call to the patient's caregiver on the next day lasts at least 15 minutes.

CHAPTER 8

Preventive Services

CPT copyright 2022 American Medical Association. All rights reserved.

Contents

Chapter 8. Preventive Services

● indicates a new code; ▲, revised; #, re-sequenced; ✚, add-on; ★, audiovisual technology; and ◀, synchronous interactive audio.

Chapter Highlights

- Specific diagnosis and procedure codes for preventive evaluation and management (E/M) services including sports preparticipation physical evaluations.
- Coding for immunization administration (IA) services.
- Assigning and linking proper diagnosis and procedure codes for all preventive services provided at an encounter.
- Reporting a significant E/M service to address a problem at the same encounter as a preventive E/M service.

Preventive Care

Preventive care is the hallmark of pediatrics. A pediatric preventive visit (also known as a health supervision visit or well-child visit) typically includes a preventive medicine E/M service and recommended screenings, tests, and immunizations. In this chapter, we discuss coding for combinations of preventive services.

Payment for Recommended Preventive Care Services

The Patient Protection and Affordable Care Act (PPACA) recognized the importance of preventive care for children and includes a critical provision that ensures that most health care plans cover, *without cost sharing*, the criterion standard of pediatric preventive care—the American Academy of Pediatrics (AAP) *Bright Futures: Guidelines for Health Supervision of Infants, Children, and Adolescents*, 4th Edition (www.aap.org/en/practice-management/bright-futures).

Coverage of and appropriate payment for these pediatric preventive services should, at a minimum, reflect the total relative value units (RVUs) outlined for the current year under the Medicare Resource-Based Relative Value Scale Physician Fee Schedule, inclusive of all separately reported codes for these services. Section 2713 of the PPACA includes the following 2 sets of services that must be provided to children without cost sharing:

1. The standard set of immunizations recommended by the Advisory Committee on Immunization Practices (ACIP) of the Centers for Disease Control and Prevention (CDC) with respect to the individual involved
2. Evidence-informed preventive care and screenings provided for in the comprehensive guidelines supported by the Health Resources and Services Administration (HRSA), which include
   - The AAP/Bright Futures periodicity schedule, "Recommendations for Preventive Pediatric Health Care" (www.aap.org/en/practice-management/care-delivery-approaches/periodicity-schedule)
   - Recommendations of the Advisory Committee on Heritable Disorders in Newborns and Children

The AAP/Bright Futures periodicity schedule is a great tool to identify recommended age-appropriate services, including many that may be reported with their own *Current Procedural Terminology* (*CPT*®) or Healthcare Common Procedure Coding System (HCPCS) code, when provided in conjunction with a comprehensive preventive service or on a separate date of service. This tool can be found as an insert in this book and can be accessed online at www.aap.org/en/practice-management/care-delivery-approaches/periodicity-schedule.

Although all recommended preventive services are covered, physicians and practice managers should be aware of health plan policies that may affect payment.

- Specific diagnosis codes may be required to support claims adjudication under preventive medicine benefits. Be sure to link the appropriate diagnosis to each service provided (eg, code **Z71.3**, dietary counseling, may be linked to code **99401** for a risk-factor reduction counseling visit).
- Some payers bundle certain services when the services are provided on the same date. For instance, some plans will not allow separate payment for obesity counseling on the same date as a well-child examination (at a health supervision visit) but will cover obesity counseling when no other E/M service is provided on the same date.
  - It is beneficial to monitor and maintain awareness of the payment policies of the plans most commonly billed by your practice.
  - Most policies are available on payers' websites with notification of changes provided in payer communications, such as electronic newsletters.

● indicates a new code; ▲, revised; #, re-sequenced; ✛, add-on; ★, audiovisual technology; and ◀, synchronous interactive audio.

Chapter 8. Preventive Services

Preventive Medicine Evaluation and Management Services

Well-child or preventive medicine services are a type of E/M service and are reported with codes **99381–99395**. Most health plans provide a 100% benefit (no patient out-of-pocket cost) for the 31 recommended preventive medicine service encounters when provided by in-network providers. The selection of the pediatric-specific codes **99381–99395** is based simply on the age of the patient and whether the patient is new or established to the practice (**Table 8-1**).

Table 8-1. New and Established Preventive Medicine Codes		
Code Description **Comprehensive preventive medicine evaluation and management**	**New Patient Code**	**Established Patient Code**
infant (age <1 year)	**99381**	**99391**
early childhood (age 1–4 years)	**99382**	**99392**
late childhood (age 5–11 years)	**99383**	**99393**
adolescent (age 12–17 years)	**99384**	**99394**
age 18–39 years	**99385**	**99395**

In brief, an established patient has been seen (face-to-face, including via real-time audiovisual telehealth) by the physician or another physician of the same specialty and group practice within the past 3 years. Generally, other qualified health care professionals (QHPs; eg, advanced practice nurses, physician assistants/associates) are considered to be working in the same specialty as the physicians with whom they work. Refer to **Chapter 7** for more information about *new* versus *established* patients.

> A neonate who received hospital newborn care by the same physician or a physician of the same specialty and same group practice will be an established patient for post-discharge care in the office or other outpatient setting.

- Most health plans limit the benefits for preventive medicine E/M services covered in a year on the basis of the patient's age. See **Figure 8-1** for an illustration of recommended preventive visits by age.
- Immunizations, laboratory tests, and other special procedures or screening tests (eg, vision, hearing, or developmental screening) that have their own specific *CPT* codes are reported separately *in addition to* preventive medicine E/M services.
- Most payers will require reporting modifier **25** with the preventive medicine service when immunizations or other services are also performed and reported. Some payers do not pay for preventive screenings but may allow a physician to bill the patient. Contracts with payers may limit what may be billed to the patient.
- A comprehensive history and physical examination must reflect an age- and a gender-appropriate history and examination.
- The comprehensive history performed as part of a preventive medicine visit requires a comprehensive age-appropriate review of systems (ROS) with an updated past, family, and social history. The history should also include a comprehensive assessment or history of age-pertinent risk factors.
- Generally, the ROS of a preventive medicine service is not a list of systems with pertinent positive and negative responses but, rather, a list of inquiries and patient

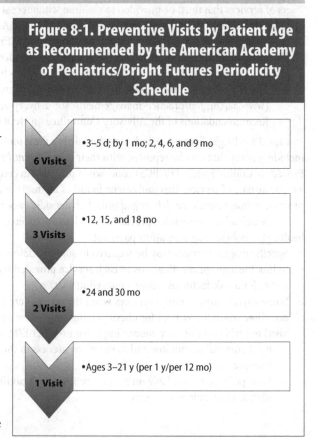

Figure 8-1. Preventive Visits by Patient Age as Recommended by the American Academy of Pediatrics/Bright Futures Periodicity Schedule

6 Visits • 3–5 d; by 1 mo; 2, 4, 6, and 9 mo

3 Visits • 12, 15, and 18 mo

2 Visits • 24 and 30 mo

1 Visit • Ages 3–21 y (per 1 y/per 12 mo)

responses for those areas of risk identified in preventive medicine guidelines as pertinent for patients of that age and gender. However, some payers may require review of all systems regardless of age and gender (eg, required by some Medicaid plans under Early and Periodic Screening, Diagnostic, and Treatment [EPSDT] benefits).

> The American Academy of Pediatrics (AAP) has developed an initial history questionnaire that promotes good documentation of preventive medicine services. Examples can be ordered from the AAP by calling 888/227-1770 or visiting https://shop.aap.org/initial-history-questionnaire-documentation-form. Additionally, some Medicaid programs have developed documentation templates for preventive services delivered in their Early and Periodic Screening, Diagnostic, and Treatment program.

- Routine counseling on and management of contraception are considered part of the comprehensive preventive medicine E/M service when they are provided during the preventive visit. Contraceptive procedures (eg, insertion or removal of a device or implant, injection) are separately reported. See *International Classification of Diseases, 10th Revision, Clinical Modification* (*ICD-10-CM*) category **Z30** for diagnosis codes for contraceptive counseling and/or management.
- A comprehensive physical examination is a multisystem examination that may include a routine pelvic and breast examination (when performed in the absence of specific symptoms of a problem) depending on the age of the patient and/or sexual history. If the pelvic examination is performed because of a gynecologic problem during a routine preventive medicine service, it may be appropriate to report a problem-oriented E/M service in addition to the preventive medicine service when additional physician work and requirements of the E/M code are met.
- Medicaid programs have requirements for performing, documenting, and reporting certain services in their EPSDT programs. Modifier **52** (reduced services) may be required when the complete EPSDT service cannot be completed. Review your Medicaid policies for the specific documentation and reporting requirements for services to patients in these programs.

ICD-10-CM Codes for Preventive Care Visits

ICD-10-CM well-care diagnosis codes should be linked to the appropriate preventive medicine code (**99381–99395**). *ICD-10-CM* codes for well-child examinations include developmental, hearing, and vision screening.

Z00.110	Health examination for newborn <8 days
Z00.111	Health examination for newborn 8–28 days old
Z00.121	Routine child health examination (≥29 days) with abnormal findings
Z00.129	Routine child health examination (≥29 days) without abnormal findings
Z00.00	Encounter for general adult medical examination without abnormal findings
Z00.01	Encounter for general adult medical examination with abnormal findings

- For the purpose of assigning codes from this category, an *abnormal finding* is a newly discovered condition on a screening or a known or chronic condition that requires attention (eg, uncontrolled, acutely exacerbated). Assign additional codes for any abnormal findings. A stable chronic condition is not considered an abnormal finding.
- An abnormal finding *ICD-10-CM* code (eg, **Z00.121**) can be linked to the procedure code for a normal screening test result; the abnormality will be identified with the appropriate *ICD-10-CM* code elsewhere on the claim so the payer will be aware that the abnormality is unrelated to the screening.
- *ICD-10-CM* does not specify an age at which codes **Z00.00** and **Z00.01** are reported in lieu of codes **Z00.121–Z00.129**. The age of majority varies by state and payer, who may or may not adopt the Medicare Outpatient Code Editor assignment of age limitations (29 days–17 years) to codes **Z00.121–Z00.129**, as indicated in many *ICD-10-CM* references.
- Link routine health examination codes (eg, **Z00.129**) and code **Z23** (encounter for immunization) to the IA and vaccine product codes when immunizations are administered at the preventive medicine encounter. *ICD-10-CM* instructs to report code **Z00.-** first, followed by code **Z23**.
- When an existing problem is addressed at the preventive medicine service but is not a newly discovered condition or a known or chronic condition that has increased in severity, report a routine child health examination without abnormal findings and also code the condition addressed.

> **Preventive Services for Children With Chronic and Complex Health Care Needs**
>
> Like all children, children with chronic and complex health care needs must also receive periodic preventive care visits. Preventive medicine evaluation and management (E/M) services may take longer for children who are medically complex. However, preventive E/M services are not reported on the basis of time and prolonged service does not apply. Only report a separate E/M service on the date of a preventive E/M service when a problem is addressed that requires significant physician work (ie, medical decision-making [MDM] or time) and is separately identifiable in the documentation. A chronic medical condition that is not separately addressed with documentation of the required MDM or time spent addressing the condition does not support reporting both preventive care and a separate E/M service (eg, 99213).
>
> See Chapter 10 for information on care management for children with complex health care needs.

Examples

➤ **A 9-year-old is seen for an established patient preventive medicine service.** The child was seen 1 month ago for mild persistent asthma and reports no increase in asthma symptoms. However, the child's mother notes that the child's rescue inhaler, which is carried to and from school, is nearing the expiration date. An age- and gender-appropriate preventive service is provided and documented. A refill prescription is ordered for the rescue inhaler. Diagnoses are well-child visit and stable mild persistent asthma.

ICD-10-CM	CPT
Z00.129 (routine child health exam without abnormal findings) **J45.30** (uncomplicated mild persistent asthma)	**99393** (preventive medicine visit; age 5–11)

Teaching Point: Because the asthma is not newly identified or failing to respond adequately to treatment, this is not an abnormal finding. However, it is appropriate to report the code for the asthma that is still present in addition to code **Z00.129**. In this example, the work of prescribing the asthma medication refill did not equate to a significant, separately identifiable E/M service.

➤ **A 9-year-old was diagnosed 8 weeks ago with mild persistent asthma.** The child presents today for a scheduled preventive service and follow-up visit. The child complains of increasing asthma symptoms and use of rescue inhaler. The patient's medications and asthma control plan are revised, and the physician provides counseling to reinforce the avoidance of asthma triggers and management adherence. The age- and gender-appropriate preventive service is also provided and documented. The diagnoses are well-child visit with abnormal findings and mild persistent asthma with increasing symptoms.

ICD-10-CM	CPT
Z00.121 (routine child health exam with abnormal findings) **J45.31** (mild persistent asthma with acute exacerbation)	**99393** (preventive medicine visit; age 5–11)
J45.31	**99214 25** (established patient office visit with moderate level medical decision-making [MDM])

Teaching Point: Because the asthma was inadequately controlled, the routine health examination included an abnormal finding. A significant E/M service was provided to address the patient's asthma control. For more on this topic, see Reporting a Preventive Medicine Visit With a Problem-Oriented Visit section later in this chapter. Code **J45.31** is reported once on the claim but linked to each procedure code.

If a vaccine had been administered at this encounter, modifier **25** would have also been appended to code **99393** to signify that the preventive E/M service was significant and separately identifiable from the IA service.

Quality Initiatives and Preventive Care

Quality initiatives and measurement are becoming standard practice in health care. Many physicians have participated in quality measurement through programs such as the Centers for Medicare & Medicaid Services (CMS) Promoting Interoperability Programs and medical home recognition programs. In pediatrics, many quality measures are associated with preventive care (eg, provision of one meningococcal vaccine on or between the patient's 11th and 13th birthdays).

● indicates a new code; ▲, revised; #, re-sequenced; ✦, add-on; ★, audiovisual technology; and ◀, synchronous interactive audio.

Quality measurement is also required of health plans funded by government programs or offered through health exchanges created to support health insurance adoption under the PPACA. These health plans must collect and submit Quality Rating System measure data to the CMS. This entails collecting clinical quality measures, including a subset of the National Committee for Quality Assurance Healthcare Effectiveness Data and Information Set (HEDIS) measures and a Pharmacy Quality Alliance measure. Physicians contracting with these plans may be asked to provide evidence that quality measures were met through claims data or medical records. Examples of HEDIS measures related to preventive care include

- Percentage of members who turned 15 or 30 months old during the measurement year and who had 6 or more well-child visits with a primary care provider during the first 15 months after birth *and* 2 or more well-child visits from 1 day after the child turned 15 months old to turning 30 months old
- Percentage of members 3 to 21 years of age who had at least 1 comprehensive well-care visit with a primary care provider or obstetrician-gynecologist during the measurement year
- Members 3 to 17 years of age who had an outpatient visit with a primary care provider and who had the following services in the current year:
  — Body mass index (BMI) percentile documentation
  — Counseling for nutrition
  — Counseling for physical activity

Certain preventive services, such as anticipatory guidance on healthy diet (**Z71.3**) and exercise (**Z71.82**), are components of the preventive medicine service and require no additional procedure coding for payment purposes. However, associated diagnosis and procedure codes may be reported to support quality reporting initiatives.

ICD-10-CM guidelines instruct that codes for BMI are reported when the there is an associated, reportable diagnosis (eg, overweight, obesity). However, some health plans still require this code to support quality measures in lieu of *CPT* performance measurement code **3008F** (BMI, documented). Pediatric BMI codes in category **Z68** include

Z68.51	BMI <5th percentile
Z68.52	BMI 5th–<85th percentile
Z68.53	BMI 85th–95th percentile
Z68.54	BMI ≥95th percentile

> *International Classification of Diseases, 10th Revision, Clinical Modification (ICD-10-CM)* codes for pediatric body mass index (BMI) percentiles (Z68.51–Z68.54) are reported only in conjunction with physician documentation of a related condition (eg, overweight, obesity). If reporting codes Z68.51–Z68.54 on the basis of a payer's written guidance for reporting quality measures, it is advisable to keep a copy of the payer's guidance. An alternative method for reporting that the patient's BMI was documented is to report *Current Procedural Terminology* Category II code 3008F (BMI, documented) in lieu of *ICD-10-CM* codes for BMI.

Any chronic conditions reported may also support quality measurement and/or risk adjustment. See **chapters 3** and **10** to learn more about risk adjustment and reporting chronic conditions.

Certain other procedure codes also support quality measurement. For example, submission of claims containing codes for meningococcal (**90734**, **#90619**); tetanus, diphtheria, and acellular pertussis (**90715**); and 2 or 3 doses of human papillomavirus (HPV) vaccine (**90651**) provided to an adolescent before the patient's 13th birthday is indicative of meeting the measure for the immunization of adolescents.

Some quality measures include information on reporting that a patient is ineligible for inclusion in the measure. For example, screening for depression (**Z13.31**) is recommended for patients 12 years and older who were seen during the measurement year. However, patients already diagnosed with depression or bipolar disorder are not included in the measurement.

Example

> ➤ **A 13-year-old currently under a pediatrician's care for depression returns for a well-child visit.** A preventive service is provided including documentation of the child's BMI and counseling for healthy diet and exercise. The physician also counsels for booster immunization against COVID-19. The vaccine is administered at the encounter. The patient is not screened for depression because of an active diagnosis of depression, but the physician briefly inquires about whether the patient or parents have any concerns regarding current management. The physician issues a refill of the medication prescribed for the depression as requested by the patient's mother because the previous pharmacy is no longer in network with the patient's health plan.

Chapter 8. Preventive Services

ICD-10-CM	CPT
Z00.129 (routine child health examination without abnormal findings) **Z71.3** (anticipatory guidance on healthy diet) **Z71.82** (exercise counseling) **F32.9** (major depressive disorder, single episode, unspecified)	**99394** **3008F** (BMI, documented)
Z00.129 (routine child health examination without abnormal findings) **F32.9** (major depressive disorder, single episode, unspecified)	**G9717** (documentation stating the patient has had a diagnosis of depression or has had a diagnosis of bipolar disorder)
Z00.129 **Z23** (encounter for immunization) *Note:* See the Coding for COVID-19 Immunization section later in this chapter for more information.	**0004A** (IA by intramuscular injection of severe acute respiratory syndrome coronavirus 2 [SARS-CoV-2] [coronavirus disease (COVID-19)] vaccine, mRNA-LNP, spike protein, preservative free, 30 mcg/0.3 mL dosage, diluent reconstituted; booster dose) **91300** (severe acute respiratory syndrome coronavirus 2 [SARS-CoV-2] [coronavirus disease (COVID-19)] vaccine, mRNA-LNP, spike protein, PF, 30 mcg/0.3mL dosage, diluent reconstituted, for IM use)

Teaching Point: Reporting code **G9717** removes this patient from the population measured for screening for depression and a follow-up plan. If the physician uses a structured screening instrument to briefly assess the patient's depression status, code **96127** is reported for the use of the instrument with documentation and scoring. Codes **G9717** and **3008F** are only informational and should have no charge or, if required for claims processing, a charge of $0.01.

Codes **Z13.41** (encounter for autism screening) and **Z13.42** (encounter for screening for global developmental delays [milestones]) may be used to track developmental screening measures of the Child Core Set for patients receiving benefits through their Medicaid and Children's Health Insurance Program. Use of the Child Core Set is optional for state programs and physicians. Codes **Z13.41** and **Z13.42** may be reported at any encounter where screening is performed (eg, with or without a preventive E/M service).

It is important to note that a request for medical records is less likely when claims are submitted with procedure and diagnosis codes associated with pediatric quality measures.

See Chapter 3 for more information on Healthcare Effectiveness Data and Information Set and quality reporting.

Sports/Camp Preparticipation Physical Evaluations

CPT guidelines recommend that preventive medicine service codes (**99381–99395**) be reported, when possible, for physical evaluations performed to determine participation eligibility. These codes most accurately describe the services performed in that they are preventive and age appropriate in nature and physicians offer counseling on topics such as appropriate levels of exercise or injury prevention. However, the need for these services often arises after the child has had a yearly preventive medicine service, thereby rendering this service non-covered by some health plans, which allow only 1 preventive service per year. In this case, the parent may be billed if the payer contract allows because the service is non-covered.

ICD-10-CM code **Z02.5** is reported for an encounter for examination for participation in sports. If the preparticipation physical evaluation is incorporated into the annual health supervision visit, use code **Z00.121** or **Z00.129** in lieu of **Z02.5**. Any problems or conditions that are addressed during the course of the visit would also be reported.

Codes in category **Z02** are not reported in conjunction with codes for routine child health examination (category **Z00**).

● indicates a new code; ▲, revised; #, re-sequenced; ✚, add-on; ★, audiovisual technology; and ◀, synchronous interactive audio.

When reporting sports or camp preparticipation physical evaluations for patients who have already received a recommended preventive medicine service, check the health plan's policy on payment for these services and instructions for coding and billing. Under some plans (especially Medicaid plans), school and preparticipation physical evaluations may be covered even when the child has already had an annual preventive medicine service.

Office visit codes (**99212–99215**) may be used if a problem is discovered during the service. Outpatient consultation codes (**99242–99245**) might be considered (when the health plan allows payment for these codes) if the coach or school nurse requested the physician's opinion of a suspected problem (eg, exercise cough associated with reduced performance in cold weather). The medical record must include documentation of the written or verbal request as well as a copy of the written report with the physician's opinion or advice that was sent back to the coach or school nurse when reporting a consultation.

Learn more about reporting preparticipation physical evaluations, including those for return to activity after COVID-19, in the July 2021 *AAP Pediatric Coding Newsletter* article, "Coding for 2021 Preparticipation Physical Evaluations" (https://doi.org/10.1542/pcco_book207_document001).

Immunizations

Vaccine services are reported by using 2 families of *CPT* codes—one for the vaccine serum (the product) and one for the services associated with the administration of the vaccine. Exceptions to this fall under those patients receiving vaccines through the Vaccines for Children (VFC) program. See the Vaccines for Children Program section later in this chapter for more details on VFC coding.

Vaccines and Toxoids

> The administration of immunoglobulins (including palivizumab [Synagis]) is not reported using the immunization administration codes. See codes 96365–96368, 96372, 96374, and 96375. Medications, including birth control, are reported with 96372 (therapeutic, prophylactic, or diagnostic subcutaneous or intramuscular injection).

Codes **90476–90758** and **91300–91307** are used to report the vaccine or toxoid product only. They do not include the administration of a vaccine.

- **Appendix III** provides a quick reference to codes, descriptors, and the number of vaccine components for each vaccine linked to the brand and manufacturer for each.
- The exact vaccine product administered needs to be reported to meet the requirements of immunization registries, vaccine distribution programs, and reporting systems (eg, Vaccine Adverse Event Reporting System), as well as for payment.
- Codes may be specific to the product manufacturer and brand, schedule (ie, number of doses or timing), chemical formulation, dosage, and/or route of administration. When a vaccine code descriptor includes "when administered to" patients of certain ages, this is not an indication of the ages for which the product is licensed.
- Codes for combination vaccines (eg, **90697**, diphtheria, tetanus toxoids, acellular pertussis vaccine, inactivated poliovirus vaccine, Haemophilus influenza type b PRP-OMP conjugate vaccine, and hepatitis B vaccine [DTaP-IPV-Hib-HepB]) are available, as are separate codes for single-component vaccines (eg, **90744**, Hep B).
- It is not appropriate to code each component of a combination vaccine separately by using separate vaccine product codes when a combination vaccine is administered. However, if a combination vaccine is commercially available but a physician elects to administer the component vaccines due to unavailability or other clinical reason, each vaccine product administered would be separately reported.

> The word *component* refers to an antigen in a vaccine that prevents disease(s) caused by 1 organism.

New Vaccines/Toxoids

The *CPT* Editorial Panel, in recognition of the public health interest in vaccine products, has chosen to publish new vaccine product codes before US Food and Drug Administration (FDA) approval. The American Medical Association (AMA) uses its *CPT* site (www.ama-assn.org/practice-management/cpt/category-i-vaccine-codes) to provide updates of *CPT* Editorial Panel actions on new vaccine products. Once approved by the *CPT* Editorial Panel, vaccine/toxoid product codes are typically made available for release on a semiannual basis (July 1 and January 1). As part of the electronic distribution, there is

● indicates a new code; ▲, revised; #, re-sequenced; ✚, add-on; ★, audiovisual technology; and ◀, synchronous interactive audio.

a 6-month implementation period from the initial release date (ie, codes released on January 1 are eligible for use on July 1; codes released on July 1 are eligible for use on January 1). Codes for products pending FDA approval are indicated with a lightning bolt symbol (⚡) and will be tracked by the AMA to monitor FDA approval status. The lightning bolt symbol will be removed once the FDA status changes to "approved." Refer to the AMA *CPT* site indicated earlier for the most up-to-date information on codes with this symbol. More rapid code release and implementation may occur when a government agency has identified an urgent need for a vaccine to address an emergent health issue and the FDA has granted that vaccine an expedited review process. In such cases, codes may be approved and released on an *immediate* (ie, outside the normal code consideration schedule) or *rapid* (ie, within the normal code consideration schedule but released shortly after approval with an implementation date within 3 months of release) basis.

Before administering any new vaccine product or an existing vaccine product with new recommendations, make certain that the CDC, in the *Morbidity and Mortality Weekly Report,* or the AAP, in *Pediatrics,* has endorsed the use or recommendations of the vaccine. You may also want to verify with a patient's health plan that the vaccine is covered.

In the rare event that a vaccine enters the market this year and is FDA approved, recommendations for use are published by the CDC or AAP, and no code exists for the specific vaccine, use code **90749** (unlisted vaccine/toxoid) and list the specific vaccine given.

National Drug Code

Many payers, specifically Medicare, Medicaid, other government payers (eg, Tricare), and some private payers, require the use of the National Drug Code (NDC) when reporting vaccine product codes. The NDCs are universal product identifiers for medications, including vaccines. NDCs are found on outer packaging, product labels, and/or product inserts. Report the NDC from the outer packaging or product labels/inserts as required by the payer. This is discussed more fully in **Chapter 1**.

NDCs are 10-digit, 3-segment numbers that identify the product, labeler, and trade package size. The Health Insurance Portability and Accountability Act of 1996 standards require an 11-digit code. See **Chapter 1** and **Table 1-3** for more information including how 10-digit codes are converted to the 11-digit format for reporting.

If you are not currently reporting vaccines with NDCs, be sure to coordinate the requirements with your billing software company. For more information on NDCs, visit www.fda.gov/Drugs/InformationOnDrugs/ucm142438.htm.

Immunization Administration

CPT codes for IA are reported *in addition to* vaccine/toxoid code(s) **90476–90758** and **91300–91307**. There are 3 sets of IA codes.
- **0001A–0104A** (administration of COVID-19 vaccine products)
- **90460** and **90461** (immunization administration with counseling by a physician or QHP to child from birth through 18 years of age)
- **90471–90474** (immunization administration to adult or to a child, from birth through 18 years of age, without counseling by a physician or QHP)

Administration of childhood immunizations for COVID-19 are discussed separately from other immunizations, as the administration codes for these services are structured differently from the codes for routine immunization.

Coding for COVID-19 Immunization

During the public health emergency (PHE) declared in response to COVID-19, a specific set of codes was developed for COVID-19 vaccines and their administration. Codes for the COVID-19 vaccine products and their administration were assigned specific codes by product and dose (eg, administration of first, second, third, or booster dose) and have been updated with each new authorized use of a specific product.

CPT Appendix Q provides a quick reference guide to codes for COVID-19 vaccine products and administration.

Administration of COVID-19 vaccines includes counseling and time spent monitoring the patient after vaccine administration.

> **COVID-19 vaccine products and codes were still evolving at the time of this publication. See the American Academy of Pediatrics web page, "COVID-19 Vaccine Administration: Getting Paid," for an up-to-date discussion of coding for COVID-19 vaccines and administration (https://services.aap.org/en/pages/2019-novel-coronavirus-covid-19-infections/covid-19-vaccine-for-children/covid-19-vaccine-administration-getting-paid).**

● indicates a new code; ▲, revised; #, re-sequenced; ✚, add-on; ★, audiovisual technology; and ◀, synchronous interactive audio.

Example

➤ **A 5-year-old established patient with no symptoms presents to be tested for COVID-19 caused by suspected exposure at school.** The child tests negative for COVID-19. The parent is counseled regarding benefits of immunization and agrees to have the child immunized. The first dose of the Pfizer-BioNTech COVID-19 vaccine is administered.

CPT: appropriate code for the COVID-19 test performed (eg, **87635 QW** [infectious agent detection by nucleic acid (DNA or RNA); severe acute respiratory syndrome coronavirus 2 (SARS-CoV-2) (coronavirus disease [COVID-19]), multiplex amplified probe technique])

ICD-10-CM: **Z20.822** (contact with and [suspected] exposure to COVID-19) linked to code for COVID-19 test, **Z23** (encounter for immunization) linked to codes for vaccine and IA

CPT: **91307** (SARS-CoV-2 [coronavirus disease (COVID-19)] vaccine, mRNA-LNP, spike protein, PF, 10 mcg/0.2 mL dosage, diluent reconstituted, tris-sucrose formulation, for IM use)

CPT: **0071A** (immunization administration by intramuscular injection of severe acute respiratory syndrome coronavirus 2 [SARS-CoV-2] [coronavirus disease (COVID-19)] vaccine, mRNA-LNP, spike protein, preservative free, 10 mcg/0.2 mL dosage, diluent reconstituted, tris-sucrose formulation; first dose)

Teaching Point: Only the administration of the first dose of the vaccine is reported with code **0071A**. Code **0072A** is reported for administration of the second dose of this vaccine product. Code **0073A** will be reported for administration of a third dose, when indicated.

A clinically indicated separate E/M service to address a patient's signs, symptoms, or diagnosed illness may be reported with modifier **25** appended to the E/M code when the service is significant and separately identifiable from the other services reported. Immunization counseling is included in the IA and is not a separately reportable service.

Note that, unlike other IA codes (**90460, 90461; 90471–90474**), codes for administration of a COVID-19 vaccine identify the specific product administered. This has been in part caused by federal government provision of vaccine products at no charge to the physician or other provider during the COVID-19 PHE. Some payers require reporting of the COVID-19 vaccine code with a $0.00 or $0.01 charge and the appropriate administration code, while others require only the appropriate IA code. As with any vaccine, always follow the ACIP recommendations.

Codes 90460 and 90461

90460   Immunization administration through 18 years of age via any route of administration, with counseling by physician or other qualified health care professional; first or only component of each vaccine or toxoid administered

✚90461   each additional vaccine or toxoid component administered (report only in addition to **90460**)

When reporting codes **90460** and **90461**,

- Physicians or QHPs must provide *face-to-face* counseling to the patient and/or family (patient aged ≤18 years) at the time of the encounter for the administration of a vaccine. (See the Codes **90471–90474** section later in this chapter for IA without physician counseling or to patients >18 years. Also see the Coding for Counseling When Immunizations Are Not Carried Out section later in this chapter.)
- *CPT* defines a physician or other QHP as follows:

   A "physician or other qualified health care professional" is an individual who by education, training, licensure/regulation, facility credentialing (when applicable), and facility privileging (when applicable) performs a professional service within his/her scope of practice and independently reports that professional service. These professionals are distinct from "clinical staff."

- Clinical staff will not qualify to perform the counseling reported under codes **90460** and **90461**. While state scope of practice may allow certain clinical staff to perform the service, it will not qualify them to report these codes. In the absence of counseling by a physician or QHP, administration services by clinical staff are reported with codes **90471–90474**. *CPT* defines clinical staff as follows:

   A clinical staff member is a person who works under the supervision of a physician or other qualified health care professional and who is allowed by law, regulation, and facility policy to perform or assist in the performance of a specified professional service, but who does not individually report that professional service. Other policies may also affect who may report specific services.

- When a private payer contract does not allow QHPs to report services under their own name and National Provider Identifier, check with the payer to determine the eligibility of these professionals to report immunization counseling (**90460, 90461**) and report under the name and number of the supervising physician.

- Documentation of immunization counseling should include a listing of all vaccine components with notation that counseling was provided for all listed components with authentication (electronic or written signature and date) by the physician or other QHP. Supply of the Vaccine Information Statement (VIS) without discussion of risks and benefits does not constitute counseling. Some payers require documentation of parent or caregiver questions or concerns that were addressed during counseling.
- Code **90460** is reported for the *first (or only) component of each vaccine administered* (whether single or combination) on a day of service and includes the related vaccine counseling.
- Code **90461** is reported only in conjunction with **90460** and is used to report the work of counseling for *each additional component(s) beyond the first* in a given combination vaccine. (See the Vaccines for Children Program section later in this chapter for reporting administration of vaccines containing multiple components to this program.)
- Combination vaccines are those vaccines that contain multiple vaccine components. Refer to **Appendix III** for the number of components in the most commonly reported pediatric vaccines.
- Immunization administration codes include the physician or other QHP discussing risks and benefits of the vaccines, providing parents with a copy of the appropriate CDC VIS for each vaccine given, giving the vaccine, and observing and addressing reactions or side effects, as well as the cost of clinical staff time to record each vaccine component administered in the medical record and statewide vaccine registry and the cost of supplies (eg, syringe, needle, bandages).

Code **90460** is reported for each individual vaccine administered because every vaccine will have, at minimum, 1 vaccine component. For combination vaccines, code **90461** is additionally reported for counseling on each additional component. No modifier is typically required for reporting multiple units of the IA codes. Most payers advise reporting multiple units of the same service on a single line of the claim. However, individual payer guidance may vary. The AAP continues to advocate to the CMS for increased RVUs for codes **90460** and **90461**.

Append modifier **25** when a significant, separately identifiable E/M service (eg, office or other outpatient service, preventive medicine service) is performed in addition to the vaccine and toxoid administration codes. If vaccines are given during the course of a preventive medicine E/M service and another E/M service, both E/M services will need modifier **25** if required by the payer. See also the Reporting a Preventive Medicine Visit With a Problem-Oriented Visit section later in this chapter.

Examples

➤ **An adolescent presents for an influenza immunization.** After you counsel the patient, clinical staff administer an intranasal quadrivalent influenza vaccine (LAIV) at the same encounter.

Report code **90460** with 1 unit in addition to **90672** (LAIV). Code **90461** is not reported because the vaccine contains only 1 component (ie, protects against 1 disease). Link the vaccine and administration *CPT* codes to *ICD-10-CM* code **Z23** on health insurance claims.

➤ **A 6-month-old patient presents for an established patient well-baby visit.** The physician (or QHP) provides and documents the preventive medicine E/M service. The physician counsels the caregivers about recommended immunization with diphtheria and tetanus toxoids and acellular pertussis vaccine, inactivated poliovirus vaccine, and *Haemophilus influenzae* type b vaccine (DTaP-IPV/Hib); pneumococcal vaccine (PCV13); and influenza (IIV4) vaccine. The parent/guardian is given the CDC VIS and consents; the nurse prepares the vaccine. The nurse administers each vaccine, charts the required information, and accesses and enters vaccine data into the statewide immunization registry. The patient is discharged home after the nurse confirms that there are no serious immediate reactions.

ICD-10-CM	*CPT*
Z00.129 (encounter for routine child health examination without abnormal findings)	**99391 25** (preventive E/M service, established patient; infant [age younger than 1 year])
Z00.129 **Z23** (encounter for immunization)	**90700** (DTaP-IPV/Hib, for IM use) **90670** (PCV13, for IM use) **90685** (IIV4, split virus, preservative free, 0.25ml dose, for IM use) **90460** × 3 **90461** × 4

● indicates a new code; ▲, revised; #, re-sequenced; ✦, add-on; ★, audiovisual technology; and ◀, synchronous interactive audio.

Teaching Point: Because the physician personally performed the counseling, code **90460** is reported for the initial component of the DTaP-IPV/Hib vaccine and each of the 2 single-component vaccines. Code **90460** is appropriate regardless of the route of administration. Code **90461** is reported for the 4 secondary components of the DTaP-IPV/Hib vaccine.

Payers who have adopted the Medicare National Correct Coding Initiative (NCCI) edits will require that modifier **25** be appended to code **99391** to signify that it was significant and separately identifiable from the IA. (For more information on NCCI edits, see **Chapter 2.**) *ICD-10-CM* code **Z00.129** is reported first, followed by code **Z23**.

Codes 90471–90474

90471	Immunization administration (includes percutaneous, intradermal, subcutaneous, or intramuscular injections); one vaccine (single or combination vaccine/toxoid)
+90472	each additional vaccine (single or combination vaccine/toxoid)
	(List separately in addition to code for primary procedure.) (Use code **90472** in conjunction with **90460**, **90471**, or **90473**.)
90473	Immunization administration by intranasal or oral route; one vaccine (single or combination vaccine/toxoid)
+90474	each additional vaccine (single or combination vaccine/toxoid)
	(List separately in addition to code for primary procedure.) (Use code **90474** in conjunction with **90460**, **90471**, or **90473**.)

Codes **90471–90474** will be reported when criteria for reporting the 2 pediatric IA codes (**90460** and **90461**) have not been met. This occurs when either of the following circumstances are true:

- The physician or QHP does not counsel the patient or family or does not document that the counseling was personally performed.
- The patient is 19 years or older.

The CMS assigned 0.49 RVUs to codes **90460**, **90471**, and **90473** and 0.37 RVUs to codes **90461**, **90472**, and **90474** in 2022 (2023 RVUs were not established at the time of this publication).

- Appropriate reporting of codes **90460** and **90461** in lieu of codes **90471–90474** should result in higher payment based on reporting of multiple units of code **90461** for *each additional vaccine component* versus reporting of codes **90472** and **90474** for *each additional vaccine product.*
- Individual payers may or may not assign payment values based on the RVUs published by the CMS. (Administration of vaccines provided through the VFC program is paid differently. For more about the VFC program, see the Vaccines for Children Program section later in this chapter.)

When reporting codes **90471–90474**,

- Codes **90471–90474** are reported for each vaccine administered, whether single or combination vaccines.
- *Only one* "first" IA code (**90460**, **90471**, or **90473**) may be reported per date of service.

The "first" IA code can be reported from either family or either route of administration (eg, when a patient receives an immunization via injection and a second one via intranasal route, IA services can be reported with codes **90471** and **90474** or with codes **90473** and **90472**).

- If a physician personally performs counseling on one vaccine but not on another when given during the same encounter, IA will be reported by using codes **90460** (and **90461** if appropriate) and either **90472** (IA, each additional vaccine via injection) or **90474** (IA, each additional vaccine via intranasal or oral route). The Medicare NCCI edits pair code **90460** with codes **90471** and **90473** and, therefore, do not allow codes from the pairs to be reported on the same day of service by the same physician or physician of the same group and specialty.

For more information on vaccine administration, please see the following examples and **Appendix III**:

Examples

➤ **A 4-year-old patient who was recently seen as a new patient for clearance to attend preschool returns for influenza immunization, which was not available at the time of the previous visit.** The service is scheduled with clinical staff only. The patient is noted to be in good health with no contraindications to the immunization per CDC guidelines. Next, the VIS and the antipyretic dosage for weight are reviewed with the father, who provides consent for the immunization. The influenza vaccine is administered, and the child is observed for immediate reactions before discharge.

● indicates a new code; ▲, revised; #, re-sequenced; ✚, add-on; ★, audiovisual technology; and ◄, synchronous interactive audio.

ICD-10-CM	CPT
Z23 (encounter for immunization)	**90686** (influenza vaccine [IIV4], preservative free, 0.5 mL, IM) **90471** (IA, first injection)

Teaching Point: Because counseling by a physician or QHP is not provided at this encounter, code **90471** is reported in lieu of **90460**.

➤ **A 5-year-old established patient presented 2 weeks ago for her 5-year checkup and vaccines.** At that appointment, her physician provided counseling for each recommended vaccine component and corresponding VISs. The patient's mother asked that the vaccines be split, so only the DTaP and IPV vaccines were given at that encounter. The patient returns today and sees a nurse for an immunization-only visit to get the measles-mumps-rubella (MMR) and varicella vaccines.

ICD-10-CM	CPT
Z23 (encounter for immunization)	**90707** (MMR, live) **90471** (IA, first injection) **90716** (varicella vaccine) **90472** (IA, subsequent injection)

Teaching Point: Services at this second visit did not include physician counseling, which is required to support use of **90460** and **90461**. Counseling for all vaccines occurred at the most recent encounter and all VISs were handed out, so only administration occurred today. Immunization administration of DTaP and IPV vaccines at the previous encounter would be reported with *CPT* codes **90460** × 2 and **90461** × 2 (in addition to the code for the 5-year preventive service) for services completed on that date.

Only report codes 90460 and 90461 when physician counseling is provided on the date of vaccine administration. If vaccine administration is delayed to another date when physician counseling is not provided, report codes 90471–90474 as appropriate. There is no separate procedure code for counseling without administration during a preventive medicine service.

➤ **A 19-year-old established patient presents for a college entrance examination.** In addition to providing a preventive medicine service, the physician counsels the patient on the need for meningococcal serogroup B (MenB-4C) immunization. The vaccine is administered, and a medical history and physical examination form provided by the college are completed.

ICD-10-CM	CPT
Z02.0 (encounter for examination for admission to educational institution)	**99395 25** (preventive medicine service, established patient, 18–39 years old)
Z23 (encounter for immunization)	**90620** (MenB-4C) **90471** (IA, first injection)

Teaching Point: Because the patient is older than 18 years, code **90460** cannot be reported even though the physician provided counseling for the vaccine provided. Code **Z02.0** is appropriate as the reason the patient presented for the encounter. Code **Z00.00** (encounter for general adult medical examination without abnormal findings) is not reported because *ICD-10-CM* excludes reporting of code **Z00.00** in conjunction with codes in category **Z02**. Code **Z00.00** is reported in lieu of **Z02** when the patient receives a routine age- and gender-appropriate preventive medicine E/M service.

● indicates a new code; ▲, revised; #, re-sequenced; ✚, add-on; ★, audiovisual technology; and ◀, synchronous interactive audio.

Coding for Counseling When Immunizations Are Not Carried Out

Pediatricians may counsel patients and caregivers on the need for immunization but either decide that immunization is contraindicated or decide not to obtain consent to immunize.

> When immunization counseling takes place at the time of a preventive evaluation and management service (well-child visit) and does not result in administration, the counseling is not separately reported.

- When the purpose of the encounter is immunization counseling and immunizations are not administered, preventive medicine counseling codes **99401–99404** (for further discussion, see the Counseling and/or Risk-Factor Reduction section later in this chapter) may be reported on the basis of the time spent in face-to-face counseling with the patient and/or caregivers.
  - Codes for E/M services to address health problems (eg, **99202**) may be reported in addition to **99401–99404** when preventive counseling is provided at the same encounter. Append modifier **25** (significant, separately identifiable E/M service) to the problem-oriented code (eg, **99202 25**) when reporting both services at the same encounter.

> When a payer does not pay for immunization safety counseling services reported with codes 99401–99404, another evaluation and management (E/M) service (eg, office E/M service) may be reported on the basis of the time spent on that date of service.

  - Report *ICD-10-CM* code **Z71.85** (encounter for immunization safety counseling) as the primary diagnosis. In addition, report the reason that an immunization was not carried out, beginning with a code from *ICD-10-CM* category **Z28**, immunization not carried out, and under-immunization status.
- Under-immunization is reported with codes in subcategory **Z28.3-**.
Z28.310	Unvaccinated for COVID-19
Z28.311	Partially vaccinated for COVID-19
Z28.39	Other underimmunization status

> Codes in subcategory Z28.3- should not be used for individuals who are ineligible for the COVID-19 vaccines, as determined by the health care professional. Additional codes in category Z28 are reported to indicate the reason for under-immunization status.

- Contraindications to immunization are captured with codes in subcategory **Z28.0-**.
Z28.01	Immunization not carried out because of acute illness of patient
Z28.02	chronic illness or condition of patient
Z28.03	immune compromised state of patient
Z28.04	patient allergy to vaccine or component
Z28.09	other contraindication
- Other codes in category **Z28** provide for reporting of immunization not carried out due to patient reasons, caregiver refusal, or other specified reason.
Z28.1	Immunization not carried out because of patient decision for reasons of belief or group pressure
Z28.20	because of patient decision for unspecified reason
Z28.21	because of patient refusal
Z28.29	because of patient decision for other reason
Z28.81	due to patient having had the disease
Z28.82	because of caregiver refusal
Z28.83	due to unavailability of vaccine

> The American Academy of Pediatrics offers additional resources for addressing refusal to vaccinate, including vaccine refusal forms in English and Spanish (https://downloads.aap.org/DOPCSP/SOID_RTV_form_01-2019_English.pdf and https://downloads.aap.org/DOPCSP/SOID_RTV_form_01-2019_Spanish.pdf).

Chapter 8. Preventive Services

Examples

➤ **Parents of a 2-month-old established patient come to their physician's office to discuss immunizations.** To date, they have refused to have their infant immunized. Although the physician has discussed the need for vaccines during the infant's previous visits, the parents indicate they have further questions. The physician spends 20 minutes counseling the parents about current recommendations, safety and efficacy of vaccines, and their importance in preventing disease.

ICD-10-CM	CPT
Z71.89 (other specified counseling) **Z28.3** (personal history of under-immunization status) **Z28.82** (vaccination not carried out because of caregiver refusal)	**99401** (risk-factor reduction counseling) or **99213** (office E/M, 20–29 minutes)

Teaching Point: Because the *CPT* midpoint rule applies, code **99401** is reported for service times between 8 and 22 minutes. Alternatively, when a payer does not pay for code **99401**, established patient office E/M code **99213** is reported for 20 to 29 minutes of a physician's or QHP's total time on the date of the encounter that was directed to care of the individual patient.

➤ **An 11-year-old girl (new patient) presents to a pediatrician for a preventive medicine service.** In addition to the preventive E/M service with no abnormal findings, the physician discusses risks of the HPV vaccine and the disease for which it provides protection. The parent/guardian is given the CDC VIS. The parent/guardian consents; the nurse prepares to administer the vaccine. However, the patient refuses to be immunized. The physician returns to the examination room and provides additional counseling, but the patient continues to refuse the vaccine. The patient's mother wishes to discuss the decision with the child's father and return on a later date. A follow-up appointment is scheduled.

ICD-10-CM	CPT
Z00.129 **Z28.21** (immunization not carried out because of patient refusal)	**99383**

Teaching Point: Because no vaccine was administered, no charge for the product or the administration would be reported. Written procedures for documentation and reporting of expired and wasted vaccine doses may be required for vaccines provided under the VFC program.

When the patient returns for follow-up, the codes reported will depend on the outcome of the encounter. If the vaccine is administered after additional physician counseling at the same encounter, code **90460** will be reported in addition to the appropriate vaccine product code. If the patient returns for administration by clinical staff without additional counseling by a physician, code **90471** will be reported in lieu of **90460**.

Additional counseling at the follow-up physician visit that does not result in immunization may be reported with a preventive medicine counseling code (**99401–99404**) based on the physician's face-to-face time with the patient. Do not report codes **99401–99404** on the same date as a preventive medicine E/M service (eg, **99383**).

Note that modifier **JW** (drug amount discarded/not administered to any patient) is typically inappropriate when no vaccine is administered to the patient. Modifier **JW** is used to report waste from a single-dose vial/package when the required patient dose is less than the available single-dose amount. Two claim lines report the amounts administered and wasted. Follow payer instructions for reporting wasted vaccines and use of modifier **JW**.

For more information, see the July 2020 *AAP Pediatric Coding Newsletter* article, "Coding for Vaccines Not Administered," (https://doi.org/10.1542/pcco_book195_document007).

Vaccines for Children Program

The VFC program makes vaccines available to children, teens, and young adults up to 19 years of age who meet any of the following criteria: are enrolled in the Medicaid program (depending on the Medicaid managed care), do not have health insurance, have no coverage of immunizations under their health plan, or are American Indians or Alaska Natives. Vaccines are provided at no cost to the participating physician or patient, and payment is made only for administration of the vaccine.

● indicates a new code; ▲, revised; #, re-sequenced; ✚, add-on; ★, audiovisual technology; and ◀, synchronous interactive audio.

If reporting the VFC vaccine with administration codes and not the product code, data for the vaccine products administered must be captured for registry and quality initiatives. This can be accomplished by entering the vaccine codes with a $0 charge (if your billing system allows) and appending modifier **SL** (state-supplied vaccine) to the vaccine code. However, follow individual payer rules for reporting.

Providers are encouraged to use code **90460** for administration of a vaccine under the VFC program unless otherwise directed by a state program. If code **90461** is used for a vaccine with multiple antigens or components, it should be given a $0 value for a child covered under the VFC program. This applies to Medicaid-enrolled VFC-entitled children as well as non–Medicaid-enrolled VFC-entitled children (ie, uninsured, underinsured, and American Indian or Alaska Native children not enrolled in Medicaid).

Please be aware that some Medicaid programs do have reporting rules that differ from those of VFC. *Be sure to get this policy in writing from your Medicaid program* and follow it to prevent denied payment. The AAP continues to advocate to the CMS to allow for recognition and payment for component-based vaccine counseling and administration (ie, code **90461**). Under the current statute, administration can be paid only "per vaccine" and not per component.

Participants in the VFC program should be aware of program-specific guidance, including storage of VFC vaccine separate from privately purchased vaccines. For more information on the VFC program, visit www.cdc.gov/vaccines/programs/vfc/index.html.

See "FAQ: Immunization Administration" at www.aap.org/cfp2023 for more discussion of coding for IA.

Screening Tests and Procedures

Recommendations for age-appropriate screening services are outlined in the AAP/Bright Futures periodicity schedule, "Recommendations for Preventive Pediatric Health Care" (www.aap.org/en/practice-management/care-delivery-approaches/periodicity-schedule) or in your state's EPSDT plan.

When routine vision, developmental, and/or hearing screening services are performed in conjunction with a preventive medicine visit, the diagnosis code for a routine infant or child health checkup should be linked to the appropriate screening service. The services/codes listed as follows are examples of services that could be used to screen a patient. Some payers have specific policies that outline covered screening tools based on age; know your payer policies. For example, past a certain age, code **92567** (tympanometry) may not be covered under preventive services.

Hearing Screening

92551	Screening test, pure tone, air only
92552	Pure tone audiometry (threshold); air only (full assessment)
#92558	Evoked otoacoustic emissions, screening (qualitative measurement of distortion product or transient evoked otoacoustic emissions), automated analysis
92567	Tympanometry (impedance testing)
92568	Acoustic reflex testing, threshold portion
92583	Select picture audiometry

Audiometric tests require the use of calibrated electronic equipment, recording of results, and a written report with interpretation (eg, chart of hertz and decibels with pass/fail result for each ear tested and overall pass/fail result). Services include testing of both ears. If the test is applied to only 1 ear, modifier **52** (reduced services) must be appended to the code.

When hearing screening is performed in the physician office because of a failed screening in another setting (eg, school), report *ICD-10-CM* codes from category **Z01.11-**. Code **Z01.110** is reported for a normal screening result following a failed screening. Code **Z01.118** indicates a failed repeated screening. An additional code is reported to identify the abnormality found following the failed repeated screening.

> Medicaid plans may provide specific hearing screening/testing coverage information and documentation forms/requirements. Follow the individual plan's guidance for reporting these services and any failed attempts to screen (eg, an attempt to screen an uncooperative child).

- Code **92551** (screening test, pure tone, air only) is used when the patient wears earphones and is asked to respond to tones of different pitches and intensities. This is a limited study.
- Code **92552** (full pure tone audiometric assessment; air only) is used when the patient wears earphones and is asked to respond to tones of different pitches and intensities. The threshold (lowest intensity of the tone heard by the patient 50% of the time) is recorded for a number of frequencies.

- Code **92558** (evoked otoacoustic emissions [OAEs] screening) is used when a probe tip is placed in the ear canal to screen for normal hearing function. Sounds that bounce back in low-intensity sound waves (ie, OAEs) are recorded and analyzed by computerized equipment and the results are automated.
- Code **92583** (select picture audiometry) is typically used for younger children. The patient is asked to identify different pictures with the instructions given at different sound intensity levels.
- Other commonly performed procedures include codes **92567** (tympanometry [impedance testing]) and **92568** (acoustic reflex testing, threshold portion). However, both codes may have limited coverage; check with payers.
- Automated audiometry testing is reported with Category III codes **0208T–0212T**. Verify individual payer payment policy before providing these services.

Examples

➤ **George is a 16-year-old established patient presenting for a preventive service and clearance to participate in school sports.** A complete preventive E/M service (**99394**) is provided. George has not received a hearing screening since he was 13 years old, so pure tone, air-only screening audiometry is performed (**92551**). No abnormalities are found, and George receives clearance to participate in sports. The *ICD-10-CM* code reported for each of the services is **Z00.129** (encounter for routine child health examination without abnormal findings).

➤ **Sally is a 6-year-old who failed a hearing screening at school and is referred to her pediatrician for additional evaluation.** Sally's parents indicate no prior concerns about her hearing, and risk-factor assessment is negative. The pediatrician chooses to perform screening audiometry (**92551**), which produces typical results. The *ICD-10-CM* code reported is **Z01.110** (encounter for hearing examination following failed hearing screening). If the MDM or total physician time (not including time of testing) supports a separate office or other outpatient E/M service, this is separately reported (eg, **99212**).

Vision Screening

99173	Screening test of visual acuity, quantitative, bilateral
99174	Instrument-based ocular screening (eg, photoscreening, automated-refraction), bilateral; with remote analysis and report
99177	with on-site analysis
0333T	Visual evoked potential, screening of visual acuity, automated, with report
0469T	Retinal polarization scan, ocular screening with on-site automated results, bilateral

- Screening test of visual acuity (**99173**) must use graduated visual stimuli that allow a quantitative estimate of visual acuity (eg, Snellen chart).
  - Code **99173** is reported only when vision screening is performed in association with a preventive medicine visit.
  - Medical record documentation must include a measurement of acuity for both eyes, not just a pass or fail score.

> Do not report code 99173 when it is performed as part of an evaluation for an eye problem or condition (eg, examination to rule out vision problems in a patient presenting with problems with schoolwork) because the assessment of visual acuity is considered an integral part of the eye examination.

- Instrument-based ocular screening (**99174, 99177**) is used to report screening for a variety of conditions, including esotropia, exotropia, isometropia, cataracts, ptosis, hyperopia, myopia, and others, that affect or have the potential to affect vision. These tests are especially useful for screening infants, preschool patients, and those older patients whose ability to participate in traditional acuity screening is limited or very time intensive.
  - Code **99177** specifies screening with an instrument that provides an on-site (ie, in-office) pass or fail result. The result should be documented.
  - Code **99174** specifies the use of a screening instrument that incorporates remote analysis and report (by a physician located elsewhere).
  - These screenings cannot be reported in conjunction with codes **92002–92700** (general ophthalmologic services), **99172** (visual function screening), or **99173** (screening test of visual acuity, quantitative) because ocular screening is inherent to these services. An AAP policy statement on instrument-based pediatric vision screening is available at https://doi.org/10.1542/peds.2012-2548.

● indicates a new code; ▲, revised; #, re-sequenced; ✚, add-on; ★, audiovisual technology; and ◀, synchronous interactive audio.

- Vision screening performed by using an automated visual evoked potential system is reported with code **0333T**. This code applies to automated screening via an instrument-based algorithm with a pass or fail result. A report of the result must be documented. Report code **95930** only for comprehensive visual evoked potential testing with physician interpretation and report.
- Retinal polarization scanning (**0469T**) is used to detect amblyopia due to strabismus and defocus. As with code **99177**, results of each scan are generated on-site.

Developmental Screening and Health Assessment

Standardized screening instruments (ie, validated tests that are administered and scored in a consistent or "standard" manner consistent with their validation) are used for screening and assessment purposes as reported by codes **96110** and **96127**.

Health risk assessments that are patient focused (**96160**) are differentiated from those such as maternal depression screening that are caregiver focused (**96161**) for the benefit of the patient.

Developmental Screening

96110   Developmental screening, with scoring and documentation, per standardized instrument

Structured screening for developmental delay is a universal recommendation of the "Recommendations for Preventive Pediatric Health Care." At 18- and 24-month visits, specifically screen for autism spectrum disorder (ASD). Global developmental screening is recommended at 9-, 18-, and 30-month visits. When reporting these screenings, code **96110** represents developmental screening with scoring and documentation per standardized instrument. (*Note:* Screening results should be documented in the patient medical record.)

ICD-10-CM codes **Z13.40–Z13.49** (eg, **Z13.42**, screening for global developmental delays [milestones]) may be reported to indicate screening for developmental disability in children when the screening is performed with or without a well-child visit at the same encounter.

Code **96110**

- Is reported only for standardized developmental screening instruments. It is not reported when the pediatrician conducts an informal survey or surveillance of development as part of a comprehensive preventive medicine service (which is considered part of the history and is not separately billed).
- Does not require interpretation and report (ie, includes scoring and documentation only).
- Is *not* reported for brief emotional or behavioral assessment; see code **96127**.
- May be reported for each standardized developmental screening instrument administered. Medicaid Medically Unlikely Edits (MUEs) allow reporting of 3 screening instruments per date of service. If use of more than 3 instruments is clinically indicated and performed, code **96110** is reported with 3 units billed on the first claim line and **96110 59** is billed with 1 unit for each additional instrument reported on a separate claim line.

Example

➤ **An 18-month-old girl presents to her primary physician for an established patient well-child examination.** The mother is given standardized screening instruments for developmental status and ASD by clinical staff, who explain their purpose and how they should be completed. The nursing assistant scores the completed forms and attaches them to the child's medical record. The physician interprets and documents the normal results of the instruments. The physician provides the recommended 18-month preventive E/M service (**99392**). The child will return for a scheduled 2-year-old preventive service.

   Teaching Point: Code **99392** is reported and linked on the claim form to *ICD-10-CM* code **Z00.129**. Code **96110** is reported with 2 units of service linked to *ICD-10-CM* codes **Z13.41** (autism screening) and **Z13.42** (screening for delayed milestones) to identify the reason for 2 units of service. Or, if required by a health plan, code **96110** linked to code **Z13.41** and code **96110 59** linked to code **Z13.42** are reported on 2 separate claim lines (1 unit per claim line). (For an illustration of how codes are linked on a claim form, see **Chapter 1, Figure 1-1**.)

Emotional/Behavioral Assessment

96127   Brief emotional/behavioral assessment (eg, depression inventory, ADHD scale), with scoring and documentation, per standardized instrument

Chapter 8. Preventive Services

• indicates a new code; ▲, revised; #, re-sequenced; ✚, add-on; ★, audiovisual technology; and ◀, synchronous interactive audio.

Code **96127**

- Is reported for standardized emotional/behavioral assessment instruments.
- Represents the practice expense of administering, scoring, and documenting each standardized instrument. No physician work value is included. Physician interpretation is included in a related E/M service.
- Is *not* reported in conjunction with preventive medicine counseling/risk-factor reduction intervention (**99401–99404**) or psychiatric or neurologic testing (**96130–96139** or **96146**).
- Can involve 2 or more separately reported completions of the same form (eg, attention-deficit/hyperactivity disorder [ADHD] rating scales by teacher and by parent). Note that MUEs limit reporting to 2 units per claim line. When reporting to payers adopting MUEs, additional units beyond the first 2 must be reported on a separate claim line with an NCCI modifier (eg, **59**, distinct procedural service). As always, documentation should support the appropriateness of the additional units of service. Note at the time of this publication, the AAP was working on increasing the MUE.
- Can be reported for standardized depression instruments that are required under US Preventive Services Task Force (USPSTF) and Bright Futures recommendations (see AAP/Bright Futures "Recommendations for Preventive Pediatric Health Care" [periodicity schedule] insert).
- Alternatively, there is a HCPCS code for depression screening that some payers (particularly Medicaid or managed Medicaid plans) prefer in lieu of **96127** for annual depression screenings. If required, report **G0444** (annual depression screening, 15 minutes) to those payers.

> The code descriptor for G0444 includes "15 minutes." Verify the payment policies of Medicaid plans that require G0444, specifically noting any requirement to document time spent providing the depression screening service. Some health plans may require documentation of either 8 to 15 minutes (ie, passing the midpoint between 0 and 15 minutes) or no less than 15 minutes of time spent in the screening and discussion of screening results.

Example

> **A 12-year-old boy is seen for an established patient well-child examination at a health supervision visit.** In addition to the preventive medicine service, the physician's staff administers and scores a standardized depression screening instrument. The physician reviews the score, documents that the screening result is negative for symptoms of depression, and completes the preventive medicine service.
>
> The preventive medicine service code (**99394**) would be reported in addition to code **96127**. The diagnosis codes reported are **Z00.129** (encounter for routine child health examination without abnormal findings) and **Z13.31** (encounter for screening for depression). Link **Z00.129** and **Z13.31** to the claim service line for code **96127**. Inclusion of codes may support claims-based data collection for quality measurement (ie, number of adolescent patients screened for depression).
>
> When the physician performs further evaluation of positive screening results, leading to a diagnosis of depression, report the preventive service with abnormal findings (**Z00.121**) followed by the appropriate code for the diagnosed depression (eg, **F32.0**, major depressive disorder, single episode, mild). When appropriate, a significant and separately identifiable E/M service to evaluate and manage depression may be reported by appending modifier **25** to an office or other outpatient E/M code (eg, **99214 25**). Documentation should clearly support the MDM of the separate service or, if billing based on time, the physician's total time (not including the time spent providing the separately reported preventive medicine service and screening for depression) and a summary of the service provided (eg, education on the condition, questions answered, patient and/or caregiver concerns, management options discussed, plan of care). Link the diagnosis code for the depression to the office or other outpatient E/M code.

Health Risk Assessment

96160   Administration of patient-focused health risk assessment (eg, health hazard appraisal) with scoring and documentation, per standardized instrument

96161   Administration of caregiver-focused health risk assessment (eg, depression inventory) for the benefit of the patient, with scoring and documentation, per standardized instrument

Codes **96160** and **96161** are reported with 1 unit for each standardized instrument administered. Payer edits may limit the number of times codes **96160** and **96161** may be reported for an individual patient and/or on the same date of service. Medically Unlikely Edits are set to 3 units for **96160** and 1 unit for **96161** per claim line. Append modifier **59** to the code for additional units on a second claim line.

> Sparse coverage for codes 96160 and specifically 96161 has been noted by the American Academy of Pediatrics, and advocacy efforts are being made.

Code **96160** is reported for administration of a patient-focused health risk assessment with scoring and documentation. This is differentiated from code **96161**, which is used to report a health risk assessment focused on a caregiver for the benefit of the patient (eg, maternal depression screening).

- Code **96160** cannot be used in conjunction with assessment and brief intervention for alcohol/substance abuse (**99408, 99409**).
- Check individual payer guidance to determine if and for what purposes code **96160** is included as a covered and payable service under the payer's policies (eg, some Medicaid plans pay for adolescent health questionnaires reported with **96160**).

Code **96161** is reported for administration and scoring of a health risk assessment to a patient's caregiver. Examples are a postpartum depression inventory administered to the mother of a newborn and administration of a standardized caregiver strain instrument to parents of a child who is seriously injured or ill.

- Screening for postpartum depression is caregiver focused (sign/symptoms of depression in mother) but performed in this setting for the benefit of the infant. This service is reported as a service provided to the infant with code **96161** and the appropriate *ICD-10-CM* code for the infant's routine child health examination (eg, **Z00.129**).
- Check payer policy on adoption of code **96161** versus a requirement to report as a service to the mother (ie, to mother's health plan) with code **96127** (brief emotional/behavioral assessment [eg, depression inventory, ADHD scale], with scoring and documentation, per standardized instrument). Many Medicaid plans provide separate payment for maternal depression screening at well-child visits, but specific reporting instructions may apply. Vaccines and administration services would also be reported.

> Prevent denials! National Correct Coding Initiative (NCCI) edits bundle codes 96160 and 96161 with code 96110 and with immunization administration (90460–90474) services, but a modifier is allowed when each code represents a distinct service and is clinically appropriate. Append modifier 59 (distinct procedure) to the bundled code (second column of NCCI edits) when these services are reported on the same date to a payer that has adopted NCCI edits.

Example

➤ **As part of a health supervision visit for a 9-month-old established patient, the physician directs clinical staff to administer a screening for postpartum depression that was not performed at the infant's 6-month visit.** Clinical staff explain the purpose of the instrument to the infant's mother. After the mother has completed the screening instrument, clinical staff score and document the result in the patient record. The mother is also asked to complete a developmental screening instrument, which is scored and documented. The physician completes the preventive medicine service with no abnormal findings and counsels the patient's mother about influenza immunization. With the mother's consent, clinical staff administer 0.25 mL of a preservative-free split-virus vaccine. Anticipatory guidance that advises the mother that her screening indicates no current signs of postpartum depression is included, along with a list of symptoms that should prompt a call to her physician. The patient is scheduled to return for a second dose of influenza vaccine in 1 month.

ICD-10-CM	CPT
Z00.129 (encounter for routine child health examination without abnormal findings)	**99393 25** (preventive medicine visit) **96110 59** (developmental screening) **96161 59** (administration of caregiver-focused health risk assessment [eg, depression inventory] for the benefit of the patient, with scoring and documentation, per standardized instrument) **90460** (IA with physician counseling) **90685** (IIV4 vaccine, split virus, preservative free, 0.25 ml dose for IM use)

Chapter 8. Preventive Services

Teaching Point: National Correct Coding Initiative edits bundle the codes shown with a modifier appended to other codes reported for this encounter (eg, **99393** is bundled to **90460**). For each of the bundled code pairs, a modifier is allowed to override the edit when both services are provided and clinically appropriate. Electronic claim scrubbers are useful for identifying and addressing NCCI edit pairs before claim submission. See **Chapter 2** for more on NCCI edits.

Never report *International Classification of Diseases, 10th Revision, Clinical Modification* code **Z13.32** (encounter for maternal depression screen) on the baby's medical record/bill.

Prevention of Dental Caries

Application of Fluoride Varnish

99188   Application of topical fluoride varnish by a physician or other qualified health care professional

- Topical fluoride application by primary care physicians is a recommended preventive service for children from birth through 5 years of age (Grade B rating by the USPSTF). This service may be covered when provided alone or in conjunction with other services. Coverage is usually limited to once every 6 months.
- *ICD-10-CM* code **Z29.3** is reported to identify an encounter for prophylactic fluoride administration. When applicable, diagnosis of dental caries may be reported as a secondary diagnosis with codes in category **K02**. Encounter for prophylactic fluoride administration is reported separately from the encounter for routine child health examination (**Z00.121** or **Z00.129**) when both services are provided at the same encounter.

Example

➤ **A 4-year-old established patient undergoes a routine preventive medicine service without abnormal findings.** In addition, a medical assistant who has been qualified by a required online training and assessment program applies fluoride varnish to the child's teeth under supervision of the pediatrician, who remains in the office suite.

    The pediatrician reports diagnosis code **Z00.129** (routine child health examination without abnormal findings) linked to code **99392** (established patient routine child health examination, age 1–4) and diagnosis code **Z29.3** linked to code **99188** (application of fluoride varnish).

    Teaching Point: Although code **99188** specifies application by a physician or QHP, payers may allow billing of services by trained clinical staff under direct physician supervision (incident to). Some Medicaid plans require training of clinical staff through specific programs and documentation of training and/or certification. It is important to identify the requirements of individual payers before providing this service and maintain documentation demonstrating that all coverage requirements were met.

Counseling to Prevent Dental Caries

Some payers will provide coverage for oral evaluation and health risk assessment or other dental preventive services when provided on the same day as a preventive medicine visit; other payers will allow services only when they are provided at an encounter separate from a preventive medicine visit. It is important to know payer requirements for reporting.

- Preventive counseling for oral health may be included as part of the preventive medicine service (**99381–99395**) or, if performed at a separate encounter, reported under the individual preventive medicine counseling service codes (**99401–99404**) or with an office or outpatient E/M service code (**99202–99215**). *ICD-10-CM* code **Z13.84** may be reported for an encounter for screening for dental disorders.

Other Codes for Prevention of Dental Caries

- *Code on Dental Procedures and Nomenclature* (CDT) codes also exist for topical application of fluoride varnish and fluoride. In addition, *CDT* codes exist for nutrition counseling to prevent dental disease, oral hygiene instruction, and oral evaluations. However, acceptance of these codes by health plans may be limited to Medicaid plans.
- For those carriers (particularly Medicaid plans under EPSDT) that cover oral health care, some will require a modifier. These modifiers are payer specific and should be used only as directed by your Medicaid agency or other private payer.
  - **SC**   Medically necessary service or supply
  - **EP**   Services provided as part of Medicaid EPSDT program
  - **U5**   Medicaid Level of Care 5, as defined by each state

Chapter 8. Preventive Services

Screening Laboratory Tests

- A test performed in the office laboratory should be billed by using the appropriate laboratory code and, if performed, the appropriate blood collection code (**36400–36416**). See the Blood Sampling for Diagnostic Study section in **Chapter 12**.
- Laboratories and physician offices performing waived tests may need to append modifier **QW** to the *CPT* code for Clinical Laboratory Improvement Amendments (CLIA)–waived procedures. The use of modifier **QW** is payer specific. To determine if a test is a CLIA-waived procedure, go to www.accessdata.fda.gov/scripts/cdrh/cfdocs/cfCLIA/search.cfm.
- *ICD-10-CM* allows separate reporting of special screening examinations (codes in categories **Z11–Z13**) in addition to the codes for routine child health examinations when these codes provide additional information. A screening code is not necessary if the screening is inherent to a routine examination. Payer guidelines for reporting screening examinations may vary. When specific *ICD-10-CM* codes are required to support payment for a screening service, be sure to link the appropriate *ICD-10-CM* code to the claim line for the screening service.

> A positive finding on a screening test does not change the test to a diagnostic test. When a screening test results in an abnormal finding that has been identified at the time of code assignment, list first the code for the screening or preventive service followed by a code for the abnormal finding. Failure to list the screening code first may affect the patient's out-of-pocket costs for preventive services. Please see Chapter 12 for information on coding for diagnostic tests in non-facility settings.

- To meet the HEDIS measure for percentage of children who turned 2 years of age in a measurement year and who had 1 or more capillary or venous lead blood test(s) for lead poisoning by their second birthday, a laboratory report of lead screening test result, or a note indicating the date the test was performed and the result or finding must be documented. See **Chapter 3** for more information on HEDIS measures.

> Follow payer instructions for reporting that patients were referred to an outside laboratory for lead screening (eg, report a code for the appropriate lead screening test with modifier 90, reference [outside] laboratory, and no charge).

- A table of common pediatric screening laboratory tests and codes is included at www.aap.org/cfp2023 ("Screening Laboratory Tests and Codes").

Preventive Care Provided Outside the Preventive Visit

Counseling and/or Risk-Factor Reduction

Codes **99401–99404**, **99411**, and **99412** are used to report risk-factor reduction services provided for the purposes of promoting health and preventing illness or injury in persons without a specific illness.

Preventive medicine service codes (**99381–99395**) include counseling, anticipatory guidance, and/or risk-factor reduction interventions that are provided at the time of the periodic comprehensive preventive medicine examination. *CPT* states to "refer to codes **99401–99404**, and **99411–99412** for reporting those counseling/anticipatory guidance/risk-factor reduction interventions that are provided at an encounter separate from the preventive medicine examination." Therefore, according to *CPT*, do not report **99401–99404** or **99411** or **99412** in addition to **99381–99397**.

- Risk-factor reduction services will vary with age and address issues such as diet, exercise, sexual activity, dental health, immunization safety counseling, injury prevention, safe travel, and family problems.
- Services are reported on the basis of time, and time should be distinctly documented (eg, 15 minutes spent in counseling about diet and exercise to reduce risk of developing diabetes).
- Counseling, anticipatory guidance, and risk-factor reduction interventions provided at the time of an initial or periodic comprehensive preventive medicine examination are components of the periodic service and not separately reported.
- Risk-factor reduction may be reported separately with other E/M services.
  - Evaluation and management services (other than preventive medicine E/M services) reported on the same day must be separate and distinct.
  - Time spent in the provision of risk-factor reduction may not be used as a basis for the selection of the other E/M code.
- When reporting a distinct E/M service, append modifier **25** to the code for the distinct E/M service.

Chapter 8. Preventive Services

Payment policies for preventive medicine counseling may vary by health plan. Ideally, recommended preventive medicine counseling provided outside a preventive evaluation and management (E/M) service (99381–99385, 99391–99395) is a covered preventive service paid with no out-of-pocket cost to the patient/caregiver. It is important to know if a payer considers preventive medicine counseling bundled to a problem-oriented E/M service when provided on the same date of service. Plans may require that the preventive counseling be included in the level of problem-oriented E/M service reported in lieu of reporting the appropriate preventive counseling code. Written copies of payment policies should be documented to support billing for preventive medicine counseling as part of a problem-oriented E/M service rather than separately reporting as directed by *Current Procedural Terminology*.

Preventive Medicine, Individual Counseling Codes

Codes **99401–99404** are time-based codes. See **Table 8-2** for code descriptors, required time, and RVUs for these services.

Table 8-2. Preventive Medicine Counseling Codes and Relative Value Units

Preventive medicine counseling and/or risk-factor reduction intervention(s) provided to an individual (separate procedure);

Code	Time Required	Total NF-RVUs[a]	Total F-RVUs[a]
99401	approximately 15 minutes (8–22)	1.14	0.71
99402	approximately 30 minutes (23–37)	1.89	1.45
99403	approximately 45 minutes (38–52)	2.57	2.13
99404	approximately 60 minutes (≥53)	3.31	2.87

Abbreviations: F, facility; NF, non-facility; RVU, relative value unit.

[a] 2022 RVUs, not geographically adjusted.

Report codes **99401–99404**
- On the basis of a physician's or other QHP's face-to-face time spent providing counseling
- For a new or an established patient
- When the medical record includes documentation of the total counseling time and a summary of the issues discussed

Time for codes 99401–99404 is met when the midpoint is passed (eg, 8 minutes of service required to report a 15-minute service).

Codes **99401–99404** may be reported when expectant parents request a consultation with a pediatric physician regarding risk reduction for the fetus. However, consultation or office and other outpatient E/M services are reported when the service is requested by another physician, another QHP, or an appropriate source (eg, genetic counselor). See the Consultations section in **Chapter 16** for information on reporting *ICD-10-CM* and *CPT* codes for expectant parent consultation services to the mother's health insurance.

Examples

➤ **A 7-week-old girl (established patient) is presented to a pediatrician with a scaly rash on her scalp.** The infant is examined and found to have seborrheic infantile dermatitis of the scalp and skinfolds on the extremities. The pediatrician provides information on home management and risk of yeast infection and takes the opportunity to again counsel the mother about the need for immunization against hepatitis B, which the mother has previously refused. The indications, safety, and risks are discussed for 10 minutes and the mother agrees to revisit the issue with her husband, who has been strongly opposed in the past. The pediatrician documents the separate time and context of the counseling.

ICD-10-CM	CPT
L21.0 (seborrheic infantile dermatitis)	**99212 25** (MDM: 1 self-limited problem; assessment requiring an independent historian; and minimal risk of morbidity from treatment)

Z28.3 (under-immunization status) Z28.21 (immunization not carried out because of patient refusal)	99401

Teaching Point: The pediatrician's time of 10 minutes spent in preventive counseling supports reporting code **99401** because the midpoint was passed (8 minutes are required for reporting a code assigned 15 minutes). Distinct documentation of the time and work of the preventive counseling is important to support payment for both services provided.

➤ **Parents of a 6-year-old request counseling for an upcoming move to Puerto Rico.** The pediatrician spends 25 minutes reviewing CDC recommendations for immunizations and counseling for potential health hazards for the child. Any recommended vaccines are administered, and the pediatrician recommends an appointment at a travel clinic for vaccines not available in the practice (eg, dengue, typhoid).

ICD-10-CM	CPT
Z71.84 (encounter for health counseling related to travel) **Z23** (encounter for immunization), if applicable	**99402** (risk-factor reduction counseling) Codes for vaccine products and administration, as applicable

Teaching Point: The pediatrician's time of 25 minutes spent in preventive counseling supports reporting code **99402** because the midpoint between the typical times of **99401** and **99402** was passed (23 minutes). Time spent in counseling for immunizations administered at the encounter would be reported with the IA code and not included in the time of the risk-factor reduction counseling.

Preventive Medicine, Group Counseling Codes

99411   Preventive medicine counseling and/or risk factor reduction intervention(s) provided to individuals in a group setting (separate procedure); approximately 30 minutes

99412   approximately 60 minutes

● Risk-factor reduction services provided to a group are reported on the basis of time. The *CPT* midpoint rule for time applies (ie, time is met when the midpoint between the 2 codes is passed), as shown in **Table 8-3**.

● See code **99078** for reporting physician counseling to groups of patients with symptoms or an established illness. This service is reported for each participating child.

Table 8-3. Group Preventive Medicine Counseling Codes and Relative Value Units

Preventive medicine counseling and/or risk-factor reduction intervention(s) provided to an individual (separate procedure);

Code	Time Required	Total NF-RVUs[a]	Total F-RVUs[a]
99411	approximately 30 minutes (16–45)	0.61	0.22
99412	approximately 60 minutes (≥46)	0.75	0.37

Abbreviations: F, facility; NF, non-facility; RVU, relative value unit.

[a] 2022 RVUs, not geographically adjusted.

Example

➤ **A group of 10 patients aged 14 to 16 years attend a 50-minute session in the physician's office to discuss contraception and sex-related health risks.** The physician conducts the session. The session includes a 10-minute break that is not included in the time of service. Services are documented in each patient's medical record and are reported for each child.

● indicates a new code; ▲, revised; #, re-sequenced; ✚, add-on; ★, audiovisual technology; and ◀, synchronous interactive audio.

ICD-10-CM	CPT
Z30.09 (encounter for other general counseling and advice on contraception)	**99412** (risk-factor reduction counseling, group, 60 minutes)

Teaching Point: Although 10 minutes of break time is not included in the time of the counseling service, code **99412** is supported because the midpoint between the 30 minutes assigned to **99411** and the 60 minutes assigned to **99412** is passed. Services provided to a group of patients may not be reported as individual office E/M visits (**99202–99215**) because only face-to-face time spent counseling the individual patient may be reported on the basis of time.

Behavior Change Intervention

Behavior change interventions are for persons who have a behavior that is often considered an illness, such as tobacco use and addiction or substance use or misuse. Behavior change services may be reported when performed as part of the treatment of conditions related to or potentially exacerbated by the behavior or when performed to change the harmful behavior that has not yet resulted in illness. **Table 8-4** shows the codes and RVUs assigned to behavior change intervention codes.

Behavior change interventions involve validated interventions shown in **Figure 8-2**.

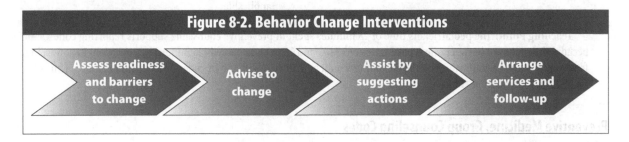

Figure 8-2. Behavior Change Interventions

Assess readiness and barriers to change → Advise to change → Assist by suggesting actions → Arrange services and follow-up

- Behavior change intervention codes **99406–99409** are reported when
  — Services are provided by a physician or QHP for patients who have a behavior that is often considered an illness (eg, tobacco use and addiction, substance use or misuse).
  — Services involve specific validated interventions, including assessing readiness for and barriers to change, advising change in behavior, providing specific suggested actions and motivational counseling, and arranging for services and follow-up care.

Table 8-4. Behavior Change Intervention Codes

Code	Description	TNF RVUs[a]	TF RVUs[a]
99406	Smoking and tobacco use cessation counseling visit; intermediate, >3 min up to 10 min	0.45	0.35
99407	intensive, >10 min	0.83	0.74
99408	Alcohol and/or substance (other than tobacco) abuse structured screening (eg, AUDIT, DAST), and brief intervention services; 15–30 minutes	1.04	0.95
99409	>30 minutes	2.00	1.91

Abbreviations: AUDIT, Alcohol Use Disorders Identification Test; DAST, Drug Abuse Screening Test; RVU, relative value unit; TF, total facility; TNF, total non-facility.

[a] 2022 RVUs, not geographically adjusted.

- Codes **99406–99409** include specific time requirements that must be met (eg, at least 15 minutes must be spent in counseling to support reporting of code **99408**). The *CPT* midpoint rule does not apply to codes **99406–99409**.
- Do not separately report code **96160** for screening instruments used in conjunction with codes **99408** and **99409**.
- Medical record documentation supports the total time spent in the performance of the service, and a detail of the behavior change intervention is provided.

> Behavior change intervention services cannot be performed on a parent or guardian of a patient and reported under the patient's name.

- Behavior change interventions may be reported separately with preventive medicine or other E/M services.
  - Evaluation and management services reported on the same day must be separate and distinct.
  - Time spent in the provision of behavior change intervention may not be used as a basis for the selection of the other E/M code.
- When reporting a distinct E/M service, append modifier **25** to the code for the distinct E/M service (eg, **99213 25**).

> See the Physician Group Education Services section in Chapter 12 for an example of how code **99078** is used.

Examples

➤ **During an office visit for a 17-year-old new patient for an unrelated problem, it is learned that he has been smoking for 2 years but would like to quit.** The physician spends 15 minutes discussing specific methods to overcome barriers, pharmacological options, behavioral techniques, and nicotine replacement. The patient is referred to a community support group and a follow-up visit is scheduled in 2 weeks to provide additional encouragement and counseling as needed. Diagnosis is tobacco use.

ICD-10-CM	CPT
Use the code appropriate for problem addressed.	**99202–99205 25** (based on service performed and documented)
Z72.0 (tobacco use) **Z71.6** (tobacco abuse counseling)	**99407**

Teaching Point: If only general advice and encouragement to stop smoking had been provided, it would be considered part of the new patient office visit. Counseling time must be documented. *ICD-10-CM* does not include a code for use of vaping products without a diagnosis of abuse or a vaping-related illness. Report **Z71.89** (other specified counseling) when counseling is focused on risks associated with vaping. See **F17.29-** for codes for nicotine dependence and vaping.

➤ **A 14-year-old established patient with primarily hyperactive ADHD presents for a preventive E/M service.** The patient and parents report no problems in school and no concerns with current ADHD management. During time alone with the patient, the physician uses a structured screening tool to interview the patient about substance use. The result is positive, and the physician spends a total of 20 minutes interviewing the patient about substance use history and counseling the patient about risks associated with alcohol and drug use, not driving or riding with someone under the influence, and seeking an agreement to avoid future use.

ICD-10-CM	CPT
Z00.129 (routine child health examination without abnormal findings) **F90.1** (attention-deficit hyperactivity disorder, predominantly hyperactive type)	**99394 25** (preventive medicine visit)
Z71.89 (other specified counseling)	**99408**

Time of counseling should be specifically documented as beginning after conclusion of the preventive medicine service.

> *International Classification of Diseases, 10th Revision, Clinical Modification* guidelines state that substance use codes (eg, **F10.99**, alcohol use, unspecified with unspecified alcohol-induced disorder) should be assigned only when the use is associated with a mental or behavioral disorder and such a relationship is documented by the provider.

● indicates a new code; ▲, revised; #, re-sequenced; ✚, add-on; ★, audiovisual technology; and ◄, synchronous interactive audio.

Preventive Medicine Services Modifier

33   Preventive services

Modifier **33** is used to differentiate services provided as recommended preventive care when the service might also be provided for diagnostic indications. Some payers provide a listing of services for which modifier **33** is required when provided as a preventive service.

- The appropriate use of modifier **33** will reduce claim adjustments related to preventive services and corresponding payments to members.
- Modifier **33** should be appended only to codes represented in 1 or more of the following 4 categories:
  - Services rated A or B by the USPSTF
  - Immunizations for routine use in children, adolescents, and adults as recommended by ACIP
  - Preventive care and screenings for children as recommended by Bright Futures (AAP) and newborn testing (American College of Medical Genetics and Genomics)
  - Preventive care and screenings provided for women supported by HRSA

> **The US Preventive Services Task Force (USPSTF) grades A and B are defined as follows:**
>
> - **Grade A: The USPSTF recommends the service. There is high certainty that the net benefit is substantial.**
> - **Grade B: The USPSTF recommends the service. There is high certainty that the net benefit is moderate or there is moderate certainty that the net benefit is moderate to substantial.**
>
> **Most health plans cover preventive services with grade A or B without cost to the patient (ie, no deductible, co-payment, or coinsurance).**

- **DO *NOT* USE MODIFIER 33**
  - **When the *CPT* code(s) is identified as inherently preventive (eg, preventive medicine counseling)**
  - **When the service(s) is not indicated in the categories noted previously**
  - **With an insurance plan that continues to implement the cost-sharing policy on preventive medicine services (legacy health plan)**
- Check with your payers before fully implementing the use of modifier **33** to verify any variations in reporting requirements. Modifier **33** *is not used for benefit determination by some payers* and may be required by others only for services that may be either diagnostic/therapeutic or preventive.

Example

➤ **A 12-year-old established patient is seen for behavioral intervention for obesity due to excess calorie intake and family history of type 2 diabetes.** The patient and her parents previously received counseling on the health risks associated with obesity and requested assistance with lifestyle changes to help the patient recover and maintain a healthy weight. The physician uses shared decision-making to develop a plan for adopting a healthier lifestyle that will lead to weight loss and improve the health status of the patient. The physician's total time on the date of service is 35 minutes.

ICD-10-CM	CPT
E66.9 (obesity, unspecified) **Z68.54** (BMI ≥95th percentile) **Z83.3** (family history of diabetes mellitus)	**99214 33** (level 4 established patient office visit, total time 30–39 minutes)

Teaching Point: Modifier **33** is appended to code **99214** to indicate the preventive nature of the service, based on the USPSTF Grade B recommendation that clinicians screen for obesity in children and adolescents 6 years and older and offer to refer them for comprehensive, intensive behavioral interventions to promote improvements in weight status.

Other Preventive Medicine Services

99429   Unlisted preventive medicine service

Code **99429** may be reported if these options are not suitable. If the unlisted code is used, most payers will require a copy of the progress notes filed with the claim.

● indicates a new code; ▲, revised; #, re-sequenced; ✚, add-on; ★, audiovisual technology; and ◀, synchronous interactive audio.

Reporting a Preventive Medicine Visit With a Problem-Oriented Visit

When a problem or an abnormality is addressed, *requires significant additional work* (eg, symptomatic atopic dermatitis, exercise-induced asthma, migraine headache, scoliosis), and is medically necessary, it may be reported by using the office or other outpatient services codes (**99202–99205, 99212–99215**) in addition to the preventive medicine services code.

> ### Know Payer Policies for Same-Day Preventive and Problem-Oriented Evaluation and Management Services
>
> Some payers have adopted policy that problem-oriented evaluation and management (E/M) services provided on the same date as a preventive medicine E/M service will be paid at 50% of the contractual amount agreed on under the health plan contract. When reporting to these payers, be sure to include all work related to the problem-oriented encounter in determining the level of service provided. Physicians should not reduce the level of service reported.

- The presence of a chronic condition(s) in and of itself neither changes a preventive medicine visit to a problem-oriented visit nor unilaterally supports a separate problem-oriented E/M service (**99202–99205, 99212–99215**) with the well visit, unless it is significant and has been separately addressed.
- An insignificant problem or condition (eg, minor diaper rash, stable chronic problem, renewal of prescription medications) that does not require significant MDM or time cannot be reported as a separate E/M service.
- Although a separate E/M service is not reported when a minor problem or chronic condition requires less than significant additional work, the diagnosis code for the problem or chronic condition may be reported in addition to code **Z00.121** (routine child health examination with abnormal findings).
- It is important to make parents aware of any additional charges that may occur at the preventive medicine encounter. This includes, but is not limited to, a significant, separately identifiable E/M service.
  - Some patients will be required to provide a co-payment for the non–preventive medicine visit code under the terms of their plan benefit even when there is no co-payment required for the preventive medicine visit. Legally, this co-payment cannot routinely be written off.

  When reporting both E/M services,
- The documentation of the problem-oriented service must be distinct from that of the preventive service (even if included in the same encounter note) and clearly support the level of service reported.
- When the level of service is selected on the basis of the physician's total time (on the date of the encounter) spent addressing the problem (not including any time spent providing the preventive service), the physician's total time spent addressing the problem must be distinctly documented in addition to documentation of the problem workup (eg, history of present illness, examination, records or test results reviewed), assessment, and plan.
- Documentation might indicate, "My total time of XX minutes was directed to activities of evaluating and managing X condition after I provided the preventive service."

> ### Coding Conundrum: Reporting Evaluation and Management Services With Immunization Administration
>
> Evaluation and management (E/M) services most often reported with the vaccine product and immunization administration (IA) include new and established patient preventive medicine visits (*Current Procedural Terminology* [*CPT*] codes **99381–99395**), problem-oriented visits (**99202–99215**), and preventive medicine counseling services (**99401–99404**).
>
> If a patient is seen only for the administration of a vaccine, it is not appropriate to report an E/M visit if it is not medically necessary, significant, and separately identifiable. The E/M service must be clinically indicated.
>
> Payers may require modifier **25** (significant, separately identifiable E/M service by the same physician on the same day of the procedure or other service) to be appended to the E/M code to distinguish it from the administration of the vaccine.
>
> Do not report *CPT* code **99211** (established patient E/M, minimal level, not requiring physician presence) when the patient encounter is for vaccination only because Medicare Resource-Based Relative Value Scale (RBRVS) relative values for IA codes include administrative and clinical services (ie, greeting the patient, measuring routine vital signs, obtaining a vaccine history, presenting the Vaccine Information Statement and responding to routine vaccine questions, preparing and administering the vaccine, and documenting and observing the patient following administration of the vaccine). However, if the service is medically necessary, significant, and separately identifiable, it may be reported with modifier **25** appended to the E/M code (**99211**). The medical record must clearly state the reason for the visit, the brief history, the physical examination, the assessment and plan, and any other counseling or discussion items. The progress note must be signed, and a physician's countersignature may be required. For more information and clinical vignettes on the appropriate use of E/M services during IA, see "FAQ: Immunization Administration" at www.aap.org/cfp2023. Payers who do not follow the Medicare RBRVS may allow payment of code **99211** with IA. Know your payer guidelines, and if payment is allowed, make certain that the guidelines are in writing and maintained in your office. Be aware that a co-payment may be required when the "nurse" visit is reported.
>
> The same guidelines apply to physician visits (**99202–99215**).

● indicates a new code; ▲, revised; #, re-sequenced; ✚, add-on; ★, audiovisual technology; and ◀, synchronous interactive audio.

- Modifier **25** (significant, separately identifiable E/M service by the same physician on the same day of the procedure or other service) should be appended to the problem-oriented service code (eg, **99212**). If vaccines are given at the same encounter, append modifier **25** to the problem-oriented E/M service code and to the preventive medicine service code to prevent payer bundling edits that may allow payment only for IA.
- ICD-10-CM well-care diagnosis codes (for the code list, see *ICD-10-CM* Codes for Preventive Care Visits earlier in this chapter) should be linked to the appropriate preventive medicine service code (**99381–99395**) and the sick-care diagnosis code linked to the problem-oriented service code (**99202–99205**, **99212–99215**).

Examples

➤ **A 10-year-old boy receives health supervision at a well-child visit.** This established patient also has previously diagnosed anxiety that is now exacerbated by health concerns of the grandmother who is his only caregiver. The grandmother notes she too is fearful about being too ill to care for her grandchild. Counseling with a licensed clinical social worker is recommended and arranged. The physician documents 20 minutes spent in counseling and coordinating care related to the patient's anxiety and the family's need for social support.

ICD-10-CM	CPT
Z00.121 (well-child check with abnormal findings) **F41.96** (anxiety) **Z63.79** (other stressful life events affecting family and household)	**99393** (preventive medicine visit)
F41.96 (anxiety) **Z63.79** (other stressful life events affecting family and household)	**99213 25** (office E/M service, total physician time 20–29 minutes)

Teaching Point: Documentation should clearly support the separate time of the problem-oriented E/M service, discussion topics, and plan of care for the problems addressed.

Codes for preventive counseling and risk-factor reduction intervention (eg, **99401**) are not appropriate for this example. Risk-factor reduction services are used for persons without a specific illness for which the counseling might otherwise be used as part of treatment. This patient has increased anxiety that prompts the counseling.

➤ **A 7-year-old boy with previously repaired patent ductus arteriosus is seen for a preventive medicine visit.** There are no new abnormal findings at the encounter.

ICD-10-CM	CPT	
Z00.129 (well-child check without abnormal findings) **Z87.74** (personal history of [corrected] congenital malformations of heart and circulatory system)	Preventive medicine visit	
	New Patient 99382	**Established Patient** 99392

Teaching Point: Because there were no current problems addressed at the encounter, only the preventive E/M code is reported. The diagnosis code for history of a congenital malformation of the heart and circulatory system may be reported as an additional diagnosis to the code for the well-child checkup but is not a finding of the well-child checkup.

See the Preventive and Problem-Oriented Services: Coding Continuum section later in this chapter for additional examples of coding for problems addressed at a preventive encounter.

To test your knowledge of coding for preventive services, complete the quiz found at the end of this chapter, after the resources. Answers to each quiz are found in **Appendix IV**.

Preventive and Problem-Oriented Services: Coding Continuum

Continuum Model for Problem-Oriented and Preventive Evaluation and Management on the Same Date			
Code selection may be based on the level of MDM or the total time[a] spent by the physician or QHP devoted to the problem-oriented E/M on the date of the encounter.			
CPT Code With Time and Vignette (Appropriate preventive E/M service codes are also reported.)	Medical Decision-making (2 of 3 Elements Required)		
	No. and Complexity of Problems Addressed	Amount and/or Complexity of Data Reviewed and Analyzed	Risk of Complications and/or Morbidity or Mortality of Patient Management
99212 (10–19 minutes) An infant is evaluated and found to have seborrheic capitis.	**Minimal:** Self-limited problem	**Limited:** Assessment requiring an independent historian(s)	**Minimal**
99213 (20–29 minutes) A 14-year-old presents today for a rash on their forearms. Diagnosis is poison ivy.	**Low:** 1 acute, uncomplicated illness or injury	**Minimal or none**	**Low:** Home management with over-the-counter products
99214 (30–39 minutes)[b] A child presents with new-onset rash and history of fever and sore throat in the past week.	**Moderate:** Acute illness with systemic symptoms and high risk of morbidity without treatment	**Moderate:** Streptococcal test performed and specimen sent to outside laboratory for culture. Assessment requiring an independent historian(s).	**Moderate:** Prescription of antibiotic for treatment of streptococcal sore throat
99215 (40–54 minutes)[b] A 14-year-old presents today for a previously scheduled preventive service and with concern of recent-onset anxiety with palpitations and depression for which they are seeing a therapist. Patient describes suicidal ideation without plan or intent. Mother provides family history, which is negative for bipolar disorder and positive for anxiety disorders.	**High:** 1 acute or chronic illness or injury that poses a threat to life or bodily function	**High:** Independent historian. Tests ordered are CBC, thyroid function tests, comprehensive metabolic panel, and electrocardiography. Phone discussion with therapist regarding prescription of SSRI.	**Moderate:** Prescription drug management

Abbreviations: CBC, complete blood cell count; *CPT, Current Procedural Terminology;* E/M, evaluation and management; MDM, medical decision-making; QHP, qualified health care professional; SSRI, selective serotonin reuptake inhibitor.

[a] Time-based E/M: Time is the total time spent in activities related to the problem-oriented E/M service by the physician or QHP on the date of the encounter. Do not include time of the preventive medicine service or time of other separately reported services.

[b] In many cases, a problem that requires higher levels of E/M service (ie, **99214** or **99215**) may warrant delay of the preventive E/M service.

● indicates a new code; ▲, revised; #, re-sequenced; ✚, add-on; ★, audiovisual technology; and ◀, synchronous interactive audio.

Chapter Takeaways

In this chapter, common pediatric preventive services and reporting for a combination of preventive and problem-oriented services have been discussed. Following are takeaways from this chapter:

- Well-child or preventive medicine services are a type of E/M service and are reported with codes **99381–99395**.
- Appropriate diagnosis coding for preventive medicine is based on the patient's age and, for infants and children, on whether an abnormality is identified during the service.
- Vaccine services are reported by using 2 families of *CPT* codes, one for the vaccine serum (the product) and one for the services associated with the administration of the vaccine.
- Codes **99401–99404**, **99411**, and **99412** are used to report risk-factor reduction services provided for the purposes of promoting health and preventing illness or injury in people without a specific illness.
- An insignificant problem or condition (eg, a minor diaper rash, stable chronic problem, or renewal of prescription medications) that does not require significant MDM or time cannot be reported as a separate E/M service.

Resources

AAP Coding Assistance and Education

AAP *Bright Futures: Guidelines for Health Supervision of Infants, Children, and Adolescents,* 4th Edition (www.aap.org/en/practice-management/bright-futures)

AAP/Bright Futures periodicity schedule, "Recommendations for Preventive Pediatric Health Care" (also see insert) (www.aap.org/en/practice-management/care-delivery-approaches/periodicity-schedule)

AAP "COVID-19 Vaccine Administration: Getting Paid" (https://services.aap.org/en/pages/2019-novel-coronavirus-covid-19-infections/covid-19-vaccine-for-children/covid-19-vaccine-administration-getting-paid)

AAP "Immunizations: Refusal to Vaccinate," including a vaccine refusal form in English and in Spanish (www.aap.org/en/patient-care/immunizations/implementing-immunization-administration-in-your-practice/refusal-to-vaccinate)

AAP "Payment for Oral Health Services" (www.aap.org/en/patient-care/oral-health/payment-for-oral-health-services)

AAP *Pediatric Vaccines: Coding Quick Reference Card 2023* (https://shop.aap.org/pediatric-vaccine-coding-quick-reference-card-2023)

AAP Section on Ophthalmology and Committee on Practice and Ambulatory Medicine, American Academy of Ophthalmology, American Association for Pediatric Ophthalmology and Strabismus, and American Association of Certified Orthoptists "Instrument-Based Pediatric Vision Screening Policy Statement," *Pediatrics* (https://doi.org/10.1542/peds.2012-2548)

Oral Health Coding Fact Sheet for Primary Care Physicians (https://downloads.aap.org/AAP/PDF/coding_factsheet_oral_health.pdf)

"Vaccine Financing and Coding" (www.aap.org/en/practice-management/practice-financing/coding-and-valuation/vaccine-financing-and-coding)

AAP Pediatric Coding Newsletter™

"Coding for 2021 Preparticipation Physical Evaluations," July 2021 (https://doi.org/10.1542/pcco_book207_document001)

"Coding for Vaccines Not Administered," July 2020 (https://doi.org/10.1542/pcco_book195_document007)

"Preparing for Preparticipation Physical Evaluations," July 2018 (https://doi.org/10.1542/pcco_book171_document001)

Immunization and Vaccines

Appendix III

AMA Category I vaccine codes (www.ama-assn.org/practice-management/cpt/category-i-vaccine-codes)

CDC VFC program (www.cdc.gov/vaccines/programs/vfc/index.html)

Laboratory Testing

FDA CLIA test category database (www.accessdata.fda.gov/scripts/cdrh/cfdocs/cfCLIA/search.cfm)

● indicates a new code; ▲, revised; #, re-sequenced; ✚, add-on; ★, audiovisual technology; and ◀, synchronous interactive audio.

National Drug Codes

FDA National Drug Code Directory (www.fda.gov/drugs/drug-approvals-and-databases/national-drug-code-directory)

Online Exclusive Content at www.aap.org/cfp2023

"FAQ: Immunization Administration"

"Preventive Medicine Encounters: What's Included? (Letter Template)"

"Screening Laboratory Tests and Codes"

Quality Measurement Information

Agency for Healthcare Research and Quality, US Department of Health and Human Services, National Guideline Clearinghouse (www.qualitymeasures.ahrq.gov)

CPT Category II codes (www.ama-assn.org/practice-management/cpt-category-ii-codes)

Test Your Knowledge!

1. **Which of the following examples supports an abnormal finding during a routine health examination for the purpose of** *International Classification of Diseases, 10th Revision, Clinical Modification* **code selection?**
   a. A child has epilepsy that is stable on the date of the encounter.
   b. A child is recovering from acute otitis media requiring no further management.
   c. A newborn is found to have ankyloglossia that requires release.
   d. A patient has a history of COVID-19 with no residual problems.

2. **Which of the following services is reported with code 90460?**
   a. Influenza immunization of an 18-year-old patient with physician counseling
   b. Immunization administration on a date different from the date that physician counseling was provided
   c. Immunization of a 19-year-old patient with physician counseling
   d. Administration of a monoclonal antibody

3. **Which of the following administration codes are reported for administration of a COVID-19 vaccine?**
   a. 94060–90461
   b. 90471–90474
   c. 0001A–0104A
   d. 91300–91307

4. **Which of the following codes is reported for 25 minutes spent in preventive medicine counseling provided to a patient when no comprehensive preventive evaluation and management services are provided?**
   a. 99401
   b. 99402
   c. 99411
   d. 99408

5. **Which of the following statements is true for reporting an office visit (eg, 99214) in addition to a preventive medicine evaluation and management (E/M) service (eg, 99393)?**
   a. The problem-oriented service must be separately identifiable in the documentation.
   b. The problem must require physician work significantly beyond the work of the preventive service.
   c. Modifier 25 is appended to the code for the problem-oriented E/M service.
   d. All of the above.

● indicates a new code; ▲, revised; #, re-sequenced; ✚, add-on; ★, audiovisual technology; and ◀, synchronous interactive audio.

Chapter 8. Preventive Services

‖‖‖

Telephone and Online Digital Evaluation and Management Services

‖‖‖

CPT copyright 2022 American Medical Association. All rights reserved.

Contents

● indicates a new code; ▲, revised; #, re-sequenced; ✚, add-on; ★, audiovisual technology; and ◀, synchronous interactive audio.

Chapter Highlights

Identify the following types of non–face-to-face evaluation and management (E/M) services and the reporting guidelines for each:

- Telephone services (**99441–99443**)
- Virtual check-in services (**G2012, G2252**)
- Online digital E/M services (**99421–99423**)
- Remote evaluation of recorded video and/or images (**G2010**)
- Interprofessional telephone/Internet/electronic health record assessment and management service (**99446–99452**)

Selecting the Appropriate Evaluation and Management (E/M) Codes

This chapter includes information on coding for non–face-to-face E/M services provided by a physician or other qualified health care professional (QHP) by using asynchronous communications (eg, by telephone or online digital communication). This chapter does not discuss temporary policies in effect only for a specified period because of the COVID-19 public health emergency. Temporary policies may allow a physician or QHP flexibility in reporting certain non–face-to-face services with codes typically restricted to face-to-face or telemedicine (synchronous real-time audiovisual) services. Follow current guidance from each individual payer when reporting these services.

> Services discussed in this chapter are not typically reported with modifier **95** (synchronous telemedicine service via synchronous [real-time] audio and video telecommunications system) or place of service code **02** (telehealth provided other than in a patient's home) or **10** (telehealth provided to a patient at home). See Chapter 20 for information on reporting evaluation and management services provided via telemedicine (ie, through synchronous audiovisual technology).

> See Chapter 13 for assessment and management services (**98966–98971**) provided by qualified health care professionals whose scope of practice does not include evaluation and management services (eg, licensed clinical social workers, occupational therapists).

When codes indicate services provided for new and established patients, a new patient is one who has not received any *face-to-face* professional services within the past 3 years from the physician or another physician of the same exact specialty who belongs to the same group practice. When a service is limited to established patients, it is necessary to verify the patient's status of new or established before provision of services.

> Most of the services described in this chapter can either be a separately reportable service or represent preservice or post-service work that is included in the relative value units assigned to either another evaluation and management service or a procedure when provided within a specified period. Each category of codes includes specific reporting instructions. See Chapter 4 for additional information on how services are valued to include preservice and post-service work.

Verification of the payer's benefit policy for these services is recommended before service; if non-covered, an *advance beneficiary notice* (ABN) or *waiver* should be signed by the patient. This is a written notice to the patient of noncoverage and/or potential out-of-pocket costs that is provided *before delivery of a service*. Verify payer requirements and applicable state regulations before using waivers in your practice. When used, a copy of the signed notice should be kept on file with the practice's billing records. One reference for creating your own ABN is the Medicare program's ABN (www.cms.gov/Medicare/Medicare-General-Information/BNI/ABN).

Telephone E/M Services (99441–99443)

99441   Telephone E/M service by a physician or other qualified health care professional who may report evaluation and management services provided to an established patient, parent, or guardian not originating from a related E/M service provided within the previous 7 days nor leading to an E/M service or procedure within the next 24 hours or soonest available appointment; 5–10 minutes of medical discussion

---

● indicates a new code; ▲, revised; #, re-sequenced; ✚, add-on; ★, audiovisual technology; and ◀, synchronous interactive audio.

99442	11–20 minutes of medical discussion
99443	21–30 minutes of medical discussion

Telephone services (**99441–99443**) are non–face-to-face E/M services provided by a telephone call between a patient and/or caregiver/parent and a physician or other QHP who may report E/M services (eg, nurse practitioner, clinical nurse specialist, physician assistant). See the following "Coding Conundrum: Telephone or Other E/M Service?" box for discussion of use of modifier **93** (synchronous telemedicine service rendered via telephone or other real-time interactive audio-only telecommunications system) to report other services when provided via telephone or other audio-only synchronous communication:

Coding Conundrum: Telephone or Other Evaluation and Management Service?

In 2022, *Current Procedural Terminology* (*CPT*) introduced modifier **93** (full description follows) for indicating that a service was provided via audio-only communication (eg, telephone).

93 Synchronous telemedicine service rendered via telephone or other real-time interactive audio-only telecommunications system: Synchronous telemedicine service is defined as a real-time interaction between a physician or other qualified health care professional and a patient who is located away at a distant site from the physician or other qualified health care professional. The totality of the communication of information exchanged between the physician or other qualified health care professional and the patient during the course of the synchronous telemedicine service must be of an amount and nature that is sufficient to meet the key components and/or requirements of the same service when rendered via a face-to-face interaction.

Appendix T of the *CPT* manual lists the codes to which modifier **93** may be appended and does not include codes for evaluation and management (E/M) services provided by a telephone call or for E/M services typically performed face to face with a patient. Check the payment policies of Medicaid and other payers before reporting an audio-only service by using modifier **93** appended to E/M codes not included in Appendix T.

Codes **99441–99443** may be reported when

- The call was initiated by an established patient or the caregiver of an established patient.
- The service includes physician management of a new problem that does not result in an office visit within 24 hours from the telephone call or at the next available urgent visit appointment.
- The service includes physician management of an existing problem for which the patient was not seen in a face-to-face encounter within the previous 7 days from the telephone call (physician request or unsolicited patient follow-up) or within the postoperative period of a performed and reported procedure.
- The physician documentation of telephone call(s) includes the date(s) of the call(s), name and telephone number of the patient, name of and relationship of the caller, type of service provided (eg, evaluation of an acute or chronic problem, initiation or adjustment of therapy), and time spent in the encounter.

Codes **99441–99443** are *not* reported when

- The call includes less than 5 minutes of medical discussion.
- The call results in a face-to-face encounter within 24 hours or the next available urgent appointment. The call is considered preservice work included in the face-to-face encounter.
- There was a face-to-face encounter (including a telemedicine service) related to the problem within the previous 7 days from the telephone call. The call is considered post-service work included in the face-to-face encounter.
- The call occurs within the postoperative period of a reported procedure.

Figure 9-1 illustrates reporting decisions for telephone evaluation and management services in relation to other services.

- Time of the call is included as part of care plan oversight (CPO; **99374–99380**) or care management services (**99487–99490, 99439, 99491, 99424–99427, 99437**).
- The call is provided during the service period of transitional care management (**99495, 99496**) services.
- Non–face-to-face communication is between the physician and other health care professionals. If applicable, the services may be reported through non–face-to-face prolonged physician service codes **99358** and **99359** or as part of CPO or care management services (**99374–99380; 99439, 99487–99490; 99491, 99437; 99424–99427; 99495, 99496**).
- The call is performed by clinical staff or a provider who may not report E/M services. (See codes **98966–98968** for services by QHPs who may not report E/M services.) Telephone calls between clinical staff and the patient/caregiver are generally not reportable.

● indicates a new code; ▲, revised; #, re-sequenced; ✚, add-on; ★, audiovisual technology; and ◀, synchronous interactive audio.

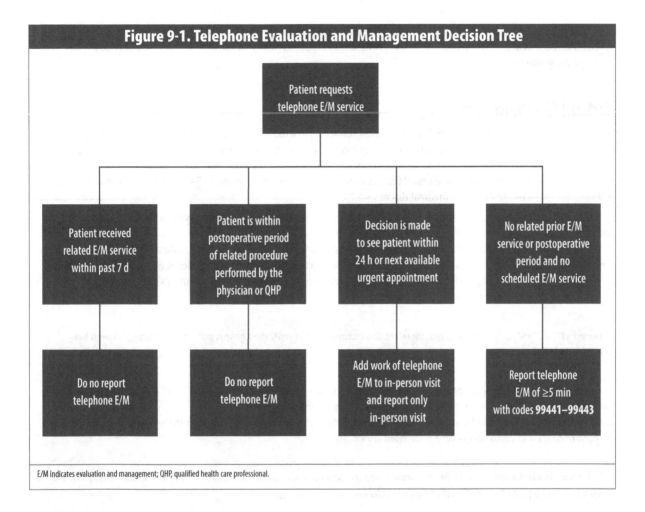

Figure 9-1. Telephone Evaluation and Management Decision Tree

E/M indicates evaluation and management; QHP, qualified health care professional.

Examples

➤ **On January 1, a pediatrician provides a telephone E/M service to an established patient whose parent is concerned about the child's upper respiratory tract symptoms.** The child has not received an E/M service from the same or other physician or QHP of the same specialty and group practice within the prior 7 days. The physician obtains a history of the patient's illness and then provides counseling regarding home care and advises the patient's parent to telephone if the child's symptoms worsen or there are additional questions. The time of service is 10 minutes and is reportable with code **99441**.

Teaching Point: The telephone service is reported because it was not provided within 7 days of another E/M service and did not lead to an E/M service within the next 24 hours or soonest available appointment.

➤ **On January 3, a pediatrician provides a telephone E/M service to a patient with concern of upper respiratory tract symptoms including sore throat.** The pediatrician advises the patient to be seen in the office later that day. The patient is seen in the office on that day. Because the diagnosis is pharyngitis likely caused by postnasal drip, the parent is instructed to begin administering an over-the-counter allergy medication according to the product instructions.

Teaching Point: Only the office E/M service (eg, **99213**) is reported for the combined medical decision-making (MDM) or time of the telephone and in-person E/M services.

➤ **On January 3, a physician spends 20 minutes on a telephone call with a patient's parent who was absent at an encounter that took place 2 days before the call to discuss treatment options recommended at an office visit.** The service is not separately reported.

● indicates a new code; ▲, revised; #, re-sequenced; ✚, add-on; ★, audiovisual technology; and ◀, synchronous interactive audio.

Teaching Point: Because the telephone call refers to an E/M service performed and reported by the physician within the previous 7 days (either requested or unsolicited patient follow-up), the telephone E/M service is not separately reported.

Virtual Check-in Services (G2012, G2252)

G2012	Brief communication technology-based service, eg, virtual check-in, by a physician or other qualified health care professional who can report evaluation and management services, provided to an established patient, not originating from a related E/M service provided within the previous 7 days nor leading to an E/M service or procedure within the next 24 hours or soonest available appointment; 5–10 minutes of medical discussion
G2252	11–20 minutes of medical discussion

The Centers for Medicare & Medicaid Services (CMS) and some other payers allow payment for what CMS terms *communication technology-based services* or virtual check-ins in lieu of telephone E/M services (**99441–99443**). These services are furnished via telecommunications technology and considered virtual care but not telemedicine services (ie, services rendered via real-time audiovisual technology). Per the CMS, virtual check-ins are for patients with an established (or existing) relationship with a physician or other QHP who communicate with their physician or QHP regarding a problem to potentially avoid unnecessary face-to-face visits.

> The use of G2012 and G2252 varies by payer; therefore, it is recommended to verify the payment policies of the individual payer before provision of services.

Payers that adopt Medicare policies for coverage of services reported with codes **G2012** and **G2252** may apply the following guidelines. The service reported with **G2012** or **G2252** must
- Be initiated and agreed to by an established patient or their caregiver/parent (although the practice may inform the patient of the option to access care via virtual check-in)

> A plan may require documentation of the agreement to receive and be billed for the services represented by codes G2012 and G2252. The agreement can typically be verbal but must be given before receipt of the service.

- Be unrelated to a medical visit within the previous 7 days and not lead to a medical visit within the next 24 hours (or soonest appointment available)
- Be provided by a physician or QHP by using communication technology such as a telephone, a patient portal, secure text messaging, or secure email to determine whether a face-to-face service is indicated
- Be reported on the basis of time spent personally by a physician or QHP, not clinical staff

Example

➤ **On January 1, a pediatrician provides a telephone E/M service to a patient whose parent is concerned about the child's nasal congestion.** The time of service is 10 minutes and is reportable with code **99441**, but the child's health plan does not pay for services reported with that code.

Teaching Point: The physician reports **G2012** according to the plan's payment policy for E/M services provided by telephone.

Online Digital E/M Services (99421–99423)

#99421	Online digital evaluation and management service, for an established patient, for up to 7 days, cumulative time during the 7 days; 5–10 minutes
#99422	11–20 minutes
#99423	21 or more minutes

Digital communication technology (eg, a patient portal, secure email) that supports only asynchronous communication is increasingly used to provide online digital E/M services.

● indicates a new code; ▲, revised; #, re-sequenced; ✚, add-on; ★, audiovisual technology; and ◀, synchronous interactive audio.

Online digital E/M services differ from telemedicine services. The required delivery mechanism for telemedicine (ie, synchronous [real-time] audiovisual communication) is not required for online digital E/M services. Communication for online digital E/M services may be an exchange of messages through technology such as secure email, secure text messaging, or a patient portal.

Verify individual health plan policies for payment for digital E/M services.

Codes **99421–99423** are reported by physicians and other QHPs whose scope of practice includes E/M services as described by codes **99202–99499**. Online assessment and management codes **98970–98972** are reported by health care professionals (eg, speech or physical therapists) whose scope of practice does not include E/M services as described by codes **99202–99499**.

Online digital E/M services must be patient or caregiver initiated. Online digital E/M services include

- *Cumulative physician or other QHP time* devoted to the patient's care over 7 days whether the time is spent addressing *single or multiple different problems* within the 7-day period
- Cumulative service time beginning at the physician's personal review of the patient's initial inquiry, including
  - Review of patient records or data pertinent to assessment of the patient's problem
  - Physician's or QHP's personal interaction with clinical staff focused on the patient's problem
  - Development of management plans including physician or QHP generation of prescriptions or ordering of tests
  - Subsequent communication with the patient through online, telephone, email, or other digitally supported communication that does not otherwise represent a separately reported E/M service

> A physician or qualified health care professional (QHP) may instruct clinical staff to relay a response to a patient and/or caregiver, but only the physician's or QHP's time is included in the service time used to select a code for the online digital evaluation and management service.

- Permanent documentation storage (electronic or hard copy) of the encounter

  Document but do not report online digital services
- ✖ Of less than 5 minutes' total time
- ✖ Based on any time spent by clinical staff
- ✖ During the postoperative period of a procedure
- ✖ If another E/M service (in person or via telemedicine) for the same or related problem occurred within 7 days before the online digital service

> If a patient generates the initial online digital inquiry for a new problem within 7 days of a previous evaluation and management (E/M) visit that addressed a different problem, the online digital E/M service may be reported separately. Figure 9-2 illustrates reporting instructions for **99421–99423** with or without additional services within a 7-day period.

- If a separately reported E/M visit occurs within 7 days following the initiation of the online service, only report 1 code. Combine the work of the online digital E/M service into selection of the code for the other E/M service.

Learn more about online digital and telephone services in the December 2020 *AAP Pediatric Coding Newsletter* article, "General Documentation Requirements for Digital and Telephone Evaluation and Management Services" (https://doi.org/10.1542/pcco_book200_document004).

Examples

➤ **On January 1, a pediatrician provides an online digital E/M service to a patient with a rash, which includes obtaining history, reviewing digital photographs of the rash, and advising the parent/caregiver on home treatment.** The time of service is 10 minutes and is reportable with code **99421**. The service is reported when the 7-day service period is complete and no face-to-face E/M service has been rendered during that period.

  Teaching Point: The time of any *subsequent* online E/M service within the 7-day service period is added to the time of the first service and 1 code is reported (eg, **99422**) for the combined services.

Chapter 9. Telephone and Online Digital Evaluation and Management Services

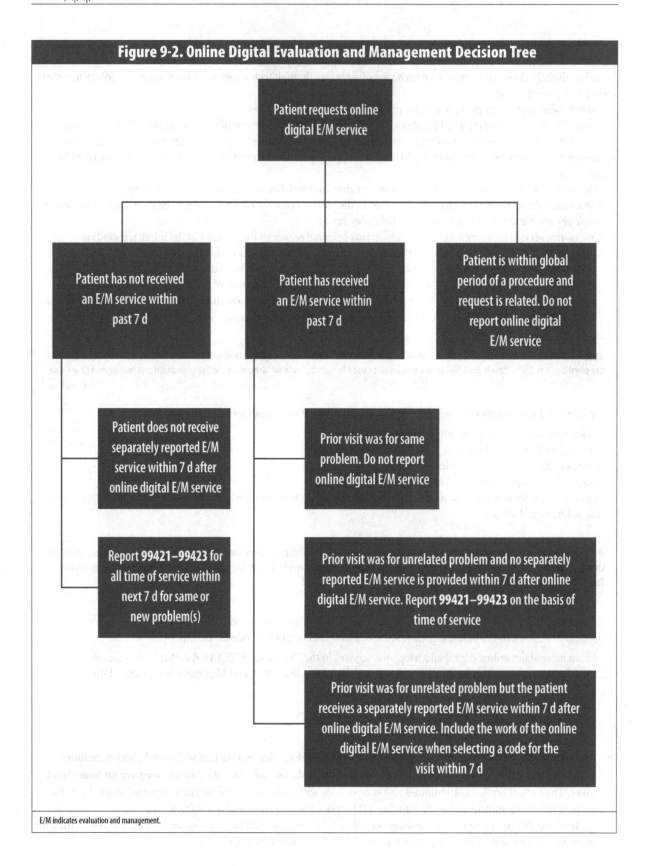

Figure 9-2. Online Digital Evaluation and Management Decision Tree

Patient requests online digital E/M service

Patient has not received an E/M service within past 7 d

Patient has received an E/M service within past 7 d

Patient is within global period of a procedure and request is related. Do not report online digital E/M service

Patient does not receive separately reported E/M service within 7 d after online digital E/M service

Prior visit was for same problem. Do not report online digital E/M service

Report **99421–99423** for all time of service within next 7 d for same or new problem(s)

Prior visit was for unrelated problem and no separately reported E/M service is provided within 7 d after online digital E/M service. Report **99421–99423** on the basis of time of service

Prior visit was for unrelated problem but the patient receives a separately reported E/M service within 7 d after online digital E/M service. Include the work of the online digital E/M service when selecting a code for the visit within 7 d

E/M indicates evaluation and management.

➤ **For the same patient as in the previous example, the parent/caregiver sends a new photograph on January 3 because they are concerned that the rash is not responding to treatment.** The pediatrician sees the patient in the office later that day.

    Teaching Point: Code **99421** is not reported for the prior online digital E/M services, but the level of service reported for the office encounter (eg, **99213**) includes the MDM of the online encounters.

➤ **A patient is seen in the office by a pediatrician for concern of a foreign body in the ear on January 9.** On January 14, the same patient receives an online digital E/M service for advice on managing fear of sleeping in their own bed. Because the problem addressed by the online service is unrelated to the problem addressed at the office encounter, the online service is separately reported (eg, **99422**).

    Teaching Point: Follow payer instructions for reporting an unrelated online service within 7 days of an office E/M service (eg, append modifier **XU** [unusual nonoverlapping service]).

➤ **A 10-year-old patient is seen in the office by a pediatrician for concern of (serous) otitis media on January 9.** On January 11, a parent/caregiver contacts the pediatrician via secure email with concern that the patient's symptoms have worsened, so the pediatrician prescribes an antibiotic.

    Teaching Point: Only the office encounter (eg, **99213**) is reported because the online digital E/M service is provided within 7 days for the same problem addressed at the in-person visit.

➤ **A patient receives an online digital E/M service on January 9.** The physician's total time spent providing the service is 10 minutes. On January 15, the same patient receives an online digital E/M service for an unrelated problem with a total physician time of 15 minutes.

    Teaching Point: The 2 services occurring within 7 days are combined (even though each service addressed different problems) and reported with code **99423**.

Do not include the time of separately reported online digital E/M services in the time attributed to other services (eg, CPO [**99374, 99375, 99377–99380**] or chronic or principal care management services [**99487, 99489, 99490, #99439, 99491, 99424–99427**]).

Remote Evaluation of Recorded Video and/or Images

G2010   Remote evaluation of recorded video and/or images submitted by an established patient (eg, store and forward), including interpretation with follow-up with the patient within 24 business hours, not originating from a related E/M service provided within the previous 7 days nor leading to an E/M service or procedure within the next 24 hours or soonest available appointment

The CMS created code **G2010** as a virtual check-in service allowing payment for evaluation of patient images and/or recorded video sent via digital technology (eg, secure email or text messaging, a patient portal) to a physician or QHP by an established patient or their caregiver and the physician's or QHP's response regarding recommended management. This is not a time-based service and includes review of the patient-submitted images and/or video and communications with the patient/caregiver in response to the findings.

    Report **G2010** when the service

- Is initiated and agreed to by an established patient (although the practice may inform the patient of the option to access care via virtual check-in)
- Is unrelated to a medical visit within the previous 7 days and does not lead to a medical visit within the next 24 hours (or soonest appointment available)
- Is a physician or QHP service in response to receipt of images and/or video from an established patient and/or caregiver
- Is reported on the basis of time spent personally by a physician or QHP, not clinical staff, in review of images and/or video and response to the patient and/or caregiver

---

● indicates a new code; ▲, revised; #, re-sequenced; ✚, add-on; ★, audiovisual technology; and ◀, synchronous interactive audio.

Example

> ➤ **A physician receives images of a rash on a 9-month-old's trunk.** The patient's mother sent the images in a secure email asking whether this rash is likely roseola. The physician reviews the images and telephones the patient's mother to obtain history. The patient was feverish earlier in the week but does not act or appear ill. The patient is not showing any signs of itching or discomfort. The physician agrees with the mother that the rash is likely caused by roseola and encourages follow-up if any new symptoms develop. The service is reported to a payer that allows payment when reported with code **G2010**.
>
> **Teaching Point:** This service is defined as including any additional service required by the patient. However, if the patient required an in-person or telemedicine E/M service on the same date or at the next available appointment in response to the review of images/video, **G2010** would not be separately reported.

Remote Interprofessional Consultations

> In 2023, codes 99446–99451 have been revised to include qualified health care professionals as potential consultants for these services.

Remote interprofessional consultations include a request by a patient's attending or primary care physician or other QHP for an opinion and/or treatment advice by telephone, internet, or electronic health record (EHR) from a physician or other QHP with specialty expertise (ie, consultant). This consultation does not require face-to-face contact with the patient by the consultant. The patient may be in the inpatient or outpatient setting.

- When the purpose of communication is to arrange a transfer of care or face-to-face patient encounter, interprofessional consultation codes are not reported.
- As with all consultations, the request for advice or an opinion, including what advice or opinion was sought, should be documented in the patient record. For a new patient with no record, the consultant should create a record to document this service.

Interprofessional Consultation Reporting by an Attending/Primary Care Physician

#99452   Interprofessional telephone/Internet/electronic health record referral service(s) provided by a treating/requesting physician or qualified health care professional, 30 minutes

The treating/requesting physician or other QHP may report code **99452** or prolonged service (outpatient [**99417**] or inpatient/observation [**99418**]).

- Code **99452** may be reported when 16 to 30 minutes is spent by the requesting individual in a service day preparing for the referral and/or communicating with the consultant.
- Time spent in discussion with the consultant may also be reported with prolonged service codes (in lieu of **99452**) *if the requirements for the appropriate prolonged service codes are met.*
  - Prolonged service code **99417** may be reported when the requesting physician has had a face-to-face encounter with the patient in the office or other outpatient setting on the same day and the physician's total time on that date extends at least 15 minutes beyond the total time of the highest-level E/M service (ie, ≥75 minutes when reporting **99205**, ≥55 minutes when reporting **99215** or **99245**).
  - Prolonged service provided in conjunction with an inpatient, observation, or nursing facility E/M service on the same date may be reported with code **99418** when the physician's total time on that date extends at least 30 minutes beyond the total time of the highest-level E/M service (ie, **99223**, **99233**, **99236**, **99255**, **99306**, **99310**).
  - Prolonged service of greater than 30 minutes in a day without the patient present is reported with codes **99358** and **99359**.

> For more information on prolonged outpatient evaluation and management services, see Chapter 7. Coding for prolonged service in a facility setting is reviewed in Chapter 17.

Interprofessional Consultation Reporting by a Consultant

▲99446 Interprofessional telephone/Internet/electronic health record assessment and management service provided by a consultative physician or other qualified health care professional including a verbal and written report to the patient's treating/requesting physician/qualified health care professional; 5–10 minutes of medical consultative discussion and review

▲99447   11–20 minutes of medical consultative discussion and review

▲99448   21–30 minutes of medical consultative discussion and review

▲99449   31 minutes or more of medical consultative discussion and review

▲#99451 Interprofessional telephone/Internet/electronic health record assessment and management service provided by a consultative physician or qualified health care professional including a written report to the patient's treating/requesting physician or other qualified health care professional, 5 or more minutes of medical consultative time

Guidelines for the consultant reporting interprofessional telephone/internet/EHR consultations include

- Telephone/internet/EHR consultations of less than 5 minutes are not reported. For codes **99446–99449**, *more than 50% of the time* reported as interprofessional consultation must have been spent in medical consultative verbal or internet discussion rather than review of data (eg, medical records, test results).
- Code **99451** is reported on the basis of the total time of review and interprofessional consultation.
- Both verbal and written reports are required for completion of the services represented by codes **99446–99449**. Only a written report is required for code **99451**.
- A single interprofessional consultation code is reported for the cumulative time spent in discussion and information review regardless of the number of contacts necessary to complete the service.
- Codes **99446–99451** are not reported more than once in a 7-day interval.
- Time spent in telephone or online consultation directly with the patient and/or family may be reported by using codes **99441–99443** (telephone E/M) or **99421–99423** (online digital E/M), and the time related to these services is not included in the time attributed to interprofessional consultation services. Qualified nonphysician health care professionals (eg, therapists) report codes **98966–98968** or **98970–98972** for these services.
- Interprofessional consultation services are not reported if the consultant has provided a face-to-face service to the patient within the past 14 days or when the consultation results in scheduling of a face-to-face service within the next 14 days or at the consultant's next available appointment date.
- Time spent by the consultant reviewing pertinent medical records, studies, or other data is included in the time of the interprofessional consultation and not separately reported.
- ✖ Do not report prolonged E/M service before and/or after direct patient care (**99358**, **99359**) for any time within the service period if reporting codes **99446–99451**.
- As with all consultations, the request for advice or opinion should be documented in the patient record. For a new patient with no record, create a record to document this service.

Example

➤ **A 10-year-old girl who has predominantly inattentive attention-deficit/hyperactivity disorder (ADHD) presents to her pediatrician to discuss new behavioral concerns that are resulting in poor academic performance and discord at home.** History and examination indicate increased anxiety and related behavioral changes since returning to in-person school after homeschooling the previous year. The patient sees a psychologist who has indicated that a change in medication may be necessary for this patient. The girl and her mother complete structured screening instruments for anxiety disorders. The girl scores just below the score, a finding indicating a generalized anxiety disorder. The diagnosis for the visit is anxiety with increased symptoms of ADHD. The physician's total time on the date of the visit is 30 minutes, including time spent arranging for a telephone consultation with the patient's psychologist to discuss the patient's diagnosis and management of anxiety in the patient with preexisting ADHD.

On the next day, the psychologist spends 5 minutes reviewing the pediatrician's documentation of the patient's evaluation. Later that day, the pediatrician and psychologist spend a total of 21 minutes discussing the pediatrician's findings, diagnosis, and appropriate treatment options. The psychologist provides the pediatrician with a written report of the recommendations discussed. The diagnosis is adjustment disorder with anxiety complicating management of ADHD.

On a third date, the pediatrician provides an E/M service via secure real-time audiovisual communications technology to the patient and her parents to discuss recommendations based on the prior interprofessional consultation. A diagnosis of adjustment reaction with anxiety exacerbating ADHD and related management options are discussed. The pediatrician's total time on the date of the visit is 25 minutes.

Service	ICD-10-CM	CPT
First date of service (pediatric E/M visit)	**F41.9** (anxiety disorder, unspecified) **F90.0** (ADHD, predominantly inattentive type)	**99214** (established patient office or other outpatient visit E/M, 30–39 minutes of total time) **96127** × 2 (brief emotional/behavioral assessment using a structured instrument)
Second date (interprofessional consultation)	The pediatrician and psychologist each report **F43.22** (adjustment disorder with anxiety) and **F90.0** (ADHD, predominantly inattentive type).	The pediatrician reports **99452** for the 21 minutes spent in interprofessional referral service. The psychologist reports **99448** (21–30 minutes of medical discussion and review).
Third date (pediatric E/M visit via telemedicine)	**F43.22** and **F90.0**	**99213 95** (established patient office or other outpatient visit E/M, 20–29 minutes of total time, provided via telemedicine)

Teaching Points: In this vignette, the patient and parents are not present for the interprofessional consultation. The consultation service by the psychologist included 5 minutes of record review and 21 minutes of conversation with the pediatrician. If less than 50% of the psychiatrist's time was devoted to the medical consultative verbal or internet discussion, an interprofessional consultation would not be reported. The pediatrician may report code **99452** for 16 to 30 minutes of interprofessional consultation.

Modifier **95** is appended to **99213** because the service took place via real-time audiovisual communication technology. Place of service code **10** (telehealth provided to a patient at home) is appropriate on the claim for this service.

Use the resources and quiz that follow to enhance your knowledge of when and how E/M services provided via telephone or online digital communication are reported.

Chapter Takeaways

This chapter reviews codes for reporting services that are not provided in a face-to-face visit or by telemedicine (real-time audiovisual communication). Following are some takeaways from this chapter:

- Time spent in a telephone (**99441–99443**) or online E/M (**99421–99423**) service requested by an established patient and/or caregiver/family may be reported when all reporting requirements are met.
- Some payers allow payment for what CMS terms *communication technology-based services* or virtual check-ins (**G2012**, **G2252**, or **G2010**) in lieu of or addition to other non–face-to-face E/M services.
- Both a requesting physician and a consultant may report codes (**99446–99452**) for time spent in interprofessional consultation.
- Codes discussed in this chapter have specific guidelines regarding reporting in relation to other services provided within a specific period (eg, within 7 days of a prior E/M service or in advance of the next available urgent face-to-face appointment).
- Only time spent by a physician or QHP whose scope of practice includes E/M services is reported with codes discussed in this chapter.

● indicates a new code; ▲, revised; #, re-sequenced; ✚, add-on; ★, audiovisual technology; and ◄, synchronous interactive audio.

Resources

AAP Pediatric Coding Newsletter™

"General Documentation Requirements for Digital and Telephone Evaluation and Management Services," December 2020 (https://doi.org/10.1542/pcco_book200_document004)

"Reporting Evaluation and Management Services Provided Through Online Digital Communication," May 2022 (https://doi.org/10.1542/pcco_book217_document005)

ABN of Noncoverage Form

Medicare program ABN form and instructions for use as an example for creating a practice-specific form (www.cms.gov/Medicare/Medicare-General-Information/BNI/ABN)

Test Your Knowledge!

1. **Which of the following services is reportable with 99441–99443?**
   a. A physician telephones a patient to advise that results of tests ordered at a recent office evaluation and management (E/M) service are normal and no further testing is recommended.
   b. A physician provides a telephone E/M service that results in scheduling the patient for the first available urgent care appointment.
   c. On the day after performing a procedure that includes 10 days of post-procedural care, the physician returns a call to the patient's parent, who has a question about the patient's activities.
   d. A nurse practitioner telephones an adolescent patient who requested a telephone E/M service because their anxiety has escalated since the most recent visit, 2 weeks ago.

2. **Which of the following technologies can be used to provide communication technology-based services or virtual check-in reported with G2012 or G2252?**
   a. Secure email
   b. A patient portal
   c. A telephone
   d. All of the above

3. **Which of the following services includes the cumulative time spent by a physician or qualified health care professional caring for a patient and/or caregiver during a 7-day service period?**
   a. Telephone evaluation and management (E/M) service
   b. Online digital E/M service
   c. All E/M services
   d. No E/M services

4. **Which of the following services is appropriately reported with G2010?**
   a. Remote evaluation by a physician or qualified health care professional of an image or video submitted by a patient or caregiver/parent
   b. Evaluation of a patient's problem via telephone
   c. Review of a patient's radiological imaging
   d. An evaluation and management service provided via secure text messaging

5. **Which of the following statements is true for remote interprofessional consultation services?**
   a. Only the consultant reports their time spent providing the service.
   b. The service may be requested by a patient or caregiver.
   c. When the reporting requirements are met, the requesting physician may report 99452 for time spent preparing for and participating in the consultative service.
   d. A consultant may report an interprofessional consultation service when the sole purpose of the communication is to arrange a transfer of care.

Indirect Management of Chronic and Complex Conditions

CPT copyright 2022 American Medical Association. All rights reserved.

Contents

Chapter 10. Indirect Management of Chronic and Complex Conditions

● indicates a new code; ▲, revised; #, re-sequenced; ✚, add-on; ★, audiovisual technology; and ◀, synchronous interactive audio.

Chapter Highlights

- Options for reporting evaluation and management (E/M) services provided without direct patient contact
- Tracking time of services provided within a 30-day or calendar-month period
- Related but separately reported services

Children with chronic and complex health care needs require greater levels and amounts of multidisciplinary medical, psychosocial, rehabilitation, and habilitation services than their same-aged peers. The child with special health care needs will require extra services, such as prolonged services and care management, with an increased frequency of E/M visits.

In addition to codes for services provided on a single date of service, *Current Procedural Terminology* (*CPT*®) includes categories of codes created to recognize episodes of care for complex health care needs that go beyond the work included in preservice, intraservice, and post-service values of the traditional E/M service provided directly (in person or by telecommunications technology) by a physician or other qualified health care professional (QHP). Several code categories include codes for reporting care management services performed by clinical staff under the supervision of a physician or QHP and for reporting a combination of physician or QHP and clinical staff services.

Indirect Management of Chronic and Complex Conditions

Management of complex medical conditions may be reported with multiple codes for individual services and/or single codes that describe a combination of direct and indirect services or a period of indirect services reported with 1 or more codes based on time of service.

Five key categories of E/M services that include indirect services are discussed in this chapter.

1. Transitional care management (TCM) (**99495, 99496**) includes a combination of 1 direct service and indirect services, over a 30-day period, as needed, to help patients transition from a stay in a facility to their home environment without gaps in their care management. The reporting physician or QHP provides or oversees the management and/or coordination of services, as needed, for all the patient's health care needs.

2. Chronic care management (**99490, 99439, 99491, 99437**) and complex CCM (CCCM) (**99487, 99489**) are monthly services provided by a single physician to manage or coordinate services for patients with 2 or more complex chronic conditions. The reporting individual provides or oversees the management and/or coordination of services, as needed, for all the patient's health care needs.

3. Principal care management (PCM) (**99424–99427**) is a monthly service provided by a physician with a focus on the medical and/or psychological needs manifested by a single complex chronic condition (eg, poorly controlled diabetes). Principal care management services do not require management and coordination of services for all of a patient's health care needs.

> Care management services cannot be reported when provided during a postoperative portion of the global period of a service reported by the same physician or other physician of the same specialty and same group practice. For example, a surgeon would not report transitional care management (TCM) during a postoperative period, but a primary pediatrician may report TCM when managing all the patient's medical conditions following hospital discharge. Care management services are not reported for postoperative care alone (eg, when reporting a surgical service code with modifier **55** only for postoperative management).

4. Care plan oversight (CPO) (**99374, 99375; 99377, 99378; 99379, 99380**) is another monthly service provided by a single physician in supervision of health care services typically delivered by qualified nonphysician health care professionals (QNHCPs) (eg, therapists), home health, or hospice services. Care plan oversight is reported by only 1 individual who has the sole or predominant supervisory role with a particular patient.

5. Psychiatric collaborative (**99492–99494**) or general behavioral health integration (**99484**) care management services are monthly services provided by a treating physician or QHP and are focused on psychiatric and behavioral health issues. Services are provided in collaboration with a psychiatrist (**99492–99494**) or provided by clinical staff under the supervision of a treating pediatrician or QHP (**99484**).

Chapter 10. Indirect Management of Chronic and Complex Conditions

> Please see Chapter 11 for information on reporting psychiatric collaborative care management services and general behavioral health integration care management services.

Each of these categories of service is reported on the basis of time and/or specified levels of service devoted to care of the individual patient in a specified period. *CPT* instructions for each category of services specify the service requirements, eligible service providers, required time (when applicable), and whether or not certain other services may be separately reported within the period of each service. A table comparing requirements for reporting CCM, PCM, and CPO services is included at www.aap.org/cfp2023 ("Monthly Care Management and Care Plan Oversight Services: A Comparison").

- Review the codes for these services and the related coding instructions to take advantage of opportunities to be paid for providing and/or coordinating comprehensive care for all children.
- To take advantage of opportunities to be paid for providing and reporting services related to managing chronic conditions and complex health care needs, identify the services that practice capabilities will support. For instance, provision of TCM services requires timely identification of patients discharged from an inpatient or observation stay so contact may be made with the patient or caregiver within 2 business days of facility discharge.
- Payers may require specific electronic capabilities (eg, an electronic health record [EHR] that meets specifications required by the Medicaid Promoting Interoperability Programs and/or Merit-based Incentive Payment System).
- Codes and payment policy for many of these services continue to evolve. Be sure to review reporting instructions for any changes that will take place on January 1 of each year.
- Report these services and the diagnosis codes representing the patient's chronic and complex conditions to demonstrate the higher-quality, lower-cost care that is a key element of emerging payment methodologies.

> See Chapter 4 for information on emerging payment methodologies such as value-based purchasing.

- Payers that have adopted value-based or enhanced payment initiatives, such as per-member-per-month (PMPM) payment models, may consider certain care management services bundled into the services for which the enhanced payment is made. However, practices may choose to assign codes for use in internal calculations of the cost to provide enhanced care in comparison to any enhanced payments.

For more information on preparing your practice to care for patients with complex health care needs, see the American Academy of Pediatrics (AAP) policy statement, "Patient- and Family-Centered Care Coordination: A Framework for Integrating Care for Children and Youth Across Multiple Systems" (https://doi.org/10.1542/peds.2014-0318).

- This policy statement, coauthored by the AAP Council on Children With Disabilities and the Medical Home Implementation Project Advisory Committee, outlines the essential partnerships that are critical to this framework.
- To further augment and facilitate the recommendations in this policy statement, refer to the freely accessible Boston Children's Hospital Care Coordination Curriculum (www.pcpcc.org/resource/care-coordination-curriculum). This curriculum provides content that can be adapted to the needs of any entity (eg, a single practice, a network of practices, parent and family organizations, a statewide organization). By design, most of the content is universally relevant, but the curriculum is optimally used when it is adapted and customized to reflect local needs, assets, and cultures.

> Services such as chronic care management do not prevent separate reporting of preventive services when provided to children with complex health care needs. See Chapter 8 for more information on reporting preventive evaluation and management services and separately reportable services on the same date.

Tracking Time of Periodic Services

Care management services, other than TCM, are reported only when a specific amount of time is spent providing the service during 1 calendar month. Care plan oversight also requires specified amounts of time spent within a calendar month. Services typically occur on multiple days within the month. *Each segment of time must be documented.*

> Be sure to identify the reporting period of care management services. Transitional care management services (99495, 99496) are reported for a 30-day period beginning with the date of discharge from a facility setting. Other services are reported per calendar month of service, including all chronic and principal care management, care plan oversight, psychiatric collaborative care management, and care management for behavioral health conditions.

Documentation and tracking of time for services that are reported periodically, such as time spent in CCM activities in a calendar month, require establishment of routine processes to capture all billable services. Failure to track the time and activities may result in practice expense that does not yield revenue.

Practice and system capabilities vary. Potential tracking mechanisms include

- Electronic health record flow sheets designed to capture each activity and the related time throughout a period of service and provide a report of time per patient within each period of service.
- Stand-alone time-tracking software, which may also offer a solution for documenting time of service.
- Manual systems, such as spreadsheets, that are updated at the time of each activity.
- Work-arounds in existing electronic systems, such as EHR templates for clinical staff appointments that are assigned pseudocodes to track time (see example that follows). Pseudocodes are never used on claims; instead, they provide a basis for tracking time-based services.

> **Collaboration with system vendors, professional colleagues, and practice management consultants may be invaluable to successful delivery, documentation, and reporting of time-based services.**

The following example illustrates one semiautomated method of using pseudocodes:

Example

➤ **A physician is providing PCM services to a child with a single high-risk disease.** The physician's clinical staff spend 35 minutes over the course of a month in PCM activities in support of the patient's plan of care. On the date of each activity, clinical staff document the nature of the activity as well as the time spent. They also select a pseudocode (COORD) and 1 unit of service for each minute spent providing a service. No charge is generated by entry of COORD. However, billing staff will generate a report of the patients for whom COORD was entered during a calendar month.

Because the PCM service to this child was 35 minutes of clinical staff time, the pediatrician reports code **99426** (PCM, first 30 minutes of clinical staff time directed by physician or QHP, per calendar month).

Coding for Episodes of Care

It is important to understand the *CPT* instructions that explain requirements and guide which activities are included in each service and which are separately reported. Many inclusion and exclusion rules are applied to the services discussed in this chapter.

- Certain niche services (eg, management of end-stage renal disease) may be considered components of or an alternative to comprehensive or PCM.
- The same time and activity are never used to support multiple codes (eg, time used to support reporting of an online digital E/M service code is not included in time of CCM).

Transitional Care Management Services

Transitional care management (**99495, 99496**) includes services provided to a new or an established patient whose medical and/or psychosocial problems require moderate- or high-level medical decision-making (MDM) during the transition from the following settings to the patient's community setting (eg, home, domiciliary, rest home, or assisted living facility):

- Inpatient hospital including partial, acute, rehabilitation, and long-term acute stays
- Observation care
- Skilled nursing or nursing facility

Transitional care management commences on the date of discharge and continues for the next 29 days. There are no specific requirements for time spent in TCM services. However, TCM activities should be documented on the dates provided.

Moderate to high MDM is a requirement for TCM. Follow-up care that includes low-intensity services such as discussion of improving or normal laboratory results, which require only straightforward or low MDM, are not reported with codes for TCM. **Box 10-1** includes code descriptors for TCM services.

Transitional care management includes a combination of patient care activities by a physician or other QHP and clinical staff working under supervision of a physician or QHP.

Chapter 10. Indirect Management of Chronic and Complex Conditions

● indicates a new code; ▲, revised; #, re-sequenced; ✚, add-on; ★, audiovisual technology; and ◀, synchronous interactive audio.

Non–face-to-face services provided by the physician or other QHP may include
- Obtaining and reviewing the discharge information
- Reviewing, ordering, or following up on pending diagnostic tests and treatments
- Communicating with or educating the family and/or other caregivers
- Interacting with other QHPs who will assume/reassume care of the patient's system-specific problems
- Scheduling assistance for necessary follow-up services
- Arranging referrals and community resources as necessary

Box 10-1. Transitional Care Management at a Glance

Patient Population

New or established patients whose medical and/or psychosocial problems require moderate- or high-level MDM during a 30-day transition period beginning with the date of discharge from a facility setting to the patient's home, domiciliary, rest home, or assisted living facility.

★**99495** Transitional care management services with the following required elements:	★**99496** Transitional care management services with the following required elements:
• Communication (direct contact, telephone, electronic) with the patient and/or caregiver within 2 business days of discharge • At least moderate level of MDM during the service period • Face-to-face or telemedicine visit, within 14 calendar days of discharge[a]	• Communication (direct contact, telephone, electronic) with the patient and/or caregiver within 2 business days of discharge • High level of MDM during the service period • Face-to-face or telemedicine visit, within 7 calendar days of discharge[a]

Abbreviation: MDM, medical decision-making.

[a] Medication reconciliation and management must occur no later than the date of the face-to-face visit.

Licensed clinical staff time (under the direction of the physician or other QHP) may include face-to-face and non–face-to-face time spent
- Communicating with the patient and/or family or other caregivers about aspects of care and with other agencies and community services used by the patient
- Educating the patient and/or family or other caregivers to support self-management, independent living, and activities of daily living
- Assessing and supporting adherence to the treatment plan and medication management
- Facilitating access to care and other services needed by the patient and/or family, including identifying community and health resources

The 2022 Medicare Physician Fee Schedule values for TCM services were 6.04 total non-facility relative value units (RVUs), not adjusted for geographic practice cost index for code **99495** and 8.14 RVUs for **99496**. Total non-facility RVUs include values for physician work, practice expense, and liability. Values for 2023 were unavailable at the time of this publication.
- This equated to $241.60 and $325.60, respectively, for providing TCM services over a 30-day period (calculated at $40.00 per RVU and not adjusted for geographic practice cost index).
- 2022 physician work RVUs assigned were 2.78 for **99495** and 3.79 for **99496**. Work RVUs are often used in salary calculations for employed physicians.

For more information on how relative value units affect payment, see Chapter 4.

Transitional care management services are not limited to the attending provider of the related facility stay (eg, hospitalist) or to physicians of any specific specialty.
- The individual reporting TCM provides or oversees the management and/or coordination of services necessary *for all* the patient's medical conditions, psychosocial needs, and activities of daily living.
- Only 1 individual may report TCM for each qualifying patient within 30 days of discharge. Another TCM service may not be reported by the same individual or group for any subsequent discharge(s) within those 30 days.
- Hospital or observation discharge services (ie, **99238**, **99239**, or **99217**) may be reported by the same individual reporting TCM services. Discharge services do not qualify as the required face-to-face visit for TCM.

The TCM services begin on the date of discharge (day 1 of 30-day period) and continue for the next 29 days.

● One face-to-face visit (in person or by telemedicine) with the reporting physician or QHP is included in addition to indirect services performed by the physician/QHP and/or licensed clinical staff under the direction of the physician/QHP. Any additional face-to-face visits during the service period are separately reported.

Codes **99495** and **99496**

● Require initial patient contact, a face-to-face visit with the reporting physician or QHP, and medication reconciliation *within specified time frames.*

> To provide direct patient contact within 2 business days of discharge and to schedule appointments within 7 or 14 days, practices must have a process for receiving notification of observation and inpatient hospital discharges. Failure to make contact within 2 business days of discharge or to provide a face-to-face visit within 14 days of discharge eliminates the possibility of reporting transitional care management services.

● Medication management must occur *no later than* the date of the face-to-face visit.
  — *Medication reconciliation* refers to the process of avoiding inadvertent inconsistencies across transitions in care by reviewing the patient's complete medication regimen at the time of admission, transfer, and discharge and comparing it with the regimen being considered for the new setting of care.
  — Clinical staff may perform and document medication reconciliation under general supervision of the physician or QHP.

> When medication management occurs in conjunction with a face-to-face visit, code **1111F** (discharge medications reconciled with the current medication list in outpatient medical record) may be reported in addition to the code for the service provided. Code **1111F** is a Category II *Current Procedural Terminology* code used for performance measurement in some quality initiatives and is not associated with fee-for-service payment.

● Code selection is based on the level of MDM and the date of the first face-to-face visit, as shown in **Table 10-1**. Note that all 3 components (communication within 2 business days, type of MDM, and timing of face-to-face visit) must be met to report TCM services, although only the MDM and time of the face-to-face visit differentiate code selection.

Table 10-1. Levels of Transitional Care Management		
Level of Medical Decision-making	**Face-to-face Visit Within 7 Days**	**Face-to-face Visit Within 8 to 14 Days**
Moderate	**99495**	**99495**
High	**99496**	**99495**

● The first face-to-face visit is included in the TCM service and is not reported separately.

Additional face-to-face E/M services (eg, **99212–99215**) during the 30-day TCM period but provided on dates subsequent to that of the first included face-to-face visit may be separately reported.

● Documentation includes the timing of the initial post-discharge communication with the patient or caregivers, date of the face-to-face visit, and elements supporting moderate- or high-level MDM over the 30-day service period. *Medical decision-making is defined by the office and other outpatient E/M service guidelines.*

● Follow payer guidelines for reporting. The Centers for Medicare & Medicaid Services (CMS) allows reporting of TCM services following completion of the required face-to-face visit (ie, before the end of the service period). Other payers may not allow billing until the complete service period has elapsed.

Examples

To help illustrate the use of codes for management of complex medical conditions, examples in this chapter focus on Patient A, an adolescent who was recently diagnosed with major depression because of distress caused by hemoglobin SS disease and asthma.

Chapter 10. Indirect Management of Chronic and Complex Conditions

● indicates a new code; ▲, revised; #, re-sequenced; ✚, add-on; ★, audiovisual technology; and ◀, synchronous interactive audio.

➤ **A patient with hemoglobin SS disease and asthma is discharged from the hospital after a 3-day admission for asthma symptoms and concern for acute chest syndrome.** One day after discharge, the patient's primary care pediatrician reviews records from the hospital stay and notes concerning issues with mental health. The pediatrician telephones the parent, who shares a concern about a new diagnosis of depression because the recommended follow-up appointment with a psychologist cannot be scheduled sooner than 3 weeks from discharge. The patient is seen by the pediatrician in follow-up later that day. Asthma symptoms are improved, and his pain is currently controlled. The depression is reassessed, and the patient is determined to have suicidal thoughts, although there is no current intent. The pediatrician telephones the sickle cell program at the children's hospital 130 mi away, where the patient has received behavioral health care in the past. After speaking with a psychiatrist specializing in caring for children with chronic illness, it is agreed that the patient will receive care from the clinic rather than wait to meet with the local psychologist. Although admission for psychiatric care is discussed as an option, intensive telemedicine treatment is scheduled. The patient is also advised to keep an in-person follow-up appointment with the pulmonologist the following week. The pediatrician and clinical staff closely monitor and coordinate ongoing treatment for the duration of the 30-day period that began on the date of discharge. The MDM is highly complex because of the management of depression with suicidal ideation and a decision regarding hospitalization.

Code **99496** is reported. Because the MDM is highly complex and the visit occurred within 7 days of discharge, this service meets the requirements for code **99496**. Diagnosis codes may include **R45.851** (suicidal ideations), **F32.2** (major depressive disorder, single episode, severe without psychotic features), **J45.31** (mild persistent asthma with [acute] exacerbation), and **D57.1** (sickle-cell disease without crisis).

➤ **Patient A has hemoglobin SS disease and asthma and is discharged from the hospital after an admission for asthma symptoms and concern for acute chest syndrome.** One day after discharge, Patient A's primary care pediatrician reviews a discharge summary and learns that the patient was diagnosed with depression and an antidepressant medication was started during the stay. The pediatrician telephones the patient's mother, who shares that she is especially concerned about her child's depression because the recommended follow-up appointment with a psychologist could not be scheduled sooner than 3 weeks from discharge. Clinical staff assist with arranging an earlier follow-up appointment via telemedicine with a psychiatrist who specializes in caring for children with chronic medical conditions instead of the local psychologist. Patient A is seen by the pediatrician in follow-up 6 days after discharge. The pediatrician and clinical staff monitor and coordinate the child's ongoing treatment through the 29th day following discharge. The MDM is moderately complex.

Code **99495** is reported because the MDM was moderate even though the face-to-face visit occurred within 7 days and would have supported **99496** if the MDM were high. Diagnoses are **F32.A** (depression, unspecified), **J45.31** (mild persistent asthma with [acute] exacerbation), and **D57.1** (sickle-cell disease without crisis).

Care Management After Transitional Care Management

A patient may require ongoing care management services after the 30-day TCM service period has ended. When a TCM service period begins or ends in the same month that other care management services are provided, each service may be reported by the same physician or QHP as long as the same period is not attributed to more than one service (ie, time during the TCM service period cannot be attributed to another care management service).

Example

➤ **Patient A is discharged on January 4, 2023. Transitional care management is provided through a period ending on February 2, 2023.** The pediatrician provides CCM services for the remainder of the month of February. Only the time spent in CCM services provided from February 3, 2023, through February 28, 2023, may be considered for that calendar month per *CPT*.

Transitional care management services are valued significantly higher than other care management services. If the dates and/or time for TCM and other care management services overlap, it is advantageous to report TCM, provided all required elements of service have been provided.

● indicates a new code; ▲, revised; #, re-sequenced; ✚, add-on; ★, audiovisual technology; and ◀, synchronous interactive audio.

Monthly Care Management Services

Monthly care management services are management and support services that are not limited to the period following discharge from a facility stay. These services are provided by physicians or QHPs or by clinical staff under the direction of a physician or QHP to individuals who reside at home or in a domiciliary, rest home, or assisted living facility. The goals of care management services are to improve care coordination, reduce avoidable hospital services, improve patient engagement, and decrease care fragmentation.

CPT includes 3 types of continuous care management services. Details of patient eligibility, providers of service, and time requirements vary for these services and are discussed in detail in the sections for Chronic Care Management (CCM) and Complex CCM and for Principal Care Management later in this chapter.

1. *Chronic care management services*—provision or supervision of the management and/or coordination of services, as needed, *for all the patient's medical conditions, psychosocial needs, and activities of daily living*
2. *Complex CCM services*—CCM services that require at least 60 minutes of clinical staff time under the direction of a physician or QHP and moderate or high MDM
3. *Principal care management services*—provision or supervision of the management and/or coordination of services, as needed, for a patient's single complex chronic condition

Boxes 10-2 and **10-3** list requirements for reporting care management services.

Time, activities (eg, patient education), and identification of the individual conducting each activity must be documented. An example of a worksheet for tracking care management activities and service times is included at www.aap.org/cfp2023 ("Care Management Tracking Worksheet Template").

- Each minute of time is counted only once and only for 1 service.
- A physician or QHP may separately report a distinct time-based service (eg, an online digital E/M service) provided to the same patient during the same calendar month that other distinct time is used to report care management services.
- Only time spent by clinical staff employed directly by or under contract and clinically integrated with the reporting professional's practice is included in the time of care management services.

Box 10-2. Chronic Care Management Services

A comprehensive care plan for all the patient's medical conditions, psychosocial needs, and activities of daily living must be developed, revised, or monitored and shared with the patient/caregivers for each type of CCM service.

Patient Population for All CCM Services

Patients have multiple (≥2) chronic or episodic conditions expected to last ≥12 months, or until the death of the patient, that present significant risk of death, acute exacerbation/decompensation, or functional decline.

#99490 Chronic care management services by clinical staff

Work Required

- ≥20 minutes of clinical staff activity directed by a physician/QHP, per calendar month
- May combine physician or QHP time of <30 minutes personally spent in CCM services with clinical staff time as long as ≥20 minutes is spent within a calendar month

#+99439 each additional 20 minutes of clinical staff time directed by a physician or QHP, per calendar month (List up to 2 units separately in addition to **99490**)

#99491 Chronic care management services by physician/QHP, first 30 minutes (≥30–59 minutes)

+99437 each additional full 30-minute period (eg, 60–89 minutes equals 1 unit)

Work Required

- ≥30 minutes personally spent by a physician or QHP, per calendar month

---

99487 Complex chronic care management services by clinical staff/physician/QHP

Work Required

- Moderate- or high-level MDM
- ≥60 minutes of clinical staff activity directed by a physician/QHP, per calendar month (may include time spent personally by a physician or QHP)

+99489 each additional 30 minutes per calendar month (List separately in addition to **99487**)

Abbreviations: CCM, chronic care management; MDM, medical decision-making; QHP, qualified health care professional.

Chapter 10. Indirect Management of Chronic and Complex Conditions

Box 10-3. Principal Care Management Services

A care plan specific to the single disease must be developed, revised, or monitored and shared with the patient/caregivers for each type of PCM service. Ongoing communication and care coordination with relevant practitioners furnishing care is also required. PCM services of <30 minutes' duration in a calendar month are not reported separately.

Patient Population for All PCM Services

Patients have a single complex chronic condition expected to last ≥3 months that presents significant risk of death, acute exacerbation/decompensation, or functional decline. The condition requires frequent adjustments in the medication regimen, and/or the management of the condition is unusually complex because of comorbidities.

#99424 Principal care management services by a physician/QHP

Work Required

● ≥30 minutes of physician or QHP time, per calendar month

#✚99425 each additional 30 minutes of physician or QHP time, per calendar month (List separately in addition to **99424** for each full 30 minutes beyond the first 30 minutes)

#99426 Principal care management services by clinical staff/physician/QHP

Work Required

● ≥30 minutes of clinical staff activity directed by a physician or other QHP, per calendar month (may include time spent personally by a physician or other QHP)

#✚99427 each additional 30 minutes per calendar month (List up to 2 units separately in addition to **99426**)

Abbreviations: PCM, principal care management; QHP, qualified health care professional.

The midpoint rule commonly applied for coding based on time does not apply to care management services (99424–99427, 99437, 99439, 99487, 99489, 99490, 99491).

● When provided during the same calendar month as care management services, behavioral or psychiatric collaborative care management (PCCM) services (**99484, 99492–99494**) may be separately reported. Do not count the same minutes (eg, 1:00–1:15 pm) toward care management and behavioral or PCCM services.
● Care management services are not reported by the same individual for services to the same patient in the same calendar month as end-stage renal disease services (**90951–90970**), CPO (**99374–99380**), or other care management services (eg, do not report both CCM and CCCM).

Required Practice Capabilities

A practice providing CCM, CCCM, or PCM services must have all the following specific capabilities:
● Use of an EHR system that supports timely access to clinical information.
● Ability to provide access to care providers or clinical staff 24 hours a day, 7 days a week, including providing patients and caregivers with a means to contact health care professionals in the practice to address urgent needs, regardless of the time of day or day of the week.
● Ability to provide continuity of care through scheduling of the patient's successive routine appointments with a designated member of the care team.
● Provision of timely access and management for necessary follow-up when a patient is discharged from the emergency department or hospital.
● Patient and caregiver engagement and education and integration of care among all service professionals, as appropriate for each patient.
● The individual reporting care management services oversees activities of the care team.
● All care team members providing services are clinically integrated.

CPT no longer requires use of a standardized methodology to identify patients who may qualify for care management services. However, such processes may be beneficial in identifying and offering care management services to patients. Processes may involve developing checklists or processes for identifying characteristics of patients with complex health care needs (eg, any patient with chronic or episodic conditions that are expected to last at least 12 months and increase the risk of morbidity and mortality, acute exacerbation or decompensation, or functional decline may require CCM services). Examples of such characteristics (*examples only; not a practice guideline*) include

---

● indicates a new code; ▲, revised; #, re-sequenced; ✚, add-on; ★, audiovisual technology; and ◀, synchronous interactive audio.

- Number of chronic conditions
- Number of visits for nonroutine care in the past year
- Number of days the child did not attend school due to the health condition
- Emergency department visits or hospitalizations in the past 6 months
- Number of current medications or medications prescribed or revised in the past 6 months
- Number of physicians and other providers (eg, home health care provider, nutritionist)
- Lack of resources (eg, housing, health plan coverage, access to care in community)
- Assistance required for activities of daily living
- Other psychosocial considerations (eg, language barriers, multiple family members with complex care needs)

Activities of Care Management Services

Services include all clinical staff time spent in face-to-face and non–face-to-face services or a physician's time personally spent in care management activities. Time spent in other reported services (eg, time of prolonged clinical staff service [**99415, 99416**] or time of collection and interpretation of physiologic data [**99091**]) may not be included to meet requirements for reporting care management services.

Care management activities include

- Face-to-face and non–face-to-face time spent communicating with and engaging the patient and/or family, caregivers, other professionals, community services, and agencies
- Developing, revising, documenting, communicating, and implementing a comprehensive (CCM, CCCM) or disease-specific (PCM) care plan
- Collecting health outcomes data and registry documentation
- Teaching the patient and/or family/caregiver to support patient self-management, independent living, and activities of daily living
- Identifying community and health resources
- Facilitating access to care and other services needed by the patient and/or family
- Management of care transitions not reported as part of TCM (**99495, 99496**)
- Ongoing review of patient status, including review of laboratory and other studies not reported as part of an E/M service
- Assessment and support for adherence to the care plan

The American Academy of Pediatrics *Pediatric Care Management: Coding Quick Reference Care 2023* outlines these codes and includes decision trees to help guide users to the correct codes (https://shop.aap.org/pediatric-care-management-coding-quick-reference-card-2023).

Development of a Plan of Care

A plan of care must be developed or revised *and a copy provided to each patient* receiving care management services. For CCM and CCCM services, the plan of care addresses all the patient's health care needs. For PCM, the plan of care is focused on management of the patient's single complex chronic health condition.

- A plan of care for health problems is based on a physical, mental, cognitive, social, functional, and environmental evaluation. It is intended to provide a simple and concise overview of the patient and the patient's medical conditions and to be a useful resource for patients, caregivers, and providers. See **Figure 10-1** for an example of a plan of care.
- Creation, monitoring, or revision of a plan of care must be documented. Plans created by other entities (eg, home health agencies) cannot be substituted for a care plan established by the individual reporting CCM services.

Chronic Care Management (CCM) and Complex CCM (CCCM)

The appropriate CCM or CCCM code(s) is reported once per calendar month by only 1 individual who has assumed the management role for all the patient's care. This may be a primary pediatrician or a subspecialist, but only the 1 individual may report CCM or CCCM services in a calendar month. Face-to-face E/M services may be separately reported by the same individual during the same calendar month.

> Time spent by physicians and other qualified health care professionals of the same specialty in the same group practice (eg, covering physician) may be combined to meet the time requirements for care management services, but the service must be reported by the individual who is overseeing the patient's care.

● indicates a new code; ▲, revised; #, re-sequenced; ✚, add-on; ★, audiovisual technology; and ◀, synchronous interactive audio.

Defining a Plan of Care

Current Procedural Terminology defines a *care plan* or *plan of care* as required for care management services (ie, chronic care management [CCM], complex CCM, and principal care management) as

- Based on a physical, mental, cognitive, social, functional, and environmental assessment
- Comprehensive for all health or a single complex chronic health problem, as applicable
- Typically not limited to but possibly including
  —Problem list
  —Expected outcome and prognosis
  —Measurable treatment goals
  —Cognitive assessment
  —Functional assessment
  —Symptom management
  —Planned interventions
  —Medical management
  —Environmental evaluation
  —Caregiver assessment
  —Interaction and coordination with outside resources and other health care professionals and providers
  —Summary of advance directives

These elements are intended to be a guide for creating a meaningful plan of care rather than a strict set of requirements. They should be used only as appropriate for the individual.

The plan should be updated periodically on the basis of status or goal changes. The entire care plan should be reviewed at least annually.

Figure 10-1. Example Plan of Care

This plan of care has been written by A Great Pediatric Practice to help us work with you to be as healthy as possible. This plan will allow you to share with us what is important to you and will let you know what to expect from us.

We will keep a copy of this plan and make changes as necessary. We will share this with other people who care for you (like other doctors or therapists), as needed, to help them care for you. You can also share this with others, such as family members, who help you care for yourself.

Date	01/15/2023		Primary pediatrician		Dr J		Page 1 of 2

About Me

Name	Patient A		I like to be called	Patient A		Date of birth	12/25/2008
Primary caregivers							
Preferred contact information							
Secondary contact information							
Preferred pharmacy	Family Drug Store		Preferred hospital			Children's Hospital-Main	

Who Do I Call When I Need Care or Have Questions?

My care coordinator	

Important Health Information

I am allergic to	No known allergies
I have difficulty with	Pain episodes, asthma symptoms in late summer/fall, missing school for medical appointments
Equipment I need (like a wheelchair)	Nebulizer, inhaler
Community assistance	No food or housing insecurity (as described by mother)

My Health Concerns (Include concerns from patient and caregiver perspectives.)

Concerns	What I can expect for each concern
Asthma	Coordinated care with pulmonologist

Figure 10-1 (*continued*)	

My Health Concerns (Include concerns from patient and caregiver perspectives.)

Sickle cell disease	Coordinated care with team at Children's Hospital for hematology, pulmonary, pain management, and behavioral health Assistance with obtaining prompt and appropriate care in the emergency department, when needed
Depression	Coordination with behavioral health team of Children's Hospital

My Health Goals

Goals	Plans of action
Asthma: Maintain symptom control.	Continue daily control medication and follow action plan when symptomatic.
Sickle cell disease:	Continue current medications for control and pain management; get annual transcranial Doppler ultrasound; maintain hydration daily; alert Dr J of any fever or increased fatigue, pain, or other symptoms; go to emergency department if there are signs of stroke, uncontrolled pain, or asthma symptoms that are unresponsive to home treatment.
Depression:	Continue medication and telemedicine appointments with behavioral health team at Children's Hospital; call Dr J for any side effects of management or escalation of symptoms.

My Planned Care

Specialty care	Children's Hospital Sickle Cell Program for periodic hematology, pulmonary, pain medicine, and behavioral health care
Preventive care	Next preventive visit on 04/14/2023 at 4:00 pm; annual transcranial Doppler ultrasound on 06/2023 (Children's Hospital will schedule for same date as visit with hematologist.)
Scheduled follow-up visit	On 02/20/2023 at 4:00 pm—Call for urgent appointment as needed.
School counselor	Coordinates IEP (individualized education program) changes, available at 555/555-1234

Other: School nurse is available only 2 days a week. School plan addresses physical limitations with accommodations for medication, hydration, frequent restroom trips, and rest. School requires physician signature annually on chronic illness form because of potential for missed school.	
Notes	
Patient signature	
Parent signature	
Care coordinator signature	

Chronic care management and CCCM services are performed personally by a physician or QHP (**99491**, **99437**) or by clinical staff under supervision by an employing (direct or contractual) physician or QHP (**99490**, **99439**, **99487**, **99489**). Refer to **Box 10**-2, which provides requirements for CCM and CCCM services.

Chronic care management

- Is provided to patients with 2 or more chronic continuous or episodic health conditions expected to last 12 months or longer, or until the death of the patient, and that place the patient at significant risk of death, acute exacerbation/decompensation, or functional decline.
- Addresses *all* the patient's medical conditions, psychosocial needs, and activities of daily living.
- Requires creation, implementation, monitoring, and revision (as needed) of a comprehensive care plan for all the patient's health-related problems.
- Codes **99491** and **99437** are not reported for time spent by a physician or QHP on the date of a face-to-face E/M visit.

In addition to requirements for CCM, CCCM (**99487**, **99489**)

- Requires moderate- or high-level MDM during the calendar month
- Requires at least 60 minutes of clinical staff time, under the direction of a physician or other QHP (may include time spent by the physician or QHP)

● indicates a new code; ▲, revised; #, re-sequenced; ✚, add-on; ★, audiovisual technology; and ◄, synchronous interactive audio.

Reporting CCM and CCCM

There are significant differences in work and practice expense required for each type of CCM and CCCM service. It is important to consider the amount and type of time (clinical staff and/or physician/QHP) and type of MDM required to determine the most appropriate code for each calendar month. A patient who requires CCM in January may require CCCM in February, or vice versa, as clinical circumstances change.

- Only 1 type of CCM or CCCM service is reported per calendar month.
  - No combination of codes **99487** and **99490** or **99491** may be reported for the same month.
  - One of these codes is reported in any calendar month when the requirements of the code descriptor are met.
- For **99491**, only count the time personally performed by the physician or other QHP. Time spent by clinical staff is not counted toward the time to support **99491** or **99437**.
- More than one clinical staff member may spend time in CCM activities on a single date. Count all time that is not overlapping, but do not count the same period more than once.

    If multiple clinical staff members meet about 1 patient, count the time for only 1 staff member (eg, 3 staff members spend 5 minutes discussing a patient; the total time of the CCM activity is 5 minutes).

- Do not count any time of the clinical staff spent as part of a separately reported service (eg, rooming a patient on the date of a physician or QHP visit).
- If the physician personally performs clinical staff activities, their time may be counted toward the required clinical staff time to meet the elements of codes **99487**, **99489**, **99490**, and **99439**. If a physician or QHP personally performs at least 30 minutes of CCM services, see codes **99491** and **99437**.

    See examples for each level of CCM in **Table 10-2**.

Principal Care Management Services

Principal care management services are focused on the medical and/or psychological needs manifested by a single complex chronic condition with all the following characteristics:

- Is expected to last at least 3 months.
- Requires frequent adjustments in the medication regimen, and/or the management of the condition is unusually complex due to comorbidities.
- Places the patient at significant risk of hospitalization, acute exacerbation/decompensation, functional decline, or death.
- Requires development, monitoring, or revision of disease-specific care plan.

    Refer to **Box 10-3** for codes and work descriptions for PCM services.

    The patient may have multiple chronic conditions that may warrant provision of CCM or CCCM services, but the focus on the single condition differentiates PCM from these services (eg, Patient A, the patient in earlier examples, may require ongoing CCM by a pediatrician but also require a period of PCM by a pulmonologist or hematologist focused solely on a single condition). The same individual(s) of the same group practice *and same specialty* cannot report PCM in conjunction with CCM or CCCM.

    A patient's primary care pediatrician may provide PCM services to a patient who does not have the 2 or more chronic or episodic health conditions required to report CCM services. For example, a pediatrician may provide PCM to a patient with asthma who has had severe exacerbation until the patient's condition stabilizes. Principal care management does not, however, require the reporting individual to address, as needed, all medical conditions, psychosocial needs, and activities of daily living, as required for CCM and CCCM.

    Principal care management services include

- Establishing, implementing, revising, or monitoring a care plan specific to a single disease
- Thirty minutes or longer of time personally spent by a physician or QHP (**99424**, **99425**) or by clinical staff under the supervision of an employing (direct or contractual) physician or QHP (**99426**, **99427**)

    If a physician or QHP spends less than 30 minutes in a calendar month providing PCM services, codes **99426** and **99427** may be reported for 30 or more minutes of combined time of the physician and clinical staff.

- Ongoing communication and care coordination between relevant practitioners furnishing care

    Unlike CCM or CCCM services, PCM services may be provided by more than one physician or QHP in the same calendar month for the same patient. Documentation in the patient's medical record should reflect coordination among relevant managing clinicians.

    Table 10-3 includes examples of PCM services.

● indicates a new code; ▲, revised; #, re-sequenced; ✚, add-on; ★, audiovisual technology; and ◀, synchronous interactive audio.

Table 10-2. Chronic Care Management Coding Examples	
The patient in each example is Patient A, who has hemoglobin SS disease, asthma, and new-onset depression with suicidal thoughts and has just completed a 30-day period of TCM. *ICD-10-CM* diagnosis codes may include **F32.2** (major depressive disorder, single episode, severe without psychotic features), **J45.31** (mild persistent asthma with [acute] exacerbation), and **D57.1** (sickle-cell disease without crisis), in addition to codes for any other conditions addressed.	
Each activity included in the CCM service must be documented in the patient record with the date and description of the activity and authenticated with the performing clinician's signature (electronic or written) and date signed.	
Example	**Code Assignment**
Patient A is receiving CCM services. Time begins the day after the 30-day period of TCM was completed. Clinical staff spend 65 minutes in the remainder of the calendar month implementing the care plan and responding to questions and concerns. MDM is moderate.	Code **99487** (CCCM of at least 60 minutes with moderate to high MDM) is reported by supervising physician Dr J. *Tip:* No time spent during the TCM period is counted toward the time of CCM or CCCM.
Patient A is receiving continued CCM services. During the calendar month, MDM includes management of increased asthma symptoms and a decision to prescribe a new asthma control medication. A total of 95 minutes of combined physician and clinical staff time is spent in CCM activities in the calendar month.	Dr J reports code **99487** for the first 60 minutes and **99489** (CCCM, each additional 30 minutes) for the additional 35 minutes. One unit of **99489** is reported for each full 30 minutes after the first 60 minutes of CCM in a calendar month.
Patient A is receiving continuing CCM services. Dr J spends 40 minutes revising the plan of care following review of records from a visit with specialists at the Children's Hospital Sickle Cell Program. Clinical staff also spend 15 minutes in CCM activities during the calendar month.	Dr J reports **99491** (CCM, personally performed by a physician or QHP, at least 30 minutes in the calendar month). Only Dr J's time is counted toward **99491**. If Dr J's total time in the month is at least 60 minutes, codes **99491** and **99437** are reported.
Patient A is receiving CCM services for symptom monitoring and management. Dr J's clinical staff spend 15 minutes in CCM activities. Dr J also personally spends 10 minutes in CCM activities.	Dr J reports **99490** (CCM with at least 20 minutes of clinical staff time). Dr J and the clinical staff's combined time is counted toward **99490**. *Tip:* Dr J did not personally spend 30 minutes in CCM activities to support **99491**.
Patient A is receiving continued CCM services. Dr J personally spends 10 minutes in CCM activities in addition to 30 minutes spent by clinical staff.	**99490, 99439** × 1 (CCM of at least 20 minutes and at least 20 minutes beyond the first 20 minutes in a calendar month) are reported for 40 minutes' combined time of Dr J and clinical staff.
Abbreviations: CCM, chronic care management; CCCM, complex CCM; *ICD-10-CM, International Classification of Diseases, 10th Revision, Clinical Modification;* MDM, medical decision-making; QHP, qualified health care professional; TCM, transitional care management.	

Care Plan Oversight Services

Care plan oversight is recurrent physician or QHP supervision of a complex patient or a patient who requires multidisciplinary care and ongoing physician or QHP involvement. Transitional care management or CCM/CCCM/PCM services would not be reported in conjunction with CPO services. (See the "Coding Conundrum: Chronic Care Management or Care Plan Oversight?" box later in this chapter to compare CPO with CCM services.) Care plan oversight services are not face-to-face and reflect the complexity and time required to supervise the care of the patient. The codes are reported separately from E/M office visits.

Box 10-4 compares CPO services, including patient population served, work included, and services not separately reported. (Work included and services not separately reported are the same for all CPO services.)

● indicates a new code; ▲, revised; #, re-sequenced; ✚, add-on; ★, audiovisual technology; and ◄, synchronous interactive audio.

Box 10-4. Care Plan Oversight Service Codes at a Glance

Activity by clinical staff is not included in the time of CPO service.

Codes by Patient Population

All patients receiving CPO require complex and multidisciplinary care modalities involving regular development and/or revision of care plans by the physician. The patient is not present at the time of service.

Supervision of a *patient under care of home health agency* (not in hospice or nursing facility) **99374** 15–29 min **99375** ≥30 min	Supervision of *hospice patient* **99377** 15–29 min **99378** ≥30 min	Supervision of a *nursing facility patient* **99379** 15–29 min **99380** ≥30 min

Work Included in CPO Services

- At least 15 min by physician in regular development and/or revision of care plans
- Review of subsequent reports of the patient's status and related laboratory or other diagnostic studies
- Communication (including telephone calls) for assessment or care decisions with individuals (eg, family, caregivers, health care professionals) involved in the patient's care
- Integration of new information into the medical treatment plan or adjustment of medical therapy

May Be Separately Reported When the Time of Each Service Is Distinct and Nonoverlapping

98966–98968, 99441–99443 Telephone services
98970–98972, 99421–99423 Online digital services
99358, 99359 Prolonged E/M service before and/or after direct patient care

May Not Be Reported in the Same Calendar Month as CPO

94005 Home ventilator management care plan oversight
99091 Collection and interpretation of physiologic data
99487, 99490, 99491 Care management services
99424–99427 Principal care management services

Abbreviations: CPO, care plan oversight; E/M, evaluation and management.

Table 10-3. Principal Care Management Coding Examples

The patient in each example is Patient A, who has hemoglobin SS disease, asthma, and new-onset depression with suicidal thoughts and has just completed a 30-day period of TCM. *ICD-10-CM* diagnosis codes may include (when addressed) **F32.2** (major depressive disorder, single episode, severe without psychotic features), **J45.31** (mild persistent asthma with [acute] exacerbation), and **D57.1** (sickle-cell disease without crisis), in addition to codes for any other conditions addressed.

Example	Code Assignment
Patient A is receiving PCM services. A hematologist spends 35 minutes in the calendar month implementing a care plan focused on managing hemoglobin SS disease in coordination with the other physicians and caregivers.	Code **99424** (PCM of ≥30 minutes by a physician or QHP) is reported by the hematologist. If time in the calendar month exceeds 59 minutes, code **99425** is reported for each additional period of ≥30 minutes in addition to code **99424**.
Patient A is receiving PCM services. A hematologist spends 35 minutes in the calendar month implementing a care plan focused on managing hemoglobin SS disease in coordination with the other physician's and caregivers. A nurse practitioner in the same hematology practice spends 30 minutes coordinating care with the behavioral health team and student's school nurse.	The hematologist reports code **99424** (PCM of ≥30 minutes by a physician or QHP) and **99425** (each additional 30 minutes) for the combined services during the calendar month. No overlapping time is counted. If the hematologist and nurse practitioner meet to discuss the patient's care, only 1 person counts the time spent in the meeting.
Patient A is also receiving PCM services focused on pain management. During the calendar month, clinical staff of a pain management specialist spend 25 minutes in PCM activities. The pulmonologist also spends 20 minutes in the same calendar month in PCM activities.	The pulmonologist reports code **99426** for combined clinical staff and physician time (45 minutes). If the combined time were 60–89 minutes in a calendar month, code **99427** would also be reported with 1 unit. For any time ≥90 minutes, 2 units of service may be reported with **99427**.

Abbreviations: *ICD-10-CM, International Classification of Diseases, 10th Revision, Clinical Modification;* PCM, principal care management; QHP, qualified health care professional; TCM, transitional care management.

● indicates a new code; ▲, revised; #, re-sequenced; ✛, add-on; ★, audiovisual technology; and ◀, synchronous interactive audio.

Medicare requires the use of Level II Healthcare Common Procedure Coding System codes for CPO services provided to patients under the care of a home health agency (**G0181**) or hospice (**G0182**). To report these **G** codes, Medicare requires a minimum of 30 minutes of physician supervision per calendar month. Because some Medicaid programs may follow suit, check with your payer to learn its requirements for reporting these services.

Coding Conundrum: Chronic Care Management or Care Plan Oversight?

Chronic care management (CCM) or principal care management (PCM) services personally performed by a physician or other qualified health care professional (QHP) (**99491, 99424, 99425, 99437**) are like care plan oversight (CPO) for patients under the care of home health (**99374, 99375**) or hospice (**99377, 99378**). Which should be reported for a physician's or QHP's personally provided services?

There are differences in code selection, as shown in this conundrum. Additionally, practices reporting CCM/PCM must meet certain qualifications (eg, provide patients and caregivers with a means to contact health care professionals in the practice to address urgent needs, regardless of time of day or day of week). Specific practice qualifications are not required for CPO.

CPO	CCM/PCM
Time Requirement in Calendar Month Require ≥15 min **99374, 99377** Require ≥30 min **99375, 99378**	**Time Requirement in Calendar Month** <30 min not separately reported Require ≥30 min CCM: **99491, 99437** PCM: **99424, 99425**
No. of Chronic Conditions ≥1	**No. of Chronic Conditions** CCM: ≥2 PCM: 1 (complex)
Care Plan Work Regularly develop and/or revise.	**Care Plan Work** Establish, implement, revise, or monitor. CCM: comprehensive care plan PCM: focus on a single complex disease

Care plan oversight services
- Are reported only by the individual (ie, physician/QHP) who has the predominant supervisory role in the care of the patient or is the sole provider of the services.
- Cannot be assumed until a face-to-face service with the patient has been provided by the physician. The CMS requires a face-to-face visit within 6 months before CPO services. Verify individual payer policies for similar requirements and possible inclusion of telemedicine services in support of a face-to-face visit requirement.
- Include
  — Regular development and/or revision of care plans
  — Review of subsequent reports of the patient's status
  — Review of related laboratory or other diagnostic studies
  — Communication (including telephone calls) for the purpose of assessment or care decisions with health care professionals, family members, surrogate decision-makers (eg, legal guardians), and/or key caregivers involved in the patient's care
  — Integration of new information into the medical treatment plan or adjustment of medical therapy
  — Team conferences
  — Prolonged E/M service before and/or after direct patient care when the same time is attributed to CPO
- Are reported once per month on the basis of the amount of time spent by the physician during that calendar month.

Unlike care management services, time included in care plan oversight is only that of the physician or other qualified health care professional and not that of clinical staff.

- Include all cumulative time within the same calendar month.
- Are reported on the basis of the patient's location or status (eg, nursing facility, hospice) and the total time spent by the physician within a calendar month. Less than 15 minutes' cumulative time within a calendar month cannot be reported.

● indicates a new code; ▲, revised; #, re-sequenced; ✚, add-on; ★, audiovisual technology; and ◀, synchronous interactive audio.

- Are reported separately from other office or other outpatient, hospital, home, or nursing facility E/M services.
- Do not require specific practice capabilities as are defined for CCM services.
- Require recurrent supervision of therapy.

  Time spent on the following activities may not be considered CPO:
- Travel time to or from the facility or place of domicile
- Services furnished by clinical staff (ancillary or incident-to staff)
- Very low-intensity or infrequent supervision services included in the pre- and post-encounter work for an E/M service

Example

➤ **A physician reviews a final report from a home health nurse on a patient who no longer requires home health after the first week of the calendar month.** These low-intensity services are considered part of the pre- and post-encounter work of related E/M services and are not reported as CPO services.

- Interpretation of laboratory or other diagnostic studies associated with a face-to-face E/M service
- Informal consultations with health professionals not involved in the patient's care
- Routine postoperative care provided during the global surgery period of a procedure
- Time spent on telephone calls or online digital E/M or in medical team conferences if they are separately reported with codes **99441–99443**, **99421–99423**, or **99367**

A CPO billing worksheet can be used to track time of CPO services based on documentation in the patient's medical record and used to support billing when time in a calendar month supports reporting a CPO service. A template is included at www.aap.org/cfp2023 ("Care Plan Oversight Billing Worksheet Template"). An example of a completed CPO log follows. Electronic time-tracking software may be used in lieu of a worksheet.

Home Ventilator Management

94005   Home ventilator management care plan oversight of a patient (patient not present) in home, domiciliary or rest home (eg, assisted living) requiring review of status, review of laboratories and other studies and revision of orders and respiratory care plan (as appropriate), within a calendar month, 30 minutes or more

  Services include determining ventilator settings, establishing a plan of care, and providing ongoing monitoring.
- Code **94005** is used to report home ventilator management CPO. It may be reported only when 30 or more minutes of CPO is provided within a calendar month.
- Home ventilator management CPO is distinct from CPO to patients under care of a home health care or hospice agency (**99374–99378**) when provided and reported by a separate physician or QHP (eg, pulmonologist reports **94005** and primary physician reports **99374**).

Medical Team Conferences

Medical team conference codes are used to coordinate or manage care and services for established patients with chronic or multiple health conditions (eg, child who experienced a stroke caused by sickle cell disease and requires physical and occupational therapy, speech therapy, pain management, and scheduled transfusions).

  Box 10-5 provides an overview of the patient population, code descriptors, and services not separately reported with medical team conference services.

Care Plan Oversight Billing Worksheet Template

Physician: Dr J   Patient Name: Patient A   Month: February 2023

Supporting documentation is found in patient's medical record. Patient A is receiving home health care at home under a wound care plan approved by Dr J.

Date of Service	Documented Service	Start Time	End Time	Total Minutes	Monthly Subtotal
02/04/2023	Development of wound care plan and order for home health	12:00 pm	12:20 pm	20	20
02/04/2023	Discussion with wound care nurse concerned about drainage from wound	12:15 pm	12:21 pm	6	26
02/15/2023	Discussion with pain management physician	5:15 pm	5:25 pm	10	36
02/16/2023	Review of report from wound care nurse	5:30 pm	5:35 pm	5	41

Time Requirements per Calendar Month	Patient Under the Care of a Home Health Care Agency	Hospice Patient		Nursing Facility Patient
15–29 min	99374	99377		99379
≥30 min	99375	99378		99380
≥30 min Medicare code	G0181	G0182		

Code Supported: **99375**

An online version of this worksheet is included at www.aap.org/cfp2023.

ª Follow individual payer guidelines for reporting care plan oversight for a pediatric-prescribed extended care facility. Codes **99374** and **99375** (home health care plan oversight) are required by some plans.

Box 10-5. Medical Team Conference Services

Patient Population
Established patients with chronic and multiple health conditions or with congenital anomalies (eg, cleft lip and palate, craniofacial abnormality)

Physician or Qualified Health Care Professional Service
99367 Medical team conference with interdisciplinary team of health care professionals, patient and/or family not present, 30 minutes or more; participation by physician

(When patient or caregivers attend conference, report other E/M codes.)

Nonphysician Service
99366 Medical team conference with interdisciplinary team of health care professionals, face-to-face with patient and/or family, 30 minutes or more; participation by nonphysician qualified health care professional

99368 Medical team conference with interdisciplinary team of health care professionals, patient and/or family not present, 30 minutes or more; participation by nonphysician qualified health care professional

Work Required
- At least 30 minutes of face-to-face services from different specialties or disciplines
- Performed face-to-face evaluations or treatments of the patient, independent of any team conference, within the previous 60 days
- Presentation of findings and recommendations
- Formulation of a care plan and subsequent review/proofing of the plan

Do not report during the service time of
99437, 99439, 99487, 99489, 99490, 99491 Chronic care management services

Abbreviation: E/M, evaluation and management.

Medical team conferences require

- *Face-to-face participation* by a minimum of 3 physicians and/or QHPs or QNHCPs from different subspecialties or disciplines (eg, speech pathologists, dietitians, social workers), with or without the presence of the patient, family member(s), community agencies, surrogate decision-maker(s) (eg, legal guardian), and/or caregiver(s).
  - Participation by telephone is not reported.
  - Verify payer policies for participation via interactive audiovisual communication (telemedicine). Participation in team conferences via telemedicine *has not yet been added* to the lists of services reported with modifier **95** or the Medicare list of services approved for provision via telehealth.
- Active involvement in the development, revision, coordination, and implementation of health care services needed by the patient by each participant.
- Face-to-face evaluations and/or treatments within the previous 60 days, by the participant, that are separate from any team conference.
- Only 1 individual from the same specialty reporting codes **99366–99368** for the same encounter. However, physicians of different specialties may each report their participation in a team conference.
- Medical record documentation supporting the reporting physician's or QHP's contributed information and subsequent treatment recommendations and the time spent from the beginning of the review of an individual patient until the conclusion of the review.
- Medical team conferences may not be reported if the facility or organization is contractually obligated to provide the service, they are informal meetings or simple conversations between physicians and other QHPs and QNHCPs, or less than 30 minutes of conference time is spent in the team conferences.

Codes differentiate reporting provider (physician or other QHP who may report E/M services vs other health care professional) and face-to-face versus non–face-to-face (patient and/or family is or is not present) team conference services.

- *CPT* instructs that physicians *or other QHPs* who may report E/M services should report their participation in a team conference with the patient and/or family present by using E/M codes for the place of service based on the instructions for the E/M service provided.
- Code **99367** is the only code that may be reported by a physician or other QHP who may report E/M services, and it can be reported only when the patient and/or family is not present at the team conference.
- Time reported with code **99367** may not be used in the determination of time for CPO (**99374–99380**), CCM services (**99487–99491**), prolonged services (**99358, 99359**), psychotherapy (**90832–90853**), or any E/M service.

Examples

For each of the following examples, a team meets to discuss the care of Patient A, a child with **D57.1** (sickle-cell disease without crisis), **F32.2** (major depressive disorder, single episode, severe without psychotic features),and **J45.31** (mild persistent asthma with [acute] exacerbation). Each participant in the conference has completed their evaluation of the patient within 60 days before the conference.

➤ **A primary care pediatrician, a hematologist, a pulmonologist, a pain medicine specialist, and a psychiatrist participate in discussion and planning, including plans for transitioning Patient A's care from pediatric to adult care.** The conference lasts 60 minutes and neither patient nor parents attend.

CPT	
99367	Each participating physician (if they are different specialties and/or from different practices [ie, separate tax identification numbers])
99368	Each QNHCP (eg, psychologist, clinical social worker)

Physicians who provide a face-to-face visit (eg, consultation, **99242–99245**) on the same date as a *medical team conference without the patient/family present* should report codes for the individual services provided. A payer may require modifier **25** (significant, separately identifiable E/M service) on the code for the face-to-face visit.

➤ **A primary care pediatrician, hematologist, pulmonologist, and licensed clinical social worker participate in discussion and planning with Patient A and his parent present.** The conference lasts 60 minutes. No other E/M services are provided by the physicians on this date.

CPT	
99366	Each nonphysician QHP (eg, licensed clinical social worker)
99202–99499	Each participating physician (if they are different specialties and/or from different practices [ie, separate tax identification numbers]) reports an E/M service based on the place of service and applicable time-based coding instructions.

Physicians who provide a face-to-face visit on the same date as a medical team conference *with the patient/family present* should report the appropriate E/M code for the site of the visit and may also report an appropriate prolonged service code (eg, **99418** for inpatient or observation services or, for E/M services in office or outpatient settings, **99417**) for time extending beyond the parameters designated by the E/M code and to the minimum time of the appropriate prolonged service code.

If licensed QHPs (including clinical nurse specialists and clinical nurse practitioners) participated in a conference without direct physician supervision, they may report the service (**99367**) if it is within the state's scope of practice and they use their own National Provider Identifier. Medicaid and commercial payers may follow these Medicare requirements or have their own specific rules.

Advance Care Planning

★**99497**   Advance care planning including the explanation and discussion of advance directives such as standard forms (with completion of such forms, when performed), by the physician or other qualified health care professional; first 30 minutes, face-to-face with the patient, family member(s) and/or surrogate

★**+99498**   each additional 30 minutes (List separately in addition to code for primary procedure)

Advance care planning includes
- A face-to-face service by a physician or QHP (including telemedicine services) to a patient, family member, or surrogate spent in counseling and discussion of advance directives
- Completion of forms, when applicable (eg, Health Care Proxy, Durable Power of Attorney for Health Care, Living Will, and Medical Orders for Life-Sustaining Treatment)

> Active management of problems is not included in advance care planning. Other evaluation and management (E/M) services provided on the same date as advance care planning may be separately reported *with the exceptions of* hourly critical care services (99291, 99292), inpatient neonatal and pediatric critical care (99468, 99469; 99471–99476), and initial and continuing intensive care services (99477–99480). Append modifier **25** to the E/M code for active management of problems.

Because the *CPT* prefatory language and code descriptors for advance care planning do not include other instruction on the time required for reporting, these services may be reported on the basis of general *CPT* instruction to report when the midpoint is passed (eg, 1 unit of **99498** may be reported for services of 46–75 minutes).

✖ Do not report code **99497** for less than 16 minutes of physician face-to-face time. Exceptions may apply for payers with policy requiring that the time be met or exceeded.

Advance care planning services may be considered bundled to enhanced payment methodologies (eg, patient-centered medical home receiving PMPM care coordination fees) and not separately paid. However, *CPT* requires reporting of the code that is specific to the service provided regardless of payment policy. Advance care planning services should not be reported as another service (eg, office visit) in an effort to prevent denial as a bundled service.

Relative value units assigned for a non-facility site of service are 2.47 for **99497** and 2.14 for **99498** ($82.99 versus $71.90, respectively, when paid at the 2022 Medicare conversion factor of $33.5983 per RVU).

CPT instructs that codes reported accurately describe the service rendered and physicians not report a code that merely approximates the service provided, so it would be inappropriate to report another service that may have higher RVUs and payment values.

However, when a payer does not recognize advance care planning codes or the main reason for an encounter is other than advance care planning, consultation codes **99242–99245** or other E/M service codes (eg, **99212–99215**) may be appropriately reported.

Examples

➤ **A child and his parents, who have learned at a recent visit that the child's prognosis is poor, return for advance care planning.** The physician spends 50 minutes face-to-face with the patient and parents, assesses their understanding of the diagnosis, and confirms and documents the desire to limit lifesaving measures and decisions about palliative care. A plan of care is developed and documented, and an appointment with the supportive care team at the hospital is scheduled.

CPT
99497   Advance care planning, initial 30 minutes
99498 × 1   each additional 30 minutes
The physician's face-to-face time of 50 minutes spent providing the advance care planning supports reporting **99497** with 1 unit of **99498** for the final 20 minutes of service.

➤ **An adolescent with cystic fibrosis wishes to discuss and be involved in planning her care after learning she will require a lung transplant.** The pulmonologist spends 80 minutes face-to-face with the patient and her parents, assessing their understanding of the diagnosis and prognosis, their continued hope that treatment is successful, and the patient's wishes to be included in decisions about her care. A plan of care is developed and documented, and an appointment with the supportive care team at the hospital is scheduled to provide additional counseling and support services to the patient and family.

The physician may report codes **99497** and **99498** × 2 for the 80 minutes of face-to-face time spent providing the advance care planning. Per *CPT* instruction, an additional unit of **99498** is reported because the midpoint between the time reported with the first unit (31–60 minutes) and the starting time of the second unit (61 minutes) was passed.

Indirect Prolonged Service on Date Other Than the Face-to-face E/M Service

Prolonged services without direct patient contact (**99358, 99359**) are reported when a physician or QHP provides prolonged service *on a date other than* the date of a face-to-face E/M service. Codes **99358** and **99359** are not reported for services provided on the same date as a face-to-face E/M that uses total time to select the service on the date of the encounter. Indirect prolonged services may be reported in relation to any E/M service that was provided on another date of service regardless of whether time was used to select the level of the face-to-face service.

See codes **99417** and **99418** for prolonged service on the date of a face-to-face E/M service.

Prolonged service must relate to a service during or patient for which direct (face-to-face) patient care has occurred or will occur and to ongoing patient management. The primary service may be an E/M service (with or without an assigned time), a procedure, or another face-to-face service.

The place of service does not affect reporting.

Guidelines for reporting non-direct prolonged services include
- Prolonged service before and/or after direct patient care does not include time spent by clinical staff.
- Time is met when the midpoint is passed.
  - Less than 30 minutes' total duration on a given date cannot be reported.
  - Less than 15 minutes beyond the first hour or beyond the final 30 minutes is not reported separately. Use code **99359** to report the final 15 to 30 minutes of prolonged service on a given date. **Table 10-4** breaks down the time requirements.

Table 10-4. Non–face-to-face Prolonged Services at a Glance	
99358 Prolonged evaluation and management service before and/or after direct patient care; first hour	
✚99359 each additional 30 minutes (Use in conjunction with code **99358**.)	
Prolonged service must be related to another service provided by the same individual.	
Total Duration of Prolonged Service Without Direct Face-to-face Contact	**Code(s) and Unit(s) of Service Reported**
<30 min	Not separately reported
30–74 min	**99358** × 1
75–104 min	**99358** × 1 and **99359** × 1
≥105 min	**99358** × 1 and **99359** × 2

- May be reported on a different date than the related primary service. *CPT* does not specify a time frame (eg, within 1 week of related service) for provision of prolonged service before and/or after direct patient care.

● indicates a new code; ▲, revised; #, re-sequenced; ✚, add-on; ★, audiovisual technology; and ◄, synchronous interactive audio.

- Cannot be reported for time spent in provision of and reported with codes for
  - Care plan oversight services (**99374–99380**)
  - Chronic care management (**99491**, **99437**)
  - Principal care management (**99424**, **99425**)
  - Medical team conferences (**99366–99368**)
  - Online medical evaluations (**99421–99423**)
  - Interprofessional telephone/Internet/EHR consultations (**99446–99452**)
  - Anticoagulant management for a patient taking warfarin (**93792**, **93793**)

Example

➤ **A physician requested and received medical records from multiple sources for a child with hemoglobin SS disease who has been placed into foster care and has had multiple hospitalizations and inconsistent care over the past 3 years.** On a day before the date of the initial consultation service, the physician spends 35 minutes reviewing and summarizing the medical records and documents his time in the medical record. The physician reports

CPT
99358   Prolonged physician services without direct patient contact; 30–74 minutes

ICD-10-CM
D57.1   Sickle-cell disease without crisis

> See Chapter 7 for prolonged service on the same date as an evaluation and management (E/M) service provided in an office or other outpatient setting (eg, office visit, consultation) and for discussion of prolonged clinical staff services.
>
> See Chapter 16 for discussion of prolonged services on the same date as an E/M service provided in a facility setting such as inpatient hospital or observation services.

Related Services Discussed in Other Chapters

Online Digital E/M Services

An online digital medical evaluation (**99421–99423**) is a non–face-to-face E/M service by a physician or other QHP who may report E/M services to a patient by using internet resources in response to a patient's online inquiry.

This is in contrast with telemedicine services, which represent interactive audio and video telecommunications systems that permit real-time communication between the physician, at the distant site, and the patient, at the originating site.

Codes **98970–98972** are used by a QNHCP to report an online assessment and management service. The reporting guidelines for codes **98970–98972** are the same as those for online services provided by the physician or QHP.

> See Chapter 9 for more information about online digital medical services.

Remote Physiologic Monitoring

#99457   Remote physiologic monitoring treatment management services, 20 minutes or more of clinical staff/physician/other qualified health care professional time in a calendar month requiring interactive communication with the patient/caregiver during the month
#✚99458   each additional 20 minutes

Code **99457** is reported for time spent managing care when the results from a monitoring device(s) are used for treatment management services. This code requires 20 or more minutes of time spent using the results of physiologic monitoring to manage a patient under a specific treatment plan. When the time of service extends a full 20 minutes beyond the first 20 minutes (ie, at least 40 minutes total), report code **99458** in addition to **99457**.

> Please see Chapter 21 for more information on remote physiologic monitoring services.

Chapter 10. Indirect Management of Chronic and Complex Conditions

● indicates a new code; ▲, revised; #, re-sequenced; ✚, add-on; ★, audiovisual technology; and ◀, synchronous interactive audio.

Telephone E/M Services

Telephone services (**99441–99443**) are non–face-to-face E/M services provided at the request of a patient or caregiver by a physician or other QHP who may report E/M services provided to a patient through the telephone.

Codes **98966–98968** are used to report telephone assessment and management services by health care professionals who may not report E/M services (eg, occupational therapists, speech pathologists).

> See Chapter 9 for more details on reporting telephone and consultation services.

Interprofessional Telephone/Internet Consultations

Patients with chronic conditions may often require collaboration between their primary pediatrician and a subspecialist or between subspecialists.

A consultation request by a patient's attending or primary physician or QHP soliciting opinion and/or treatment advice *by telephone, internet, or EHR* from a physician with specialty expertise (consultant) is reported by the consultant with interprofessional consultation codes **99446–99449** or **99451**. These consultations do not require face-to-face contact with the patient by the consultant.

The physician requesting the consultation may report code **99452** when 16 to 30 minutes is spent preparing for the referral and/or communicating with the consultant in a service day. Alternatively, prolonged service codes may be reported by the requesting individual when supported by the time of service. When separately reported, the time attributed to preparing for and communicating in an interprofessional consultation is not counted toward the time of another service (eg, CCM).

After-hours and Special Services

Codes **99050–99060** are used to report services that are provided after hours or on an emergency basis and are an adjunct to the basic E/M service provided.

> See Chapter 7 for more details on after-hours and special services codes.

Reporting a Combination of Complex Medical Management Services

Services such as CCM and TCM offer a means of reporting many activities of care management with 1 or 2 codes that describe the complexity and period of care. However, when these codes do not apply (eg, patient does not meet criteria) or a payer does not provide benefits for care management services, it may be necessary to report a combination of codes for non–face-to-face services provided to a child with complex health care needs. These may include CPO, online or telephone E/M services, prolonged services, and team conference services. Some of these services may also be reported in addition to care management services when the time of each service is distinct.

- Be sure to review payer guidance on reporting of these services, as National Correct Coding Initiative edits or other payment policy may require appending modifiers to indicate that distinct periods were spent in the provision of each service. For instance, prolonged E/M service is bundled to CPO, but a modifier may be appended to indicate distinct services within the same reporting period. Guidance for reporting and coverage may vary.
- Practices with the capabilities required for reporting CCM services in lieu of CPO may still report the CPO codes when the service provided and nature of the patient presentation support reporting CPO services. Physicians must determine the appropriate code selection based on the practice capabilities, services rendered, and nature of the patient presentation.

To test your knowledge of the information presented in this chapter, complete the quiz found at the end of it, after the resources.

Chapter 10. Indirect Management of Chronic and Complex Conditions

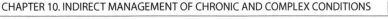

Chapter Takeaways

This chapter discusses codes for periods of indirect care management for all of a patient's health care needs, for a single serious chronic condition, or for direction of home health or hospice services. Following are takeaways from this chapter:

- Transitional care management is reported by a single physician or QHP who assumes management of all a patient's health care needs following discharge from a facility stay during a 30-day period.
- Chronic care management and CCCM services are reported for services provided to a patient with 2 or more chronic conditions that are expected to last at least 1 year. They include ongoing coordination of care for all the patient's health care needs.
- Principal care management is a service provided to a patient with a single serious chronic condition. Principal care management does not require management of all a patient's health care needs, and more than one physician may provide PCM services when provided for distinct conditions.
- Care plan oversight is like other care management services but includes only time spent by a physician or QHP and does not have the practice requirements of CCM or PCM.
- Although other services may be provided and separately reported during the service period of an indirect care management service, times of service cannot be overlapping.

Resources

AAP Coding Assistance and Education

AAP *Pediatric Care Management: Coding Quick Reference Care 2023* (https://shop.aap.org/pediatric-care-management-coding-quick-reference-card-2023)

AAP policy statement, "Patient- and Family-Centered Care Coordination: A Framework for Integrating Care for Children and Youth Across Multiple Systems" (https://doi.org/10.1542/peds.2014-0318)

AAP Pediatric Coding Newsletter™

"Chronic Care Management for 2 or More Conditions: 2022 Changes," October 2021 (https://doi.org/10.1542/pcco_book210_document004)

"Principal Care Management: Care Management Services for a Single Disease," October 2021 (https://doi.org/10.1542/pcco_book210_document003)

Online Exclusive Content at www.aap.org/cfp2023

"Care Management Tracking Worksheet Template"
"Care Plan Oversight Billing Worksheet Template"
"Monthly Care Management and Care Plan Oversight Services: A Comparison"

Patient- and Family-Centered Care Coordination

Boston Children's Hospital Care Coordination Curriculum (www.pcpcc.org/resource/care-coordination-curriculum)

Chapter 10. Indirect Management of Chronic and Complex Conditions

---

Test Your Knowledge!

1. **Which of the following statements is true of transitional care management?**
   a. The period of service is a calendar month.
   b. The patient must have only 1 complex chronic condition.
   c. A care plan must be established, implemented, revised, or monitored.
   d. The period of service begins on the date of discharge and continues for the next 29 days.

2. **Which of the following statements is true of chronic care management (CCM) services reported with code 99490?**
   a. Clinical staff time is not included in the time of service.
   b. At least 30 minutes of clinical staff time spent in CCM activities must be documented.
   c. At least 20 minutes of clinical staff time spent in CCM activities must be documented.
   d. Medical decision-making during the month must be at least moderate.

3. **Which of the following statements describes the type of condition that may be addressed with principal care management (PCM)?**
   a. The condition must require a high level of medical decision-making.
   b. The complex chronic condition is expected to last at least 12 months.
   c. Any chronic condition qualifies for PCM services.
   d. The complex chronic condition is expected to last at least 3 months.

4. **Which of the following examples of services is never reported by the same individual in the same calendar month?**
   a. Transitional care management (TCM) and chronic care management (CCM)
   b. TCM and office evaluation and management services (eg, **99213**)
   c. Principal care management and care plan oversight
   d. CCM and online digital services (**99421–99423**)

5. **When are prolonged services without direct patient contact (99358, 99359) reported?**
   a. When the prolonged service is provided on the same date as another evaluation and management (E/M) service
   b. Only when the prolonged service is provided on a date other than the date of a face-to face E/M service
   c. Only when time was used to select the level of the face-to-face service
   d. When the time spent is also counted toward the time of chronic care management or principal care management services

---

● indicates a new code; ▲, revised; #, re-sequenced; ✚, add-on; ★, audiovisual technology; and ◀, synchronous interactive audio.

‖‖‖‖‖

Mental and Behavioral Health Services

‖‖‖‖‖

CPT copyright 2022 American Medical Association. All rights reserved.

Contents

● indicates a new code; ▲, revised; #, re-sequenced; ✚, add-on; ★, audiovisual technology; and ◀, synchronous interactive audio.

Chapter Highlights

- Who may provide mental and behavioral health services
- Important payment considerations
- Diagnosis coding guidelines for mental and behavioral health services
- Options for reporting psychiatric services, substance use treatment, and behavioral health integration in primary care practices
- Testing for developmental, neuropsychological, and psychological conditions
- Adaptive behavior assessment and treatment
- Psychiatric services, substance use treatment, and behavioral health integration into primary care practices

Mental and Behavioral Health Services

This chapter focuses on services that are provided to diagnose, manage, or treat mental and behavioral health conditions. Mental and behavioral health services are an important part of pediatric medicine. The public health emergency (PHE) caused by COVID-19 increased the need for pediatric mental health care, as evidenced by the American Academy of Pediatrics (AAP) October 2021 joint declaration of a national emergency, "AAP-AACAP-CHA Declaration of a National Emergency in Child and Adolescent Mental Health" (www.aap.org/en/advocacy/child-and-adolescent-healthy-mental-development/aap-aacap-cha-declaration-of-a-national-emergency-in-child-and-adolescent-mental-health). This joint declaration includes a list of proposed actions to improve the access to and quality of care across the continuum of pediatric mental health promotion, prevention, and treatment. However, obtaining and/or providing mental and behavioral health services to children currently involves complexities that physicians must understand to help their patients access needed services.

Physicians and Other Mental/Behavioral Health Providers

Services included in this chapter may be provided by

- Physicians and other qualified health care professionals (QHPs) and qualified nonphysician health care professionals (QNHCPs), including licensed clinical psychologists and licensed clinical social workers (State regulations and payment policies are often least restrictive for these providers.)
- Allied health care professionals, such as technicians and developmental specialists, who provide services ordered by and under the general supervision of physicians and QHPs (State regulations and payment policies are often somewhat restrictive for these providers.)
- Clinical staff working under direct physician supervision (State regulations and payment policies are typically most restrictive for these providers.)

Including Nonphysician Providers in Your Practice

Services such as behavioral health assessment by a licensed clinical social worker or licensed psychologist may be provided within a general pediatric group practice and can be an integral part of providing a full scope of care in the medical home. However, billing and coding of these services must align not only with coding guidelines but also state scope of practice and individual payer policies on credentialing, contracting, and billing for services of the specific QNHCP.

Payment and Coverage Issues for Mental/Behavioral Health Services

Behavioral health services may be covered through a plan and provider network separate from other health care services. When arranging for or providing behavioral health services, it is very important to explore the patient's health plan policy options.

- Failure to credential and, when applicable, contract with behavioral health plans may lead to unpaid or underpaid charges.
- Payer policies may allow specific licensed professionals, such as licensed clinical psychologists and licensed clinical social workers, to directly provide and report certain services. Other QNHCPs (eg, licensed master social workers) may be limited to providing services under direct supervision and reporting in the name of the participating health care professional (eg, licensed clinical psychologist or psychiatrist).

● indicates a new code; ▲, revised; #, re-sequenced; ✦, add-on; ★, audiovisual technology; and ◀, synchronous interactive audio.

- General pediatricians and other QHPs may be ineligible to participate in the behavioral health plan network and limited to reporting evaluation and management (E/M) services to the health plan on the basis of time.

The AAP Council on Early Childhood, Committee on Psychosocial Aspects of Child and Family Health, and Section on Developmental and Behavioral Pediatrics included the following information about coverage of treatment of emotional and behavioral health problems in the policy statement, "Addressing Early Childhood Emotional and Behavioral Problems" (https://doi.org/10.1542/peds.2016-3023):

American Academy of Pediatrics Policy Statement

"Without adequate payment for screening and assessment by primary care providers and management by specialty providers with expertise in early childhood mental health, treatment of very young children with emotional and behavioral problems will likely remain inaccessible for many children. Given existing knowledge regarding the importance of early childhood brain development on lifelong health, adequate payment for early childhood preventive services will benefit not only the patients but society as well and should be supported. Mental health carve-outs should be eliminated because they provide a significant barrier to access to mental health care for children. Additional steps toward equal access to mental health and physical health care include efficient prior authorization processes; adequate panels of early childhood mental health providers; payment to all providers, including primary care providers, for mental health diagnoses; sustainable payment for co-located mental health providers and care coordination; payment for evidence-based approaches focused on parents; and payment for the necessary collection of information from children's many caregivers and for same-day services. Advocacy for true mental health parity must continue."

Integration of psychiatric and/or developmental/behavioral health care professionals into the primary care practice may also require an understanding of health plan payment policies. Payer edits may not allow separate payment for mental and behavioral health services when E/M services are provided in the same practice on the same date. Verify coverage and billing options before provision of services.

Learn more about payer edits in Chapter 2 and about American Academy of Pediatrics payer advocacy in Chapter 4.

- Payers often place limitations on the diagnoses that may be paid under a patient's health benefits versus a separate behavioral health benefit.
  - Pediatricians may be required to report codes for symptoms rather than diagnosed conditions (eg, sadness in lieu of depression). This conflicts with *International Classification of Diseases, 10th Revision, Clinical Modification* (*ICD-10-CM*) guidelines.
  - *ICD-10-CM* guidelines instruct, "Codes that describe symptoms and signs, as opposed to diagnoses, are acceptable for reporting purposes when a related definitive diagnosis has not been established (confirmed) by the provider."
  - Adherence to these guidelines when assigning *ICD-10-CM* diagnosis codes is required under the Health Insurance Portability and Accountability Act of 1996. Payers are required to accept codes reported in compliance with the official guidelines for code selection and reporting.
  - When payers deny claims appropriately reported with codes **F01–F99** (mental, behavioral and neurodevelopmental disorders), pediatricians may report the issue by using the AAP Coding Hotline (https://form.jotform.com/ Subspecialty/aapcodinghotline) or seek the assistance of an AAP pediatric council (www.aap.org/en/practice-management/practice-financing/payer-contracting-advocacy-and-other-resources/aap-payer-advocacy/aap-pediatric-councils).
- Healthcare Common Procedure Coding System (HCPCS) modifiers identifying the type of health care professional (eg, **AJ**, clinical social worker) may be necessary to override edits that bundle E/M services provided by a physician/QHP and mental/behavioral health services provided by a QNHCP on the same date.
- Relevant HCPCS modifiers include

AH	Clinical psychologist
AJ	Clinical social worker
AM	Physician, team member service
FQ	Furnished using audio-only communication technology
GT	Via interactive audio and video telecommunication systems
HA	Child/adolescent program
HN	Bachelor's degree level
HO	Master's degree level
HP	Doctoral level

Chapter 11. Mental and Behavioral Health Services

HQ	Group setting
TL	Early intervention/individualized family service plan (IFSP)
UN	Two patients served
UP	Three patients served
UQ	Four patients served
UR	Five patients served
US	Six or more patients served

Telemedicine for Mental Health Services

> In January 2022, modifier 93 (audio-only telemedicine service) was added to *Current Procedural Terminology* (*CPT*). In *CPT 2023*, a new symbol (◀) precedes codes that may be reported with modifier 93. See chapters 2 and 20 for additional information on reporting codes with modifier 93 or 95 (synchronous audiovisual telemedicine service).

Access to health care services via electronic communication technology has advanced significantly since the COVID-19 PHE. Although many advances were temporary on the basis of short-term amendments to payer policies, payment policies for services provided for mental health and substance use diagnoses have changed permanently in many areas. It is important for physicians and other providers of these services to maintain an awareness of changing regulations and payment policies that may support greater use of telemedicine.

See **chapters 2** and **20** for discussion of coding and documentation for telemedicine services. Some plans also pay for E/M services provided via telephone or online digital communication technology (eg, secure messaging through a patient portal). See **Chapter 9** for information on reporting telephone and online digital E/M services.

Reporting Codes F01–F99

Diagnosis of behavioral and mental health conditions is typically based on the criteria set forth in the *Diagnostic and Statistical Manual of Mental Disorders, 5th Edition* (*DSM-5*) classification system.

- Often, a simple crosswalk from the *DSM-5* diagnosis to the *ICD-10-CM* code supporting the diagnosis can be made. However, the classifications are not always equivalent.

  DSM-5 does not differentiate Asperger syndrome from autism spectrum disorder (ASD). *ICD-10-CM* provides a specific code for Asperger syndrome (**F84.5**) in addition to codes for autistic disorder (**F84.0**) and other pervasive developmental disorders (eg, Rett syndrome, **F84.2**).
- It is important that documentation clearly reflects a diagnostic statement separate from the assignment of an *ICD-10-CM* code as required by official guidance for *ICD-10-CM*.
  - Documentation should include the findings supporting the diagnosis (eg, observations made during the appointment, history, standardized rating scale results, pertinent physical examination findings).
  - Failure to document the information supporting the diagnostic statement could affect the patient's access to care and the physician's payment for services provided.
- *ICD-10-CM* includes codes for specifying how an accident or injury happened (eg, unintentional or accidental; intentional, such as suicide or assault).
  - Treatment of patients who have sustained injury or illness (eg, poisoning) due to intentional self-harm are reported with codes signifying the intent (eg, **T52.92XA**, toxic effect of unspecified organic solvent, intentional self-harm, initial encounter, and **R45.88**, nonsuicidal self-harm).
  - If the intent of the cause of an injury or another condition is unknown or unspecified, code the intent as accidental intent. All transport accident categories assume accidental intent.
  - Codes for events of undetermined intent are for use only if the documentation in the record specifies that the intent cannot be determined at the encounter (eg, suspected abuse under investigation).

> To fully report conditions such as poisoning, follow *International Classification of Diseases, 10th Revision, Clinical Modification* instructions in the tabular list. For example, instructions for code T52.92XA include "Use additional code(s) for all associated manifestations of toxic effect, such as: respiratory conditions due to external agents (J60–J70)."

Chapter 11. Mental and Behavioral Health Services

Current Procedural Terminology Add-on Codes

Many mental and behavioral health services are described by a combination of a base code with add-on codes representing extended services. Add-on codes (marked with a ✚ before the code) are always performed in addition to a primary procedure and are never reported as a stand-alone service. Like most other codes, add-on codes describe additional intraservice work and are not valued to include preservice and post-service work.

Behavioral Health Integration

One strategy promoted in the previously discussed "AAP-AACAP-CHA Declaration of a National Emergency in Child and Adolescent Mental Health" (www.aap.org/en/advocacy/child-and-adolescent-healthy-mental-development/aap-aacap-cha-declaration-of-a-national-emergency-in-child-and-adolescent-mental-health) is accelerating the adoption of effective and financially sustainable models of integrated mental health care in primary care pediatrics, including clinical strategies and models for payment. Following are 2 sets of codes that describe integrated behavioral health services:

1. Psychiatric collaborative care management (PCCM) services (**99492–99494**) include a defined team of health care professionals providing care by using a specific care method.
2. General behavioral health integration (GBHI; **99484**) services do not include specific types of providers or a specified method of delivery.

These behavioral health integration services are differentiated by the required elements of service.

Psychiatric Collaborative Care Management Services

99492   Initial psychiatric collaborative care management, first 70 minutes in the first calendar month of behavioral health care manager activities, in consultation with a psychiatric consultant, and directed by the treating physician or other qualified health care professional, with the following required elements:
- outreach to and engagement in treatment of a patient directed by the treating physician or other qualified health care professional,
- initial assessment of the patient, including administration of validated rating scales, with the development of an individualized treatment plan,
- review by the psychiatric consultant with modifications of the plan if recommended,
- entering patient in a registry and tracking patient follow-up and progress using the registry, with appropriate documentation, and participation in weekly caseload consultation with the psychiatric consultant, and
- provision of brief interventions using evidence-based techniques such as behavioral activation, motivational interviewing, and other focused treatment strategies.

99493   Subsequent psychiatric collaborative care management, first 60 minutes in a subsequent month of behavioral health care manager activities, in consultation with a psychiatric consultant, and directed by the treating physician or other qualified health care professional, with the following required elements:
- tracking patient follow-up and progress using the registry, with appropriate documentation,
- participation in weekly caseload consultation with the psychiatric consultant,
- ongoing collaboration with and coordination of the patient's mental health care with the treating physician or other qualified health care professional and any other treating mental health providers,
- additional review of progress and recommendations for changes in treatment, as indicated, including medications, based on recommendations provided by the psychiatric consultant,
- provision of brief interventions using evidence-based techniques such as behavioral activation, motivational interviewing, and other focused treatment strategies,
- monitoring of patient outcomes using validated rating scales, and
- relapse prevention planning with patients as they achieve remission of symptoms and/or other treatment goals and are prepared for discharge from active treatment.

✚**99494**   Initial or subsequent psychiatric collaborative care management, each additional 30 minutes in a calendar month of behavioral health care manager activities, in consultation with a psychiatric consultant, and directed by the treating physician or other qualified health care professional (List separately in addition to code for primary procedure)

        (Use **99494** in conjunction with **99492** or **99493**.)

Psychiatric collaborative care management includes use of validated rating scales in monitoring patient outcomes. Do not separately report use of standardized rating scales (eg, **96127**).

● indicates a new code; ▲, revised; #, re-sequenced; ✚, add-on; ★, audiovisual technology; and ◀, synchronous interactive audio.

Psychiatric collaborative care management services are reported by a physician or QHP who supervises a behavioral health care manager (BHM) who delivers the services. Psychiatric collaborative care management services are provided to patients who have a new or existing psychiatric disorder that requires a behavioral health assessment; care plan implementation, revision, or monitoring; and provision of brief interventions. The treating physician or QHP reports codes **99492–99494** when all requirements for reporting are met. Evaluation and management and other services may be reported separately by the same physician or QHP during the same calendar month.

Each team member's role is defined in *Current Procedural Terminology* (*CPT*) as follows:

- The treating physician or QHP
  - Directs the BHM and continues to oversee the patient's care, including prescribing medications, treating medical conditions, and making referrals to specialty care when needed.
  - Engages the services of the psychiatric consultant who does not directly bill for PCCM services (ie, the treating physician's or QHP's practice contracts with the psychiatric consultant for this component of the PCCM service).
  - Acts in a supervisory role to the BHM (may be a direct employee or contractual employee but should represent a practice expense as other clinical staff and QNHCPs do).
  - May personally perform behavioral health care management activities. When those activities are not used to meet criteria for a separately reported service (eg, office E/M), their time may be counted toward the required time for PCCM.
  - Is ultimately responsible for delivery, documentation, and billing of PCCM services in compliance with *CPT* and payer policies.
- The BHM is a QNHCP or clinical staff member with master- or doctoral-level education *or* specialized training in behavioral health who provides behavioral health care management services under the treating physician's or QHP's supervision and in consultation with a psychiatric consultant. The BHM provides the following services, as needed:
  - Assessment of needs, including the administration of validated rating scales.
  - Development of a care plan.
  - Provision of brief face-to-face and non–face-to-face interventions.
  - Ongoing collaboration with the treating physician or QHP.
  - Consultation with the psychiatric consultant at least weekly (typically non–face-to-face).
  - Maintenance of a registry.
  - Sometimes, provision and reporting of other services (within the BHM's scope of practice) in the same calendar month as PCCM. These may include psychiatric diagnosis, psychotherapy, smoking and tobacco use cessation counseling (**99406**, **99407**), and alcohol and/or substance use structured screening and brief intervention services (**99408**, **99409**).
- The psychiatric consultant is a medical professional trained in psychiatry or behavioral health *and qualified to prescribe a full range of medications.* The psychiatric consultant does not typically see the patient or prescribe medications, except in rare circumstances. The psychiatric consultant advises and makes recommendations to the treating physician or QHP (typically via consultation with the BHM). The psychiatric consultant's services include recommending the following services, as needed:
  - Psychiatric and other medical differential diagnosis
  - Treatment strategies addressing appropriate therapies
  - Medication management
  - Medical management of complications associated with treatment of psychiatric disorders
  - Referral for specialty services
    The psychiatric consultant may directly provide and separately report E/M or psychiatric services, such as psychiatric evaluation (**90791**, **90792**), to a patient within a calendar month when the same patient receives PCCM services.

Reporting requirements for PCCM services include

- Time of service is met when the midpoint is passed. Documentation must support provision of PCCM services for the required time.
  - When service time does not meet the midpoint (ie, ≥36 minutes for **99492**, ≥31 minutes for **99493**, ≥16 minutes beyond most recent full period for **99494**), do no report PCCM.
- Services are provided for an episode of care defined as beginning when the treating physician or QHP directs the patient to the BHM and ending with
  - The attainment of targeted treatment goals, which typically results in the discontinuation of care management services and continuation of usual follow-up with the treating physician or other QHP
  - Failure to attain targeted treatment goals culminating in referral to a psychiatric care provider for ongoing treatment

— Lack of continued engagement with no PCCM services provided over a consecutive 6-month calendar period (break in episode)

- A new episode of care starts after a break in episode of 6 calendar months or more.
- Medical necessity of PCCM services may be supported by documentation such as
  — A newly diagnosed condition
  — A patient's need for help engaging in treatment
  — A patient who has not responded to standard care delivered in a nonpsychiatric setting or who requires further assessment and engagement before consideration of referral to a psychiatric care setting
      These are typical patient scenarios. Other reasons for services may support medical necessity.
  — Documentation of the patient's behavioral health conditions, psychosocial needs, and other factors influencing patient care may help support the necessity of services when health plans implement specific coverage criteria and/or prior authorization for PCCM services.

Psychiatric collaborative care management services do not require establishment of a care plan for *all* the patient's health care needs. The services are directed to behavioral health needs. Patients may or may not have comorbid conditions that affect treatment and management.

- Psychiatric collaborative care management services may be reported in the same month as chronic care management (CCM) or principal care management (PCM) services (**99439**, **99487**, **99489–99491**, **99424–99427**, **99437**) when the requirements for each service are met without overlap.
- Remote therapeutic monitoring treatment management services for cognitive behavioral therapy (**98980**, **98981**) are separately reported when they are provided and the time is not overlapping with that of PCCM.

> **See Chapter 21 for discussion of codes 98980 and 98981.**

- Provision of PCCM services may support quality initiatives such as use of an electronic clinical data system to track care and administration of a validated rating scale (eg, depression screening instrument) during a 4-month period for patients diagnosed with major depression or dysthymia.

Example

➤ **A pediatrician orders PCCM services for a 15-year-old patient diagnosed with moderate depression, single episode.** A licensed clinical social worker acting as the BHM discusses PCCM services with the patient and performs an initial assessment. Standardized assessment instruments are used in the assessment, and a treatment plan including psychotherapy is agreed on. Later, the BHM enters the patient information into a registry that will be used to track medication adherence and progress. At a regularly scheduled conference call between the BHM and a consulting psychiatrist, the patient's assessment is reviewed and the treatment plan approved. The supervising pediatrician is also consulted and approves the treatment plan. The BHM, whose scope of practice includes psychotherapy, provides 3 separately reportable individual psychotherapy sessions within the calendar month in addition to PCCM services. During the calendar month, the BHM documents 60 minutes of time spent in PCCM services.

ICD-10-CM	CPT
F32.1 (major depressive disorder, single episode, moderate)	**99492** (initial month PCCM service, first 70 minutes)
	90832, **90834**, or **90837** (psychotherapy without E/M based on time of service; 30, 45, or 60 minutes)

Teaching Point: Time of services for PCCM is met when the midpoint is passed. In this example, the 60 minutes spent by the BHM supports reporting of code **99492**, which includes the first 70 minutes of PCCM services in the initial month of service.

Psychotherapy services may be reported on a separate claim before fulfilling the time requirement for PCCM. No time spent in providing separately reported psychotherapy may be attributed to the time of PCCM services. If psychotherapy services were not within the scope of practice for the BHM, the patient might be referred to another provider (eg, the consulting psychiatrist), who would report the services rendered.

● indicates a new code; ▲, revised; #, re-sequenced; ✚, add-on; ★, audiovisual technology; and ◀, synchronous interactive audio.

General Behavioral Health Integration Care Management

#99484   Care management services for behavioral health conditions, at least 20 minutes of clinical staff time, directed by a physician or other qualified health care professional, per calendar month, with the following required elements:

● Initial assessment or follow-up monitoring, including the use of applicable validated rating scales,
● Behavioral health care planning in relation to behavioral/psychiatric health problems, including revision for patients who are not progressing or whose status changes,
● Facilitating and coordinating treatment such as psychotherapy, pharmacotherapy, counseling and/or psychiatric consultation, and
● Continuity of care with a designated member of the care team

General behavioral health integration care management (**99484**) is reported by a physician or QHP for supervision of clinical staff who provide at least 20 minutes of outpatient GBHI services within a calendar month to a patient with a behavioral health condition (includes substance use). A treatment plan must be documented and address the patient's behavioral health condition(s), but a comprehensive health care plan is not required. Code **99484** does not include requirements for a BHM or collaboration with a psychiatrist.

Clinical staff providing GBHI services are not required to have qualifications that would permit them to separately report services (eg, psychotherapy), but, if they are qualified and they perform such services, they may report such services separately. The time of the separately reported service is not used to support reporting **99484**.

Services must be provided under general physician supervision and in accordance with the licensing and scope of practice requirements of the state where services are provided. The individual supervising and reporting GBHI care management services must be able to report E/M services.

All the required elements of service listed in the code descriptor must be provided and documented.

Example

➤ **A 15-year-old established patient presents to a primary care pediatrician with concerns of social anxiety and lack of interest in previously enjoyed activities.** The primary care physician diagnoses the patient with a behavioral health disorder and prescribes a medication. The physician also recommends that the patient receive behavioral health care management as part of the treatment plan. The physician reports the appropriate code for the E/M service (eg, **99214**) provided on that date.

A few days later, clinical staff (eg, a nurse with specialized training in behavioral health services) meets with the patient and parent(s) to develop a behavioral health plan of care based on the physician's orders. During the calendar month, clinical staff, working under the physician's supervision, provide coordination of care with a psychologist in another practice and with a school counselor. At least 20 minutes of clinical staff time is documented for activities of GBHI during the calendar month to assess adherence to the plan of care, assess progress through standardized rating scales, and coordinate care, including facilitating access to community resources, as needed.

Teaching Point: If clinical staff time of less than 20 minutes is documented in a calendar month, code **99484** is not reported. Use of standardized rating scales is not separately reported. Physician services are separately reportable when the time and activities of those services are not included toward meeting the criteria of code **99484**.

● *Use of validated rating scales is required and is not separately reported* (ie, do not report code **96127** for rating scales administered during the period of behavioral health care management services).
● Time may be face-to-face but more typically may be non–face-to-face. Clinical staff must be available to provide face-to-face services to the patient when requested.
● Evaluation and management and/or psychiatric services may be reported on the same date or in the same calendar month as GBHI services when performed, but the time of separately reported services is not counted toward the time of GBHI services.
● General behavioral health integration (**99484**) may be reported in the same month as CCM or PCM services (**99439, 99487, 99489–99491, 99424–99427, 99437**) when the requirements for each service are met without overlap. Psychiatric collaborative care management (**99492–99494**) may not be reported by the same provider in the same month as GBHI.
● The reporting individual may personally provide elements of GBHI services and combine the time of service with that of clinical staff to support reporting code **99484**. However, the time of services that are separately reported (eg, 20 minutes' total time spent providing an E/M service reported with code **99213**) cannot be included in the time supporting **99484**.

- Clinical staff time spent coordinating care with the ED may be reported by using **99484**, but time spent while the patient is an inpatient or is admitted to observation status may not be reported by using **99484**.

Evaluation and Treatment of Alcohol and Substance Use

The initial evaluation of a child for alcohol and/or substance use is often in the context of an E/M service (eg, office and other outpatient E/M **99202–99205** or **99212–99215**). Evaluation and management codes may be selected on the basis of the total time spent by the physician or QHP in care of the individual patient on the date of service.

Additionally, codes **99408** and **99409** are reported for a brief assessment and intervention for alcohol or substance use. This behavior change service involves specific validated interventions of assessing readiness for change and barriers to change, advising a change in behavior, assisting by specifically suggesting actions and motivational counseling, and arranging for services and follow-up. Services are time based and may be separately reported when provided on the same date as other non-preventive E/M services (eg, office or emergency department [ED] visit for illness or injury related to substance use). Append modifier **25** (significant, separately identifiable E/M service) to other E/M codes (eg, **99214 25**) when a significant E/M service is provided on the same date as the service described by codes **99408** and **99409**.

★◀**99408**   Alcohol and/or substance (other than tobacco) abuse structured screening (eg, AUDIT, DAST), and brief intervention (SBI) services; 15 to 30 minutes

★◀**99409**   greater than 30 minutes

Codes **99408** and **99409** are included in the lists of codes that may be reported with telemedicine modifiers **93** (audio-only telemedicine service) and **95** (synchronous audiovisual telemedicine service), when applicable.

ICD-10-CM Coding for Use, Abuse, and Dependence

The guidelines for *ICD-10-CM* offer specific guidance for reporting diagnoses of mental and behavioral disorders caused by psychoactive substance use.

- Code **Z71.41** is reported as the first-listed code when an encounter is primarily focused on alcohol abuse counseling and surveillance. A code for alcohol abuse or dependence (**F10.-**) is additionally reported.
- Code **Z71.51** is reported as the first-listed code when an encounter is primarily for counseling on drug abuse and surveillance of a person with drug abuse. Codes for drug abuse or dependence (**F11–F16**, **F18**, or **F19**) are reported in addition to code **Z71.51**.
- When substance use is addressed and/or affects patient management during an encounter that is primarily for management or treatment of other conditions, report a code for management of the other condition(s) first, followed by a code for substance use.
- The codes for psychoactive substance *use* disorders (**F10.9-**, **F11.9-**, **F12.9-**, **F13.9-**, **F14.9-**, **F15.9-**, **F16.9-**) are to be used only when the psychoactive substance use is associated with a physical, mental, or behavioral disorder and such a relationship is documented by the provider. Note that codes for inhalant use (**F18.9-**) and polysubstance or indiscriminate drug use (**F19.9-**) are not included in this instruction.

> For a diagnosis of nicotine vaping, assign code **F17.29-**, nicotine dependence, other tobacco products. Electronic nicotine delivery systems are noncombustible tobacco products.

- Subcategories of codes for mental and behavioral disorders caused by psychoactive substance use indicate *use* and *abuse* of and *dependence* on various psychoactive substances. These categories do not include abuse of nonpsychoactive substances such as antacids, laxatives, or steroids that are reported with category **F55**. Each subcategory offers a spectrum of use, abuse, and dependence with extended information such as *with intoxication, with withdrawal*, and *with delusions*.
- For each encounter, only 1 code should be assigned to identify the pattern of use (use, abuse, or dependence) based on the hierarchy shown in **Figure 11-1**. Report a code for the condition farthest to the right in the figure.

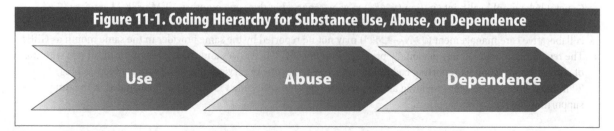

Figure 11-1. Coding Hierarchy for Substance Use, Abuse, or Dependence

Use → Abuse → Dependence

● indicates a new code; ▲, revised; #, re-sequenced; ✚, add-on; ★, audiovisual technology; and ◀, synchronous interactive audio.

- Selection of codes for mental and behavioral disorders caused by psychoactive substance use for substance abuse or dependence in remission (categories **F10–F19** with **-.11, -.21**) requires the provider's clinical judgment. The appropriate codes for in remission are assigned only on the basis of provider documentation unless otherwise instructed by the classification.
- Mild substance use disorders in early or sustained remission are classified to the appropriate codes for substance abuse in remission, and moderate or severe substance use disorders in early or sustained remission are classified to the appropriate codes for substance dependence in remission.

Management/Treatment of Alcohol and/or Substance Use Disorders

Treatment of alcohol and/or substance use disorders may be covered only when provided by physicians with certification in addiction medicine or by other licensed health care professionals whose scope of practice includes treating substance use disorders. Verify health plan benefits and eligible providers before beginning treatment services. Prior authorization of services is often required.

Coding for management/treatment of alcohol and/or substance use disorders is largely payer driven. Psychotherapy codes may be applicable, or E/M codes may be selected on the basis of time of counseling and/or coordination for ongoing counseling on alcohol and/or substance use disorders. However, many health plans and Medicaid programs require use of HCPCS codes and/or modifiers for reporting assessments and management/treatment of alcohol and/or substance use disorders.

Examples of HCPCS codes include

H0016   Alcohol and/or drug services; medical/somatic (medical intervention in ambulatory setting)

T1007   Alcohol and/or substance abuse services, treatment plan development and/or modification

Modifiers **HF–HI** provide details such as whether the program is an integrated mental health/substance abuse program. See payer guidelines for use of these modifiers.

Opportunities may exist to treat alcohol and substance use through integrated behavioral health such as PCCM services (for a discussion of these, see the Psychiatric Collaborative Care Management Services section earlier in this chapter).

Central Nervous System Assessments/Tests

The following codes are used to report the services provided during testing of central nervous system functions. Central nervous system assessments include, but are not limited to, memory, language, visual/motor responses, and abstract reasoning/problem-solving abilities. The mode of completion can be by a person (eg, paper and pencil) or via automated means. The administration of these tests will generate material that will be interpreted and formulated into a report by a physician or other QHP or an automated result.

> Standardized instruments are used in the performance of central nervous system assessment/testing services. Standardized instruments are validated tests administered and scored in the consistent or "standard" manner performed during their validation. Informal checklists created by a physician or an electronic health record developer are not considered standardized instruments.

Claims for testing are typically reported after the final date of testing services, with the appropriate codes for each date of service reported on the single claim. However, payer instructions may vary, and some require reporting with only the date on which testing services are completed (for an example, see discussion of **96112** and **96113** in the Developmental Testing section later in this chapter).

Payers may require prior authorization of tests. Practices should adopt procedures for verifying coverage and obtaining prior authorization, when required.

Central nervous system assessments and tests are not reported in conjunction with adaptive behavior treatment (**97151–97158, 0362T, 0373T**).

Developmental Testing

96112   Developmental test administration (including assessment of fine and/or gross motor, language, cognitive level, social, memory and/or executive functions by standardized developmental instruments when performed), by physician or other qualified health care professional, with interpretation and report; first hour

+96113   each additional 30 minutes (List separately in addition to code for primary procedure)

Chapter 11. Mental and Behavioral Health Services

> Developmental screening services are described by code 96110. Developmental screening using an objective standardized instrument, including scoring and documentation, is typically done by clinical staff. Interpretation and counseling on the score are included in the related evaluation and management service.

Codes **96112** and **96113**

- Allow reporting of developmental testing in which the child is observed doing standardized tasks that are then scored, with interpretation and report.
- Include assessment of motor, language, social, and/or cognitive function by standardized developmental instruments (eg, scales of infant and toddler development) and include objective assessments as well.
- Billing time includes both face-to-face time spent in testing and time of interpretation and report.
  - Although not specifically stated in the code descriptor, interpretation and report is included as intraservice work in the assignment of work relative value units (RVUs) for these services.
  - Payer policies may vary on reporting of time spent in interpretation and report. Check the policies of individual health plans when reporting.
- Code selection is based on time spent per hour by the physician or QHP.
    The midpoint rule applies to developmental testing; time is met *when the midpoint is passed* (≥31 minutes to report 1 hour of service and ≥16 minutes to report a service assigned a time of 30 minutes).
- If a developmental instrument does not meet the criteria of being an objective instrument with the subjective element and does not take a minimum of 31 minutes to complete including interpretation and report, refer to code **96110** instead.
    Do not report **96110** if also reporting code **96112** or **96113** on the same day for the same patient.

Example

➤ **A 7-year-old boy presents for extended developmental testing due to long-standing social and learning difficulties at school.** Developmental tests are administered, with total testing time on this date of 75 minutes. The child returns and spends a total of 60 minutes to complete testing 1 week later. After testing is completed, the developmental pediatrician spends another 60 minutes on the same date interpreting the test results and 60 minutes formulating a report of the findings and recommendations.

Code **96112** is reported for the 75 minutes of service on the first date. **96113** is not reported because the midpoint between 60 and 90 minutes (76 minutes) was not passed. On the second date of service, codes **96112** (first 60 minutes of testing) and **96113** with 4 units of service (2 hours interpreting the testing results and developing the report) are reported. On the final date of service (ie, the day of the feedback session), submit 1 claim for all cumulative services detailed *by separate dates of service*.

Teaching Point: Some payers may require the entire service be reported on a single claim and single date of service. For these payers, report code **96112** (for the 60 minutes of testing on the first day) and 6 units of **96113** (for the remaining 195 minutes) on the date of the second session. It is important that staff are trained to submit the records for all dates that testing services were provided, when necessary, in response to a payer's request for records.

Remember, the midpoint must be passed for the additional units to be billed. In this case, the remaining time was only 15 minutes.

Neuropsychological and Psychological Testing

Neuropsychological and psychological testing evaluation services typically include integration of patient data with other sources of clinical data, interpretation, clinical decision-making, treatment planning, and report.

- Interactive feedback, conveying the implications of psychological or neuropsychological test findings and diagnostic formulation, is included when performed.
- Testing by a physician or QHP is separately reportable as an evaluation service on the same or a different date.
- Testing codes differentiate tests administered by a physician or other QHP, by a technician, or via an electronic platform.

> Mini mental status examination performed by a physician is included as part of the central nervous system physical examination of an evaluation and management service and is not separately reportable.

Neurobehavioral Status Examination

★◄96116   Neurobehavioral status examination (clinical assessment of thinking, reasoning and judgment [eg, acquired knowledge, attention, language, memory, planning and problem solving, and visual spatial abilities]), by physician or other qualified health care professional, both face-to-face time with the patient and time interpreting test results and preparing the report; first hour

✚96121   each additional hour

> Code 96116 is included in Appendix T, indicating that this service may be reported with modifier 93 when provided through interactive telecommunications equipment that includes, at a minimum, audio. For further discussion of telemedicine modifiers, see chapters 2 and 20.

- Documentation of these services includes scoring, informal observation of behavior during the testing, and interpretation and report. Include the date and time spent in testing, time of interpretation and report, reason for the test, and titles of all instruments used.
- Report neurobehavioral status examination based on the time of face-to-face testing and include time interpreting test results and preparing a report.
- The unit of time is 60 minutes and time is met when the midpoint is passed (ie, at least 31 minutes of time is required for the first or last unit of service).
- These services may be provided via telemedicine; append modifier 95 to indicate a service provided via real-time audiovisual technology or modifier 93 to indicate a service provided via audio-only communication.

Example

➤ **An 8-year-old boy, previously diagnosed with attention-deficit/hyperactivity disorder (ADHD), predominantly inattentive type, is being evaluated for gradual problems with remembering directions, organizing his school materials and his room at home, and other behavior concerns.** The physician or QHP performs a neurobehavioral status examination, which involves clinical assessments and observations for impairments in acquired knowledge, attention, learning, and memory. The results indicate the need for further standardized language, memory, and intelligence testing. The total time for testing, scoring, and report writing is 3½ hours.

This service is reported with codes 96116 (neurobehavioral status examination) and 96121 with 2 units for the additional 2½ hours of testing, scoring, and report writing. The diagnosis code would be *ICD-10-CM* code F90.0 (ADHD, predominantly inattentive type). Additional *ICD-10-CM* codes may be assigned for specific developmental disorders diagnosed following testing (eg, F81.2, mathematics disorder).

Psychological and Neuropsychological Testing Services

Codes for psychological and neuropsychological testing differentiate test administration by physicians and QHPs, technicians, or automated systems. A combination of testing evaluation and test administration and scoring services is typically reported on a single claim.

The tests selected, test administration, and method of testing and scoring are the same regardless of whether the testing is performed by a physician, QHP, or technician.

Testing Evaluation Services by a Physician or Other Qualified Health Care Professional With Interpretation and Report

96130   *Psychological* testing evaluation services by physician or other qualified health care professional, including integration of patient data, interpretation of standardized test results and clinical data, clinical decision making, treatment planning and report, and interactive feedback to the patient, family member(s) or caregiver(s), when performed; first hour

✚96131   each additional hour (List separately in addition to code for primary procedure)

96132   *Neuropsychological* testing evaluation services by physician or other qualified health care professional, including integration of patient data, interpretation of standardized test results and clinical data, clinical decision making, treatment planning and report, and interactive feedback to the patient, family member(s) or caregiver(s), when performed; first hour

✚96133   each additional hour (List separately in addition to code for primary procedure)

● indicates a new code; ▲, revised; #, re-sequenced; ✚, add-on; ★, audiovisual technology; and ◄, synchronous interactive audio.

- Report codes **96130–96133** on the basis of the face-to-face time with the patient and the time spent integrating and interpreting data. The standard *CPT* time definitions (ie, a minimum of 31 minutes must be provided to report a 1-hour unit of service) apply.
- *Time spent in test administration and scoring is not included in time used to support codes* **96130–96133**. Separately report psychological/neuropsychological test administration and scoring services (**96136–96139**) on the same or different days (ie, each service is separately reported on the same claim). Report the total time of evaluation and testing services at the completion of the entire episode of evaluation on a single claim with each date of service listed separately.

> Time of 30 minutes or less would not be reported with codes 96132 and 96133.

- Documentation of these services includes scoring, observation of behavior, and interpretation and report. It should include the date and time spent in testing and the time spent integrating and interpreting data, reason for the testing, and titles of all instruments used.

> The time reported in codes 96130–96133 is a combination of the *documented* face-to-face time with the patient and the time spent integrating and interpreting data. An itemization of time for each activity is preferable.

Example

➤ **An adolescent patient with history of brain surgery is referred for neuropsychological evaluation due to difficulties with memory and reading.** A physician spends 2 hours reviewing the patient's medical records, interpreting data from tests administered and scored on an earlier date by a technician, and creating a report (copied to the referring physician) of the diagnosis and recommendations for treatment. Another 40 minutes was spent providing interactive feedback to the patient and caregivers.

Code **96132** and 2 units of **96133** are reported for 160 minutes spent in data interpretation, interactive feedback, and report writing. If the physician had also personally administered and scored tests, codes **96136** and **96137** would have also been reported on the basis of the time of testing and scoring. Test administration and scoring by a technician would be reported separately with codes **96138** and **96139** on the basis of the time of service (for discussion of codes **96138** and **96139**, see the Technician-Administered Testing section later in this chapter).

Teaching Point: Report code **96133** with 1 unit of service in addition to **96132** for time of 91 to 150 minutes. Time of 151 minutes or more supports additional units of service for code **96133** (include 1 unit for 31–59 minutes beyond the last full hour).

Testing Administration Services

Test administration and scoring services are selected on the basis of time of service. The midpoint rule applies. Separate codes are reported on the basis of whether testing and scoring are personally performed by a physician or QHP or are performed by a technician.

> At least 2 distinct tests must be administered and scored to report codes 96136–96139. Do not separately count subtests in a multifaceted test (eg, Wechsler Preschool and Primary Scale of Intelligence is 1 test with 14 subtests). Code 96127 (brief emotional/behavioral assessment, with scoring and documentation, per standardized instrument) may be reported for administration and scoring of a single standardized test.

Physician or Qualified Health Care Professional Administration and Scoring

96136	Psychological or neuropsychological test administration and scoring by physician or other qualified health care professional, two or more tests, any method; first 30 minutes
✚96137	each additional 30 minutes after first 30 minutes (List separately in addition to code for primary procedure)

Services include administration of a series of tests, recording of behavioral observations made during testing, scoring, and transcription of scores to a data summary sheet.

- Codes are selected on the basis of time of testing and scoring. Time is met when the midpoint is passed (ie, a minimum of 16 minutes for 30-minute codes). Refer to **Table 11-1** for more details.
- *Do not include* time spent in integration of patient data or interpretation of test results in the time reported with codes **96136** and **96137**. This time is included with psychological and neuropsychological test evaluation services (**96130–96133**).
- Psychological or neuropsychological test administration *through a single test/instrument,* with interpretation and report by a physician or QHP, is reported with code **96127** (brief emotional/behavioral assessment [eg, depression inventory, ADHD scale], with scoring and documentation, per standardized instrument).

Table 11-1. Calculating Units of Service for Time of Test Administration and Scoring				
Total Minutes of Administration and Scoring Performed By	First 30 min (16–45 min)	First Additional 30 min (46–75 min)	Second Additional 30 min (76–105 min)	Each Additional 30 min or Last 16 min Beyond Final Full 30-min Period (>106 min)
Physician/QHP	**96136** (1 unit)	**96136** and **96137** (1 unit each)	**96136** (1 unit) and **96137** (2 units)	**96136** (1 unit) and units of **96137** for each 30 min or last 16 min beyond final full 30-min period
Technician	**96138** (1 unit)	**96138** and **96139** (1 unit each)	**96138** (1 unit) and **96139** (2 units)	**96138** (1 unit) and units of **96139** for each 30 min or last 16 min beyond final full 30-min period

Abbreviation: QHP, qualified health care professional.

Examples

➤ **A physician spends 80 minutes administering tests, recording observations, scoring, and transcribing results to a data summary sheet.** Codes **96136** × 1 unit and **96137** × 2 units are reported.

Teaching Point: Code **96136** is reported for the first 30 minutes. Two units of code **96137** are also reported for the remaining 50 minutes (1 full period of 30 minutes and the final 20 minutes). If the final period of service were less than 16 minutes, only 1 unit of **96137** would be reported.

➤ **An adolescent is referred for psychological testing evaluation.** The patient undergoes physician-administered psychological testing to evaluate emotionality, intellectual abilities, personality, and psychopathology and to make a mental health diagnosis and treatment recommendations as applicable. The total time of face-to-face testing is 45 minutes. The physician's total time of evaluation and data integration and interpretation is 75 minutes. Codes **96136** and **96130** are reported.

Teaching Point: Test administration and scoring time of 45 minutes is reported with code **96136**. Seventy-five minutes of physician testing evaluation service is reported with code **96130**.

Technician-Administered Testing

Testing and administration services performed by a technician are reported with codes **96138** and **96139**.

96138   Psychological or neuropsychological test administration and scoring by technician, two or more tests, any method; first 30 minutes

✚96139   each additional 30 minutes (List separately in addition to code for primary procedure)

 Codes **96138** and **96139** do not include the work of a physician or QHP. These codes are valued only for practice expense and medical liability.

- Evaluation services by the physician or QHP are reported with codes **96130–96133** whether provided on the same or a different date. Do not include time for evaluation services (eg, integration of patient data or interpretation of test results in the time of technician-administered testing) in time of test administration and scoring.

● indicates a new code; ▲, revised; #, re-sequenced; ✚, add-on; ★, audiovisual technology; and ◀, synchronous interactive audio.

Example

➤ **An adolescent patient is referred for neuropsychological testing.** A technician spends 40 minutes administering and scoring tests. The technician also notes any behavioral observations. Code **96138** is reported with 1 unit of service.

Teaching Point: When a physician or QHP provides evaluation services, including integration and interpretation of data from tests administered by a technician, on the same or different date, see codes **96132** and **96133** for those services.

Automated Testing and Result

When a single test instrument is completed by the patient via an electronic platform without physician, QHP, or technician administration and scoring, report code **96146**.

96146   Psychological or neuropsychological test administration, with single automated, standardized instrument via electronic platform, with automated result only

Code **96146** does not include scoring by a health care professional or interpretation and report. Results are generated via the electronic platform.

● If a test is administered by a physician, QHP, or technician, do not report **96146**. For brief emotional/behavioral assessment, see code **96127**.

Example

➤ **A child who is recovering from a concussion is provided a single computerized test for postconcussion symptoms.** The patient completes the test and the automated result is included in the patient's medical record.

Code **96146** is reported in addition to the code representing the physician's related E/M service (eg, **99213**). Append modifier **25** (significant, separately identifiable E/M service) if the payer uses National Correct Coding Initiative edits.

Behavior Management Services

New in 2023! Codes 96202 and 96203 are used to report group behavior management/modification training services provided to parents/caregivers of children with a behavior that affects an identified mental or physical health diagnosis.

●**96202**   Multiple-family group behavior management/modification training for parent(s)/guardian(s)/caregiver(s) of patients with a mental or physical health diagnosis, administered by physician or other qualified health care professional (without the patient present), face-to-face with multiple sets of parent(s)/guardian(s)/caregiver(s); initial 60 minutes

✚●**96203**   each additional 15 minutes

Behavior management/modification training is provided to a multiple-family group of parent(s)/guardian(s)/caregiver(s), without the patient present. The physician or QHP provides a *face-to-face service* to train parent(s)/guardian(s)/caregiver(s) to use skills and strategies to address behaviors affecting the patient's mental or physical health diagnosis and to support adherence to the patient's treatment and the plan of care.

Training may include
● Verbal instruction
● Video and live demonstrations
● Feedback from a physician/other QHP or other parents in group sessions

The time of service is the physician's/other QHP's face-to-face time with multiple sets of parent(s)/guardian(s)/caregiver(s). Code **96202** requires at least 31 minutes of service. No specific instruction for the required time to report **96203** is included in *CPT* instructions. On the basis of the midpoint rule, time is met when the midpoint is passed (ie, at least 8 minutes for a service time of 15 minutes). *Time must be documented to support the service provided.*

The qualified health care professionals (QHPs) who may provide this service may be those who can provide evaluation and management (E/M) services (eg, nurse practitioners, clinical nurse specialists) or may be other QHPs whose scope of practice does not include E/M services (eg, licensed clinical social workers, psychologists, occupational therapists).

● indicates a new code; ▲, revised; #, re-sequenced; ✚, add-on; ★, audiovisual technology; and ◀, synchronous interactive audio.

The services reported with **96202** and **96203**
- Must take place without the patient present
- Are provided to a multiple-family group of parent(s)/guardian(s)/caregiver(s)
- Emphasize active engagement and involvement of the parent(s)/guardian(s)/caregiver(s) in the treatment of a patient with a mental or physical health diagnosis

Do not report **96202** and **96203**
- ✖ For preventive medicine counseling (**99401–99404**; **99410, 99411**)
- ✖ For risk-factor reduction interventions (**99406–99409**)
- ✖ For services to the patient and the parent(s)/guardian(s)/caregiver(s) during the same session (Report with appropriate E/M code[s] for site of service.)
- ✖ For educational services rendered to patients in a group setting (eg, prenatal, obesity, or diabetic instructions) (Report with code **99078**.)

Example

➤ **A pediatric clinical nurse specialist provides behavior management services to a group of parents and caregivers whose children have diagnosed illnesses and behaviors that affect their illnesses and management or treatment.** The group participates in activities to learn interventions that participants can independently use to effectively manage their children's illnesses/diseases. The clinical nurse specialist documents a total of 45 minutes spent face-to-face providing the behavior management services to the group.

Codes reported to the health plan for each child include diagnosis codes for the child's illness/disease.

●**96202** Multiple-family group behavior management/modification training for parent(s)/guardian(s)/caregiver(s) of patients with a mental or physical health diagnosis, administered by physician or other qualified health care professional (without the patient present), face-to-face with multiple sets of parent(s)/guardian(s)/caregiver(s); initial 60 minutes

Teaching Point: The clinical nurse specialist reports **96202** for each patient whose parent(s)/guardian(s)/caregiver(s) participated in the service. If the time of service had exceeded the first 60 minutes by at least 8 minutes (the midway point between 60 minutes and 75 minutes), code **96203** would have been reported in addition to **96202**.

Adaptive Behavior Assessment and Treatment Services

Adaptive behavior services address
- Deficient adaptive behaviors, such as impaired social, communication, or self-care skills
- Maladaptive behaviors, such as repetitive and stereotype behaviors
- Behaviors that risk physical harm to the patient, others, and/or property

Codes for adaptive behavior services are a combination of Category I and Category III (emerging technology) *CPT* codes. Adaptive behavior services may be delivered by a physician or QHP, behavioral analyst, and/or licensed psychologist working with assistant behavior analysts or technicians. Services are typically reported for conditions that present with maladaptive behaviors such as ASD.

It is important to verify health plan policies for coverage and payment of adaptive behavior services, including any required provider qualifications (eg, certification, licensure) before provision of services.

Most states mandate coverage of adaptive behavior services for patients diagnosed with autism spectrum disorder (ASD). Some states require that behavior analysts providing ASD-related assessment and/or treatment be certified by the Behavior Analyst Certification Board as a Board-Certified Behavior Analyst.

- In the discussion of adaptive behavior services, the QHP includes behavior analysts and licensed psychologists who can independently report these services.

See your procedure coding reference (eg, *CPT* coding manual) for specific instructions for reporting these services, including definitions of functional behavioral assessment, functional analysis, standardized instruments and procedures, and non-standardized instruments and procedures.

The general rule that time is met when the midpoint is passed applies because *CPT* doesn't include category-specific instructions on the time of service for adaptive behavior services (eg, at least 8 minutes of service is required to support a service specified as 15 minutes).

● indicates a new code; ▲, revised; #, re-sequenced; ✚, add-on; ★, audiovisual technology; and ◀, synchronous interactive audio.

Adaptive Behavior Assessment

#97151 Behavior identification assessment, administered by a physician or other qualified health care professional, each 15 minutes of the physician's or other qualified health care professional's time face-to-face with patient and/or guardian(s)/caregiver(s) administering assessments and discussing findings and recommendations, and non-face-to-face analyzing past data, scoring/interpreting the assessment, and preparing the report/treatment plan

#97152 Behavior identification supporting assessment, administered by one technician under the direction of a physician or other qualified health care professional, face-to-face with the patient, each 15 minutes

0362T Behavior identification supporting assessment, each 15 minutes of technicians' time face-to-face with a patient, requiring the following components:

- administration by the physician or other qualified health care professional who is on site;
- with the assistance of two or more technicians;
- for a patient who exhibits destructive behavior;
- completion in an environment that is customized to the patient's behavior

Behavior identification assessment (**97151**) is conducted by a physician or other QHP and may include

- Analysis of pertinent past data (including medical diagnosis)
- A detailed behavioral history
- Patient observation
- Administration of standardized and/or non-standardized instruments and procedures
- Functional behavior assessment
- Functional analysis
- Guardian/caregiver interview to identify and describe deficient adaptive behaviors, maladaptive behaviors, and other impaired functioning secondary to deficient adaptive or maladaptive behaviors

Documentation should include a report of the assessment and a person-centered treatment plan.

If the physician or other QHP personally performs the technician activities, their time engaged in these activities should be included as part of the required technician time to meet the components of the code.

- Codes **97151**, **97152**, and **0362T** may be repeated on the same or different days until the behavior identification assessment (**97151**) and, if necessary, supporting assessment(s) (**97152**, **0362T**) are complete.
- Code **97152** is reported for assessment by a technician. The reporting physician or QHP is not required to be on-site during the assessment. See code **0362T** when multiple technicians and a customized assessment environment are required due to destructive behavior(s) of the patient.
- Code **0362T** represents testing of a patient who demonstrates destructive behavior (ie, maladaptive behaviors associated with a high risk of medical consequences or property damage) and requires multiple technicians and an environment customized to the patient and behavior. The reporting physician or QHP is required to be on-site (ie, immediately available and interruptible to provide assistance and direction throughout the performance of the procedure). The reporting physician or QHP is not required to be in the room during testing.
- Count the time of only 1 technician when 2 or more technicians are present. Code **0362T** is reported on the basis of a single technician's face-to-face time with the patient and not the combined time of multiple technicians (eg, 1 hour with 3 technicians equals 1 hour of service) despite the expectation that more than one technician will be needed.

Examples

➤ **A 3-year-old boy with symptoms of ASD presents for assessment.** The physician/QHP spends 1 hour face-to-face with the patient and/or guardian(s)/caregiver(s) administering assessments and discussing findings and recommendations and 38 minutes of non–face-to-face time analyzing past data, scoring/interpreting the assessment, and preparing the report/treatment plan. The total time of service is 98 minutes. Code **97151** is reported with 7 units (1 for each full 15 minutes of service and 1 for the last 8 minutes).

Teaching Point: If less than 8 minutes past the last full 15 minutes of service were provided, only the number of 15-minute periods of service would be reported (eg, 1 hour 37 minutes equals 6 units).

● indicates a new code; ▲, revised; #, re-sequenced; ✚, add-on; ★, audiovisual technology; and ◀, synchronous interactive audio.

Chapter 11. Mental and Behavioral Health Services

➤ **An additional assessment of the 3-year-old from the previous example is required to assess behavior that interferes with acquisition of adaptive skills.** A technician, under the physician's or QHP's direction, observes and records occurrence of the patient's deficient adaptive and maladaptive behaviors and the surrounding environmental events several times in a variety of situations. The physician/QHP reviews and analyzes data from the technician's observations. The face-to-face time of the technician is 1 hour.

Code **97152** is reported with 4 units of service.

➤ **An 11-year-old boy with ASD requires evaluation due to increased self-injury and aggression toward others.** A team of technicians conducts the assessment session in a room that is devoid of any objects that might cause injury. A physician/QHP is on-site and immediately available throughout the session. The technicians implement functional analysis (ie, they systematically present and withdraw events to the patient multiple times while observing and measuring occurrence of a target behavior) as directed by the physician/QHP and record data. Graphed data are reviewed and analyzed by the physician/QHP to identify the environmental events in whose presence the level of behavior was highest and lowest. The technicians spend a total of 90 minutes face-to-face with the patient during the assessment.

Code **0362T** is reported with 6 units of service.

Adaptive Behavior Treatment

Adaptive behavior treatment services address specific treatment targets and goals based on results of previous assessments and include ongoing assessment and adjustment of treatment protocols, targets, and goals. Codes describe services to an individual patient, groups of patients, families, and an individual patient who exhibits destructive behavior.

Codes for adaptive behavior treatment specify services provided by protocol (**97153**, **97154**) or with protocol modification (**97155**, **97158**, **0373T**). Behavior treatment with protocol modification requires adjustments be *made in real time* rather than for a subsequent service.

Adaptive Behavior Treatment by Protocol

#**97153**   Adaptive behavior treatment by protocol, administered by technician under the direction of a physician or other qualified health care professional, face-to-face with one patient; each 15 minutes

#**97154**   Group adaptive behavior treatment by protocol, administered by technician under the direction of a physician or other qualified health care professional, face-to-face with two or more patients, each 15 minutes

● Adaptive behavior treatment by protocol to a single patient (**97153**) and group adaptive behavior treatment by protocol (**97154**) are administered by a technician under the direction of a physician/QHP, with a treatment protocol *designed in advance* by the physician or other QHP, who may or may not provide direction during the treatment.
  — The service described by code **97153** is face-to-face with only 1 patient.
  — Code **97154** is reported for services delivered face-to-face with 2 or more patients but not more than 8 patients.
● Codes **97153** and **97154** do not include protocol modification.
● If the physician/QHP personally performs the technician activities, their time spent engaged in these activities should be reported as technician time. The physician is not required to be on-site during the provision of these services.

Examples

➤ **A 4-year-old girl with ASD presents with deficits in language and social skills and emotional outbursts in response to small changes in routines or when preferred items are unavailable.** A QHP directs a technician in the implementation of treatment protocols and data collection procedures. The technician conducts a treatment session in the family home with multiple planned opportunities for the patient to practice target skills. The QHP reviews the technician's recorded and graphed data to assess the child's progress and determine if any treatment protocol needs adjustment. The technician spends 1 hour at the patient's home with face-to-face time of the treatment session lasting 50 minutes. Code **97153** is reported with 3 units of service.

Teaching Point: Only the technician's face-to-face time with the patient is used to determine the units of service. This service may also be conducted in a community setting (eg, playground, store).

Chapter 11. Mental and Behavioral Health Services

➤ **Peer social skills training in a small group is recommended for a 7-year-old girl with deficits in social skills due to ASD.** A technician conducts the group session by using treatment protocols and data collection procedures as previously designed by a QHP. The QHP reviews the technician's recorded and graphed data to assess the child's progress and determine if treatment protocols need adjustment. The total face-to-face time of the session is 60 minutes.

Code **97154** is reported with 4 units.

Adaptive Behavior Treatment With Protocol Modification

#97155	Adaptive behavior treatment with protocol modification administered by physician or other qualified health care professional, which may include simultaneous direction of technician, face-to-face with one patient, each 15 minutes
#97158	Group adaptive behavior treatment with protocol modification, administered by physician or other qualified health care professional, face-to-face with multiple patients, each 15 minutes
0373T	Adaptive behavior treatment with protocol modification, each 15 minutes of technicians' time face-to-face with a patient, requiring the following components:

- administration by the physician or other qualified health care professional who is on site;
- with the assistance of two or more technicians;
- for a patient who exhibits destructive behavior;
- completion in an environment that is customized to the patient's behavior.

- Adaptive behavior treatment with protocol modification (**97155**) is administered by a physician/QHP *face-to-face with a single patient.*
  - The physician/QHP resolves 1 or more problems with the protocol and may simultaneously direct a technician in administering the modified protocol *while the patient is present.*
  - Physician/QHP direction to the technician without the patient present is not reported separately.
- Group adaptive behavior treatment with protocol modification (**97158**) is reported when a physician/QHP provides *face-to-face* protocol modification services with up to 8 patients in a group. The physician/QHP monitors the needs of individual patients and adjusts treatment techniques during the group sessions, as needed.
- Adaptive behavior treatment with protocol modification (**0373T**) is reported for services to a patient who presents with 1 or more destructive behavior(s).
  - The service time is based on a single technician's face-to-face time with the patient and not the combined time of multiple technicians.
  - The physician/QHP must be on-site and immediately available during the service described by code **0373T**.

Examples

➤ **A 5-year-old boy previously showed steady improvements in language and social skills at home as a result of one-to-one intensive applied behavior analysis intervention, but skill development seems to have recently reached a plateau.** A QHP modifies the previously used written protocols to incorporate procedures designed to build the child's language and social skills into daily home routines (eg, play, dressing, mealtimes). The QHP demonstrates the procedures to the technician and directs the technician to implement the protocols with the child. The QHP then observes and provides feedback as the technician implements the procedures with the child. The technician's face-to-face time with the patient is 45 minutes. Code **97155** is reported with 3 units of service.

Teaching Point: Time spent by the technician and QHP without the patient present is not included in the time of service.

➤ **A 13-year-old girl is reported to be isolated from peers due to poor social skills and odd behavior.** The child attends a group treatment session that focuses on peer social skills. A QHP begins the group session by asking each patient to briefly describe 2 of their recent social encounters with peers, one that went well and one that did not. The information is used to develop a group activity in which each patient has the opportunity to practice the skills they used in the encounters that went well and to problem-solve the interactions that did not go well. The QHP helps each patient identify social cues that were interpreted correctly and incorrectly and what they could have done differently. The QHP also provides prompts and feedback individualized to each patient's skills. The QHP ends the session by summarizing the discussion. The total time of the session was 70 minutes, including a 10-minute break (ie, 60 minutes of group session). Code **97158** is reported with 4 units of service.

Teaching Point: Only the QHP's face-to-face time spent providing the service is reported.

● indicates a new code; ▲, revised; #, re-sequenced; ✚, add-on; ★, audiovisual technology; and ◀, synchronous interactive audio.

➤ **A 16-year-old boy has had 2 surgeries to relieve esophageal blockages due to pica involving repeated ingestion of small metal objects (eg, paper clips, pushpins).** The patient's pica behavior has not responded to previous treatment. The QHP supervising the patient's treatment plan has previously developed written protocols for reducing the patient's pica. A technician carefully inspects the room before the session to make sure there are no potential pica items on the floor. Two technicians are present, with one presenting the patient with a series of trials in which the patient is presented with a food item and a nonhazardous item that resembles a pica item. The second technician prompts the patient to choose the food item and blocks attempts to choose the pica item. The patient's response to each trial is recorded. The QHP is on-site and available to assist as needed. The total session lasts 40 minutes. Code **0373T** is reported with 3 units.

    Teaching Point: Although 2 technicians were present, time is counted only once. The midpoint rule allows reporting a unit of service for the final 10 minutes of service.

Family Adaptive Behavior Treatment Guidance

Family adaptive behavior treatment guidance (**97156**) and multiple-family group adaptive behavior treatment guidance (**97157**) are administered by a physician or QHP face-to-face with guardian(s)/caregiver(s) and involve identifying potential treatment targets and training guardian(s)/caregiver(s) to implement treatment protocols designed to address deficient adaptive or maladaptive behaviors.

#97156   Family adaptive behavior treatment guidance, administered by physician or other qualified health care professional (with or without the patient present), face-to-face with guardian(s)/caregiver(s), each 15 minutes

#97157   Multiple-family group adaptive behavior treatment guidance, administered by physician or other qualified health care professional (without the patient present), face-to-face with multiple sets of guardians/caregivers, each 15 minutes

● Family adaptive behavior treatment guidance (**97156**) provided to the caregiver(s) of one patient may be performed with or without the patient present.

    Adaptive behavior treatment where the parent(s) or guardian(s) are present but not part of the therapy would not qualify as family adaptive behavior treatment.

● Family adaptive behavior treatment guidance provided to the caregiver(s) of multiple patients (**97157**) is performed without the patients present. The group must be no larger than the caregiver(s) of 8 patients. *CPT* does not include a code for reporting services to a group of 9 or more patients.

Examples

➤ **The parents of a 6-year-old boy seek training on procedures for helping the child communicate by using picture cards during typical family routines (a skill he previously developed in adaptive behavior treatment therapy sessions with technicians).** A physician/QHP trains the parents. The service includes reviewing the written treatment and data collection protocols with the parents, demonstrating how to implement the cards in role-playing and with the child, and having the parents implement the protocols with the child while the provider observes and provides feedback. The time of service is 1 hour.

    Code **97156** is reported with 4 units of service.

➤ **The parents of a 3-year-old boy who has pervasive hyperactivity and no functional play, social, or communication skills seek training on how to manage his hyperactive and disruptive behavior and help him develop appropriate play, social, and communication skills.** The parents attend a group session (without the patient) led by a physician who asks each set of parents to identify 1 skill to be increased or 1 problem behavior to be decreased in their own child. The physician describes how behavior analytic principles and procedures could be applied to the behavior identified by the parents of this 3-year-old patient. The physician demonstrates a procedure (eg, prompting the child to speak instead of whining when he wants something; not giving him preferred items when he whines). The parents then role-play, implementing that procedure. Other group participants and the physician provide feedback and make constructive suggestions. That process is repeated for skills/behaviors identified by other sets of parents. The group session ends with the physician summarizing the main points, answering questions, and giving each set of parents a homework assignment to practice the skills they worked on during the session. The session lasts 110 minutes. Code **97157** is reported with 7 units.

Teaching Point: The last 5 minutes is not reported because the midpoint of 8 minutes beyond the last full 15-minute period (105 minutes) was not passed.

Habilitative and Rehabilitative Modifiers

Adaptive behavior services may be either habilitative or rehabilitative. *Habilitative* services are those provided to help an individual learn skills not yet developed and to keep and/or improve those skills. *Rehabilitative* services help a patient keep, get back, or improve skills that have been lost or limited due to illness, injury, and/or disability. Because the Patient Protection and Affordable Care Act requires that certain health plans provide equal coverage for habilitative and rehabilitative services and count each type of service separately, it may be necessary to indicate that a service is habilitative or rehabilitative. Modifiers **96** (habilitative services) and **97** (rehabilitative services) are appended to procedure codes to designate the nature of a service. Modifiers **96** and **97** may not be adopted for use by all payers or may have limited utility. Verify payer policies for these modifiers when providing habilitative and rehabilitative services.

Health and Behavior Assessments/Interventions

Health and behavior assessment and intervention procedures (**96156**, **96158**, **96159**, and **96164–96171**) are provided by QNHCPs who cannot report E/M services. These services are used to identify and address psychosocial, behavioral, emotional, cognitive, and interpersonal factors important to the assessment, treatment, or management *of physical health problems.*

The patient's primary diagnosis must be a medical (physical) issue, and the focus of the assessment and interventions is on factors complicating medical conditions and treatments. These codes describe assessments and interventions to improve the patient's health and well-being using psychological and/or psychosocial interventions designed to ameliorate specific disease-related problems.

These services do not represent preventive medicine counseling and risk-factor reduction interventions.

- Physicians and QHPs who can provide and report E/M services do not report **96156**, **96158**, **96159**, or **96164–96171**. Evaluation and management codes including preventive medicine services are reported instead depending on the type of service provided.
- When an E/M service is provided by a physician or QHP on the same date that a QNHCP (eg, licensed clinical social worker) provides health and behavior assessment/intervention, each service is separately reported by the individual providing the service. The same provider cannot report both services.
- May be reported by psychologists, clinical social workers, licensed therapists, and other QNHCPs within their scope of practice who have specialty or subspecialty training in health and behavior assessment or intervention procedures.
- Are not reported with psychiatric codes (**90785–90899**) when provided on the same day. Only the primary service is reported (ie, **96156**, **96158**, **96159**, and **96164–96171** or **90785–90899**).
- Are not reported with adaptive behavior assessment or treatment (**97151–97158**, **0362T**, **0373T**).
- Are not used in conjunction with a primary diagnosis of mental disorder. (Payers may deny claims when a diagnosis code indicating mental disorder is included for these services.)

Health Behavior Assessment

96156   Health behavior assessment, or re-assessment (ie, health-focused clinical interview, behavioral observations, clinical decision making)

Health behavior assessment includes evaluation of the patient's responses to disease, illness or injury, outlook, coping strategies, motivation, and adherence to medical treatment. Assessment is conducted through health-focused clinical interviews, observation, and clinical decision-making.

Code **96156** is not reported on the basis of time. Report only 1 unit of service.

Example

➤ **A 13-year-old girl with multiple food allergies and newly increased anxiety is assessed for response to management of food allergies.** The patient notes feelings of social isolation at home and school due to restricted diet. She is fearful of having an allergic reaction in front of her peers. The patient is assessed with standardized questionnaires. The child's parents are also interviewed.

Code **96156** would be reported with, for example, *ICD-10-CM* code **Z91.010**, allergy to peanuts. If the patient has been diagnosed with an anxiety disorder, report also a code for the anxiety disorder (eg, **F41.9**, anxiety disorder, unspecified). However, codes for mental and behavioral health conditions should not be reported as the first-listed or primary reason for health behavior assessment. The health behavior assessment is not primarily focused on behavioral health conditions.

> When neuropsychological and/or psychological testing is performed at the same session as health behavior assessment or reassessment, payer edits may require modifier **59** to be appended to the code for the testing to indicate a distinct service.

Health Behavior Intervention

Codes **96158**, **96159**, and **96164–96171**

- Are time-based services requiring documentation of the time spent face-to-face with the patient(s) and/or family.
- ✖ Do not report **96158**, **96164**, **96167**, or **96170** for less than 16 minutes of service.
- Include promotion of functional improvement, minimizing psychological and/or psychosocial barriers to recovery, and management of and improved coping with medical conditions.
- Emphasize active patient/family engagement and involvement. These interventions may be provided individually, to a group (≥2 patients), and/or to the family, with or without the patient present.

Refer to **Table 11-2** for a breakdown of the health behavior intervention codes.

Table 11-2. Health Behavior Intervention Codes		
Health Behavior Intervention Provided To	**Initial Code**	**Add-on Code**
Individual, face-to-face;	**96158** initial 16–30 min	✚**96159** each additional 15 min (List separately in addition to code **96158**)
Group (2 or more patients), face-to-face;	#**96164** initial 16–30 min	#✚**96165** each additional 15 min (List separately in addition to code **96164**)
Family (with the patient present), face-to-face;	#**96167** initial 16–30 min	#✚**96168** each additional 15 min (List separately in addition to code **96167**)
Family (without the patient present), face-to-face;	#**96170** initial 16–30 min	#✚**96171** each additional 15 min (List separately in addition to code **96170**)

Examples

➤ **Health behavior intervention is provided to an adolescent who has morbid obesity (caused by excess calories) with familial hypercholesterolemia and who does not adhere to his plan of care.** Results from a health behavior assessment are used to develop a plan to address health risk behaviors and factors impeding adherence to a plan of care developed through shared decision-making by the patient, his parents, and his physician. Thirty minutes is spent with the patient discussing the behavior and steps to help him adhere to the plan of care.

Code **96158** with 1 unit of service would be reported with diagnosis codes for the morbid obesity due to excess calories (**E66.01**) (and body mass index, if documented) and familial hypercholesterolemia (**E78.01**).

➤ **Three patients with type 1 diabetes and identified needs for better treatment adherence take part in a group intervention.** On the basis of assessments conducted at previous encounters, the clinical psychologist works with the patients to gain understanding and acceptance of their physician's care plan, addresses barriers to adherence, and helps each patient develop goals for better adherence. A total of 55 minutes is spent face-to-face with the group of patients.

Code **96164** (1 unit for first 30 minutes) and **96165** with 2 units of service (1 full 15-minute period and 1 unit for the last 10 minutes because the midpoint of 8 minutes beyond the last full period was passed). *ICD-10-CM* codes appropriate to each patient's condition (eg, appropriate codes from category **E10**, type 1 diabetes, and codes for any manifestations) are reported.

● indicates a new code; ▲, revised; #, re-sequenced; ✚, add-on; ★, audiovisual technology; and ◀, synchronous interactive audio.

Psychiatric Services

Psychiatric services include diagnostic services, psychotherapy, and other services to an individual, a family, or a group. Comprehensive services may be provided by a multidisciplinary team (eg, a psychiatrist, developmental-behavioral pediatrician, nurse practitioner, psychologist, clinical social worker, and/or clinical counselor).

However, in many parts of the country, children's mental and behavioral health professionals are not available. General pediatricians must often take on management of minor mental health problems and, when possible, consult with a mental/behavioral health professional at a distant location or arrange for telemedicine services. (See the Payment and Coverage Issues for Mental/Behavioral Health Services section earlier in this chapter for important considerations for general pediatricians providing psychiatric services.)

> Psychiatric services described by codes 90785, 90791 and 90792, 90832–90840, and 90845–90847 are included in Appendix T and preceded by the ◄, indicating that these services may be reported with modifier 93 (audio-only telemedicine service). See chapters 2 and 20 for additional information on reporting codes with modifier 93.

Interactive Complexity

★◄✚90785   Interactive complexity

Psychiatric services to children may include interactive complexity. According to *CPT*, psychiatric procedures may be reported "with interactive complexity" when at least 1 of the following circumstances is present:

- The need to manage maladaptive communication (related to, eg, high anxiety, high reactivity, repeated questions, disagreement) among participants that complicates delivery of care
- Caregiver emotions or behavior interfering with the caregiver's understanding and ability to assist in the implementation of the treatment plan
- Evidence or disclosure of a sentinel event and mandated report to third party (eg, abuse or neglect with report to state agency) with initiation of discussion of the sentinel event and/or report with the patient and other visit participants
- Use of play equipment or other physical devices to communicate with the patient to overcome barriers to therapeutic or diagnostic interaction between the physician or other QHP and a patient who has not developed or has lost either the expressive language communication skills to explain their symptoms and response to treatment or the receptive communication skills to understand the physician or other QHP if they were to use typical language for communication

Add-on code **90785** is reported when interactive complexity complicates delivery of psychiatric services, including diagnostic psychiatric evaluation (**90791**, **90792**), psychotherapy (**90832–90834**, **90836–90838**), and group psychotherapy (**90853**). Report code **90785** in conjunction with code **90853** for the specified patient when group psychotherapy includes interactive complexity.

- Interactive complexity indicates an *increased complexity of work* as opposed to an extended duration of services. The increased complexity of the psychiatric service is due to specific communication factors that can result in barriers to diagnostic or therapeutic interaction with the patient.
- Interactive complexity is not billed in conjunction with psychotherapy for crisis (**90839**, **90840**) or with psychiatric or neuropsychiatric testing (**96130–96134**, **96136–96139**, **96146**).
- *Interactive complexity applies only to the psychiatric portion of a service* including both psychiatric and E/M components. Code **90785** is never reported alone and is not reported in conjunction with E/M services alone.

    When provided in conjunction with time-based psychotherapy services, the time spent providing interactive complexity services is reflected in the time of the psychotherapy service and must relate only to the psychotherapy service.
- ✖ Do not report code **90785** in conjunction with adaptive behavior assessment or treatment services (**97151–97158**, **0362T**, **0373T**).

Examples

➤ **A 10-year-old patient undergoes psychiatric evaluation.** The child is accompanied by separated parents who report that the child has recently demonstrated significant anxiety about abandonment and has new onset of tantrums. The child's teachers report that the child requires a plan for anxiety management during the school day and is easily influenced by peers. The parents are extremely anxious and repeatedly ask questions about the treatment process. Each parent continually challenges the other's observations of the patient.

Codes **90791** (psychiatric diagnostic evaluation) and **90785** (interactive complexity) are reported.

➤ **A 6-year-old girl is seen for psychotherapy.** The child was placed in foster care following hospitalization for injuries sustained due to physical abuse and neglect by her mother 3 years before this evaluation. The service includes the psychologist's review of the child's medical record and telephone interviews with the child's social worker and teacher. The mother refuses a request for interview. The psychologist interviews current and former foster parents, who express concerns that the child is easily offended and retaliates against perceived offenses with violent outbursts. The psychologist uses play to gain trust and evaluate the child. The psychologist and foster mother agree on a treatment plan and then discuss the plan with the child in terms she can understand. Following the service, the psychologist provides a report to the patient's social worker.

Codes **90791** (psychiatric diagnostic evaluation) and **90785** (interactive complexity) are reported.

Psychiatric Diagnostic Evaluation

★◀**90791** Psychiatric diagnostic evaluation
★◀**90792** Psychiatric diagnostic evaluation with medical services

Psychiatric diagnostic evaluation (**90791**) and psychiatric diagnostic evaluation with medical services (**90792**) include an integrated biopsychosocial assessment, including history, mental status, and recommendations. When medical services (ie, medical assessments and physical examination other than mental status, when indicated) are included, code **90792** is reported by the physician or other QHP whose scope of practice includes medical services.

● Psychiatric diagnostic evaluation or reevaluation (**90791**, **90792**) is reported once per day. Do not report psychotherapy codes (90832–90839) on the same date of service as **90791** or **90792**.

● The same individual may not separately report E/M services on the same date as psychiatric diagnostic evaluation.

● Report code **90785** for interactive complexity in addition to code **90791** or **90792**, when applicable.

Health plans may not cover mental health consultation, testing, or evaluation that is performed to assess custody, visitation, or parental rights.

- **Verify health plan contractual obligations before providing services that may lack medical necessity and determine if a waiver of liability must be signed by the patient(s) before beginning the service.**
- **A waiver of liability (eg, Medicare's advance beneficiary notice) is the patient's agreement to pay out of pocket for services not covered by their health plan.**
- **Modifier GA (waiver of liability statement issued as required by payer policy, individual case) may be appended to the code reported to indicate that the waiver is on file.**

When services are requested for purposes that a health plan may not consider medically necessary, failure to obtain the responsible party's signature on a waiver of liability *before the service* may release the patient from the obligation to pay based on contractual agreement between the provider and health plan.

Examples

➤ **A 14-year-old girl is referred by her primary care pediatrician for evaluation and treatment of depression with suicidal ideation.** The psychologist obtains information on the presenting problem and situation. A statement of need and expectations is documented. Current symptoms and behaviors are documented. The patient has no history of previous psychiatric treatment. The patient does not describe previous or current substance use. Her current medication regimen of fluoxetine at 10 mg once a day is documented. She has no current medical problems and is not allergic to any medications. The patient's family and social status (current and historical), school status/functioning, and

(side margin) **Chapter 11. Mental and Behavioral Health Services**

Chapter 11. Mental and Behavioral Health Services

resources are obtained and documented. A diagnosis of moderate major depressive disorder, single episode, and parent-child relationship problem is documented.

Code **90791** is reported in conjunction with *ICD-10-CM* codes **F32.1** (major depressive disorder, single episode, moderate) and **Z63.8** (other specified problems related to primary support group).

➤ **A 15-year-old girl was admitted through the ED for new-onset psychosis.** The girl is evaluated by a psychiatrist. The psychiatrist performs a psychiatric diagnostic evaluation of this patient, who previously attempted suicide at age 13 years and has a history of recurrent major depressive disorder. The patient also expresses fear that she may be pregnant and has been exposed to a sexually transmitted infection. Medical history includes nausea with vomiting for the past week and most recent menstrual period of 6 weeks ago. Laboratory tests are ordered to rule out pregnancy and/or infection, and consultation with a gynecologist is ordered. Diagnoses are major depressive disorder, recurrent, severe with psychotic symptoms (**F33.3**); nausea with vomiting (**R11**); and pregnancy test, unconfirmed (**Z72.40**).

Code **90792** is reported for combined psychiatric and medical evaluations.

➤ **A 17-year-old girl wishes to be evaluated for the purpose of determining her ability to accept responsibility for herself.** The girl is seeking emancipation from her mother, who is currently living with an abusive boyfriend and will not allow her to move in with her aunt while finishing high school. An attorney has advised obtaining a psychological evaluation to support the girl's claims that she is psychologically prepared to take this action. The girl's health plan considers this service not medically necessary but allows for patient payment when a waiver of liability is obtained before the service. The patient agrees to sign the waiver and pay for the service. An evaluation is completed, and a report of the evaluation is provided to the girl and her attorney.

The service is reported to the health plan with modifier **GA** (waiver of liability statement issued as required by payer policy, individual case) appended to code **90791**.

Psychotherapy

CPT defines *psychotherapy* as the treatment of mental illness and behavioral disturbances in which the physician or QHP, through definitive therapeutic communications, attempts to alleviate the emotional disturbances, reverse or change maladaptive patterns of behavior, and encourage personality growth and development.

Progress notes for psychotherapy services should include

- **Start and stop times of psychotherapy**
- **Service type**
- **Diagnosis**
- **Interval history (eg, increase/decrease in symptoms, current risk factors)**
- **Names and scores of standardized rating scales used in monitoring progress**
- **Therapeutic interventions (eg, type of therapy, medications)**
- **Summary of goals and progress**
- **An updated treatment plan**
- **Date and signature of performing provider**

These elements should be documented in the progress note in the patient record rather than the protected psychotherapy notes. Protected psychotherapy notes *are not disclosed* for the purpose of receiving or supporting accurate payment.

- Services include ongoing assessment and adjustment of psychotherapeutic interventions and may include involvement of informants in the treatment process.
- Codes differentiate psychotherapy services to individuals (with and without E/M services), an individual family or groups of families, and groups of patients. Codes for each are provided in the following discussions.
- Separate codes (**90839**, **90840**) are reported for psychotherapy for crisis (see the Psychotherapy for Crisis section later in this chapter).

Follow these instructions when selecting codes for any psychotherapy service.

- Select psychotherapy codes based on face-to-face time with a patient and/or family member.

● indicates a new code; ▲, revised; #, re-sequenced; ✚, add-on; ★, audiovisual technology; and ◀, synchronous interactive audio.

- Report family psychotherapy (**90846, 90847**) for services that involve techniques to benefit the patient (eg, attempting to improve family communication or alter family interactions that negatively affect the patient, encouraging interactions to improve family functioning).
  - Family psychotherapy includes sessions with the entire family and sessions possibly without the patient.
  - The patient must be present for all or some of the service except when reporting family psychotherapy *without the patient present* (**90846**). This allows for the participation of others in the psychotherapy session for the patient as long as the patient remains the focus of the intervention. Documentation must support that the patient was present for a significant portion of the session.
- In reporting, choose the code closest to the actual time (**Table 11-3**). Do not report psychotherapy of less than 16 minutes' duration.

Table 11-3. Reporting Psychotherapy Services	
Duration of Psychotherapy (min)	**CPT Codes**
<16	Do not report.
16–37	**90832, 90833**
38–52	**90834, 90836**
53–89	**90837, 90838**
≥26	**90846, 90847** (family psychotherapy)

Abbreviation: *CPT, Current Procedural Terminology.*

- ✖ Do not report psychotherapy codes in conjunction with codes for adaptive behavior assessment or treatment services (**97153–97158, 0362T, 0373T**).
- Psychotherapy of more than 45 minutes is often considered unusual and may require health plan precertification.

> When time spent in psychotherapy exceeds time assigned to the highest level of psychotherapy service (individual or family), see codes for psychotherapy for crisis (**90839–90840**).

Psychotherapy With Evaluation and Management

★◀✚**90833** Psychotherapy, 30 minutes with patient when performed with an evaluation and management service
★◀✚**90836** 45 minutes with patient when performed with an evaluation and management service
★◀✚**90838** 60 minutes with patient when performed with an evaluation and management service

Psychiatrists and other physicians who provide a combination of psychotherapy and E/M services (eg, **99213**) on the same date may report an E/M code and an add-on code for psychotherapy (**90833, 90836, 90838**).
- To report both E/M and psychotherapy, the 2 services must be significant and separately identifiable.
- Time may not be used as the basis of E/M code selection. Evaluation and management code selection must be based on the level of *medical decision-making (MDM) alone* when reported in conjunction with psychotherapy.
- Prolonged services *may not* be reported when psychotherapy with E/M (**90833, 90836, 90838**) is reported.

Example

➤ **An 8-year-old boy presents for psychotherapy.** The psychiatrist provides not only 20 minutes of psychotherapy services (face-to-face time) but also an E/M service to reevaluate the effectiveness and patient reaction to current medications. The office E/M service includes low-level MDM based on the low number and complexity of problems (1 stable chronic illness) with moderate risk of morbidity of prescription drug management. Codes reported are **99213** and **90833**.

The 20 minutes of psychotherapy services does not include the time of the E/M service. Because the midpoint (at least 16 minutes) was passed, code **90833** (30 minutes) is reported. No modifier is required (eg, modifier **25**) because the add-on codes were assigned values that account for the overlapping practice expense of the 2 services (eg, same clinical staff and examination room).

● indicates a new code; ▲, revised; #, re-sequenced; ✚, add-on; ★, audiovisual technology; and ◀, synchronous interactive audio.

In 2022, the total non-facility RVUs assigned to codes **99213** (2.66) and **90833** (2.06) were 4.72. In contrast, when reporting only an E/M code based on the physician's total time on the date of the encounter, **99215** (40–54 minutes) is valued at 5.29 RVUs. If the physician's total time were to exceed 54 minutes, code **99417** would be reported, adding another 0.93 RVUs for each 15-minute period beyond the 54 minutes included in code **99215**.

Psychotherapy Without Evaluation and Management

★◀**90832**   Psychotherapy, 30 minutes with patient and/or family member

★◀**90834**   45 minutes with patient and/or family member

★◀**90837**   60 minutes with patient and/or family member

★✚**90863**   Pharmacologic management, including prescription and review of medication, when performed with psychotherapy services

When psychotherapy is provided without an E/M service on the same date, codes **90832**, **90834**, and **90837** are reported on the basis of the face-to-face time of service.

- To accommodate reporting of pharmacological management by psychologists who have prescribing privileges but who cannot provide E/M services, add-on code **90863** is reported in addition to the appropriate code for psychotherapy without E/M.

  Only a psychologist with prescribing authority may provide pharmacological management. Other QHPs may provide psychotherapy but must collaborate with a physician or advance practice professional who provides pharmacological management.

- Physicians and QHPs providing pharmacological management report the service with an E/M code.

- Code **90863** is an add-on code and may be reported only in addition to one of the stand-alone psychotherapy codes (ie, **90832**, **90834**, **90837**). Time spent providing medication management is not included in the time spent in psychotherapy.

Example

➤ **An 8-year-old boy presents for psychotherapy.** The licensed clinical psychologist (whose state scope of practice includes prescribing authority) provides psychotherapy services with face-to-face time of 40 minutes and also provides a pharmacological management service to reevaluate the effectiveness and patient reaction to current medications. Codes reported are **90834** and **90863**.

  A physician or other QHP who may provide and report E/M services would report code **90836** (psychotherapy with E/M, 40 minutes) for this service.

Psychotherapy With Biofeedback

90875   Individual psychophysiological therapy incorporating biofeedback training by any modality (face-to-face with the patient), with psychotherapy (eg, insight oriented, behavior modifying or supportive psychotherapy); 30 minutes

90876   45 minutes

When psychotherapy incorporates biofeedback training, code **90875** or **90876** is reported on the basis of the face-to-face time of the combined services. Do not separately report codes for psychotherapy (**90832–90838**) or biofeedback training (**90901**).

Example

➤ **A child with frequent tension headaches is provided psychotherapy and biofeedback training to help her cope with and control her pain.** The face-to-face time of service is 45 minutes.

  Code **90876** is reported for the combined services. Were biofeedback training provided on a date when no psychotherapy was provided, code **90901** would be reported. Time of service is not a factor in reporting code **90901**.

Psychotherapy for Crisis

★◀**90839**   Psychotherapy for crisis; first 60 minutes

★◀✚**90840**   each additional 30 minutes (List separately in addition to code **90839**)

●, indicates a new code; ▲, revised; #, re-sequenced; ✚, add-on; ★, audiovisual technology; and ◀, synchronous interactive audio.

Psychotherapy for crisis is provided on an urgent basis to a patient requiring mobilization of resources to defuse a crisis and restore safety. It also incorporates implementation of psychotherapeutic interventions to minimize the potential for psychological trauma.

● This includes assessment and history of a crisis state, a mental status examination, and a disposition.

● The presenting problem is typically life threatening or complex and requires immediate attention to a patient in high distress.

● Codes **90839** and **90840** are reported on the basis of the total face-to-face time the physician or QHP spends with the patient and/or family providing psychotherapy for crisis on a single date of service. Time is cumulative for all psychotherapy for crisis on the same date even if time is not continuous.

— Code **90839** is reported for the first 30 to 74 minutes of psychotherapy for crisis on a single date of service. For psychotherapy for crisis with face-to-face time of less than 30 minutes' duration, report individual psychotherapy codes (**90832** or **90833**).

— Add code **90840** for each additional block of time (ie, 1 unit for 75–90 minutes and additional units for each period up to 30 minutes beyond 90 minutes).

✖ Do not report psychotherapy for crisis (**90839**, **90840**) for service of less than 30 minutes or on the same date as other psychiatry services (**90785–90899**).

Example

➤ **A psychologist or psychiatrist is consulted in the ED for a patient who was brought to the hospital by his parents after threatening to harm others and exhibiting paranoia.** The psychologist obtains history from the patient's parents. The psychologist examines the patient, obtains agreement for inpatient treatment, and makes arrangements for admission. The total face-to-face time of the encounter is 45 minutes.

Code **90839** is reported. Although the code descriptor states, "first 60 minutes," the instructions for reporting psychotherapy for crisis instruct that code **90839** is reported for the first 30 to 74 minutes of face-to-face service.

Family Psychotherapy

★◀**90846**   Family psychotherapy (without the patient present), 50 minutes
★◀**90847**   Family psychotherapy (conjoint psychotherapy) (with patient present), 50 minutes
90849   Multiple-family group psychotherapy

While family members may act as informants during individual psychotherapy, psychotherapy using family psychotherapy techniques is reported with codes **90846** and **90847** on the basis of whether the patient is present for the service.

● The focus of family psychotherapy is on family dynamics and/or subsystems within the family (eg, parents, siblings) and on improving the patient's functioning by working with the patient in the context of the family.

✖ Do not report family psychotherapy for services of less than 26 minutes.

● Codes for individual psychotherapy (**90832–90838**) may be reported on the same day as family psychotherapy codes **90846** and **90847** when the services are separate and distinct. Append modifier **59** (distinct procedural service) to the group psychotherapy code when both services are reported on the same date.

● When multiple families participate in family psychotherapy at the same session, code **90849** is reported once for each family.

Group Psychotherapy

90853   Group psychotherapy (other than of a multiple-family group)
● Report code **90853** with 1 unit of service for each group member. Documentation should support the individual patient's involvement in the group session, the duration of the session, and issues that were presented.

● No time is assigned to code **90853**. This service is reported with 1 unit of service regardless of the time of service.

Other Psychiatric Services

The following services are often bundled under payer contracts (ie, considered components of other services) or noncovered. However, check plan benefits, especially for Medicaid patients, as there may be circumstances in which these services are separate benefits. Plan-specific modifiers are often required when coverage of the following services is a health plan benefit:

Chapter 11. Mental and Behavioral Health Services

90882   Environmental intervention for medical management purposes on a psychiatric patient's behalf with agencies, employers, or institutions

90885   Psychiatric evaluation of hospital records, other psychiatric reports, psychometric and/or projective tests, and other accumulated data for medical diagnostic purposes

> **Code 90885 may be reported in addition to psychotherapy services (90832–90838) when both services are provided by the same individual on the same date of service.**

90887   Interpretation or explanation of results of psychiatric, other medical examinations and procedures, or other accumulated data to family or other responsible persons, or advising them how to assist patient

Do not report code **90887** in conjunction with adaptive behavior services (**97151–97158, 0362T, 0373T**).

90889   Preparation of report of patient's psychiatric status, history, treatment, or progress (other than for legal or consultative purposes) for other individuals, agencies, or insurance carriers

Code **90889** should not be reported in conjunction with psychological or developmental testing, as the codes for these services include time for report writing.

● ✚ **0770T**   Virtual reality technology to assist therapy

Code **0770T** represents the practice expense of using virtual reality technology in conjunction with specified patient therapy. Report **0770T** in addition to codes for psychotherapy (**90832–90853**); treatment of speech, language, voice, communication, and/or auditory processing disorder (**92507, 92508**); health and behavior assessment/intervention (**96158–96171**); physical therapeutic procedures (**97110–97112, 97150, 97530–97537**); therapeutic interventions that focus on cognitive function (**97129**); and adaptive behavior services (**97153–97155, 97158**).

To test your knowledge of the information presented in this chapter, complete the quiz found at the end of it, after the resources. Answers to each quiz are found in **Appendix IV**.

Chapter Takeaways

A variety of services related to diagnosis and management of behavioral and mental health have been discussed in this chapter. Following are some takeaways from this chapter:

- Services for behavioral and mental health conditions may include a variety of health care professionals working within their scope of practice.
- Billing and coding of behavioral and mental health services must align with not only coding guidelines but also state scope of practice and individual payer policies on credentialing, network participation, and contracting.
- When payers deny claims appropriately reported with codes **F01–F99**, limiting submission of these codes to providers in a mental or behavioral health network, pediatricians may report the issue by using the AAP Coding Hotline (https://form.jotform.com/Subspecialty/aapcodinghotline) or seek the assistance of an AAP pediatric council (www.aap.org/en/practice-management/practice-financing/payer-contracting-advocacy-and-other-resources/aap-payer-advocacy/aap-pediatric-councils).

Resources

AAP Coding Assistance and Education

"AAP-AACAP-CHA Declaration of a National Emergency in Child and Adolescent Mental Health" (www.aap.org/en/advocacy/child-and-adolescent-healthy-mental-development/aap-aacap-cha-declaration-of-a-national-emergency-in-child-and-adolescent-mental-health)

AAP Coding Hotline (https://form.jotform.com/Subspecialty/aapcodinghotline)

AAP pediatric councils (www.aap.org/en/practice-management/practice-financing/payer-contracting-advocacy-and-other-resources/aap-payer-advocacy/aap-pediatric-councils)

AAP *Pediatric Mental Health: Coding Quick Reference Card 2023* (https://shop.aap.org/pediatric-mental-health-coding-quick-reference-card-2023)

● indicates a new code; ▲, revised; #, re-sequenced; ✚, add-on; ★, audiovisual technology; and ◀, synchronous interactive audio.

AAP Policy Statement

"Addressing Early Childhood Emotional and Behavioral Problems" (https://doi.org/10.1542/peds.2016-3023)

Test Your Knowledge!

1. **Which of the following statements is true of health plan coverage for mental and behavioral health services?**
   a. Only psychiatrists and psychologists can provide and bill for these services.
   b. These services may be covered through a plan and provider network separate from other health care services.
   c. Health plans are required to use the same network for mental and behavioral health services as for medical services.
   d. General pediatricians and other qualified health care professionals are always eligible to participate in the behavioral health plan network.

2. **A diagnosis of substance abuse with dependence is documented. Which of the following types of codes is reported?**
   a. Use
   b. Abuse
   c. Dependence
   d. All of the above

3. **Which of the following *Current Procedural Terminology* codes or code series are reported for behavioral health care manager activities provided under physician supervision and in consultation with a psychiatric consultant?**
   a. General behavioral health integration (**99484**)
   b. Health behavior intervention (**96158** and **96159**)
   c. Psychiatric collaborative care management (**99492–99494**)
   d. Psychological/neuropsychological test administration and scoring (**96138** and **96139**)

4. **Codes 96202 and 96203 describe which of the following types of service?**
   a. Behavior management/modification training provided to a multiple-family group of parent(s)/guardian(s)/caregiver(s)
   b. Psychotherapy provided to a group
   c. Family adaptive behavior treatment guidance
   d. Behavior management/modification training provided directly to patients

5. **True or false? The patient must always be present for family psychotherapy services.**
   a. True
   b. False

● indicates a new code; ▲, revised; #, re-sequenced; ✚, add-on; ★, audiovisual technology; and ◀, synchronous interactive audio.

Common Non-facility Testing and Therapeutic Services

CPT copyright 2022 American Medical Association. All rights reserved.

Contents

● indicates a new code; ▲, revised; #, re-sequenced; ✚, add-on; ★, audiovisual technology; and ◀, synchronous interactive audio.

● indicates a new code; ▲, revised; #, re-sequenced; ✚, add-on; ★, audiovisual technology; and ◄, synchronous interactive audio.

Chapter Highlights

- Professional and technical components of services
- Supplies and medications
- In-office pathology, laboratory, and radiology services
- Respiratory testing and treatment services
- Allergy testing and allergen immunotherapy

Professional and Technical Components

This chapter includes discussion of codes for some of the most common tests and therapeutic services performed in physician offices and outpatient clinics. Certain procedures (eg, electrocardiography [ECG], radiography, diagnostic procedures) include a professional component and a technical component.

- The *professional component* includes the physician work (eg, interpretation of the test, writing of a report).
- The *technical component* includes the costs associated with providing the service (eg, equipment, salaries of technical personnel, supplies, expense of facility).

Interpretation and Report

Many tests include recording of results and a report with interpretation. *Current Procedural Terminology* (*CPT*®) instructs that

- *Results* are the technical component of a service. Testing leads to results; results lead to interpretation.
- *Reports* are the work product of the interpretation of test results.
- Certain procedures or services described in *CPT* involve a technical component (eg, tests), which produces results (eg, data, images, slides). For clinical use, some of these results require interpretation. Some *CPT* descriptors specifically require interpretation and reporting to report that code.

Do not separately report review of another physician's interpretation and report or personal review of the tracing that has been interpreted by another physician. However, these activities contribute to the medical decision-making (MDM) for any related evaluation and management (E/M) service.

Pediatricians performing services that include an interpretation of results should become familiar with the types of reports typical for each test (eg, typical report produced for the interpretation of ECG tracings). A report generated by an automated system is not typically sufficient to support reporting a service described as "with interpretation and report."

Some tests do not require interpretation and report (eg, point-of-care laboratory tests) but, rather, provide results that require analysis of how the result does or does not influence patient management or treatment. Use of the results in MDM may be credited to the amount and/or complexity of data to be reviewed and analyzed for an E/M encounter. See **Chapter 6** for more information on how tests ordered and results reviewed influence the level of MDM of an E/M service.

Professional and Technical Component Modifiers

26   Professional component: When the physician or other qualified health care professional is reporting only the professional component of a service, append modifier **26** to the procedure code.

TC   Technical component: When reporting only the technical component of a service, append modifier **TC** to the procedure code.

Modifiers are used to indicate that either the professional or the technical component was performed, but not both.

> When the physician owns the equipment and is performing the technical and professional services, the **26** or the **TC** modifier should not be appended to the code.

- If a physician is performing a service or procedure with equipment owned by a facility or another entity and the codes are written as a global service, services are reported with modifier **26** (professional component).

- *CPT* does not include a modifier for reporting the technical component. However, most payers recognize Healthcare Common Procedure Coding System (HCPCS) modifier **TC**. Facilities or an office providing use of its equipment would only report the same service by using modifier **TC**.
- Some codes were developed to distinguish between the technical and professional components (eg, routine ECG codes **93000–93010**); however, many do not.

No modifier is appended when the code descriptor for the service identifies whether the professional, technical, or global service is being reported.

Examples

➤ **A physician orders 2-view chest radiography of a child.** The child is sent to a neighboring physician's office (or outpatient department) for the radiograph (without interpretation). The radiographs are then brought back to the office and the pediatrician interprets them and creates a report of the findings.
> Physician: **71046 26** (radiologic examination, chest; 2 views)
> Neighboring physician's office: **71046 TC**

➤ **A physician orders 12-lead ECG of an adolescent patient.** The patient is sent to another office that has an ECG machine to perform the ECG. The tracings are taken back to the pediatrician for review and written interpretation and report.
> Physician: **93010** (routine ECG with at least 12 leads; interpretation and report only)
> Other office: **93005** (routine ECG with at least 12 leads; tracing only, without interpretation and report)
> Modifiers **26** and **TC** are not appended because the codes designate the professional and technical components.
> When interpreting an ECG at a location remote from the site of the tracing, follow payer guidelines for reporting. The place of service for remote interpretation and report is typically the site where the technical component of the test was performed (eg, outpatient hospital). Payer guidelines may vary.

Supplies and Medications

Supplies and Materials

99070   Supplies and materials provided by the physician over and above those usually included with the office visit or other services rendered

99071   Educational supplies, such as books, tapes, and pamphlets, for the patient's education at cost to physician or other qualified health care professional

The practice expense relative value units (RVUs) assigned to most services include the value of supplies (eg, masks, tubing, gauze, needles) that are typically required for each service.

> **If reporting code 99070, identify the supplies or materials on the claim form and be prepared to submit an invoice.**

- Supplies should be separately reported when a payer does not use a payment methodology based on the RVUs assigned to each code under the Medicare Physician Fee Schedule. However, most payers today use a payment method based on RVUs and do not provide separate payment for supplies.
- Items such as elastic wraps, clavicle splints, or circumcision and suturing trays may be reported with this code. Remember that some supplies (eg, suturing trays, circumcision trays) may be included with the surgical procedure if the payer uses RVUs as its basis for payment.
- Only the supplies purchased in an office-based practice may be reported.
- Some payers will require the use of HCPCS codes. HCPCS codes are available for a number of supplies (eg, codes **Q4001–Q4051** for cast and splint supplies). Use HCPCS codes when they are more specific than code **99070**.
- Code **99071** may be reported when the physician incurs costs for educational supplies and provides these supplies to the patient at cost. This code may be denied because of payment policies that consider supplies reported with **99071** a practice expense of a related service.

Medications

Medications used in testing or treatment (eg, albuterol) are not included in the value of service and are separately reported with HCPCS codes (eg, **J7613**, albuterol, inhalation solution, US Food and Drug Administration [FDA]-approved final product, noncompounded, administered through durable medical equipment [DME], unit dose, 1 mg).

See www.aap.org/cfp2023 for a table of the most commonly used pediatric medications, associated HCPCS **J** codes, and related administration codes.

- Report medications when the practice must have incurred a cost for the medication.
- Most payers do not cover services reported with nonspecific codes.
- Check with payers to determine if they accept these HCPCS codes or if they require reporting with code **99070**.
- Drugs are listed with a base dosage. When the dosage exceeds the amount listed, report additional units for the total dosage administered.
- Report the National Drug Code (NDC) in addition to **J** codes to provide more precise information on the medication administered. The NDC should always be reported in addition to code **99070** or **J3490** (unclassified drug). You can find a list of NDCs at www.fda.gov/drugs/drug-approvals-and-databases/national-drug-code-directory.

> **For more information on National Drug Codes, see Chapter 1.**

Some payers require modifiers **KP** (first drug of a multiple drug unit dose formulation) and **KQ** (second drug of a multiple drug unit dose formulation) when multiple NDCs are reported for *a single drug* supplied in a unit dose formulation and the total dose is greater than the amount supplied in a single-dose vial or container. Follow payer instructions for reporting these modifiers.

Blood Sampling for Diagnostic Study

Report collection of blood samples for testing (eg, venipuncture) in a physician practice regardless of whether the laboratory test is performed in the office or at an outside facility.

Venipuncture

36400	Venipuncture, younger than age 3 years, necessitating the skill of a physician or other qualified health care professional, not to be used for routine venipuncture; femoral or jugular vein
36405	scalp vein
36406	other vein
36410	Venipuncture, age 3 years or older, necessitating the skill of a physician or other qualified health care professional (separate procedure), for diagnostic or therapeutic purposes (not to be used for routine venipuncture)
36415	Collection of venous blood by venipuncture
36416	Collection of capillary blood specimen (eg, finger, heel, ear stick)
36591	Collection of blood specimen from a completely implantable venous access device

Report codes **36415** and **36416** for venipuncture performed on children of any age when the physician is not needed to perform the procedure. Some payers bundle code **36416** into the practice expense of a related service and do not pay for services reported with this code.

- When a physician's skill is required to perform venipuncture (eg, access is too difficult for other staff to attain) on a child younger than 3 years, codes **36400–36406** are reported on the basis of the anatomical site of the venipuncture as follows:
  - **36400** (femoral or jugular vein)
  - **36405** (scalp vein)
  - **36406** (another vein)
- Report code **36410** when a physician's skill is required to perform venipuncture on a child 3 years or older.

> **If the physician performs the venipuncture as a convenience or because staff is not trained in the procedure, code 36415 is reported because the physician's skill was not required.**

Some payers require that modifier **25** be appended to the E/M code if an E/M service is reported on the same day of service. This is atypical practice.

- If the *only service* provided is the obtainment of a blood specimen, only the laboratory test and/or venipuncture or capillary finger stick is reported.
  - It is inappropriate to report a nurse visit (**99211**) in these cases.
  - If a medically necessary nursing E/M service is performed in compliance with payer guidelines (eg, incident to a physician's service) on the same date as venipuncture, append modifier **25** to code **99211**.
- Report code **36591** (collection of blood specimen from a completely implantable venous access device) only when performed in conjunction with a laboratory service.

> **See Chapter 19 for discussion of arterial catheterization.**

Arterial Puncture

36600   Arterial puncture, withdrawal of blood for diagnosis

Arterial puncture (eg, radial artery) with withdrawal of blood for diagnosis is reported with code **36600**.

> **Specimen collection (eg, nasal or oral swab, urine collection), other than blood sampling, is typically not separately reported. Follow payer guidelines when exceptions are made for specimen collection (as occurred during the public health emergency caused by COVID-19).**

Pathology and Laboratory Procedures

CPT laboratory codes may either be generic for a particular analyte that is independent of testing method or have a specific *CPT* code, depending on the method used for the particular analysis.

Clinical Laboratory Improvement Amendments (CLIA)–Waived Tests

The Clinical Laboratory Improvement Amendments (CLIA) establish quality standards for all laboratory testing to ensure the accuracy, reliability, and timeliness of patient test results regardless of where the test was performed. All laboratories, including those within a physician practice, must comply with CLIA and must typically report a CLIA certificate number on claims.

- A *laboratory* is defined as any facility that performs laboratory testing on specimens derived from humans for the purpose of providing information for the diagnosis, prevention, and treatment of disease or impairment or assessment of health.
- The term *CLIA waived* refers to simple laboratory examinations and procedures that have an insignificant risk of an erroneous result when manufacturer instructions are followed. One typical test that is CLIA waived is urinalysis without microscopy (**81002**). Other tests require higher levels of CLIA certification (eg, provider-performed microscopy).
- The term *moderate complexity* refers to tests that are performed only by laboratories certified as meeting the CLIA quality system standards, such as those for proficiency testing, quality control and assessment, and personnel requirements. The difference between moderate- and high-complexity certification is the personnel required.
  - Some codes represent both CLIA-waived and higher-complexity test systems.

> **Not Sure How a Test Is Categorized?**
>
> **See the US Food and Drug Administration Clinical Laboratory Improvement Amendments database at www.accessdata.fda.gov/scripts/ cdrh/cfdocs/cfCLIA/search.cfm for tests of all categories by test system, manufacturer, or analyte. If your practice provides only waived test systems and analytes, see www.accessdata.fda.gov/scripts/cdrh/cfdocs/cfClia/analyteswaived.cfm.**

- Laboratories and physician offices performing waived tests may need to append modifier **QW** to the *CPT* code for CLIA-waived procedures. The use of modifier **QW** is payer specific.

  Only a small number of CLIA-waived tests are exempt from the use of modifier **QW** (eg, **81002**, non-automated urinalysis without microscopy; **81025**, urine pregnancy test; **82272**, occult blood by peroxidase for other than colorectal neoplasm screening).

General Guidance for Reporting Laboratory Services

- Report a test performed in the office's laboratory by using the appropriate laboratory code and, if performed, the appropriate blood collection code (**36400–36416**).

- Link the appropriate diagnosis code to the laboratory procedure and/or venipuncture and handling fee. The diagnosis must support the medical necessity or reason for the test or service.
- ✖ Do not report any laboratory test that is *not performed* in the office (eg, thyroid function, laboratory panels, phenylketonuria). Instead, report the appropriate blood-drawing code (**36415** or **36416**), when applicable, and handling fee code (**99000**).

  Exception: Follow state regulations and payer policies for physician billing of laboratory services performed by an outside laboratory. Generally, if the laboratory bills the pediatrician for the test, bill the patient by using the appropriate laboratory analysis code with modifier **90** to indicate that the procedure was performed in an outside laboratory.

Example

➤ **The physician orders a laboratory test requiring a blood sample, and the nurse obtains the blood via venipuncture.** The specimen is sent to an outside laboratory for processing.

Only the venipuncture (**36415**) and handling fee (**99000**) would be reported in addition to the E/M service and other procedures performed on that day.

Laboratory Panel Coding

All laboratory test panels in *CPT* were specifically developed only for coding purposes and should not be interpreted as clinical parameters. (See codes **80047–80076** for a component listing of these panels.) For example, the lipid panel (**80061**) includes total cholesterol (**82465**), high-density lipoprotein cholesterol (**83718**), and triglycerides (**84478**). Any additional tests performed can be coded separately from the panel code. *Do not unbundle individual laboratory tests if a laboratory panel code is available.*

Direct Optical Observation

Direct optical (ie, visual) observation is a testing platform that provides a result (ie, positive or negative) by producing a signal on the reaction chamber (eg, test strip with colored bands) that can be interpreted visually (eg, point-of-care influenza testing). (See codes **87804** [influenza], **87807** [respiratory syncytial virus], and **87880** [group A *Streptococcus*].)

Per *CPT,* when reporting tests performed by using direct optical observation, the number of unique results (eg, 2 results—positive for influenza A and negative for influenza B) determines the units of service reported.

Cultures

- Use code **87086** (culture, bacterial; quantitative colony count, urine) once per encounter for urine culture to determine the approximate number of bacteria present per milliliter of urine.
- Use of a commercial kit with defined media to identify isolates in a positive urine culture is reported with **87088** (culture, bacterial; quantitative colony count, urine with isolation and presumptive identification of each isolate).
- Code **81007** (urinalysis; bacteriuria screen, except by culture or dipstick) (CLIA waived) can be used for a bacteriuria screening by non-culture technique using a commercial kit. The type of commercial kit must be specified.
- Code **87070** (culture, bacterial; any other source except urine, blood, or stool) is reported for throat cultures.
- Use code **87045** to report culture, bacteria of the stool, aerobic, with isolation and preliminary examination (eg, Kligler [triple sugar] iron agar, lysine iron agar) for *Salmonella* and *Shigella* species. Additional pathogens are reported with code **87046** with 1 unit per plate.
- Culture, presumptive pathogenic organisms, screening only (**87081**), is reported for testing for a specific organism (eg, *Streptococcus*).
- Report services with the symptoms (eg, dysuria) or the confirmed diagnosis (eg, urinary tract infection).

Proprietary Laboratory Analyses and Multianalyte Assays With Algorithmic Analyses

To report testing performed by using a proprietary laboratory analyses (PLA) or multianalyte assays with algorithmic analyses (MAAA), see Appendix O in your *CPT* reference, and for quarterly code updates, see www.ama-assn.org/practice-management/cpt/cpt-pla-codes. Code selection for PLA and MAAA codes is based on the analysis performed and the proprietary name of the test. **Table 12-1** shows how PLA and MAAA codes are listed in Appendix O. Codes for genomic sequencing procedures are also listed in Appendix O.

Chapter 12. Common Non-facility Testing and Therapeutic Services

Table 12-1. Example of Appendix O Proprietary Laboratory Analyses Code List		
Test Name	**Code**	**Code Descriptor**
ePlex Respiratory Pathogen Panel 2, GenMark Dx, GenMark Diagnostics, Inc	0225U	Infectious disease (bacterial or viral respiratory tract infection), pathogen-specific DNA and RNA, 21 targets, including severe acute respiratory syndrome coronavirus 2 (SARS-CoV-2), amplified probe technique, including multiplex reverse transcription for RNA targets, each analyte reported as detected or not detected

Laboratory Tests Frequently Performed in the Office

COVID-19 (SARS-CoV-2 Infection) Testing

Tests for coronavirus (SARS-CoV-2) include those to detect the virus and those to detect antibodies to the virus.

Some tests for SARS-CoV-2 are designated as CLIA waived under an emergency use authorization during the public health emergency (PHE) caused by COVID-19. It is advisable to verify the current classification of a test before purchase.

Diagnosis coding for SARS-CoV-2 is based on the current *International Classification of Diseases, 10th Revision, Clinical Modification (ICD-10-CM)* codes and guidelines. During the PHE, *ICD-10-CM* guidelines were updated to provide specific advice on coding for testing of patients with and without symptoms. A table of diagnosis codes for reporting various patient indications for evaluation and testing for COVID-19 is included in the August 2021 *AAP Pediatric Coding Newsletter* article, "Table of Diagnosis Coding for Services Related to COVID-19 Exposure or Infection" (https://doi.org/10.1542/pcco_book208_document002).

SARS-CoV-2 Infection Testing

When multiple specimens are collected (eg, nasopharyngeal and oropharyngeal swabs), verify payer instructions for reporting separate assays on each specimen (eg, report **87635** and **87635 59**).

87635   Infectious agent detection by nucleic acid (DNA or RNA); severe acute respiratory syndrome coronavirus 2 (SARS-CoV-2) (Coronavirus disease [COVID-19]), amplified probe technique

87426   Infectious agent antigen detection by immunoassay technique (eg, enzyme immunoassay [EIA], enzyme-linked immunosorbent assay [ELISA], fluorescence immunoassay [FIA], immunochemiluminometric assay [IMCA]), qualitative or semiquantitative; severe acute respiratory syndrome coronavirus (eg, SARS-CoV, SARS-CoV-2 [COVID-19]) (CLIA-waived)

#87811   Infectious agent antigen detection by immunoassay with direct optical (ie, visual) observation; severe acute respiratory syndrome coronavirus 2 (SARS-CoV-2) (Coronavirus disease [COVID-19]) (CLIA-waived)

See also HCPCS codes **U0001–U0004**, which may be used to identify tests developed by the Centers for Disease Control and Prevention and/or performed via high-throughput technologies.

Combination Testing for SARS-CoV-2 and Other Infectious Agent(s)

To distinctly report testing for SARS-CoV-2 infection (COVID-19) in combination with other seasonal respiratory infections, *CPT* includes distinct combination codes for tests to detect SARS-CoV-2, influenza A and B viruses, and/or respiratory syncytial virus.

✖ Do not report **87631–87633** (multiple respiratory infectious agent detection by nucleic acid by number of targets) when one of the following codes describes the test performed:

#87428   Infectious agent antigen detection by immunoassay technique (eg, enzyme immunoassay [EIA], enzyme-linked immunosorbent assay [ELISA], fluorescence immunoassay [FIA], immunochemiluminometric assay [IMCA]), qualitative or semiquantitative; severe acute respiratory syndrome coronavirus (eg, SARS-CoV, SARS-CoV-2 [COVID-19]) and influenza virus types A and B

87636   Infectious agent detection by nucleic acid (DNA or RNA); severe acute respiratory syndrome coronavirus 2 (SARS-CoV-2) (Coronavirus disease [COVID-19]) and influenza virus types A and B, multiplex amplified probe technique

87637   Infectious agent detection by nucleic acid (DNA or RNA); severe acute respiratory syndrome coronavirus 2 (SARS-CoV-2) (Coronavirus disease [COVID-19]), influenza virus types A and B, and respiratory syncytial virus, multiplex amplified probe technique

Report **87631–87633** when testing for SARS-CoV-2 and additional pathogens beyond those described by the codes listed. Note that respiratory viral panels as described in codes **87631–87633** may have limited or no coverage in the outpatient/office setting. Verify payer policy before testing.

The most up-to-date PLA codes for detecting SARS-CoV-2 in addition to other pathogens are most easily found in *CPT* Appendix O and quarterly updates posted to www.ama-assn.org/practice-management/cpt/cpt-pla-codes. The specific test name is followed by the code and its descriptor. Remember that both the code descriptor and the proprietary name must match the test performed.

Glucose Tests

82947	Glucose, quantitative, blood (without a reagent strip) (CLIA waived)
82948	blood, reagent strip
82951	Glucose tolerance test (GTT), 3 specimens (CLIA waived)
82952	each additional beyond 3 specimens (CLIA waived)
82962	Glucose, blood by glucose monitoring device(s) cleared by the FDA specifically for home use (CLIA waived)
83036	Hemoglobin; glycosylated (A_{1c}) (CLIA waived)
83037	Hemoglobin; glycosylated (A_{1c}) by device cleared by FDA for home use (CLIA waived)

Report code **83037** for in-office hemoglobin A_{1c} measurement using a device that is cleared by the FDA for home use. This test is not limited to use in a patient's home.

Code **82962** describes the method when whole blood is obtained (usually by finger-stick device) and assayed by glucose oxidase, hexokinase, or electrochemical methods and spectrophotometry using a small portable device designed for home blood glucose monitoring. The devices are also used in physician offices, during home visits, or in clinics.

Continuous glucose monitoring is reported with codes **95249–95251** (for a discussion, see **Chapter 21**).

Hematology

85013	Spun microhematocrit (CLIA waived)
85018	Hemoglobin (CLIA waived)
85025–85027	Complete blood cell count, automated (**85025** is CLIA waived.)
88738	Hemoglobin (Hgb), quantitative, transcutaneous

If using a complete blood cell count (CBC) machine to perform only a hemoglobin test, follow these guidelines.

- If the CBC result is normal, only the hemoglobin level may be reported because that was the medically necessary test ordered.
- If the CBC reveals an abnormality and it is addressed during the course of the visit, the CBC result may be reported. The abnormality would be linked to the procedure, and the medical record would need to include documentation for the ordering of the test and to support the medical necessity of the procedure.

Influenza Point-of-Care Testing

87502	Infectious agent detection by nucleic acid (DNA or RNA); influenza virus, for multiple types or sub-types, includes multiplex reverse transcription, when performed, and multiplex amplified probe technique, first 2 types or sub-types (CLIA waived)
87804	Infectious agent antigen detection by immunoassay with direct optical (ie, visual) observation; influenza (CLIA waived)

> Code **87502** describes a test that already takes into account the first 2 types or subtypes; therefore, do not report multiple units of code **87502** for the separate testing of influenza A and B.

- Code **87804** may be reported twice with modifier **59** appended to the second code when tests performed separately detect the influenza A and B antigen, providing 2 distinct results. This applies whether the test kit uses 1 or 2 analytic chambers to deliver 2 distinct results.
  - Check with payers; some do not recognize modifier **59** and may require reporting with 2 units of service and no modifier.
  - Some payers (eg, Medicaid plans) may limit units reported to the number of separate test kits used rather than following *CPT* instruction.

Chapter 12. Common Non-facility Testing and Therapeutic Services

See also the Combination Testing for SARS-CoV-2 and Other Infectious Agent(s) section earlier in this chapter for a discussion of codes as related to combination testing of COVID-19 and other respiratory illnesses, including influenza.

Lead Testing

83655   Lead, quantitative analysis (CLIA waived)

- This test does not specify the specimen source or the method of testing. Alternative tests sometimes (although rarely) used for lead screening are **82135** (aminolevulinic acid, delta), **84202** (protoporphyrin, red blood cell count, quantitative), and **84203** (protoporphyrin, red blood cell count, screen).
- Some states provide lead testing at no cost to patients covered under the Medicaid Early and Periodic Screening, Diagnostic, and Treatment program. Check your Medicaid requirements for reporting this service.
- Report *ICD-10-CM* code **Z13.88** (encounter for screening for disorder due to exposure to contaminants) when performing lead screening. Some payers require **Z77.011**, contact with and (suspected) exposure to lead, in lieu of **Z13.88**.

> *International Classification of Diseases, 10th Revision, Clinical Modification* allows separate reporting of special screening examinations (codes in categories Z11–Z13) in addition to the codes for routine child health examinations (eg, Z00.121, Z00.129) when these codes provide additional information. A screening code is not necessary if the screening is inherent to a routine examination.

Mononucleosis Heterophile Antibodies Screening

86308   Heterophile antibodies; screening (CLIA waived)

   This code may be appropriate for rapid mononucleosis screening.

Papanicolaou Tests

- The laboratory performing the cytology and interpretation reports Papanicolaou (Pap) tests with codes **88141–88155**, **88164–88167**, or **88174** and **88175**.
- Obtaining a Pap test specimen is inherent to the physical examination performed during a preventive medicine visit or a problem-oriented office visit.
- Medicare does require reporting HCPCS code **Q0091** (screening Papanicolaou, obtaining, preparing, and conveyance of cervical and vaginal smear to laboratory) in addition to the E/M service for preventive medicine and problem-oriented office visits.
  — Some Medicaid programs and commercial payers may also recognize obtaining a Pap test as a separate service.
  — Code **Q0091** cannot be reported when a patient must return for a repeated Pap test due to inadequate initial sampling.
  — If not reporting **Q0091**, a handling fee (**99000**) can be reported in addition to an E/M service if the Pap test was obtained and sent to a laboratory.
- The appropriate *ICD-10-CM* code to link to the E/M code or code **Q0091** is either **Z01.411** (encounter for gynecological examination [general] [routine] with abnormal findings) or **Z01.419** (encounter for gynecological examination [general] [routine] without abnormal findings).
- For screening cervical Pap test not part of a gynecologic examination, report *ICD-10-CM* code **Z12.4** (encounter for screening for malignant neoplasm of cervix).
- For high-risk patients, you may also report secondary diagnosis codes to indicate personal history of other medical treatment (**Z92.89**) or other contact with and (suspected) exposures hazardous to health (**Z77.9**).

Presumptive Drug Tests

#80305   Drug test(s), presumptive, any number of drug classes, any number of devices or procedures; capable of being read by direct optical observation only (eg, utilizing immunoassay [eg, dipsticks, cups, cards, or cartridges]); includes sample validation when performed, per date of service (CLIA waived)

#80306   read by instrument assisted direct optical observation (eg, utilizing immunoassay [eg, dipsticks, cups, cards, or cartridges]); includes sample validation when performed, per date of service

#80307   by instrument chemistry analyzers (eg, utilizing immunoassay [eg, EIA, ELISA, EMIT, FPIA, IA, KIMS, RIA]), chromatography (eg, GC, HPLC), and mass spectrometry either with or without chromatography (eg, DART, DESI, GC-MS, GC-MS/MS, LC-MS, LC-MS/MS, LDTD, MALDI, TOF); includes sample validation when performed, per date of service

---

● indicates a new code; ▲, revised; #, re-sequenced; ✚, add-on; ★, audiovisual technology; and ◀, synchronous interactive audio.

- Presumptive drug class screening includes all drugs and drug classes performed by the respective methodology (eg, dipstick kit with direct optical observation) on a single date of service. Sample validation is included in presumptive drug screening service.
- Venipuncture to obtain samples for drug testing may be separately reportable with code **36415** (collection of venous blood by venipuncture).
- When testing is performed with a method using direct optical observation to determine the result, code **80305** is reported. Tests that have a waived status under CLIA may be reported with modifier **QW** (waived test).
- When a reader is used to determine the result of testing (eg, a dipstick is inserted into a machine that determines the final reading), code **80306** is reported.
- Testing that uses a chemistry analyzer or more effort than tests represented by codes **80305** and **80306** is reported with code **80307**.

Respiratory Syncytial Virus Test

87634   Infectious agent detection by nucleic acid (DNA or RNA); respiratory syncytial virus, amplified probe technique

87807   Infectious agent antigen detection by immunoassay with direct optical (ie, visual) observation; respiratory syncytial virus (CLIA waived)

For assays that include respiratory syncytial virus (RSV) with additional respiratory viruses, see **87631–87633**. Tests reported with codes **87631** and **87633** are CLIA waived. Append modifier **QW** if required. See also the Combination Testing for SARS-CoV-2 and Other Infectious Agent(s) section earlier in this chapter for a discussion of codes as related to tests for combinations of respiratory infectious agents, including SARS-CoV-2, influenza virus, and RSV.

Serum and Transcutaneous Bilirubin Testing

82247   Total bilirubin (CLIA waived)

82248   Direct bilirubin

88720   Transcutaneous total bilirubin

Streptococcal Test

87880   Infectious agent antigen detection by immunoassay with direct optical (ie, visual) observation; streptococcus group A (CLIA waived)

87651   Infectious agent detection by nucleic acid (DNA or RNA); streptococcus, group A, amplified probe technique (CLIA waived)

87081   Culture, presumptive pathogenic organisms, screening only

87430   Enzyme immunoassay, qualitative, streptococcus group A

- Report the code based on the test method rather than on the site of specimen collection.
- Culture plates by using sheep blood agar with bacitracin disks should be coded with **87081**.

Testing Stool for Occult Blood

82272   Blood, occult, by peroxidase activity (eg, guaiac), qualitative, feces, 1–3 simultaneous determinations, performed for other than colorectal neoplasm screening (CLIA waived)

- Code **82272** is reported when a single sample is obtained from a digital rectal examination or a multi-test card is returned from the patient and is tested for blood. Report **82272** with 1 unit when up to 3 cards are returned.

Tuberculin Test (Mantoux)

86580   Tuberculosis, intradermal

- This test is exempt from CLIA requirements.
- The tuberculosis (TB) skin test (Mantoux) using the intradermal administration of purified protein derivative (PPD) is the recommended diagnostic skin test for TB.
  - This is not the BCG TB vaccine.
  - The American Academy of Pediatrics (AAP) supports the use of the Mantoux test (TB, intradermal) for TB screening when appropriate.
- A separate administration code *is not reported* when the PPD is placed.

● indicates a new code; ▲, revised; #, re-sequenced; ✚, add-on; ★, audiovisual technology; and ◀, synchronous interactive audio.

Chapter 12. Common Non-facility Testing and Therapeutic Services

- Code **99211** is the appropriate code to report the reading of a PPD test when that is the only reason for the encounter.

The appropriate *ICD-10-CM* code is **Z11.1** (encounter for screening for respiratory TB). In the case of a positive test result when the physician sees the patient, the complexity may lead to a higher-level code.

- Because risk-based testing is recommended for pediatric patients, an E/M service to evaluate the need for testing may be indicated when testing is requested by a third party (eg, school, employer).
- If TB testing by cell-mediated immunity antigen response measurement, gamma interferon (**86480**), is ordered, and a specimen obtained, venipuncture (**36415**) may be separately reported.

Urine Pregnancy Test

81025 Urine pregnancy test, by visual color comparison methods (CLIA waived)

Report code **81025** with *ICD-10-CM* codes **Z32.00–Z32.02**, depending on the findings of the test (unconfirmed result, positive result, or negative result).

Urinalysis

81000 Urinalysis, by dipstick or tablet reagent for bilirubin, glucose, hemoglobin, ketones, leukocytes, nitrite, pH, protein, specific gravity, urobilinogen, any number of these constituents; nonautomated, with microscopy

81001 as per **81000** with microscopy, but automated

81002 as per **81000** but without microscopy (CLIA waived)

81003 as per **81000** but without microscopy, automated (CLIA waived)

It is important to report the correct code for the urinalysis test performed.

- Code **81000** is reported when the results are shown as color changes for multiple analytes (eg, ketone levels, specific gravity) that are compared against those on a standardized chart (nonautomated) and when microscopy (in a second step, the urine is centrifuged and examined under microscope) is performed.
- Code **81002** is reported if the test results are obtained by the same method but microscopy is not performed.
- Codes **81001** and **81003** are reported for urinalysis performed by a processor that reads the results (automated).

For urinalysis, infectious agent detection, or semiquantitative analysis of volatile compounds, use code **81099**.

✖ Do not report code **99211** for the collection of a urine specimen and/or urinalysis in the absence of a separately identifiable E/M service.

Respiratory Function Tests and Treatments

Pulmonary Function Tests

National Correct Coding Initiative (NCCI) edits exist between office-based E/M services and all pulmonology services (**94010–94799**). Append modifier **25** to the E/M service code as appropriate when reporting a pulmonology service on the same claim.

There is no code for peak flow analysis or oxygen administration. These services are considered part of the evaluation and management service and/or a component of pulmonary function testing.

- Codes include laboratory procedure(s) and interpretation of test results. If a separately identifiable E/M service is performed, the appropriate E/M service code may also be reported.
- When spirometry (**94010**) is performed before and after administration of a bronchodilator, report only code **94060** (bronchodilation responsiveness, spirometry as in **94010**, pre- and post-bronchodilator administration).
  - Code **94640** (nebulizer treatment) is inherent to (ie, included as part of) code **94060**. When an additional nebulizer treatment is performed as a distinct separate procedure on the same date as **94060**, NCCI edits allow use of a modifier (eg, **94640 59**), when applicable.
  - Relative value units assigned to codes include typical supplies (eg, masks, tubing). Report codes for supplies only if the payer does not use an RVU payment methodology.
  - Medication is separately reported with the appropriate HCPCS code (eg, **J7613**, albuterol, inhalation solution, FDA-approved final product, noncompounded, administered through DME, unit dose, 1 mg).

When a physician reports spirometry (**94010**, **94060**) on the date of an evaluation and management service, the test is not counted as ordered or reviewed for the purpose of determining the level of medical decision-making because the test includes a professional component.

- Measurement of vital capacity (**94150**) is a component of spirometry and is reported only when performed alone.
- Measurement of spirometric forced expiratory flows in an infant or child through 2 years of age is reported with code **94011**.
- Code **94012** is used to report measurement of bronchodilation spirometric forced expiratory flows (before and after bronchodilator) in an infant or a child.
- Code **94013** is used to report measurement of lung volumes (eg, functional residual capacity, expiratory reserve volume, forced vital capacity) in an infant or child through 2 years of age.

Current Procedural Terminology guidelines allow reporting of pulse oximetry (**94760**, **94761**), but health plans using the Medicare Physician Fee Schedule will pay only if no other service is paid to the same physician on the same date (ie, some plans consider this an examination component like determining blood pressure).

- Pulmonary stress testing (**94618**) includes measurement of heart rate, oximetry, and oxygen titration, when performed. If spirometry is performed before and following a pulmonary stress test, separately report 2 units of spirometry (**94010**).

Inhalation Treatment

94640   Pressurized or nonpressurized inhalation treatment for acute airway obstruction for therapeutic purposes and/or for diagnostic purposes such as sputum induction with an aerosol generator, nebulizer, metered dose inhaler (MDI) or intermittent positive pressure breathing (IPPB) device

94644   Continuous inhalation treatment with aerosol medication for acute airway obstruction; first hour (For services of less than 1 hour, use **94640**)

+94645   each additional hour (List separately in addition to code for primary procedure)

Report **94640**
- When treatment such as aerosol generator, nebulizer, MDI, or IPPB device is administered.
- With modifier **76** (repeat procedure) with the number of units when more than one treatment is given on a date of service. Some payers require reporting only with the number of units and no modifier. Follow payer guidelines for reporting these services.
- When any treatment of less than 30 minutes is performed.

Current Procedural Terminology code **94060** includes spirometry and pre- and post-bronchodilation. Report only **94060** when **94010** and/or **94640** is a component of the **94060** service.

Report codes **94644** and **94645** when
- A treatment lasts 31 minutes or longer.
- The total time spent in the provision of continuous inhalation treatments is documented in the medical record.

Codes **94644** and **94645** are not reported by physicians when services are provided in a facility setting because no physician work value is assigned to these codes.

Nebulizer Demonstration or Evaluation

94664   Demonstration and/or evaluation of patient utilization of an aerosol generator, nebulizer, metered dose inhaler or IPPB device

- Code **94664** is reported only once per date of service.
- Report code **94664** (demonstration and/or evaluation of patient utilization of an aerosol generator, nebulizer, MDI, or IPPB device) when an initial or subsequent demonstration and/or evaluation is performed and documented.
- Physicians providing nebulizer instruction in conjunction with an E/M service may include the time of nebulizer instruction in the total physician time on the date of an office E/M service (**99202–99205**, **99212–99215**) in lieu of reporting **94664**. No physician work is attributed to code **94664**.

● indicates a new code; ▲, revised; #, re-sequenced; ✚, add-on; ★, audiovisual technology; and ◄, synchronous interactive audio.

When the physician or nurse (of the same group and specialty) performs demonstration and/or evaluation of patient use of a device such as an MDI (**94664**) on the same day as a nebulizer treatment (**94640**), modifier **59** (distinct procedural service) should be appended to code **94664** to indicate to the payer that the services were separate and distinct and that both were clinically indicated.

- Per the Medicaid NCCI manual, the demonstration and/or evaluation described by code **94664** is included in code **94640** if the same device (eg, aerosol generator) is used for both services. The NCCI edits pair code **94664** with **94640** but allow an override of the edit with modifier **59** when both services are indicated (eg, treatment via nebulizer and teaching for MDI). However, some payers may not allow the use of modifier **59** in this instance if the 2 services did not occur at separate encounters. Check with your Medicaid payers.

Modifier **25** should be appended to an E/M service code reported on the same date to signify a separately identifiable service. All services must be documented in the medical record as significant, separately identifiable, and medically necessary.

Example

➤ **A 6-year-old established patient with asthma arrives to the office in acute asthma exacerbation.** Pulse oximetry is performed and indicative of moderate asthma exacerbation. One nebulizer treatment is given via a small-volume nebulizer. Physical examination after first treatment shows decreased wheezing and work of breathing. Pulse oximetry is remeasured and normal. An asthma control test is completed, scored, and documented. An order is written for continuing treatments at home, evaluation and education in use of MDI, and return to the office as needed. The nurse documents her evaluation of use and education for home use of the MDI. Later the same day, the patient returns, again in acute exacerbation. A second nebulizer treatment is given by a small-volume nebulizer. Physical examination after the second treatment shows no improvement and the patient has hypoxia on second pulse oxygen measurement. He is sent to the hospital to be admitted to observation by a hospitalist. Diagnosis is mild persistent asthma with status asthmaticus and hypoxemia.

ICD-10-CM	**J45.32** (mild persistent asthma with status asthmaticus) **R09.02** (hypoxemia)
CPT	**99215 25** (office/outpatient E/M, established patient) **94640** × 1 unit, **94640 76** × 1 unit (nebulizer treatments) **96160** (administration of asthma control test) **94664 59** (MDI demonstration) Medication (appropriate HCPCS code) **94761** (pulse oximetry, multiple determinations)

Teaching Point: Modifier **59** appended to **94664** indicates that the MDI demonstration is reported in addition to nebulizer treatments provided via a different device. Physicians should also report any medications provided at the expense of the practice. HCPCS codes describe medications such as albuterol. The documented severity of the exacerbation in combination with a decision about hospital admission will support **99215**.

Car Seat/Bed Testing

94780   Car seat/bed testing for airway integrity, for infants through 12 months of age, with continual clinical staff observation and continuous recording of pulse oximetry, heart rate and respiratory rate, with interpretation and report; 60 minutes

+94781   each additional full 30 minutes (List separately in addition to **94780**.)

To report codes **94780** and **94781**, the following conditions must be met:

- The patient must be an infant (aged ≤12 months). Reassessment after the patient is 29 days or older may be necessary.
- Continual clinical staff observation with continuous recording of pulse oximetry, heart rate, and respiratory rate is required.
- Vital signs and observations must be reviewed and interpreted and a written report generated by the physician.
- Codes are reported on the basis of the total observation time spent and documented.
- If less than 60 minutes is spent in the procedure, code **94780** may not be reported.

- Each additional full 30 minutes (ie, not <90 minutes' total) is reported with code **94781**.
- A significant, separately identifiable office or other outpatient E/M service [eg, **99213 25**]) may be reported on the same date as car seat/bed testing, when provided.

Example

➤ **A male neonate born at 34 weeks' gestation was released from the hospital 2 weeks ago with instructions to the parents to use only a car bed when transporting him until the pediatrician retests and determines that the neonate can safely ride in a car seat.** The newborn is seen in the outpatient clinic for a preventive medicine visit, and car seat testing is conducted for a period of 1 hour and 45 minutes. The physician reviews and interprets the nurse's records of pulse oximetry, heart and respiratory rates, and observations during the testing period. The interpretation is documented in a formal report and plan of care clearing the neonate to begin use of a rear-facing car seat. The plan of care is discussed with the parents, who also receive further instruction on appropriate use of the car seat.

ICD-10-CM	Codes for conditions of the newborn and **P07.37** (preterm newborn, gestational age 34 completed weeks)
CPT	**94780** (car seat/bed testing; first 60 minutes) **94781** (each additional full 30 minutes)

    Teaching Point: In this scenario, a total of 105 minutes of testing was conducted. This would be reported with 1 unit of code **94780** for the initial 60 minutes of testing and 1 unit of code **94781** for the last 45 minutes (only 1 full period of 30 minutes beyond the first 60 minutes was performed). The 15 minutes beyond the last full 30-minute period is not separately reported. An associated preventive E/M service with modifier **25** would be separately reportable.

Allergy and Clinical Immunology

Allergy Testing

95004	Percutaneous tests (scratch, puncture, prick) with allergenic extracts, immediate type reaction, including test interpretation and report, specify number of tests
95017	Allergy testing, any combination of percutaneous (scratch, puncture, prick) and intracutaneous (intradermal), sequential and incremental, with venoms, immediate type reaction, including test interpretation and report, specify number of tests
95018	Allergy testing, any combination of percutaneous (scratch, puncture, prick) and intracutaneous (intradermal), sequential and incremental, with drugs or biologicals, immediate type reaction, including test interpretation and report, specify number of tests
95024	Intracutaneous (intradermal) tests with allergenic extracts, immediate type reaction, including test interpretation and report, specify number of tests
95027	Intracutaneous (intradermal) tests, sequential and incremental, with allergenic extracts for airborne allergens, immediate type reaction, including test interpretation and report, specify number of tests
95028	Intracutaneous (intradermal) tests with allergenic extracts, delayed type reaction, including reading, specify number of tests

- *CPT* codes for allergy testing are reported by type of test.
  - Percutaneous, immediate type reaction (**95004**)
  - Intracutaneous (intradermal) with immediate (**95024**, **95027**) or delayed type reaction (**95028**)
  - Any combination of percutaneous and intracutaneous, sequential and incremental tests with venoms (**95017**) or with drugs or biologicals (**95018**)
- Specification of the number of tests applied is required for accurate reporting of the units of service provided. Medicaid NCCI edits do not allow inclusion of positive or negative controls in the number of tests reported.
- Codes **95004, 95017, 95018, 95024,** and **95027** include test interpretation and report. Code **95028** includes reading.

    When a significant, separately identifiable E/M service is performed and documented (eg, counseling on allergy avoidance, treatment and use of epinephrine auto-injector) on the same date as testing, it may be reported with modifier **25** appended to the appropriate E/M code.

Chapter 12. Common Non-facility Testing and Therapeutic Services

✖ Do not report an E/M service for the obtainment of informed consent and interpretation and report of the results of allergy testing.

Example

➤ **A patient with seasonal allergies undergoes percutaneous testing with 22 allergenic extracts and 2 controls.**
A clinician administers the extracts per the physician's order and monitors the patient for signs of reaction. For each extract administered, the reaction (eg, size of wheal) or lack of reaction is noted. The physician interprets the test and creates a report of the findings.
The physician reports code **95004** with 24 units of service or, if the payer does not allow payment for controls, with 22 units. If a significant E/M service is provided on the same date and is separately identifiable in the documentation from the preservice and post-service work of the testing (eg, interpretation and report), append modifier **25** to the code for the E/M service provided.

> For more information, see the February 2020 *AAP Pediatric Coding Newsletter* article, "Allergy Skin Testing: Codes, Unit Counts, and Tips for Reporting" (https://doi.org/10.1542/pcco_book190_document002).

- Patch and photo patch testing are reported with codes **95044–95056**.
- Specific challenge testing (**95060–95079**) is coded according to target organ (eg, ophthalmic mucous membrane, nasal, inhalation bronchial challenges without pulmonary function testing, ingestion).
- Nasal cytology, a test for allergy-type cells (eosinophils) or infection-type cells (neutrophils) on a nasal scraping, is reported with code **89190**.
- Nitric oxide–expired gas determination is reported with code **95012**. Nitric oxide determination by spectroscopy should be reported with code **94799**.

Allergen Immunotherapy

Codes for allergen immunotherapy are reported on the basis of the service provided: preparation and provision of allergen extract only, administration only, or combined provision and administration.

An appropriate office or outpatient code may be reported with allergen immunotherapy codes. Modifier **25** is appended to the E/M service when it is performed and documented.

Preparation and Provision Only of Extract

95144	Professional services for the supervision of the preparation and provision of antigens for allergen immunotherapy, single-dose vials(s) (specify number of vials)
95145	Professional services for the supervision of the preparation and provision of antigens for allergy immunotherapy (specify number of doses); single stinging insect venom
95146	2 stinging insect venoms
95147	3 stinging insect venoms
95148	4 stinging insect venoms
95149	5 stinging insect venoms
95165	Professional services for the supervision of preparation and provision of antigens for allergen immunotherapy; single or multiple antigens (specify number of doses)
95170	Professional services for the supervision of preparation and provision of antigens for allergen immunotherapy; whole body extract of biting insect or other arthropod (specify number of doses)

- Codes **95144–95170** are used to report preparation and provision of antigens for allergen immunotherapy without administration of the allergenic extract.
  - Codes **95144–95170** describe the preparation of the antigen, the antigen extract itself, the physician's assessment and determination of the concentration and volume to use based on the patient's history and results of previous skin testing, and the prospective planned schedule of administration of the extract.
  - The number of vials must be specified when reporting code **95144**.
  - Report codes **95145–95170** on the basis of the *number of doses* (eg, preparation of 2 vials that will provide 20 doses of extract containing 4 insect venoms is reported with code **95148** and 20 units of service).

● indicates a new code; ▲, revised; #, re-sequenced; ✚, add-on; ★, audiovisual technology; and ◀, synchronous interactive audio.

- Services may be reported at the time the allergenic extract is prepared because injections occur on later dates (prospectively planned) or may not occur at all.
- Administration of the allergenic extract is not included.
- Report **95146–95149** for preparation of extracts containing more than one single stinging venom (eg, code **95146** is reported for 2; code **95147** is reported for 3).

National Correct Coding Initiative Immunotherapy Edits

The Medicaid National Correct Coding Initiative (NCCI) manual instructs that for the purpose of reporting units of service for antigen preparation (ie, *Current Procedural Terminology* codes 95145–95170), the physician reports "number of doses." The NCCI program defines a dose for reporting purposes as 1 mL. Thus, if a physician prepares a 10-mL vial of antigen, the physician may report only a maximum of 10 units of service for that vial even if the number of actual administered doses is greater than 10. Verify payer policies on units of service before reporting.

Administration Only of Extract

95115   Professional services for allergen immunotherapy not including provision of allergenic extracts; single injection
95117   2 or more injections

Either code **95115** or **95117** (not both) are used to report administration only of the allergenic extract. Report on the basis of the number of injections when another health care professional (eg, the patient's allergist) has prepared and supplied the allergenic extract or when a physician (usually an allergist) administers the prospectively prepared extract (ie, prepared with the intent to administer on a planned schedule).

Example

➤ **The pediatrician administers 3 injections of allergen extract for a patient with allergic rhinitis due to pollen.** The extract was prepared and supplied by an allergist.
    The pediatrician will report code **95117** with *ICD-10-CM* code **J30.1**.

Combined Provision of Allergenic Extract With Administration

Current Procedural Terminology (CPT) recommends codes 95120–95134 be reported only when specifically required by the payer. These codes are not assigned relative value units in the Medicare Physician Fee Schedule that many payers use as a basis for physician payment. The Centers for Medicare & Medicaid Services (CMS) Medicare program will accept only codes 95115, 95117, and 95144–95170 and will not allow payment for codes 95120–95134. Medicaid and commercial payers may follow the CMS Medicare guidelines or may have their own established guidelines. Therefore, before reporting these services, research the reporting policies of your major payers.

See your *CPT* code manual or other code reference for full code descriptors for 95120–95134.

- Codes **95120–95134** are reported when the entire service of preparing, providing, and administering (injection) allergenic extract is performed at 1 patient encounter.
- Codes **95131–95134** are reported for extracts containing more than one single stinging insect venom.
- Codes **95115** and **95117** *cannot* be reported with codes **95120–95134**.
- Codes **95120** and **95125** are reported on the basis of the number of injections administered (ie, a single injection or ≥2 injections).
- Codes **95130–95134** are reported per injection. Therefore, if 2 separate injections of 2 stinging insect venoms (eg, wasp and bee) are provided, code **95131** would be reported 2 times.
- For rapid desensitization per hour, see code **95180**.

Example

➤ **An allergist prepares a 10-dose vial of allergen extract and administers 1 dose at the time of the visit (allergenic extract was prepared with the intent to administer on a planned schedule).**

● indicates a new code; ▲, revised; #, re-sequenced; ✚, add-on; ★, audiovisual technology; and ◀, synchronous interactive audio.

The allergist will report code **95165** with 10 units of service and **95115** with 1 unit of service and the specific diagnosis code. Allergic rhinitis due to pollen would be reported with *ICD-10-CM* code **J30.1** or, if due to food, code **J30.5**. Alternatively, code **95120** would describe provision of allergenic extract and a single injection if required by a payer.

Epinephrine Auto-injector Administration

Administration of epinephrine via an epinephrine auto-injector in the office or other outpatient setting is reported with code **96372** (therapeutic, prophylactic, or diagnostic injection [specify substance or drug]; subcutaneous or intramuscular). Follow payer guidance for reporting an epinephrine injector kit furnished by the practice.

● Many payers require submission of code **J0171** (injection, Adrenalin, epinephrine, 0.1 mg) with 1 unit for 1 injection.

Example

➤ **The patient has a reaction to the allergenic extract.** The physician injects epinephrine by using an auto-injector device (eg, EpiPen Jr, Adrenaclick) supplied by the physician.

The injection using an auto-injection device would be reported as an intramuscular injection with code **96372**. The HCPCS table of drugs references the epinephrine injectors to code **J0171**. The HCPCS units for **J0171** are 1 unit per 0.1 mg (eg, 0.15 mg equals 1.5 units). It is advisable to include the product NDC and NDC units to specify the exact product and dose provided.

Immunoglobulins

Note: **This information does not apply to immunization services. See Chapter 8.**

When reporting codes **90281–90399**, remember that they are only for the cost of the immunoglobulin, so the appropriate separate administration code should also be reported (eg, **96372**, **96374**).

● A significant, separately identifiable E/M service performed during the same visit may also be billed if indicated.
● *ICD-10-CM* diagnosis codes to support immunoglobulin services include codes from categories **D80–D84** for certain disorders involving the immune mechanism or codes for specific conditions, such as mucocutaneous lymph node syndrome (**M30.3**).

Example

➤ **An infant requires administration of 150 mg of palivizumab for preventing serious lower respiratory tract disease caused by RSV.** A clinical staff member administers the immunoglobulin under direct physician supervision. Two single-dose vials (one 100-mg and one 50-mg) are administered. The supervising physician reports

ICD-10-CM (Link all supporting codes to each claim line.)
Z29.11 (encounter for prophylactic immunotherapy for respiratory syncytial virus [RSV])
Other *ICD-10-CM* codes supporting the need for the service (eg, preterm birth, congenital heart disease)

CPT
96372 (intramuscular injection)
90378 × 2 units (RSV, monoclonal antibody, recombinant, for intramuscular use, 50 mg, each)
90378 × 1 unit (additional 50 mg single-dose vial)

NDC
60574411301 (100mg/1ml vial) × 1.0ml
60574411401 (50mg/0.5ml vial) × 0.5ml

The appropriate number of units reported for the dose of the RSV monoclonal antibody given is 1 unit per 50 mg (eg, 3 units for 150 mg). The NDC for each vial should be included on claims for most payers requiring submission on separate claim lines. Typically, the NDC units are reported per milliliter. When prior authorization is required, a prior authorization approval number may also be included on the claim (field 23 on a paper claim).

Review individual payer policies for reporting these services. Code **90378 KP** and **90378 KQ** may be reported when required by payer policy for a single drug reported with multiple NDCs.

> See Chapter 1 for more information on reporting National Drug Codes.

Hearing Screening and Other Audiological Function Testing Codes

(For central auditory function evaluation, see **92620**, **92621***.)*

Audiometric tests require the use of calibrated electronic equipment, recording of results, and a written report with interpretation (eg, chart of hertz and decibels with pass/fail result for each ear tested and overall pass/fail result). Services include testing of both ears. If the test is applied to only 1 ear, modifier **52** (reduced services) must be appended to the code.

> Medicaid plans may offer physician resources providing hearing screening/testing coverage information and documentation forms/requirements.

- Code **92551** (screening test, pure tone, air only) is used when earphones are placed on the patient and the patient is asked to respond to tones of different pitches and intensities. This is a limited study to identify the presence or absence of a potential hearing problem. Code **92551** is not used to report hearing screenings performed on newborns and infants.

> Report hearing tests conducted following a failed hearing screening with *International Classification of Diseases, 10th Revision, Clinical Modification* code **Z01.110** if results are normal. If findings are atypical, report code **Z01.118** and a code to identify the abnormality.

- Code **92552** (full pure tone audiometric assessment) is used when earphones are placed on the patient and the patient is asked to respond to tones of different pitches and intensities. The threshold, which is the lowest intensity of the tone that the patient can hear 50% of the time, is recorded for a number of frequencies.
- Air and bone thresholds (**92553**) may be obtained and compared to differentiate among conductive, sensorineural, or mixed hearing losses. Air and bone thresholds are obtained in a similar manner.

> Automated audiometry testing is reported with Category III codes **0208T–0212T**.

- Code **92558** is reported for evoked otoacoustic emissions, screening (qualitative measurement of distortion product or transient evoked otoacoustic emissions), with automated analysis. This is used when the results are obtained automatically (ie, no interpretation and report is required). Coverage for this is typically limited to newborn screening, including follow-up newborn screening from a failed screening in the hospital and screening on younger children. Check with your payers, however.
- Code **92583** (select picture audiometry) is typically used for younger children. The patient is asked to identify different pictures with the instructions given at different intensity levels.
- Distortion product evoked otoacoustic emissions codes are reported on the basis of the number of frequencies used. Code **92587** is used to report testing for confirmation of the presence or absence of a hearing disorder, 3 to 6 frequencies. Code **92588** is reported when a comprehensive (quantitative analysis of outer hair cell function by cochlear mapping) diagnostic evaluation with a minimum of 12 frequencies is performed. Interpretation and written report are required. Do not report these codes for automated analysis.
- Other commonly performed procedures include codes **92567** (tympanometry [impedance testing]) and **92568** (acoustic reflex testing, threshold portion). Code **92550** is reported when tympanometry and reflex threshold measurements are performed.
- Optical coherence tomography of the middle ear with interpretation and report is reported with Category III codes based on whether the service was unilateral (**0485T**) or bilateral (**0486T**). Be sure to verify payer policy before provision of services.
- Most audiological procedures are bundled with impacted cerumen removal services (**69209**, **69210**) and, therefore, will not be separately payable. Report only the audiology test to payers that bundle impacted cerumen removal services.

Chapter 12. Common Non-facility Testing and Therapeutic Services

---

● indicates a new code; ▲, revised; #, re-sequenced; ✚, add-on; ★, audiovisual technology; and ◀, synchronous interactive audio.

Example

➤ **Lilly is a 5-year-old whose hearing does not meet screening criteria at school and is referred to her pediatrician for additional evaluation.** She has a history of recurrent otitis media before the age of 3 years but no recent illness. Her parents report no family history of hearing loss and no concerns at home. Tympanometry reveals no evidence of effusion. Examination findings are negative for other abnormalities. Screening audiometry is performed, and its results are atypical, as indicated by the school screening. Lilly is referred to an audiologist for further evaluation. Diagnosis is abnormal auditory function with possible hearing loss in her right ear.

ICD-10-CM	**Z01.118** (encounter for examination of ears and hearing with other abnormal findings) **R94.120** (abnormal auditory function study)
CPT	**99213** (established patient office E/M, low medical decision-making) **92567** (tympanometry [impedance testing]) **92551** (screening test, pure tone, air only)

Teaching Point: *ICD-10-CM* instructs the physician to report **Z01.118** and an additional code for abnormal findings. Although the result of the screening was abnormal, the physician did not diagnose a hearing loss at this encounter. Code **R94.120** describes the abnormal screening result.

If the screening result at this visit had been negative, the physician would have been required to code **Z01.110** (encounter for hearing examination following failed hearing screening).

Emotional/Behavioral Assessment

96127   Brief emotional/behavioral assessment (eg, depression inventory, attention-deficit/hyperactivity disorder [ADHD] scale), with scoring and documentation, per standardized instrument

Code **96127**

- Represents the practice expense of administering, scoring, and documenting each standardized instrument. No physician work value is included. Physician interpretation is included in a related E/M service.
- May be used not only for screening but also for assessment in monitoring treatment efficacy and support of clinical decision-making.
- Not reported in conjunction with **96105**, **96125**, and **99483**.
- Two separate completions (eg, by teacher and parent) of the same form may be separately reported (ie, 2 units of service). When reporting multiple units of service, it is advisable to learn if the payer has specific guidance for reporting the total number of units as a single line item or requires splitting to multiple claim lines. Medically Unlikely Edits may apply.

Example

➤ **A 16-year-old patient receiving treatment of an initial episode of major depressive disorder returns for follow-up.** A standardized instrument is used to assess the status of the patient's depression. The physician recommends continued medication and counseling with a licensed clinical social worker. The physician's total time on the date of the encounter is 25 minutes. Diagnosis is a moderate single episode of major depressive disorder.

The established patient office E/M code **99213** is reported in addition to code **96127**. The diagnosis code **F32.1** (major depressive disorder, single episode, moderate) is reported.

> **See**
> - Chapter 11 for discussion of diagnostic testing of the central nervous system
> - Chapter 8 for discussion of developmental screening, brief emotional and/or behavioral assessment, and health risk assessment as preventive services
> - Chapter 2 for more information on Medically Unlikely Edits

Chapter 12. Common Non-facility Testing and Therapeutic Services

Radiology Services

The following general guidelines are for reporting radiology services:

- Report only the service provided. See the Professional and Technical Components section earlier in this chapter for appropriate reporting when the physician does not provide the global service.
- A signed written report of the physician's or QHP's interpretation of imaging is an integral part of the professional component of a radiological service.
- A reference to *image* in *CPT* may refer to an image on film or in digital format. Images must contain anatomical information unique to the patient for which the imaging service is provided.
- Certain health plans, including Medicaid plans, may require use of modifiers **FX** (x-ray taken using film) and **FY** (x-ray taken using computed radiography technology/cassette-based imaging) when reporting the technical component or global radiology service (ie, combined professional and technical components). Verify health plan requirements, as payment may be reduced for radiographs taken by using technology other than digital imaging.

Some commonly reported codes for radiological examination follow. See your coding reference for a full listing of codes and reporting instructions for radiology services.

Imaging Guidance

Many procedures include imaging guidance. When a code descriptor for a procedure or *CPT* instruction indicates that the procedure includes imaging guidance, do not separately report a code for supervision and interpretation of imaging (eg, radiography, fluoroscopy, ultrasonography, magnetic resonance imaging, computed tomography, nuclear medicine).

- ✖ Do not report imaging guidance when a non–imaging-guided tracking or localizing system (eg, radar, electromagnetic signals) is used.
- If you do not own or lease the equipment but are only reporting the professional service of interpreting the image and writing the report, refer to the modifier **26** discussion in the Professional and Technical Components section earlier in this chapter.

Abdominal Radiographs

74018	Radiologic examination, abdomen; 1 view
74019	2 views
74021	3 or more views
74022	Radiologic examination, complete acute abdomen series, including 2 or more views of the abdomen (eg, supine, erect, decubitus), and a single view chest

Report code **74022** when a series of radiographs are obtained to view the abdomen and chest as workup of acute abdominal illness or pain. An acute abdomen series includes 2 abdominal views and a single chest view.

Chest Radiographs

71045	Radiologic examination, chest; single view
71046	2 views
71047	3 views
71048	4 or more views

- The types of views (eg, frontal and lateral) obtained no longer affect coding of chest radiographs.
- ✖ Do not separately report a single-view chest radiograph when obtained in conjunction with an acute abdomen series (**74022**).

Hip Radiographs

73501	Radiologic examination, hip, unilateral, with pelvis when performed; 1 view
73502	2-3 views
73503	performed minimum of 4 views
73521	Radiologic examination, hips, bilateral, with pelvis when performed; 2 views
73522	3-4 views
73523	minimum of 5 views
73525	Radiologic examination, hip, arthrography, radiological supervision and interpretation
73592	Radiologic examination lower extremity, infant, minimum of 2 views

---

● indicates a new code; ▲, revised; #, re-sequenced; ✚, add-on; ★, audiovisual technology; and ◄, synchronous interactive audio.

Codes **73501–73523** include radiograph of the pelvis when performed. Do not separately report a single-view radiograph of the pelvis (**72170**) when performed in conjunction with a radiograph of the hip.

Total Spine Radiographs

72081   Radiologic examination, spine, entire thoracic and lumbar, including skull, cervical and sacral spine if performed (eg, scoliosis evaluation); one view

72082   2 or 3 views

72083   4 or 5 views

72084   minimum of 6 views

Codes **72081–72084** describe imaging of the entire thoracic and lumbar spine and, when performed, the skull, cervical, and sacral spine.

Do not separately report codes for views of the individual spinal segments or skull when performed in conjunction with radiological examination of the spine. Rather, select the code that represents the total number of views obtained.

Administrative Services

Codes in this section cover some of the administrative aspects of medical practice.

99075   Medical testimony

99082   Unusual travel (eg, transportation and escort of patient)

S9981   Medical records copying fee, administrative

S9982   Medical records copying fee, per page

Codes **99071–99082** are for administrative services.

- Code **99075** may be reported when a physician presents medical testimony before a court or other administrative body.
- None of these services are assigned Medicare RVUs.
- HCPCS codes **S9981** and **S9982** may be reported when it is appropriate to charge for copying medical records. Commercial payers and some Medicaid programs may accept **S** codes.
  - State medical insurance departments or medical associations determine the amount a practice can charge for copying medical records. Be sure to know the state charge limitations and do not overcharge.
  - The Health Insurance Portability and Accountability Act (HIPAA) of 1996 regulations, where more stringent, will override state regulations. For information on charges to patients for copying medical records, see www.hhs.gov/hipaa/for-professionals/privacy/guidance/access/index.html#newlyreleasedfaqs.

Physician Group Education Services

99078   Physician or other qualified health care professional qualified by education, training, licensure/regulation (when applicable), educational services rendered to patients in a group setting (eg, prenatal, obesity, or diabetic instructions)

Code **99078** is used to report physician educational services provided to established patients in group settings (eg, obesity or diabetes classes).

- There are no time requirements.
- Modifier **25** (significant, separately identifiable E/M service) should *not* be appended to the E/M service because **99078** is an adjunct service.
- Documentation in each medical record includes the education and training provided, follow-up for ongoing education, and total time of the education.
- Health plans and parents/caregivers of each participating child may be charged.
- Payers may require that these services be reported differently.
- For preventive medicine and risk-factor reduction counseling to patients in a group setting, see codes **99411** and **99412**.

To test your knowledge of the information presented in this chapter, complete the quiz found at the end of it, after the resources. Answers to each quiz are found in **Appendix IV**.

Chapter 12. Common Non-facility Testing and Therapeutic Services

Chapter Takeaways

This chapter covers codes and coding guidance for many diagnostic and therapeutic services when provided in an office or outpatient setting. Following are some takeaways from this chapter:

- There are many services that may be reported for the complete or global service or for only the professional or technical component, when provided.
- Obtaining a blood specimen is separately reportable in conjunction with performing a point-of-care test and/or an E/M service.
- ✖ Do not report code **99211** for services to obtain a specimen and/or perform a laboratory test in the absence of an E/M service by clinical staff.
- ✖ Do not include time spent in separately reported testing or therapeutic services in the time of an E/M service reported on the same date. Append modifier **25** to significant and separately identifiable E/M services provided on the same date as tests that include an interpretation and report or as otherwise specific in *CPT*.

Resources

AAP Pediatric Coding Newsletter™

"Allergy Skin Testing: Codes, Unit Counts, and Tips for Reporting," February 2020 (https://doi.org/10.1542/pcco_book190_document002)

"Table of Diagnosis Coding for Services Related to COVID-19 Exposure or Infection," August 2021 (https://doi.org/10.1542/pcco_book208_document002)

CLIA Test Categorization

Currently waived analytes (www.accessdata.fda.gov/scripts/cdrh/cfdocs/cfClia/analyteswaived.cfm)

FDA CLIA database (www.accessdata.fda.gov/scripts/cdrh/cfdocs/cfCLIA/search.cfm)

HIPAA Release of Patient Records

"Questions and Answers About HIPAA's Access Right" (45 CFR §164.524) (www.hhs.gov/hipaa/for-professionals/privacy/guidance/access/index.html#newlyreleasedfaqs)

National Drug Codes

FDA National Drug Code Directory (www.fda.gov/drugs/drug-approvals-and-databases/national-drug-code-directory)

Online Exclusive Content at www.aap.org/cfp2023

"Medications for Pediatrics: Most Common"

Proprietary Laboratory Analyses

CPT PLA codes (www.ama-assn.org/practice-management/cpt/cpt-pla-codes)

● indicates a new code; ▲, revised; #, re-sequenced; ✚, add-on; ★, audiovisual technology; and ◀, synchronous interactive audio.

Test Your Knowledge!

1. **Which of the following items is a professional component of a test?**
   a. Results
   b. Supplies
   c. Salaries of technical personnel
   d. Interpretation and report

2. **Which of the following statements is true for code 36415?**
   a. Report code **36415** for all venipunctures not requiring a physician's skills to perform the procedure.
   b. Report code **36415** for all finger or heel sticks.
   c. Report code **36415** for all venipunctures performed on children 3 years and older.
   d. Report code **36415** for all venipunctures requiring a physician's skills to perform the procedure.

3. **Which of the following codes is reported for a test performed by using DNA or RNA to target SARS-CoV-2, influenza A and B viruses, and respiratory syncytial virus?**
   a. **87637** × 3 units.
   b. **87631** × 4 units.
   c. **87637** × 1 unit.
   d. Individual codes are reported for tests targeting each virus.

4. **Which of the following codes is appropriate for reporting injection of epinephrine in the office through an auto-injector?**
   a. **J0171**
   b. National Drug Code for the specific product used
   c. **96372**
   d. All of the above

5. **Which of the following statements is true of code 96127?**
   a. The code is not valued to include physician work.
   b. The code includes physician interpretation of the score.
   c. The code is not reported on the same date as an evaluation and management service.
   d. The code is reported only when the instrument is used for reassessment of a diagnosed problem.

● indicates a new code; ▲, revised; #, re-sequenced; ✚, add-on; ★, audiovisual technology; and ◀, synchronous interactive audio.

Qualified Nonphysician Health Care Professional Services

CPT copyright 2022 American Medical Association. All rights reserved.

Contents

• indicates a new code; ▲, revised; #, re-sequenced; ✚, add-on; ★, audiovisual technology; and ◀, synchronous interactive audio.

Chapter Highlights

- Terminology used to differentiate qualified nonphysician health care professionals (QNHCPs) from qualified health care professionals (QHPs) and clinical staff (and explanation of why this differentiation matters)
- Identifying the scope of practice for a QNHCP
- Recognizing the various QNHCPs who may perform and report services to pediatric patients
- *Current Procedural Terminology* (*CPT*®) and Healthcare Common Procedure Coding System (HCPCS) codes and modifiers that may apply to reporting services performed by QNHCPs

Services Provided by Qualified Nonphysician Health Care Professionals

In their quest to provide comprehensive and high-quality care to patients, pediatric physicians are including more QNHCPs (eg, dieticians) in their practices and using clinical staff to their full potential.

This chapter focuses on medical services that are provided by health care professionals other than physicians and other QHPs, such as nurse practitioners and physician assistants (PAs), who are distinguished by the ability to provide and report evaluation and management (E/M) services.

Terminology

> Throughout the *Current Procedural Terminology* code set, the use of terms such as *physician, qualified health care professional,* or *individual* is not intended to indicate that other entities may not report the service. In select instances, specific instructions may define a service as limited to professionals or other entities (eg, hospital, home health agency).

To help differentiate, the following definitions apply to discussions and examples in this chapter:
- **Qualified health care professional:** Advanced practice providers, such as advanced practice nurses, clinical nurse specialists, and PAs, whose scope of practice includes E/M services beyond minimal services incident to a physician (ie, **99211** or **99281** [E/M visit not requiring physician face-to-face service]).

> See Chapter 7 for detailed discussion of incident-to services and evaluation and management services reported with code **99211**.

- **Qualified nonphysician health care professional:** A broad category of health care professionals who typically would not independently prescribe and manage, whose professional services are typically performed under the order and supervision of a physician or QHP, and whose scope of practice does not include E/M services beyond **99211**. Sometimes they are able to bill under their own National Provider Identifier (NPI). This category includes providers such as clinical psychologists, licensed counselors, dietitians/nutritionists, health educators, and lactation consultants, among others.

> See Chapter 11 for information on reporting mental and behavioral health services provided by qualified nonphysician health care professionals.

- **Clinical staff member** (as defined by *CPT*): A health care team member who works under the supervision of a physician or other QHP and who is allowed by law, regulation, and facility policy to perform or assist in the performance of a specific professional service but *does not individually report that professional service.* These include, but are not limited to, registered nurses (RNs), licensed practical nurses (LPNs), and medical assistants (MAs).

CPT references *clinical staff member* mostly in the context of staff who provide components of physician or QHP services, such as obtaining patient history, and services that are always billed by a supervising physician or QHP (eg, nurse visit, medication administration).

Chapter 13. Qualified Nonphysician Health Care Professional Services

Staff who are able to perform *only administrative functions,* such as reception, scheduling, billing, dictation, or scribing, are not clinical staff for coding purposes.

Including Qualified Nonphysician Health Care Professionals in Your Practice

Services by QNHCPs, provided under a physician's or QHP's order within a physician group practice, can be an integral part of providing a full scope of care in the medical home.

- Billing and coding must align not only with coding guidelines but also state scope of practice (see the Scope of Practice Laws section later in this chapter) and individual payer policies on credentialing, contracting, and billing for services of the specific QNHCP.
- *Before including QNHCPs within your group practice,* it is important to seek expert advice on related state regulations for scope of practice and supervision requirements, enrollment and payment policies of the group's most common payers, and best practices in employment and/or contractual agreements.
- The number of services that may be provided can be estimated on the basis of current patient diagnoses or history of referral for services. Reports from electronic health records or billing software may be used in this estimation (eg, report of the number of unique patient accounts containing a diagnosis indicating mental or behavioral health conditions).

When physicians choose to arrange for services provided within their practice by QNHCPs who are not employed or contracted with their group practice, additional counsel should be obtained to prevent conflict with anti-kickback and/or self-referral regulations.

Payment for QNHCP services begins with negotiating and contracting with payers for coverage and payment of services as described by *CPT* and/or HCPCS codes. (A list of HCPCS codes that may be used to report nonphysician education services is included in the Payer-Specific Coding for Services Under a Disease Management Program section later in this chapter.)

- Payers may pay separately for these services when your practice can demonstrate the overall cost savings (eg, decrease in physician or emergency department visits, decreased hospital care) that may be achieved through expanded care in the physician practice.

For more on quality and performance measurement, see Chapter 3.

- If payers do not agree to directly compensate for individual services, consider opportunities for shared savings and other revenue that may be realized when QNHCP services support quality improvement initiatives (eg, per-member-per-month compensation for meeting certain quality measures) and redirection of physician and QHP time to services that are restricted to or best delivered within their scope of practice.

Physicians should be especially aware of each payer's policy addressing use of E/M codes for services provided by QNHCPs or clinical staff. Medicare and payers who adopt Medicare policy do not allow reporting of E/M services other than **99211** provided by QNHCPs or clinical staff. Other services that specifically indicate work of clinical staff under physician supervision (eg, transitional care management [TCM] or chronic [long-term] care management [CCM]) are exceptions.

For more information on chronic care management and transitional care management, see Chapter 10.

Example

➤ *CPT* **describes codes 99401–99404 as representing services provided face-to-face by a physician or other QHP for the purpose of promoting health and preventing illness or injury.** However, some payers directly instruct that codes such as **99401** may be reported for specific services by specific clinical staff or by QNHCPs such as medical nutritionists or certified lactation consultants.

Teaching Point: Always keep a printed or electronic copy of payer guidance that conflicts with *CPT* or standard billing practices.

● indicates a new code; ▲, revised; #, re-sequenced; ✚, add-on; ★, audiovisual technology; and ◀, synchronous interactive audio.

Scope of Practice Laws

Scope of practice is a term used by state licensing boards for various professions to define the procedures, actions, and processes that are permitted for a licensed individual. Scope of practice may also address the delegation of health care activities to unlicensed individuals who the delegating physician or other QHP/QNHCP has ascertained have the education, training, and/or certification necessary to safely perform the activity. Additional limitations on scope of practice of QNHCPs and on delegation to clinical staff may come from Medicaid programs, health care systems, or health care professional membership organizations.

Physicians, RNs, clinical nurse practitioners, PAs, LPNs, physical therapists, and licensed nutritionists are among some of the professions for which scope of practice laws are defined. Some states limit the autonomous practice of advanced practice professionals and require these QHPs to have written collaboration agreements and require general or direct supervision by a physician. Prescribing authority may also be limited. Verify your state's requirements for all clinicians and appropriate inclusions in any collaboration/supervision agreements.

Every state has laws and regulations that describe the requirements of education and training for health care professionals. However, some states do not have different scope of practice laws for every level of professional (eg, LPN, lactation consultant). Health systems, government payers, and health care professional membership organizations may also define or limit the scope of practice or delegation to QNHCPs and clinical staff.

Scope of practice should be taken into consideration when delegating directly or through standing orders (eg, physician writes order that recommended screening instruments be completed for all patients presenting for well-baby/well-child [health supervision] examinations).

While scope of practice provides guidance on what services may be performed by QNHCPs and clinical staff, certain codes also limit who can report specific services. For instance, nurses are allowed to counsel for and administer immunizations, but administration codes **90460** and **90461** are reported only when a physician or QHP has provided immunization counseling. Likewise, E/M services are reported only by a physician or QHP, although QNHCPs and clinical staff may perform tasks included in the service (eg, obtaining vital signs and initial history).

- Payers who follow Medicare policy on reporting of E/M services will not accept codes **99202–99205**, **99212–99215**, or **99217–99499** performed by QNHCPs. Codes **99211** and **99281** describe E/M services that may not require a physician's presence. For a full discussion of code **99211**, see **Chapter 7**. Code **99281** is discussed in **Chapter 15**.

National Provider Identifier

The NPI is a unique identification number for covered health care professionals. The NPI is required on administrative and financial transactions under the Health Insurance Portability and Accountability Act (HIPAA) of 1996 administrative simplification provisions.

- Anyone who directly provides health care services (eg, physical therapist, nutritionist, audiologist) can apply for and receive an NPI.
- Usually only those who will bill for services and/or order services or prescription drugs will need an NPI.
- The NPI is included on medical claims to indicate who ordered, provided, or supervised the provision of services.

Nonphysician Assessment and Management Services

A QNHCP whose scope of practice does not include providing and independently reporting E/M services may report assessment and management services. Assessment and management services may be provided in person (as discussed for specific types of services throughout this chapter), via online digital communication or telephone, or as a participant of a team conference. Each type of assessment and management service has specific reporting guidelines.

Online Medical Assessment

98970	Qualified nonphysician health care professional online digital assessment and management service, for an established patient, for up to seven days, cumulative time during the 7 days; 5-10 minutes
98971	11-20 minutes
98972	21 or more minutes

An online electronic medical assessment (**98970–98972**) is a non–face-to-face assessment and management service by a QNHCP to an established patient using internet resources in response to a patient's online inquiry.

> Online digital evaluation and management (E/M) services by a physician or other qualified health care professional (who may report E/M services) are reported with codes 99421–99423. See Chapter 9 for information on online digital E/M services.

● indicates a new code; ▲, revised; #, re-sequenced; ✚, add-on; ★, audiovisual technology; and ◀, synchronous interactive audio.

Online assessment and management refers to use of technology such as secure email and other asynchronous digital communication.

This contrasts with *telemedicine services,* which represent interactive audio and video telecommunications systems that permit real-time communication between the QNHCP at the distant site and the patient at the originating site.

- Before providing online medical services, understand local and state laws, ensure that communications will be HIPAA compliant (eg, conducted through a secure patient portal), establish written guidelines and procedures, educate payers and negotiate for payment, and educate patients.
- Codes **98970–98972** are time-based codes used by a QNHCP to report an online assessment and management service.
- One code and 1 unit of service are reported for the sum of communications pertaining to the online encounter during a 7-day period.
- The 7-day service period begins with the initial, personal QNHCP review of the patient-generated inquiry.
- All time spent addressing the manifesting problem and any additional problems (including new unrelated problems addressed by online electronic communications) during the service period is cumulative and reported as one service.
- Online assessment and management includes
  - Review of the initial inquiry
  - Review of patient records or data pertinent to assessing the patient's problem
  - Personal QNHCP interaction with clinical staff focused on the patient's problem
  - Development of management plans
  - Timely reply to the patient's/caregiver's request for online service
  - Permanent record of the service (hard copy or electronic)
  - All related communications during a 7-day episode of care (eg, ordering laboratory or other testing, prescribing, conducting related phone calls)
  - Cumulative time of QNHCPs in the same group that is involved in the online digital E/M service
- Online digital assessment services (**98970–98972**) are *not* reported
  - For services of less than 5 minutes' cumulative time
  - For new patient inquiries (although new problems may be addressed for established patients)
  - For electronic communication of test results, scheduling of appointments, or other communication that does not include assessment and management
  - If the online digital inquiry occurs within the postoperative period of a previously completed procedure
  - If the patient generates an online digital inquiry within 7 days of a previous treatment or E/M service and both services relate to the same problem
  - If a separately reported assessment service occurs within 7 days of the initial online digital inquiry
- When care plan oversight (**99374, 99375; 99377–99380**), CCM (**99487, 99489–99491**), TCM (**99495, 99496**), or collection of physiologic data (**99091**) are provided in the same period, do not count the time of communications related to these services toward the time of online digital medical services.

Example

➤ **Parents of a patient with moderate intermittent asthma securely email a respiratory therapist who is an asthma care coordinator, requesting advice on preparing their child for adhering to the asthma care plan on a weeklong trip with a sports team.** The asthma educator responds to the request, and emails are exchanged to further clarify concerns and provide advice. The child is to be instructed to contact the asthma educator or the treating physician by phone if questions or concerns arise during travel. The cumulative time of the communication is 15 minutes.

The respiratory therapist reports code **98971**. However, if the patient had been seen within the past 7 days or scheduled for an appointment within the 7-day period, this service would not have been separately reported.

Telephone Calls

98966	Telephone assessment and management services provided by a qualified nonphysician health care professional to an established patient, parent, or guardian not originating from related assessment and management service provided within the previous 7 days nor leading to an assessment and management service or procedure within the next 24 hours or soonest available appointment; 5–10 minutes of medical discussion
98967	11–20 minutes of medical discussion
98968	21–30 minutes of medical discussion

Codes **98966–98968** are used to report telephone assessment and management services by QNHCPs. Those QHPs who may independently provide and report E/M services report codes **99441–99443**.

Report codes **98966–98968** when

- The patient or caregiver initiates a call that is not in follow-up to a service by the same QNHCP within the past 7 days.
- Five minutes or more is spent in assessment and management services (*time must be documented*).
- No decision to see the patient within 24 hours or at the next available appointment is made during the telephone service.

Services Not Reported as Telephone Assessment and Management

Most telephone services provided by clinical staff (eg, MA relaying physician instructions) are included in the practice expense value assigned to physician services and not separately reported.

Do not report telephone assessment and management services that

- ✖ Relate to a service provided by the QNHCP within the past 7 days, regardless of whether the service was planned or prompted by patient or caregiver concern.
- ✖ Result in an appointment within the next 24 hours or in the next available appointment. When telephone assessment and management result in scheduling the patient for an appointment within 24 hours or the next available appointment, the service is considered preservice work to the face-to-face encounter.
- ✖ Are within a global period of another service.

> Telephone services by clinical staff may contribute to time of chronic care management (CCM) or transitional care management (TCM) when the services meet the description of the clinical staff activities included in CCM or TCM and the services are not reported with codes 98966–98968.

Example

➤ **The parents of a patient with an anxiety disorder contact a licensed clinical social worker in their physician's practice to request advice on managing a transition from remote learning to classes in school.** The social worker spends 18 minutes on the phone with the parents discussing concerns and techniques for preparing the child for the transition.

The licensed clinical social worker reports code **98967** according to the time spent addressing the parents' concerns. This service would not have been reported had the call been provided within 7 days of a previous service by the same provider or resulted in an appointment within 24 hours or the next available face-to-face appointment.

Medical Team Conferences

99366	Medical team conference with interdisciplinary team of health care professionals, face-to-face with patient and/or family, 30 minutes or more; participation by nonphysician qualified health care professional
99368	Medical team conference with interdisciplinary team of health care professionals, patient and/or family not present, 30 minutes or more; participation by nonphysician qualified health care professional

> If qualified health care professionals who may report evaluation and management services participate in a team conference without direct physician supervision, they may report team conference participation *without the patient or caregiver present* as if provided by a physician (99367), if this type of reporting is within the state's scope of practice and they use their own National Provider Identifier. See Chapter 10 for further information.

Medical team conference codes are used to report participation by a minimum of 3 health care professionals (including physicians, QHPs, and QNHCPs) of different specialties in conferences to coordinate or manage care and services for established patients with chronic or multiple health conditions (eg, a child with ventilator dependence and developmental delays, seizures, and a gastrostomy tube for nutrition).

- Codes differentiate between face-to-face (**99366**) and non–face-to-face (patient and/or family is not present [**99368**]) team conference services.
- Medicaid and commercial payers may follow these Medicare requirements or have their own specific rules.

Chapter 13. Qualified Nonphysician Health Care Professional Services

- Medical team conferences *may not be reported* when
  - The facility or organization is contractually obligated to provide the service, or the conferences are informal meetings or simple conversations between physicians and QNHCPs (eg, therapists).
  - Less than 30 minutes of conference time is spent in a team conference.
- One unit of service is reported for each conference of 30 minutes or more.
- Medicare assigns a bundled (B) status to team conference services in the Medicare Physician Fee Schedule (MFPS) and does not allow separate payment for participation in medical team conferences. Payment policies may vary among Medicaid and private health plans.

  Medical team conferences require
- Face-to-face participation by a minimum of 3 health care professionals (any combination of QNHCPs, physicians, and/ or QHPs) from different subspecialties or disciplines (eg, speech pathologists, dietitians, social workers), with or without the patient, family member(s), community agencies, surrogate decision-maker(s) (eg, legal guardian), and/or caregiver(s)

> Verify payer policies for care team conferences. Although payment for codes 99366 and 99368 is bundled into payment for other services in the Medicare Physician Fee Schedule, some benefit plans allow separate payment when a qualified nonphysician health care professional participates either in person or virtually.

- Active involvement in developing, revising, coordinating, and implementing health care services needed by the patient by each participant
- That the participant has provided face-to-face evaluation(s) and/or treatment to the patient, separate from any team conference, within the previous 60 days
- Only one individual from the same specialty to report codes 99366–99368 for the same encounter
- Medical record documentation that supports the reporting individual's participation, the time spent from the beginning of review of an individual patient until the conclusion of review, and the contributed information and subsequent treatment recommendations

Examples

➤ **A care team meets to discuss the care plans for a 4-year-old girl with history of congenital heart disease, cerebrovascular injury with residual paraplegia, and developmental delays.** As the child nears entry to kindergarten, the pediatrician has requested input to the child's individualized education program and ongoing health care plan from all health care professionals. The pediatrician, cardiologist, physiatrist, occupational and physical therapists, speech pathologist, home care coordinator, and social worker attend the conference to discuss the child's current medical status, prognosis for the short and long term, and necessary accommodations for her education. The conference lasts 60 minutes. The patient and family are not present for the conference.

Qualified nonphysician health care professionals report participation by using code 99368 when the patient or caregivers are not present. Assign appropriate *International Classification of Diseases, 10th Revision, Clinical Modification (ICD-10-CM)* codes for the specified developmental delays (codes in categories F80–F88) and other health concerns addressed.

➤ **A patient with cerebral palsy requires coordination with multiple health care professionals (eg, physical and occupational therapists, neurologist, pediatrician).** Each participant in the conference has completed their evaluation of the patient within 60 days before the conference, and a team conference of 40 minutes is held to assess the current plan of care and therapy. The patient's family is at this conference.

Code 99366 would be reported by the physical and occupational therapists. Physicians at the conference would report an E/M code that best describes their services on this date (eg, office or other outpatient E/M service based on face-to-face time with the family spent in counseling and/or coordination of care).

Patient Self-management Training Services

Education and Training for Patient Self-management

★**98960** Education and training for patient self-management by a qualified, nonphysician health care professional using a standardized curriculum, face-to-face with the patient (could include caregiver/family) each 30 minutes; individual patient

★**98961** 2–4 patients

★**98962** 5–8 patients

Report codes **98960–98962** when

● The purpose of these services is to teach the patient and caregivers how to self-manage the illness or disease or delay disease comorbidities in conjunction with the patient's professional health care team.

> Improved patient self-management may benefit a practice through payments received for quality initiatives related to management of complex and/or chronic conditions (eg, a percentage of patients aged 5–64 years and identified as having persistent asthma had a ratio of controller medications to total asthma medications of ≥0.50 during the measurement year). To learn more about how quality measurement may influence coding and payment, see Chapter 3.

● A physician prescribes the services and a standardized curriculum is used. A standardized curriculum is one that is consistent with guidelines or standards established or recognized by a physician or QNHCP society, association, or other appropriate source (eg, curriculum established or endorsed by the American Academy of Pediatrics).

● Qualifications of the QNHCPs and the content of the program are consistent with guidelines or standards established or recognized by a physician or QNHCP society, association, or other appropriate source.

   — These codes apply to diabetic and asthma self-management training—important categories of patient self-management education and training. Such training can be provided by nurse educators or other clinicians who have received special education and/or certification from accreditation societies or state licensing panels.

   — These services could be reported by the supervising physician when the services are rendered by the appropriately certified professional and acknowledged by the payer via the payer contract or published guidance.

● Education and training services are provided face-to-face (including via audiovisual telemedicine service) to patients with an established illness or disease.

● When a standardized curriculum is not used in the provision of health behavior assessment and intervention, see codes **96156**, **96158**, **96159**, and **96164–96171**.

> Qualifications of the qualified nonphysician health care professionals (QNHCPs) and the content of patient self-management education (98960–98962) must be consistent with guidelines or standards established or recognized by a physician or QNHCP society, association, or other appropriate source.

Code selection is based on the general *CPT* instruction for reporting services based on time. Time is met when the midpoint is passed (ie, report code **98960** for ≥16 minutes of face-to-face time and with units of service for each additional full 30 minutes and the last 16–30 minutes).

Example

➤ **A 14-year-old patient was recently diagnosed with type 1 diabetes and is referred to the diabetes educator for continued training under an approved curriculum.** The certified nurse educator assesses what the patient and caregivers have learned since diagnosis and uses a standardized curriculum to provide additional education. The total documented time of service is 30 minutes.

   Code **98960** is reported for the 30 minutes of service. If the time of service extended 16 to 30 minutes beyond the first 30 minutes, an additional unit would be reported.

   The content, type, duration, and patient response to the training must be documented in the medical record.

   The payer contract will determine if services are reported under the name of the asthma educator, supervising physician, or QHP. If the payer credentials educators, report under the name and NPI of the educator. If the payer does not credential educators, follow payer guidance for reporting.

● indicates a new code; ▲, revised; #, re-sequenced; ✚, add-on; ★, audiovisual technology; and ◀, synchronous interactive audio.

HCPCS modifiers and/or codes may be required to indicate that the service was provided by a QNHCP. Code **S9441** (asthma education, non-physician provider; per session) may be accepted in lieu of **98960–98962**. However, note that code **S9441** is not assigned relative value units (RVUs) in the MFPS and payment amounts may vary significantly for services reported with this code.

Payer-Specific Coding for Services Under a Disease Management Program

HCPCS Level II codes may be reported when the narrative differs from the *CPT* code for the service. What follows is a small sample of HCPCS codes and modifiers that may be used for services by QNHCPs when a payer accepts these codes to describe services rendered as part of a specific disease management program (eg, services specific to management of sickle cell anemia).

Payment for services reported with HCPCS codes may vary, especially for codes not assigned RVUs in the MFPS, on which many payers base their fee schedules.

Note that HCPCS codes may include the term *NPP* (nonphysician practitioner) rather than *QNHCP* or *QHP*. Individual payers may define *NPP* differently. It is advisable to retain copies of a payer's written policies and guidance for reporting HCPCS codes such as

S0315	Disease management program; initial assessment and initiation of the program
S0316	Disease management program, follow-up/reassessment
S0317	Disease management program; per diem
S0320	Telephone calls by a registered nurse to a disease management program member for monitoring purposes; per month
S9460	Diabetic management program, nurse visit
S9470	Nutritional counseling, dietitian visit

Payers may also instruct certain QNHCPs to report services by appending a HCPCS modifier to the *CPT* or HCPCS code for services provided.

HA	Child/adolescent program
HN	Bachelor's degree level
HO	Master's degree level (eg, licensed master social worker)
HP	Doctoral level
HQ	Group setting
UN	Two patients served
UP	Three patients served
UQ	Four patients served
UR	Five patients served
US	Six or more patients served

See an example of how to report services as part of a disease management program for diabetes in the Payer-Specific Coding for Nutrition Assessment and Intervention section later in this chapter.

Nutritional Support Services

Breastfeeding Support/Lactation Services

Under the Patient Protection and Affordable Care Act, most health insurance plans must cover breastfeeding support, counseling, and equipment to mothers for the duration of breastfeeding. These services are not subject to a deductible, co-payment, or coinsurance. However, access to benefits for lactation counseling is not always straightforward.

In the absence of feeding problems of an infant or health problems of the mother, **Z39.1** (encounter for care and examination of lactating mother) is the diagnosis code reported for lactation counseling.

Lactation consultation services do not have a specific *CPT* code, and billing is a source of confusion for many providers. Many states do not license lactation consultants. Also, many health plans do not include lactation consultants in their networks.

Physicians and QHPs may generally use preventive medicine counseling codes **99401–99404** to report personally performed lactation counseling services. (For counseling to address a feeding problem, see a problem-oriented E/M code for the site of service.) When payer policy instructs that these codes be reported for services by an RN or a QNHCP (eg, lactation consultant), a written copy of the payer policy should be kept on file.

● indicates a new code; ▲, revised; #, re-sequenced; ✚, add-on; ★, audiovisual technology; and ◀, synchronous interactive audio.

Be aware, some plans bundle provision of breastfeeding support and counseling to the global obstetric service or postpartum care of the mother and do not pay separately for breastfeeding support or lactation counseling. It is important to understand contractual obligations that may limit a physician's ability to bill the patient for these covered services.

Clinical staff services may be reported with **99211** when provided incident to a physician's plan of care for an established patient (health plan policies may or may not align with Medicare's incident-to policy).

When a pediatrician provides services related to feeding problems or maternal health issues, report evaluation and management codes by site of service for these services (eg, office visit). Evaluation and management services provided to address maternal issues are reported to the mother's health plan. An *International Classification of Diseases, 10th Revision, Clinical Modification* code is used to identify the type of problem (eg, suppressed lactation, 092.5)

Other specific codes used to report these services when provided by QNHCPs may include

S9443   Lactation classes, nonphysician provider, per session

Code **S9443** is the code most specific to lactation services. This code is included in some health plan policies for preventive medicine services or breastfeeding/lactation counseling services.

S9445   Patient education, not otherwise classified, nonphysician provider, individual, per session
S9446   Patient education, not otherwise classified, nonphysician provider, group, per session
★98960   Education and training for patient self-management by a qualified, nonphysician health care professional using a standardized curriculum, face-to-face with the patient (could include caregiver/family), each 30 minutes; individual patient

Key considerations for reporting lactation services include

- Unless the newborn or infant has been diagnosed with a feeding problem, the mother is typically the patient, and claims are filed to her health benefit plan.
- Payer policies may not allow separate payment for lactation counseling on the same date as an E/M service.
- Challenges might be encountered in states where licensure is not yet enacted for lactation support professionals. Hurdles include credentialing and coverage by payers who cover only services provided by licensed health care professionals, although services provided incident to a physician or QHP (eg, **99211** or **S9443**) may be allowed.
- When a medical condition (eg, feeding problem) was previously diagnosed by the physician on an earlier date, a QNHCP may see the mother and patient to identify the psychological, behavioral, emotional, cognitive, and social factors important to the prevention, treatment, or management of physical health problems. Behavioral health assessment and intervention codes **96156**, **96158** and **96159**, and **96164–96171** may be reportable for these services. Again, payer policy determines who may provide these services and what is paid for.
- Lactation counseling provided by a QNHCP in conjunction with a physician's or QHP's E/M service, although not always separately reported, may reduce the physician's time spent on history taking, counseling, and education. This may also support quality initiatives.

Medicaid plans often ask that physicians refer covered breastfeeding mothers to the Special Supplemental Nutrition Program for Women, Infants, and Children for lactation counseling and other support services.

Medical Nutrition Assessment and Intervention

★◀97802   Medical nutrition therapy, initial assessment and intervention, individual, face-to-face with the patient, each 15 minutes
★◀97803   Reassessment and intervention, individual, face-to-face with the patient, each 15 minutes
★◀97804   group (2 or more individuals), each 30 minutes

Medical nutrition therapy is one of the services for which *CPT* instruction excludes reporting by a physician or QHP who may report E/M services.

- Codes are reported when provided by a QNHCP who may report medical nutrition therapy services under their individual state's scope of practice.

- Many states restrict the provision of medical nutrition therapy to certain QNHCPs (eg, registered dietitians, licensed medical nutritionists). Practices providing medical nutrition therapy services should be aware of state licensing and scope of practice regulations as well as health plan credentialing policies.
- HCPCS modifiers may be required to report the type of provider for medical nutrition therapy services, such as **AE** (registered dietitian).
- Coverage may also be limited to patients with certain conditions (eg, diabetes, kidney disease) and to a number of units of service or visits per year.
- When medical nutrition therapy is provided as a preventive service (eg, counseling a patient who has overweight), modifier **33** may be appended to codes **97802–97804**.

> For more on modifier **33**, see chapters 2 and 8.

- Services are reported according to time. Per *CPT* instruction, a unit of time is met when the midpoint is passed.
  — Report code **97802** or **97803** with 1 unit for 8 to 22 minutes of service. An additional unit may be reported for each subsequent 15 minutes and the last 8 to 22 minutes of service.
  — Certain payers may require that the time in the code descriptor (eg, 15 minutes) be met or exceeded for each unit of service reported.
- Time must be documented.

Examples

➤ **A 3-year-old girl was seen by her physician for a health supervision visit 1 week ago.** Her body mass index (BMI) has fallen below the fifth percentile, and her parents report that she is finicky about food textures and very fidgety at meals but is otherwise eating a balanced diet. After a medical evaluation does not yield an underlying cause for failure to thrive, the patient is referred to the practice's registered dietitian for assessment and counseling to optimize her diet. The dietitian meets with the child and her parents and spends 30 minutes discussing planning meals, choosing snacks, and monitoring intake and weight gain/growth.

ICD-10-CM	CPT
Z71.3 (dietary counseling and surveillance) **R62.51** (failure to thrive, child) **Z68.51** (BMI pediatric, less than 5th percentile for age)	If payer allows billing under the registered dietitian's NPI **97802** × 2 (medical nutrition therapy, initial assessment and intervention, individual, face-to-face with the patient, each 15 minutes) If payer requires billing under the NPI of the supervising physician **97802 AE** × 2 (medical nutrition therapy as above by a registered dietitian)

Teaching Point: Some Medicaid plans and/or private payers may require that medical nutrition therapy in the physician practice be provided under a physician's order and general supervision. Services are reported as if provided by the physician, but modifier **AE** indicates that the service was provided by a registered dietitian.

➤ **A group of adolescent patients with type 1 diabetes is referred to a licensed medical nutritionist for reassessment and intervention.** The patients receive both individual reassessment and group therapy services for a total time of 50 minutes.

ICD-10-CM	CPT
Z71.3 (dietary counseling and surveillance) **E10.-** (type 1 diabetes mellitus [additional characters required to indicate manifestations or lack thereof])	If payer allows billing under registered dietitian's NPI **97804** × 2 (medical nutrition therapy, reassessment and intervention, each 30 minutes) If payer requires billing under the NPI of the supervising physician **97804 AE** × 2 (medical nutrition therapy as above by a registered dietitian)

Teaching Point: The service provided to a group, even with individual reassessments in the group setting, is reported to each patient's health plan with code **97804** with 1 unit per 30 minutes. Because the time of service was 50 minutes, 2 units of service are reported (ie, the midpoint between the first and last 30-minute periods was passed).

Payer-Specific Coding for Nutrition Assessment and Intervention

HCPCS codes may be required by certain payers to provide reassessment and subsequent intervention after a change in diagnosis, medical condition, or treatment.

G0270   Medical nutrition therapy; reassessment and subsequent intervention(s) following second referral in same year for change in diagnosis, medical condition, or treatment regimen (including additional hours needed for renal disease); individual, face-to-face with the patient, each 15 minutes

G0271   group (2 or more individuals), each 30 minutes

Documentation of services should include the physician or QHP order for services, information on the medical need for services, medical nutrition therapy evaluation and plan for intervention, time, correspondence with the referring provider, date of service, and name, credentials, and signature of the provider of the medical nutrition therapy.

Payers may also offer specific benefits for nutrition assessments and counseling under specific disease management programs. HCPCS codes may be required in lieu of *CPT* codes.

G0108   Diabetes outpatient self-management training services, individual, per 30 minutes
G0109   Diabetes outpatient self-management training services, group session (2 or more), per 30 minutes
S9449   Weight management classes, NPP, per session
S9452   Nutrition class, NPP, per session
S9455   Diabetic management program, group session
S9460   nurse visit
S9465   dietitian visit
S9470   Nutritional counseling, dietitian visit

Example

➤ **A group of adolescent patients with diabetes type 1 is referred to a licensed medical nutritionist for reassessment and intervention as part of a diabetes outpatient self-management training program.** The patients receive both individual reassessment and group therapy services for a total time of 50 minutes.

ICD-10-CM	CPT
Z71.3 (dietary counseling and surveillance) **E10.-** (type 1 diabetes mellitus [additional characters required to indicate manifestations or lack thereof])	If payer allows billing with *CPT* **97804** × 2 (medical nutrition therapy, reassessment and intervention, each 30 minutes) If payer requires billing with HCPCS **G0109** × 2 (diabetes outpatient self-management training services, group session [2 or more], per 30 minutes)

Teaching Point: The service should be reported per the individual payer's policy for the program. Note also that a payer may require that the time of service be met or exceeded (ie, a second unit of service will be reported only if time meets or exceeds 60 minutes).

Other Nonphysician Qualified Health Care Professional Services

Genetic Counseling Services

◀**96040**   Medical genetics and genetic counseling services, each 30 minutes face-to-face with patient/family

● Trained genetic counselors provide services that may include obtaining a structured family genetic history, pedigree construction, analysis for genetic risk assessment, and counseling of the patient and family.
● Only face-to-face time with the patient or caregiver is used in determining the units of service reported. Do not report genetic counseling of 15 minutes or less. Report code **96040** with units of service for the first and each additional 30 minutes and the last 16 to 30 minutes.

● indicates a new code; ▲, revised; #, re-sequenced; ✚, add-on; ★, audiovisual technology; and ◀, synchronous interactive audio.

- Services may be provided during 1 or more sessions and may include review of medical data and family information, face-to-face interviews, and counseling services.
- For genetic counseling and education on genetic risks by a QNHCP to a group, see codes **98961** and **98962**.
- Genetic counseling by physicians and other QHPs who may report E/M services are reported with the appropriate E/M service code.

Medication Therapy Management Services by a Pharmacist

99605   Medication therapy management service(s) provided by a pharmacist, individual, face-to-face with patient, with assessment and intervention if provided; initial 15 minutes, new patient

99606   initial 15 minutes, established patient

✚99607   each additional 15 minutes (List separately in addition to **99605** or **99606**)

   Medication therapy management services

- Are provided only by a pharmacist face-to-face with the patient or caregiver and usually in relation to complex medication regimens or medication adherence in conditions such as asthma and diabetes.
- Are provided on request of the patient or caregiver, prescribing physician, other QHPs, or prescription drug benefit plan (not reported for routine dispensing-related activities).
- Are reported with codes selected on the basis of whether the patient is new or established and the pharmacist's face-to-face time with the patient.
- Include review of pertinent patient history (not limited to drug history).
- Include documentation of review of the pertinent patient history, medication profile (prescription and nonprescription), and recommendations for improving health outcomes and treatment adherence.
- *New patients* are those who have received no face-to-face service from the pharmacist or another pharmacist of the same clinic or pharmacy within 3 years before the current date of service.
- Unless otherwise specified by the payer policy, time is met when the midpoint is passed.
  - Report codes **99605** and **99606** for the first 8 to 22 minutes of face-to-face time with the patient.
  - When time exceeds 22 minutes, code **99607** may be reported for subsequent 15-minute periods and the last 8 to 22 minutes.
- Under the Medicare program, pharmacists may also provide services incident to a physician or QHP and report E/M services with code **99211** when allowed under the scope of practice as defined by state licensure.

Physical and Occupational Therapy

Although many physical and occupational therapy services are included in a facility's charges, some states allow therapists to practice independently. There are codes for reporting therapy evaluations, reevaluations, and therapeutic activities/modalities. Payment for physical and occupational therapy services is often defined by not only the therapist's scope of practice but also the payer's credentialing and payment policies that often restrict the number of therapy services provided within a specific time frame.

   Following are some of the codes commonly used for reporting evaluative and therapeutic services to create, revise, or carry out a therapy plan of care. Therapists use specific methods of evaluating (eg, occupational therapy profile with review of medical and therapy history and assessment of performance deficits) and providing therapeutic services based on clinical guidelines.

> **Therapeutic modalities are any physical agent applied to produce therapeutic changes to biological tissue including, but not limited to, thermal, acoustic, light, mechanical, or electric energy.**

97161–97163   Physical therapy evaluations

97164   Physical therapy re-evaluation

97165–97167   Occupational therapy evaluations

97168   Occupational therapy re-evaluation

97010–97028   Supervised therapy modalities

97032–97039   Therapy modalities requiring constant attendance (one-on-one patient contact)

97110–97546   Therapeutic procedures

   See codes **97169–97172** for athletic training evaluations and reevaluations.

● indicates a new code; ▲, revised; #, re-sequenced; ✚, add-on; ★, audiovisual technology; and ◀, synchronous interactive audio.

Modifiers for Services Provided by Therapists and Speech Pathologists

Medicaid and other payers may require specific modifiers for certain outpatient therapeutic services. Check with individual payers for guidance on reporting therapy modifiers.

GN   Services delivered under an outpatient speech language pathology plan of care
GO   Services delivered under an outpatient occupational therapy plan of care
GP   Services delivered under an outpatient physical therapy plan of care

The following modifiers may be required in addition to either GO or GP when a therapy assistant provides a therapy service under a therapist's supervision:

CO   Outpatient occupational therapy services furnished in whole or in part by an occupational therapy assistant
CQ   Outpatient physical therapy services furnished in whole or in part by a physical therapist assistant

Speech Pathology Services

Speech and language evaluation and therapy may be provided for the treatment of disorders of speech, language, voice, communication, and/or auditory processing. These services are often necessary in the care of children with developmental delay, autism, injury, or congenital anomaly (eg, cleft palate).

See the September 2021 *AAP Pediatric Coding Newsletter* article, "Pediatric Feeding Disorder and a New *ICD-10-CM* Code" (https://doi.org/10.1542/pcco_book209_document007) for examples of feeding disorders that may lead to referral to an occupational therapist or speech pathologist.

Common codes for services by speech pathology services include

◀92521   Evaluation of speech fluency (eg, stuttering, cluttering)
◀92522   Evaluation of speech sound production (eg, articulation, phonological process, apraxia, dysarthria)
◀92523   with evaluation of language comprehension and expression (eg, receptive and expressive language)
◀92507   Treatment of speech, language, voice, communication, and/or auditory processing disorder; individual
92630   Auditory rehabilitation; prelingual hearing loss
92633   postlingual hearing loss

Take the quiz found at the end of this chapter to review and confirm your understanding of some of its takeaways. Answers to each quiz are found in **Appendix IV**.

Chapter Takeaways

This chapter reviews health care services that might be provided by QNHCPs and independently reported in pediatric practice. Following are some takeaways from this chapter:

- Scope of practice is a key differentiator of physicians and QHPs whose scope of practice includes E/M service and QNHCPs for the purpose of reporting health care services.
- Qualified nonphysician health care professionals are distinct from clinical staff when regulations and payer policies allow independent reporting of services.
- Assessment and management services are reported with codes other than E/M service codes.
- It is important to understand both scope of practice and payer policies for provision and coding of the QNHCP's services before provision of services.

Resource

AAP Pediatric Coding Newsletter™

"Pediatric Feeding Disorder and a New *ICD-10-CM* Code," September 2021 (https://doi.org/10.1542/pcco_book209_document007)

● indicates a new code; ▲, revised; #, re-sequenced; ✚, add-on; ★, audiovisual technology; and ◀, synchronous interactive audio.

Test Your Knowledge!

1. **Which of the following terms is used by state licensing boards to define the procedures, actions, and processes that are permitted for a licensed individual?**
   a. Contracting
   b. National Provider Identifier
   c. Credentialing
   d. Scope of practice

2. **Qualified nonphysician healthcare professionals whose scope of practice does not include provision and independent reporting of evaluation and management (E/M) services may report which assessment and management services?**
   a. Any E/M service
   b. An assessment and management service
   c. Only services described by code **99211**
   d. Any level of E/M service beyond **99211**

3. **Which of the following components of education and training is required for patient self-management?**
   a. The service is provided face-to-face (including by telemedicine) with 1 or more patients.
   b. A physician is present when the service is provided.
   c. The service is provided to prevent an illness or injury.
   d. At least 30 minutes is spent providing the service.

4. **When medical nutrition counseling is provided as a preventive service, how is the service reported?**
   a. Medical nutrition counseling is not reported when provided as a preventive service.
   b. Report diagnosis code **Z71.3** (dietary counseling and surveillance).
   c. Append modifier **33** (preventive service) to the procedure code (**97802–97804**).
   d. Report **97802–97804** and a diagnosis for a routine child health examination.

5. **Which of the following types of providers is a qualified nonphysician health care professional as described in this chapter?**
   a. Physician
   b. Qualified health care professional who may independently report evaluation and management services
   c. Medical assistant
   d. Speech pathologist

Surgery, Infusion, and Sedation in the Outpatient Setting

CPT copyright 2022 American Medical Association. All rights reserved.

Contents

Chapter 14. Surgery, Infusion, and Sedation in the Outpatient Setting

● indicates a new code; ▲, revised; #, re-sequenced; ✦, add-on; ★, audiovisual technology; and ◀, synchronous interactive audio.

● indicates a new code; ▲, revised; #, re-sequenced; ✚, add-on; ★, audiovisual technology; and ◀, synchronous interactive audio.

Chapter Highlights

- Components included in the surgical package for services assigned a global period
- Discussion of codes for some commonly performed procedural services
- Evaluation and management (E/M) services provided in conjunction with procedures

Procedural Services in the Office or Other Outpatient Setting

This chapter reviews coding for procedural services including minor surgical procedures, fracture care, and injections and infusions.

The commonly used Medicare global periods and total non-facility relative value units (RVUs) are provided for reference for many procedures discussed in this chapter. The RVUs included are pulled from the 2022 Medicare Physician Fee Schedule (MPFS) and are not geographically adjusted (2023 RVUs were unavailable at the time of this publication). Individual payers may not use Medicare global periods and/or current-year Medicare RVUs. Check contract terms and payer policies for payer-specific information.

Surgical Package Rules

Current Procedural Terminology (*CPT*®) surgical codes (**10004–69990**) are *packaged* or *global* codes. To understand documentation and coding of procedural services, it is necessary to know what is included in each service from a coding and payment perspective. *CPT* directs that each procedure code represents a "surgical package" of service components. These include

- Evaluation and management services subsequent to the decision for surgery on the day before and/or day of surgery (including the history and physical examination)
- Local or topical anesthesia, including metacarpal, metatarsal, and/or digital block
- Immediate postoperative care
- Writing orders
- Evaluation of the patient in the recovery area
- Typical postoperative follow-up care

On the basis of the *CPT* definition of the surgical package, RVUs are assigned to each procedure on the basis of the typical preoperative, intraoperative, and postoperative physician work; practice expense (eg, procedure room, instruments, supplies, support staff); and professional liability. Payers that use RVUs to calculate payments will typically not pay separately for any components of the surgical package.

> The relative value units assigned to procedures include the typically used supplies under the practice expense component. Know your payer policies on this.

Medicare Surgical Package Definition

Most Medicaid programs follow the Medicare definition of the surgical package. The Medicare definition differs from that of *CPT*.

- Medicare defines procedures as *minor* (procedures assigned a 0- or 10-day global period or endoscopies) or *major* (procedures assigned a 90-day global period) as shown in **Table 14-1**. *The day of surgery is day 0 (zero); the postoperative period begins the next day.*

> Throughout this chapter, when an assigned global period is noted, this refers to the period assigned in the Medicare Physician Fee Schedule (MPFS). While most payers use the MPFS, individual payers may assign different global periods. In particular, some Medicaid plans assign 30-day global periods.

- *CPT* does not define global periods and minor or major surgery. Global periods are defined in the MPFS (www.cms.gov/medicare/medicare-fee-for-service-payment/physicianfeesched). Although other payers can assign different global periods, most follow the MPFS.

Learn more about the Resource-Based Relative Value Scale in Chapter 4.

- *CPT* does not include care related to surgical complications in the surgical package. Medicare considers care related to complications following surgery to be included in the surgical package unless a return to the operating/procedure room is necessary.

Most office and outpatient clinic procedures will have 0- or 10-day global periods. Exceptions are certain services such as care of fractures (discussed in the Fracture and/or Dislocation Care section later in this chapter). "Office Procedures and Global Days" is included at www.aap.org/cfp2023.

The day of surgery is day 0 (zero) of the global period; the postoperative period begins the next day.

Table 14-1. The Medicare Surgical Package

Global Periods	0-Day Global Surgical Procedures	10-Day Global Surgical Procedures	90-Day Global Surgical Procedures
Services before date of procedure	Not included		All related services 1 day before surgery if after decision for surgery
Services on date of procedure	E/M services typically included regardless of when decision for surgery is made		All related services except E/M services at which decision for surgery is made
Postoperative services	Typical postoperative care on same date	All related care on date of service and 10 days following	All related care on date of service and 90 days following, including care for complications that does not require a return to the OR

Abbreviations: E/M, evaluation and management; OR, operating/procedure room.

Supplies and Materials

99070 Supplies and materials provided by the physician over and above those usually included with the office visit or other services rendered

- Items such as elastic wraps, clavicle splints, or circumcision and suturing trays may be reported with this code. Remember that some supplies (eg, circumcision and suturing trays) are included in the value of the surgical procedure when the payment is based on RVUs.
- Only the supplies purchased in an office-based practice may be reported.

If reporting code 99070, identify the supplies or materials on the claim form and be prepared to submit an invoice.

- Some payers require the use of Healthcare Common Procedure Coding System (HCPCS) codes. More specific HCPCS codes are available for a number of supplies (eg, codes **Q4001–Q4051** for cast and splint supplies). Use HCPCS codes when they are more specific.

For more information on Healthcare Common Procedure Coding System codes, see Chapter 1.

Significant Evaluation and Management Service and Procedure

The Medicare Resource-Based Relative Value Scale is used by most private payers and Medicaid plans to determine RVUs and global periods for services. Under this payment methodology, procedural services include some preservice and postservice E/M by the performing physician. Payer edits, such as the National Correct Coding Initiative (NCCI) edits used by Medicare and Medicaid also bundle E/M services with certain procedures.

For minor procedures, separate payment for a significant, separately identifiable E/M service is allowed when modifier **25** is appended to the E/M code. However, care should be taken to use modifier **25** only when documentation supports a significant, separately identifiable E/M service.

● indicates a new code; ▲, revised; #, re-sequenced; ✚, add-on; ★, audiovisual technology; and ◀, synchronous interactive audio.

- Medicare states that an E/M code may be reported on the same day as a minor surgical procedure only when a significant, separately identifiable E/M service is performed and modifier **25** is appended to the E/M code. *CPT* does not specifically include the initial E/M service before a minor procedure when the decision for surgery occurs at the visit.

  For major procedures (typically 90-day global period), modifier **57** may be appended when the decision for surgery or a procedure is made during the E/M service on the same date as the procedure. Documentation should clearly show E/M of the problem resulting in the initial decision to perform the related procedure.

- For minor procedures, the E/M visit on the date of the procedure is considered a routine part of the procedure *regardless of whether it is prior or subsequent to the decision for surgery.* In these cases, modifier **57** (decision for surgery) is not recognized.

Coding Conundrum: Procedure, or Evaluation and Management and Procedure?

The differences in the Centers for Medicare & Medicaid Services (CMS) and *Current Procedural Terminology* (*CPT*) surgical package guidelines may lead to confusion. Try to answer the following questions when determining if you should report a procedure alone or a procedure with an evaluation and management (E/M) service:

- Did you address a problem or condition before deciding to perform the procedure (above and beyond the usual preoperative care associated with the procedure) or a significant and separately identifiable problem? If yes, report an E/M service and procedure.
- Does the medical record documentation clearly support the performance of a medically necessary E/M service (and meet code descriptor requirements), the procedure (procedure note), the clinical indications for both, and the decision to perform the surgery? If yes, report an E/M service and procedure.
- Was the purpose of the visit only for the procedure (eg, decision for surgery made at an earlier visit)? If yes, do not report an E/M service.
- Does the payer follow the *CPT* or CMS guidelines for reporting surgical procedures? If the focus of an E/M service is related to the procedure, the history and physical examination are part of preoperative service and only the surgical procedure should be reported.

Examples

➤ **A patient returns for a previously planned removal of impacted cerumen from their left ear.** On examination, the physician notes and documents that the patient has a blackhead on the left earlobe. Documentation includes notation of patient/caregiver consent, procedure including instrumentation used to remove impacted cerumen, patient tolerance, outcome, and post-procedural examination finding (eg, hearing improved).

ICD-10-CM	CPT
H61.22 (impacted cerumen, left ear)	**69210** (removal impacted cerumen requiring instrumentation, unilateral)

Teaching Point: Although the physician noted a blackhead, this did not require or affect patient care treatment or management and does not support a significant and separately identifiable E/M service beyond the preservice/postservice work of the procedure that was provided or documented.

➤ **A patient presents for reevaluation of depression.** The patient also says that they got a splinter in the sole of their right foot. After reevaluating the patient's response to current management of depression, the physician evaluates the patient's right foot. The splinter is partially visible but cannot be removed with tweezers. Removal is achieved by incision with local anesthetic. The diagnoses are a single episode of stable, moderate major depression and a foreign body in the skin on the ball of the right foot. The medical decision-making (MDM) of the encounter is low, supporting **99213**.

ICD-10-CM	CPT
F32.1 (major depressive disorder, single episode, moderate) **S90.851A** (superficial foreign body, right foot, initial encounter)	**99213 25** (office or other outpatient E/M)
S90.851A	**10120** (incision and removal of foreign body, subcutaneous tissues; simple)

Teaching Point: A significant and separately identifiable E/M service was provided to address the patient's depression. If the E/M code were selected on the basis of time, the work associated with the foreign body removal (including documentation of the procedure) would not be included in the time of the E/M service.

Reporting Postoperative Care

Postoperative Evaluation and Management

- Report *CPT* code **99024** (postoperative follow-up visit) for follow-up care provided during the global surgery period. No RVUs are assigned to **99024**, as the RVUs were included in the total value of the related procedure.
    - Payment for postoperative care is included as part of the procedure. Payers track the postoperative care provided and reported with code **99024**.
    - If a physician is not providing or reporting the postoperative care typically performed for a procedure, payers may reduce payment for the surgical service.
    - Reporting **99024** allows tracking of the number of visits performed during the postoperative period of specific procedures. A practice can use this data to calculate office overhead expenses (eg, supplies, staff, physician time) associated with the procedure and potentially use the data to negotiate higher payment rates.

> **Payment of a surgical procedure may be reduced if the physician does not report code 99024. For an example of 99024, see the Fracture and/or Dislocation Care section later in this chapter.**

- When the physician who performed a procedure provides an unrelated E/M service during the postoperative period, modifier **24** (unrelated E/M service by the same physician during a postoperative period) should be appended to the E/M service code.
- When a physician *other than the surgeon* provides unrelated services to a patient during the postoperative period, the services are reported without a modifier. Despite the use of different National Provider Identifiers and diagnosis codes, some payers with assigned follow-up surgical periods will deny the service. The claim should be appealed for payment with a letter advising the payer that the service was unrelated to surgical care.

Example

➤ **A patient returns 1 month after initial closed treatment of a non-displaced clavicle fracture with concern of runny nose and nighttime cough.** History is provided by the child's mother and father. The physician's evaluation results in diagnosis of seasonal allergic rhinitis with management via over-the-counter allergy products following instructions on product labels. The physician also reevaluates the patient's healing fracture.

ICD-10-CM	CPT
J30.2 (other seasonal allergic rhinitis)	**99213 24**
S42.024D (nondisplaced fracture of shaft of right clavicle, subsequent encounter for fracture with routine healing) A code for the external cause of injury will also be reported (eg, **W07.XXXD**, fall from chair, subsequent encounter).	**99024**

Teaching Point: Modifier **24** is reported to identify that the service provided was unrelated to the prior procedure. The MDM of the E/M service was low because of a low number and complexity of problems addressed (allergic rhinitis), limited data (history from independent historians), and low risk of complications, morbidity, or mortality from over-the-counter medication use per instructions on the label. The evaluation of the healing fracture during the postoperative period is not included in determining the level of service for the encounter because it is included in postoperative care when provided during the 90-day global period.

> **See Chapter 2 for more information on modifiers.**

• indicates a new code; ▲, revised; #, re-sequenced; ✦, add-on; ★, audiovisual technology; and ◀, synchronous interactive audio.

Suture Removal

New in 2023! *Current Procedural Terminology* code 15850 (removal of sutures under anesthesia [other than local], same surgeon) has been deleted, and code 15851 (removal of sutures under anesthesia [other than local], other surgeon) has been revised. Additionally, codes 15853 and 15854 have been added for reporting removal of sutures or staples not requiring anesthesia.

The Medicare global surgery period of 0 days indicates that payment includes the procedure or service plus any associated care provided *on the same day of service.* Therefore, practices may separately report follow-up visits and removal of sutures or staples placed as part of a procedure assigned a 0-day global period.

The Medicare global surgery periods of 10 and 90 days include the procedure or service plus any associated follow-up care for 10 or 90 days following the date of the procedure. Therefore, the charge for the procedure already includes suture or staple removal by the same physician or a physician of the same group and specialty as part of the global surgical package.

✖ Do not separately report encounters for suture or staple removal *during the global period of a procedure* performed by a physician or qualified health care professional (QHP) in the same group practice except when general anesthesia or moderate sedation is required.

Removal Requiring General Anesthesia or Moderate Sedation

▲15851   Removal of sutures or staples requiring anesthesia (ie, general anesthesia, moderate sedation)

Code **15851** is reported only when the patient requires general anesthesia or moderate sedation during suture or staple removal.

✖ Do not report **15851** for reopening a wound to perform an additional procedure.

Removal Not Requiring General Anesthesia or Moderate Sedation

#✚●15853   Removal of sutures or staples not requiring anesthesia
#✚●15854   Removal of sutures and staples not requiring anesthesia

✖ Do not report **15854** in conjunction with **15853**.

Codes **15853** and **15854** are add-on codes that are reported in addition to an E/M service at the same encounter. Report **15853** and **15854** in conjunction with E/M codes **99202–99205, 99211–99215, 99281–99285, 99341–99345,** or **99347–99350**.

Some payers may require reporting of Healthcare Common Procedure Coding System code S0630. Code S0630 is for removal of sutures by a physician other than the one who originally closed the wound. Report S0630 in lieu of 15853 and 15854 when required by payer policy.

For aftercare of an injury, assign the acute injury code with the seventh character **D** (subsequent encounter). *International Classification of Diseases, 10th Revision, Clinical Modification* (ICD-10-CM) code **Z48.02** (encounter for removal of sutures) *is not reported* for removal of sutures previously placed to repair an injury but may be reported when removal of sutures is unrelated to care for an injury (eg, removal of sutures from a wound created during excision of a skin lesion).

Examples

➤ **An 8-year-old sustained a 0.5-cm laceration on her forehead.** The wound on her face requires a simple repair. She is seen in follow-up 7 days later. The wound is clean, and the sutures are removed.

Visit	ICD-10-CM	CPT
Initial visit	**S01.81XA** (laceration without foreign body of other part of head, initial encounter)	**12011** (simple repair of the facial laceration 2.5 cm or less)
Follow-up visit	**S01.81XD** (laceration without foreign body of other part of head, subsequent encounter)	**99212–99215** (established patient E/M) on the basis of MDM or the physician's total time not including time of suture removal #✚●**15853** (removal of sutures or staples not requiring anesthesia)

● indicates a new code; ▲, revised; #, re-sequenced; ✚, add-on; ★, audiovisual technology; and ◀, synchronous interactive audio.

Teaching Point: Simple laceration repair has a 0-day global period, so any medically necessary follow-up care is separately reported. Code **15853** (removal of sutures) is reported in addition to the code for the E/M service to assess healing and provide any additional instructions for follow-up. No modifier is required on the E/M code because **15853** is an add-on code.

The seventh character **D** (ie, **S01.81XD**) is reported for encounters after the patient has been actively treated for the condition (ie, injury or other condition reported with a 7-character code) and is receiving routine care for the condition during the healing or recovery phase. This type of encounter includes one for suture and/or staple removal.

➤ **A 3-year-old with 5 sutures placed in the emergency department (ED) presents at her pediatrician's office for suture removal.** The child is hesitant to have the sutures removed, so 2 clinical staff members are required to assist the pediatrician in removing them. The physician's total time devoted to the patient's care on the date of service is 25 minutes. However, the time of the separately reported suture removal is not included in the time of the E/M service.

ICD-10-CM	CPT
Appropriate code for injury with seventh character **D** (eg, **S51.812D**, laceration of left forearm without foreign body, subsequent encounter)	**99212–99215** (established patient E/M) on the basis of MDM or the physician's total time not including time of suture removal **#✚●15853** (removal of sutures or staples not requiring anesthesia)

Teaching Point: The office and other outpatient E/M codes may be reported on the basis of the physician's or other QHP's total time on the date of the encounter but do not include the time spent in suture removal. Do not include time of clinical staff.

Reporting Terminated Procedures

When a procedure is started but cannot be completed due to extenuating circumstances, physicians should consider the individual situation, including the reason for termination of the procedure and the amount of work that was performed, when determining how to report the service rendered.

When a procedure was performed but not entirely successful (eg, portion of foreign body removed), it may be appropriate to report the procedure code that represents the work performed without modification.

● Only report reduced services (modifier **52**) or discontinued procedure (modifier **53**) when the service was significantly reduced from the typical service.

● If the work performed before discontinuation was insignificant, it may be appropriate to not report the procedure. If you choose to not report the procedure, consider whether the level of a related E/M service was increased due to the level of MDM associated with the attempted procedure, any complicating factors, and the revised management or treatment plan.

> For an example of a discontinued service, see the Removal of Impacted Cerumen section later in this chapter.

ICD-10-CM Coding for Procedures

ICD-10-CM codes linked to a procedure code should be the codes that most accurately reflect the reason for the service provided (eg, **H61.21**, impacted cerumen, right ear), and these codes may differ from ones linked to other services provided on the same date (eg, E/M service). See **Chapter 1** for information on linking diagnosis codes to service lines on a claim.

● indicates a new code; ▲, revised; #, re-sequenced; ✚, add-on; ★, audiovisual technology; and ◄, synchronous interactive audio.

Know Your A, D, and S Seventh Characters!

International Classification of Diseases, 10th Revision, Clinical Modification seventh characters A, D, and S define an encounter type for injuries and certain other diagnoses. Here are tips for remembering which character to use.
- **A**ctive management of the initial injury or complications
- **D**uring healing of an injury that does not require active management (eg, routine follow-up, suture removal)
- **S**cars and other sequelae (effects of an injury) (Always report the *sequelae code* before the injury code when the service is directed to the sequelae. Injury codes with seventh character S are never the first-listed diagnosis.)

Seventh characters are also appended to codes for external cause of injury (eg, tripping). Additional seventh characters are provided for reporting types of fractures and fracture care.

Common Pediatric Procedures

Minor Procedures That Do Not Have a Code

Some minor procedures are considered inherent to an E/M code or do not have separate *CPT* codes. However, any supplies used may be reported. The following procedures are included in an E/M service:
- Insertion or removal of an ear wick
- Removal of *nonimpacted* cerumen from the ear
- Nasal aspiration
- Nasogastric tube insertion without fluoroscopic guidance
- Removal of an umbilical clamp
- Removal of foreign bodies from skin that do not require an incision
- Puncture of abscess without aspiration
- Wound closure only with adhesive strips (eg, Steri-Strips, butterfly bandages)
- The use of fluorescein dye and a Wood lamp to examine for a corneal abrasion or foreign body of the eye

When significant time is spent performing a service that is not separately reported, documentation of the total time spent on the date of the encounter and code selection based on time may more adequately represent the level of E/M service than code selection based on MDM.

Common Procedure Values and Global Days

For other procedural services, verify separate reporting through your procedural coding reference. There is value in capturing the procedural services that are distinct from E/M services.

Example

➤ **A physician removes a foreign body from a child's nose.** If the physician reports an office E/M visit with low-level MDM (**99213**, 2.65 total non-facility RVUs) in lieu of procedure code **30300** (foreign body removal from nose, 6.06 total non-facility RVUs), the service may be significantly undervalued. (2022 RVUs, not geographically adjusted)

Reporting the appropriate code for the foreign body removal will result in more appropriate payment for the service provided. Both services are reported only if a significant, separately identifiable E/M service, beyond the preservice work of the foreign body removal, is provided.

For the number of global days and RVU values from 2022 for many commonly reported office procedures, see "Office Procedures and Global Days" at www.aap.org/cfp2023.
- Remember that when reporting any procedures containing 0, 10, or 90 global days, modifier **25** or **57** is required on any separately identifiable E/M service done on the same day (or, in some instances, the previous day before a planned major surgery).
- Those E/M services that are unrelated to the procedure that take place within the code's 10- or 90-day global period will require modifier **24**.

Chapter 14. Surgery, Infusion, and Sedation in the Outpatient Setting

Integumentary Procedures

Incision and Drainage

10060   Incision and drainage of abscess (eg, carbuncle, suppurative hidradenitis, cutaneous or subcutaneous abscess, cyst, furuncle, or paronychia); simple or single

10061   complicated or multiple

- The global period is 10 days for codes **10060** (3.69 total non-facility RVUs in 2022) and **10061** (6.32 total non-facility RVUs in 2022).
- *CPT* does not provide differentiation between simple and complicated incision and drainage (I&D) and leaves code selection to the physician's judgment.
- The simple I&D procedure typically involves local anesthesia, an incision, expression of purulent drainage, obtainment of a culture, irrigation, completely opening the cavity, and packing/dressing the wound.
- Complex I&D often typically involves a deeper incision, breakdown of multiple loculations, placement of a drain, and/or debridement of the cavity.
- The difference in 2022 total non-facility RVUs for **10060** (3.69) and **10061** (6.32) indicates the significant additional work and practice expense associated with complicated or multiple I&D procedures. Documentation should support the increased complexity when reporting **10061**.

Example

➤ **A 12-year-old presents with an abscess on his right lower leg.** The decision is made to perform I&D. The physician documents administration of local anesthetic, incision of skin above the abscess, and expression of purulent material. The wound was irrigated and packed. The patient will return in 3 days for reevaluation.

Code **10060** is reported for the procedure. All related visits (eg, follow-up visit to recheck the wound) within the 10 days following the date of surgery may be reported with code **99024** and no charge.

Removal of Skin Tags and Congenital Accessory Digits

11200   Removal of skin tags, multiple fibrocutaneous tags, any area; up to and including 15 lesions

A 10-day global period applies. The 2022 total non-facility RVUs were 2.67.

Code **11200** is used to report the removal of a sixth digit from a newborn. It is equivalent to a skin tag and would not be assigned the code for an actual digit removal. The *ICD-10-CM* code for accessory digits would be **Q69.0**, accessory fingers; **Q69.1**, accessory thumb; **Q69.2**, accessory toes; or **Q69.9**, unspecified.

Destruction of Benign Lesions (eg, Warts)

17110   Destruction (eg, laser surgery, electrosurgery, cryosurgery, chemosurgery, surgical curettement) of benign lesions other than skin tags or cutaneous vascular proliferative lesions; up to 14 lesions

17111   15 or more lesions

A 10-day global period applies to codes **17110** and **17111**. The 2022 total non-facility RVUs were 3.37 for **17110** and 3.94 for **17111**.

Report destruction of common or plantar warts, flat warts, or molluscum contagiosum with code **17110** or **17111** (with 1 unit of service), depending on the number of lesions removed. Do not report both **17110** and **17111** because they are mutually exclusive. Report *ICD-10-CM* by using code **B08.1** for molluscum contagiosum, **B07.8** for common warts, or **B07.0** for plantar warts.

Chemical Cauterization of Granulation Tissue

17250   Chemical cauterization of granulation tissue (ie, proud flesh)

A 0-day global period applies. The 2022 total non-facility RVUs were 2.68.

Code **17250** is appropriately reported for cauterization of an umbilical granuloma. Do not report **17250** with removal or excision codes for the same lesion, for achieving wound hemostasis, or in conjunction with active wound care management.

- When reporting a significant and separately identifiable E/M service on the date, append modifier **25** to the E/M code reported (eg, **99391 25**, **99213 25**).

Chapter 14. Surgery, Infusion, and Sedation in the Outpatient Setting

Example

➤ **A 2-week-old presents for her well-baby check.** On examination, a moderate-sized umbilical granuloma is noted. The physician takes a very brief history and decides to cauterize. The routine well-baby check is completed in addition to cauterization of the umbilical granuloma.

ICD-10-CM	CPT
Z00.121 (encounter for routine child health examination with abnormal findings)	**99391 25**
P83.81 (umbilical granuloma)	**17250**

Teaching Point: Preservice work includes explanation of the procedure, obtaining informed consent, positioning and draping, preparing the site, and scrubbing in. Post-service work includes discussing follow-up care with parents and/or caregivers. Supplies and equipment, such as silver nitrate and an applicator, are included in the value assigned to the code when reporting to payers using RVUs. Follow-up visits are separately reportable.

Laceration Repairs

12001–12018 Simple repair
12031–12057 Intermediate repair
13100–13160 Complex repair

● Categories of difficulty of wound repairs are described as
— *Simple:* Superficial wound and/or subcutaneous wound requiring a simple single-layer closure or tissue adhesives (eg, Dermabond). Wound closure requiring only adhesive strips is included in an E/M service. A 0-day global period applies. *When performed, local or topical anesthesia and hemostasis are not reported separately.*
— *Intermediate:* Includes the repair of wounds that, in addition to the requirements for simple repair, require layered closure of 1 or more of the deeper layers of subcutaneous tissue and superficial (non-muscle) fascia, in addition to skin (epidermal and dermal) closure. Intermediate repair includes limited undermining (defined as a distance less than the maximum width of the defect, measured perpendicular to the closure line, along at least 1 entire edge of the defect). A 10-day global period applies.

> Single-layer closure of heavily contaminated wounds that require extensive cleaning or removal of particulate matter also constitutes intermediate repair.

— *Complex:* Includes the repair of wounds that, in addition to the requirements for intermediate repair, require at least 1 of the following conditions: exposure of bone, cartilage, tendon, or named neurovascular structure; debridement of wound edges (eg, traumatic lacerations or avulsions); extensive undermining (defined as distance equal to or greater than the maximum width of the defect, measured perpendicular to the closure line, along at least 1 entire edge of the defect); involvement of free margins of helical rim, vermilion border, or nostril rim; or placement of retention sutures. Necessary preparation includes creation of a limited defect for repairs or the debridement of complicated lacerations or avulsions. A 10-day global period applies to most complex wound repairs. Late wound closure (**13160**) has a 90-day global period.

> Complex repair does not include excision of benign (11400–11446) or malignant (11600–11646) lesions, excisional preparation of a wound bed (15002–15005), or debridement of an open fracture or open dislocation.

● Codes **12001–13160** are used to report wound closure using sutures, staples, or tissue adhesives (eg, Dermabond), singly or in combination with adhesive strips.
● Wound closure using chemical cauterization, electrocauterization, or adhesive strips (eg, Steri-Strips, butterfly bandages) only is considered inherent to the E/M service. However, the supplies (eg, Steri-Strips, butterfly bandages) may be reported separately by using code **99070** (supplies and materials) or **A4450** (tape, non-waterproof, per 18 sq in). There are no specific HCPCS codes for Steri-Strips or butterfly bandages.
● Some payers may accept HCPCS code **G0168** (wound closure using tissue adhesive[s]) in lieu of simple repair codes (eg, **12001**, **12011**).

● indicates a new code; ▲, revised; #, re-sequenced; ✛, add-on; ★, audiovisual technology; and ◀, synchronous interactive audio.

- Codes are reported on the basis of the difficulty of the repair, measured length of the wound, and location. To report wound repair, measure the length of the repaired wound(s) in centimeters.
  — If multiple wounds belong to the same category of difficulty and location, add the lengths and report with a single code.
  — If multiple wounds do not belong in the same category, report each repair separately with the more complicated repair reported as the primary procedure and the less complicated repair reported as the secondary procedure. Modifier **51** (multiple procedures) should be appended to the secondary code(s) when the payer does not recommend against reporting modifier **51**.
  — Simple ligation of vessels is considered as part of the wound closure.
- Wound debridement and/or cleaning and the provision of topical or injected local anesthesia are included in the wound repair code.
  — Debridement is considered a separate procedure only when gross contamination requires prolonged cleaning, excessive amounts of devitalized tissue are removed, or debridement is performed without immediate primary closure.
  — To report extensive tissue debridement, see codes **11042–11047** for selective debridement of subcutaneous, muscle, fascial tissues, and/or bone (includes debridement of dermis and epidermis when performed) or **97597** and **97598** for debridement of skin, epidermis, and/or dermis.

Examples

➤ **A 10-year-old sustained a 1.5-cm laceration on his left knee requiring a simple (single layer) repair after a fall from playground equipment.**

ICD-10-CM	CPT
S81.012A (laceration without foreign body left knee, initial encounter) **W09.8XXA** (fall on or from other playground equipment, initial encounter) **Y92.838** (other recreation area)	**12001** (simple repair of superficial wounds of scalp, neck, axillae, external genitalia, trunk and/ or extremities [including hands and feet]; 2.5 cm or less)

    Teaching Point: Simple repair includes only the care on the date of the repair (0-day global period). Follow-up E/M visits are separately reported and do not require a modifier.

➤ **A 10-year-old fell from playground equipment and sustained a 1.5-cm laceration on his left knee and a 1.5-cm laceration on his left forearm. Each laceration required an intermediate repair.**

ICD-10-CM	CPT
S81.012A (laceration without foreign body left knee, initial encounter) **S51.812A** (laceration of left forearm without foreign body, initial encounter) **W09.8XXA** **Y92.838**	**12032** (intermediate repair, extremities, 2.6–7.5 cm)

    Teaching Point: The measurement of both wounds (3 cm) is between 2.6 and 7.5 cm, both wounds are in the same family of anatomical sites, and both require the same level of repair. If the patient returns for wound follow-up within the 10 days following the date of repair, code **99024** (postoperative follow-up visit) is reported for the encounter because intermediate repair has a 10-day global period. There is no separate charge for care within the global period.

Other Repairs

Code **11760** (repair of nail bed) is reported when part or all of the nail plate is lifted and a laceration of the nail bed is repaired. A 10-day global period applies.

    Report code **40650** (repair of lip, full-thickness, vermilion only) when a laceration of the full thickness of the lip and vermilion is repaired. A 90-day global period applies to this service. For less than full-thickness repair, see codes for repair of skin. For repair of a laceration that crosses the vermilion border, see codes **40652** (up to half vertical height) and **40654** (over half of vertical height).

Laceration repairs of the tongue (**41250–41252**) are reported on the basis of size and location (eg, repair of laceration 2.5 cm or less, anterior two-thirds of the tongue is reported by using code **41250**). These codes are assigned a 10-day global period.

> See Chapter 19 for discussion of coding for negative pressure wound therapy (**97605** and **97606** or **97607** and **97608**).

Burn Care

CPT code **16000** (initial treatment, first-degree burn, where no more than local treatment is required) is reported when initial treatment is performed for the symptomatic relief of a first-degree burn that is characterized by erythema and tenderness.

16020   Dressings and/or debridement of partial-thickness burns, initial or subsequent; small or less than 5% total body (eg, finger)

A 0-day global period applies. The 2022 total non-facility RVUs were 2.51.
Code **16020**

- Is used to report treatment of burns with dressings and/or debridement of small partial-thickness burns (second degree), whether initial or subsequent.
- An E/M visit with modifier **25** appended may be reported if a significant, separately identifiable E/M service is clinically indicated, performed, and documented in addition to the burn care.

> See Chapter 19 for coding of larger partial- or full-thickness burns.

Examples

➤ **A 9-year-old with sunburn on her shoulders is seen by the physician.** There is redness and tenderness, but no blistering. Topical treatment is applied and an over-the-counter treatment of the first-degree burn is ordered.

ICD-10-CM	CPT
L55.0 (first-degree sunburn)	**16000** (first-degree burn requiring local treatment)

Teaching Point: Code **16000** was assigned 2.25 total non-facility RVUs in 2022 and is assigned a 0-day global period.

➤ **A 4-year-old is seen in the office after sustaining a burn on the first finger of her right hand from touching a hot pan.** The area is red and blistered. Following examination by the physician, the finger is treated with a topical cream and bandaged.

ICD-10-CM	CPT
T23.221A (second-degree burn of single finger, initial encounter) **X15.3XXA** (contact with other heat and hot saucepan or skillet, initial encounter)	**16020**

Teaching Point: External cause of injury codes such as **X15.3XXA** are used to report the source, place, and/or intent of a burn injury. These codes are required only when state regulations mandate reporting cause of injury (typically applies to ED services). However, it is appropriate to report external cause of injury codes when the cause is known.

Removal of Foreign Bodies

Integumentary Foreign Bodies

10120	Incision and removal of foreign body, subcutaneous tissues; simple
10121	complex

A 10-day global period applies. The 2022 total non-facility RVUs were 4.46 (**10120**) and 7.89 (**10121**).

Incision and removal of a foreign body from within the subcutaneous tissues above the fascia is reported with a code from the integumentary system regardless of the site (eg, hand, foot).

Do not report codes **10120** or **10121** when a foreign body is removed by using forceps alone with no incision. Instead, report an E/M service. Incising of the skin can be accomplished by a scalpel or another instrument needed to "break open," or incise, the skin.

- Code **10120** includes the removal of splinters or ticks when the physician has to incise the skin to retrieve the foreign body.
- Code **10121** is used to report the complicated removal of a foreign body by incision.

The removal of an embedded earring or other jewelry requiring an incision would be reported with code **10120** or **10121**, depending on the complexity of the procedure required to remove it. If the jewelry is removed by wiggling it out or another method that does not require incision, this work is included in the E/M service.

The physician determines whether the procedure is simple or complex, but the significant difference in physician work RVUs for the procedures may be used as an indicator of the difference—1.22 for **10120** versus 2.74 for **10121**. Clearly, a procedure described by code **10121** would involve double the time and effort of the simple procedure. *CPT* does not provide examples of simple versus complex procedures.

- A complex removal may require extended exploration and removal of multiple foreign bodies (eg, pieces of glass), use of imaging to help locate the foreign body, or removal that is complicated by the anatomical site of the foreign body (eg, area that is not easily seen) and will have a greater intensity of physician work.

Musculoskeletal Foreign Bodies

Musculoskeletal codes are reported when a foreign body is removed from *within the fascia, subfascial area, or muscle.* Always check the *CPT* index to ensure you are reporting the most accurate code.

Codes in the musculoskeletal system are not reported for removal of foreign bodies within the skin and subcutaneous fat. Examples of codes for removal of foreign bodies within the musculoskeletal system are

- *Foot:* For foreign body removal *from within the fascia, subfascial area, or muscle,* code **28190** (10-day global period) is used to report the removal of a subcutaneous foreign body from the foot; code **28192** (90-day global period) is used to report removal of a foreign body from the deep tissue of the foot.
- *Upper arm or elbow:* Report removal of foreign bodies of the upper arm or elbow area from subcutaneous tissues within the fascia with **24200** (10-day global period) or from deep, below the fascia, or in the muscle with **24201** (90-day global period).

> An object that is unintentionally placed (eg, trauma, ingestion) is considered a foreign body. An object intentionally placed by a physician or other qualified health care professional for any purpose (eg, diagnostic, therapeutic) is considered an implant. A broken or misplaced implant is a foreign body for coding purposes.

Foreign Bodies of Other Body Sites

CPT includes codes for reporting removal of foreign bodies from many different body sites. **Table 14-2** summarizes foreign body removal services from areas other than skin or muscle.

Fracture and/or Dislocation Care

Fracture and Dislocation Care Codes

Fracture and dislocation care codes are reported for care that is intended to begin the course of treatment of the injury. If a physician or QHP provides casting or strapping only for stabilization pending restorative treatment by another physician or QHP, see codes **29000–29799** and discussion later in this section. A significant, separately identifiable E/M service to diagnose and manage the injury is separately reported.

Most fracture and dislocation care codes include a 90-day period of follow-up care under the Medicare global package. Modifiers are required when one physician or QHP provides initial care of a fracture or dislocation (eg, closed treatment of a fracture without manipulation in the ED) and another physician or QHP provides follow-up care.

Unrelated services that are provided during the global surgery period by the same physician (or physician of the same group and specialty) may be reported. Append modifier **24** to an unrelated E/M service.

Table 14-2. Codes for Removal of Foreign Bodies Other Than From Skin or Muscle	
Site	**Code(s)**
Anus, foreign body or fecal impaction	Use appropriate E/M code or **45999** (unlisted procedure, rectum) except when performed under anesthesia (**45915**, more than local anesthesia).
External auditory canal	**69200** (removal foreign body from external auditory canal; without general anesthesia) (For removal of impacted cerumen, see the section by the same name later in this chapter.)
Eye	**65205** (removal of foreign body, external eye; conjunctival superficial) **65220** (removal of foreign body, external eye; corneal, without slit lamp)
Nose	**30300** (removal of intranasal foreign bodies when performed in the office) **30310** (removal of intranasal foreign bodies under general anesthesia)
Vagina	Use appropriate E/M code or **58999** (unlisted procedure, female genital system) except when performed under anesthesia (**57415**, more than local anesthesia).

Abbreviation: E/M, evaluation and management.

- When a patient presents for follow-up care after initial fracture care is provided in another setting (eg, ED, urgent care), it is necessary to determine if the provider of initial fracture care reported a code for fracture care with modifier **54** (surgical care only) or reported only casting/strapping for the initial care.
- If initial fracture care has been reported with modifier **54**, the physician providing continued fracture care reports the fracture care code with modifier **55** (postoperative care only) appended.

  Codes for fracture/dislocation care
- Are listed by anatomical location.
- Are provided (in most cases) for closed or open treatment, with or without manipulation, and with or without internal fixation.

> Closed treatment of a nasal bone fracture without manipulation or stabilization is reported with an evaluation and management code (eg, **99283**, **99213**) on the basis of the site of service.

- Include the initial casting, splinting, or strapping.
- ✖ Do not include radiographs or E/M to determine the extent of injury and treatment options.

  Fractures most commonly seen in a primary care pediatric practice include closed fractures (ie, skin is intact on presentation), and treatment is typically closed (ie, fracture site is not surgically opened) without manipulation (an exception is treatment of nursemaid elbow).
- *Clavicular fracture:* Report closed treatment without manipulation with code **23500**.
- *Nursemaid elbow:* Report closed treatment of radial head subluxation (nursemaid elbow) with manipulation with code **24640**. (This code has a 10-day global period.)
- *Radial fracture:* Report code **25500** for closed treatment of radial shaft fracture without manipulation and **25600** for closed treatment of distal radius fracture without manipulation.
- *Phalanx fracture:* Closed treatment of a proximal or middle phalanx, finger, or thumb (each) without manipulation is reported with code **26720**. Closed treatment of a distal phalangeal fracture (each) without manipulation is reported with code **26750**.
- *Great toe fracture:* Code **28490** is reported for the closed treatment of a fracture of the great toe, phalanx, or phalanges without manipulation.
- *Metatarsal fracture:* Report code **28470** for closed treatment of a metatarsal fracture without manipulation.
- *Lesser toe fracture:* Closed treatment of fracture, phalanx, or phalanges, other than great toe without manipulation, is coded with **28510**.

> Fractures not specified as displaced or non-displaced are reported with an *International Classification of Diseases, 10th Revision, Clinical Modification* code for a displaced fracture. Fractures not specified as open or closed are reported with a code for a closed fracture.

"Buddy taping" of a fractured digit may be reported as fracture care. When reporting fracture care, the code includes care during the global period. Buddy taping for an injury without fracture is included in the E/M service.

Examples

➤ **An urgent care physician performs and documents a comprehensive evaluation on a child (new patient) to assess for injuries following an unwitnessed fall from the stairs in her home. The child is diagnosed with a fracture of the shaft of the left clavicle and receives closed treatment without manipulation. The child will receive follow-up care from a physician of another practice.**

ICD-10-CM	CPT
S42.022A (displaced fracture shaft of clavicle, closed, initial encounter) **W10.9XXA** (fall [on] [from] unspecified stairs and steps, initial encounter)	**99202–99205 57**
S42.022A **W10.9XXA**	**23500 54** (closed treatment clavicle fracture without manipulation)

Teaching Point: Because code **23500** is assigned a 90-day global period in the MPFS and the physician will not provide post-procedural care, modifier **54** is appended to code **23500**. A payer may require modifier **57** (decision for surgery) appended to the E/M code when performed in conjunction with a procedure that is assigned a 90-day global period. Individual payers may have different policies.

When follow-up care is provided by a physician or QHP of another group practice or specialty, code **23500 55** is reported.

➤ **A physician evaluates a 22-month-old girl (established patient) whose parents report that she will not move her left arm after falling on steps while holding her father's hand.** After obtaining history and physical examination to rule out other injuries, the physician diagnoses subluxation of the radial head that is reduced by manipulation. Reassessment after 10 minutes shows that the child uses both arms without difficulty. The parents are counseled about potential for recurrent injury and prevention. Follow-up will be at previously scheduled 2-year-old visit unless otherwise indicated.

ICD-10-CM	CPT
S53.032A (nursemaid's elbow, left, initial encounter) **W10.9XXA** (fall [on] [from] unspecified stairs and steps, initial encounter)	**99213 25** (low MDM—acute uncomplicated injury with assessment requiring an independent historian and low risk of morbidity) **24640** (closed treatment of radial head subluxation in child, nursemaid elbow, with manipulation)

Teaching Point: The physician provided a significant and separately identifiable E/M service to evaluate extent of injury in addition to treatment of nursemaid elbow. Modifier **25** is required by most payers to indicate the E/M service was significant and separately identifiable from the preservice work of the minor procedure (eg, 10-day global period) performed on the same date of service.

Casts/Strapping/Splints

● Codes for the application of casts, splints, or strapping (**29000–29590**) are reported only when they are replacements for the initial application *or performed as part of the initial E/M visit and fracture care is not reported.*
✖ Do not report codes **29000–29590** for the initial (first) application when a fracture or dislocation care code is reported because they are included as part of the global surgery package.
● *Strapping* refers to the application of overlapping strips of adhesive plaster or tape to a body part to exert pressure on it and hold a structure in place. Strapping may be used to treat strains, sprains, and dislocations, in addition to fractures.
● See the Supplies section later in this chapter for information on reporting supplies such as slings.

● indicates a new code; ▲, revised; #, re-sequenced; ✚, add-on; ★, audiovisual technology; and ◀, synchronous interactive audio.

The following codes are commonly used when treating a fracture or dislocation:
- Application of splints
    - Short arm splint (forearm to hand): static (**29125**); dynamic (**29126**)
    - Finger splint: static (**29130**); dynamic (**29131**)
    - Short leg splint (calf to foot): **29515**
- Strapping
    - Shoulder: **29240**
    - Elbow or wrist: **29260**

> **Verify payer policy for coverage of strapping procedures, as some policies prohibit payment for strapping of the shoulder, elbow, or wrist.**

Example

➤ **An established adolescent patient returns to a physician for follow-up on an injury to the left wrist.** The patient was previously examined and a cast applied for a presumed scaphoid fracture (ie, diagnosed based on examination findings) that was not found on a radiograph. The service was reported with code **25622** (closed treatment of carpal scaphoid [navicular] fracture; without manipulation) The diagnosis documented at the first visit was initial encounter for unspecified scaphoid fracture of the left wrist (**S62.001A**) due to tripping while playing soccer with friends at a soccer field. The initial cast is removed and a 3-view radiograph of the wrist is ordered and obtained in the office. The physician interprets the radiograph, which now shows a fracture of the middle third (waist) of the left proximal scaphoid. The physician applies a replacement thumb spica cast. The patient will return in 4 weeks for reevaluation.

ICD-10-CM	CPT
S62.025D (nondisplaced fracture of middle third of navicular [scaphoid] bone of left wrist, subsequent encounter for fracture with routine healing) **W01.0XXD** (fall on same level from slipping, tripping and stumbling without subsequent striking against object, subsequent encounter)	**99024** (postoperative follow-up visit) **29085 58** (application cast; hand and lower forearm [gauntlet]) **Q4013** (cast supplies, gauntlet cast [includes lower forearm and hand], adult [11 years +], plaster) or **Q4014** (same but fiberglass) **73110** (radiologic examination, wrist; complete, minimum of 3 views)

Teaching Point: Code **25622** is assigned a 90-day global period by most payers. The physician reports codes for follow-up during the global period (**99024**), radiograph, and application of the replacement cast. Diagnosis codes include the seventh character **D** to report subsequent care of this fracture, although a more specific diagnosis is now confirmed. Inclusion of codes for external cause of injury, although not required, may provide information that facilitates timely payment. Modifier **58** (staged or related procedure) is appended to **29085**, as the service is related to the procedure performed by the same physician at the previous encounter.

Cast supplies are separately reported with either *CPT* code **99070** (supplies and materials [except spectacles], provided by the physician or other QHP over and above those usually included with the office visit or other services rendered) or, as shown here, more specific HCPCS codes.

If the initial care of the fracture had included only application of a splint to stabilize and protect the injury until a definitive diagnosis could be confirmed, codes for an E/M service and application of a splint would have been appropriate in lieu of fracture care. In that case, the return visit at which the fracture was diagnosed would have been initial fracture care and code **25622** would have been reported for this encounter in lieu of **99024** and **29085**.

> **When reporting codes for radiographs, documentation should include a report of the indication for the test, number of views, findings, and, when applicable, comparison to previous radiographs.**
>
> ✕ **Do not report a charge for interpretation and report for review of images that have been or will be interpreted with creation of a formal report by a radiologist or other physician or qualified health care professional.**
> - **The independent review of previously interpreted images is included in the amount and/or complexity of data to be reviewed and analyzed of an evaluation and management service or in the follow-up during the global period of a service.**

Chapter 14. Surgery, Infusion, and Sedation in the Outpatient Setting

Supplies

- Supplies associated with fracture care may be billed with every application, including the initial casting, splinting, or strapping performed in association with the global surgery procedure code when the service is performed in the private office setting.
- HCPCS codes **A4580**, **A4590**, and **Q4001–Q4051** may be reported for cast supplies; codes **E1800–E1841** may be reported for splints. Check with your major payers and/or review their payment policies for reporting these supplies.
- HCPCS codes are accepted by many Medicaid and commercial payers and are often specific to the age of the patient and type of supply and/or material.
- A description of supplies may be required when reporting special supplies code **99070**.
- The following codes are commonly used:

99070	Supplies and materials (except spectacles)
A4565	Slings
A4570	Splint
L3650–L3678	Clavicle splints
Q4001–Q4051	Cast and splint supplies
S8450–S8452	Splint, prefabricated for finger, wrist, ankle, or elbow

Ear, Nose, and Throat Procedures

Control of Nasal Hemorrhage

30901   Control nasal hemorrhage, anterior, simple (cautery or packing)

30903   Control nasal hemorrhage, anterior, complex (extensive cautery and/or packing) any method

A 0-day global period applies. The 2022 total non-facility RVUs were 4.76 (**30901**) and 7.45 (**30903**).

- If performing cautery or packing on both sides, report **30901** with modifier **50**.
- If bleeding is controlled with manual pressure or placement of a nasal clamp (clip), only the appropriate level of E/M service is reported.
- ✖ Do not report **30901** when packing is placed in the short term to administer medication (eg, insertion of medicated gauze into the nostrils) and not to serve a hemostatic and/or tamponade role following the encounter. Illumination and instrumentation (eg, suction, nasal speculum, forceps) are typically required for placement of packing to control nasal hemorrhage.

Removal of Impacted Cerumen

69209   Removal of impacted cerumen using irrigation/lavage, unilateral

69210   Removal of impacted cerumen requiring instrumentation, unilateral

A 0-day global period applies. The 2022 total non-facility RVUs were 0.45 (**69209**) and 1.40 (**69210**).

> Removal of cerumen that is not impacted is included in an evaluation and management code regardless of how it is removed. Documentation of removal of impacted cerumen should include the indication for removal (eg, impairing examination, painful, itching, hearing loss).

Modifier **25** should be appended to a significant, separately identifiable E/M service (eg, **99213**) provided on the same date as removal of impacted cerumen on the basis of NCCI edits.

Code **69209** is used to report removal of impacted cerumen by ear wash without direct visualization and instrumentation. This service may be provided by clinical staff under supervision by a physician or other QHP.

- This code is intended to capture the practice expense associated with the service and is not valued to include physician work.
- For a bilateral procedure, report **69209** with modifier **50**.
- ✖ Do not report **69209** for removal of cerumen that is not impacted.
- ✖ Do not report **69209** in conjunction with **69210** when performed on the same ear (modifiers **LT** and **RT** may be used to identify contralateral procedures).

Code **69210** is reported *only* when the physician or QHP, under direct visualization, removes impacted cerumen by using, at a minimum, an otoscope and instruments such as wax curettes or by using an operating microscope and suction plus specific ear instruments (eg, cup forceps, right angles).

- Medical record documentation must support that the cerumen was impacted and removed by the physician and include a description of what equipment and method were used to perform the procedure. Visualization of the impacted cerumen should also be documented.
- Report code **69210** with modifier **50** when bilateral procedures are performed.
- National Correct Coding Initiative edits bundle impacted cerumen removal (**69209**, **69210**) with some hearing assessments (eg, tympanometry [**92567**]). There is no modifier to override this edit.

Note: Medicare does not recognize modifier **50** when reported with code **69210** (impacted cerumen removal); therefore, those payers that follow Medicare payment policy will not recognize it and may deny the claim outright. Check with your payers.

Coding Conundrum: Unsuccessful Removal of Impacted Cerumen

If a physician or other qualified health care professional attempts to remove impacted cerumen but finds the impaction too hard for safe removal, what code is reported for the attempt? The answer depends on the individual situation, including the amount of work that was performed and whether another procedure was successful.

If the portion of the procedure completed required insignificant work and practice expense (eg, staff time), report only the services completed on that date (eg, evaluation and management).

If the patient is instructed to use softening drops and return later for removal, consider whether the effort and practice expense were sufficient to justify reporting the removal with reduced services modifier **52**.

If the procedure was discontinued after significant effort and practice expense due to extenuating circumstances or concerns that the procedure may threaten the patient's well-being, report the procedure code with modifier **53** (discontinued procedure).

If, after attempted removal by a physician is discontinued, softening drops are administered in the office and clinical staff perform removal of the impaction by lavage (**69209**), report only the completed procedure.

Examples

➤ **A physician orders removal of impacted cerumen from the right ear by lavage.** Clinical staff perform the lavage, removing the impacted cerumen. Because the child is uncooperative, the procedure takes 10 minutes.

ICD-10-CM	CPT
H61.21 (impacted cerumen, right ear)	**99202–99215 25** (Report if appropriate and use modifier **25** if required by payer.)
	69209 RT (**RT** indicates right ear.)

Teaching Point: This procedure was unilateral. If it were bilateral, modifier **50** would be appended to code **69209**. The anatomical modifier **RT** (right) is informational and may not affect payment. The extended time of service alone is not sufficient to support reporting increased procedural service (ie, modifier **22**).

➤ **Physician documents, "Impacted cerumen removed from both ears by using an otoscope and curette," in a patient with concern of decreased hearing.** Following the procedure, the patient's hearing is assessed as normal.

ICD-10-CM	CPT
H61.23 (impacted cerumen, bilateral)	**99202–99215 25** (Report if appropriate and use modifier **25** if required by payer.)
	69210 50 (bilateral removal of impacted cerumen using instrumentation)

Teaching Point: Unless a payer instructs otherwise, modifier **50** is appended to **69210** to indicate a bilateral procedure. An E/M service is reported only if significant and separately identifiable. If selecting an E/M code based on time, do not include time spent performing the procedure. The diagnosis code for the condition(s) addressed by the E/M service is linked to the E/M code on the claim.

Digestive System Procedures

Incision in Lingual Frenulum

41010　　　Incision in the lingual frenum to free the tongue

A 10-day global period applies. The 2022 total non-facility RVUs were 6.59.

Note that code **41115** (excision of lingual frenum) is not appropriate when an incisional release of tongue-tie is performed rather than excision (removal) of the frenum.

Example

➤ **A 14-day-old is seen for feeding difficulty caused by ankyloglossia.** The physician documents obtaining informed consent, positioning and restraining of the neonate, and gentle lifting of the tongue with a sterile, grooved retractor to expose the frenulum. The frenulum, adjacent to the ventral aspect of the tongue, is divided by 2 to 3 mm by using sterile scissors. Afterward, the newborn is immediately returned to his mother for comfort and feeding. The latch appears improved. After feeding, the neonate is reevaluated with no evidence of complications. Code **41010** is reported for the procedure.

ICD-10-CM	CPT
Q38.1 (congenital ankyloglossia) **P92.5** (neonatal difficulty in feeding at breast)	**41010**

Teaching Point: If a significant and separately identifiable E/M service was provided in addition to the preservice work of the procedure, modifier **25** would be appended to the appropriate E/M code. Any related visit within the 10 days following the procedure may be reported (with no charge) with code **99024**. An unrelated E/M service within 10 days following the procedure may be reported with modifier **24** (unrelated E/M service by the same physician or QHP during a postoperative period). When reporting modifier **24**, the diagnosis code(s) reported should be indicative of an unrelated service.

Gastrostomy Tube Replacement

43762　　　Replacement of gastrostomy tube, percutaneous, includes removal, when performed, without imaging or endoscopic guidance; not requiring revision of gastrostomy tract

43763　　　requiring revision of gastrostomy tract

A 0-day global period is assigned. The 2022 total non-facility RVUs were 7.01 (**43762**) and 10.58 (**43763**).

- Report codes **43762** and **43763** only for percutaneous gastrostomy tube (G-tube) or gastrojejunal tube (GJ-tube) change without imaging or endoscopic guidance (eg, replacement GJ-tube is placed into the stomach and anchored in place by inflating the gastric balloon with water or saline, and peristalsis carries the jejunal portion of the tube into the small intestine).
- See other specific codes (eg, **49450–49452** and **43246**) for G- or GJ-tube placement, conversion, or replacement of *with imaging or endoscopic guidance.*
- A significant, separately identifiable E/M service on the same date may be reported with modifier **25** appended to the E/M code (eg, **99213 25**).
- ✖ Do not report an E/M service when the encounter is solely for replacement of the G-tube.
- Codes **43762** and **43763** include the G-tube kit.

Genitourinary System Procedures

Urinary Catheterization

51701   Urinary catheterization, straight

51702   Urinary catheterization, temporary

A 0-day global period applies. The 2022 total non-facility RVUs were 1.33 (**51701**) and 1.85 (**51702**).

- Code **51701** is reported when a non-indwelling bladder catheter (straight catheterization) is inserted (eg, for residual urine, for a urine culture collection).
- Code **51702** is reported when a temporary indwelling bladder catheter is inserted (ie, Foley).

Report code 51701 when you insert a urinary catheter to collect a clean-catch urine specimen, after which the catheter is removed.

Lysis/Excision of Labial or Penile Adhesions

If lysis of labial or penile adhesions is performed by the application of manual pressure without the use of an instrument to cut the adhesions, it would be considered part of the E/M visit and not reported separately.

54450   Foreskin manipulation including lysis of preputial adhesions and stretching

A 0-day global period is assigned. The 2022 total non-facility RVUs were 1.99.

Code **54450** does not require general anesthesia.

- This procedure is performed on the uncircumcised foreskin and the head of the penis. Adhesions are broken by stretching the foreskin back over the head of the penis onto the shaft or by inserting a clamp between the foreskin and the head of the penis and spreading the jaws of the clamp.

54162   Lysis or excision of penile post-circumcision adhesions

This service includes a 10-day global surgery period. The 2022 total non-facility RVUs were 7.64.

Code **54162** is reported only when lysis is performed under general anesthesia or regional block, with an instrument, and under sterile conditions.

- If post-circumcision adhesions are manually broken during the postoperative period by the physician or physician of the same group and specialty who performed the procedure, it would be considered part of the global surgical package.
- Report the service with *ICD-10-CM* code **N47.0**, adherent prepuce in a newborn, or **N47.5**, adhesions of prepuce and glans penis (patients aged >28 days).

56441   Lysis of labial adhesions

This procedure also includes a 10-day global surgery period. The 2022 total non-facility RVUs were 5.54.

Code **56441** is performed by using a blunt instrument or scissors under general or local anesthesia.

- *ICD-10-CM* code **Q52.5** (fusion of labia) would be reported with *CPT* code **56441**.
- When provided without anesthesia, modifier **52** may be appended to indicate reduced services. Payer guidance may vary in regard to use of modifier **52**. See **Chapter 2** for more information on use of modifier **52**.

Newborn Circumcision

When circumcisions are performed in the office

- If a payer does not base payment on a global surgical package, a supply code for the surgical tray can be reported with code **99070**. The description of the supply (circumcision tray) would need to be included on the claim form.
- Anesthetic creams (eutectic mixture of local anesthetics) are included in the circumcision code itself and should not be reported unless a third-party payer pays separately for topical anesthetic agents. In that case, they would be reported with code **99070**.
- When an E/M service (eg, well-baby visit) is provided on the same date, append modifier **25** to the E/M code.
  — Link the appropriate *ICD-10-CM* code (eg, **Z00.110**, health check for newborn under 8 days old) to the E/M service and link *ICD-10-CM* code **Z41.2** (encounter for routine and ritual male circumcision) to the circumcision code.

54150   Circumcision, using clamp or other device with regional dorsal penile or ring block

This service is assigned a 0-day global period. The 2022 total non-facility RVUs were 4.42.

- If the circumcision performed by using a clamp or other device lacks dorsal penile or ring block, append modifier **52** (reduced services) to **54150**.

See codes **54160** and **54161** for circumcision performed by using surgical excision other than a clamp, device, or dorsal split. These procedures are often provided in facility settings.

See Chapter 16 for information on reporting circumcision in a facility setting.

Hydration, Injections, and Infusions

Services included as inherent to an infusion or injection are the use of local anesthesia, starting the intravenous (IV) line, access to indwelling IV lines or a subcutaneous catheter or port, flushing lines at the conclusion of an infusion or between infusions, standard tubing, syringes and supplies, and preparation of chemotherapy agents.

These services are not assigned a global period.

- These codes are intended for reporting by the physician or other QHP in an office setting. They are not reported by a physician or other QHP when performed in a facility setting because the physician work associated with these procedures involves only affirmation of the treatment plan and direct supervision of the staff performing the services.
- If a significant, separately identifiable E/M service is performed, the appropriate code may be reported with modifier **25** appended. The diagnosis may be the same for the E/M service and codes **96360–96379**.

Documentation of medications administered in the outpatient pediatric practice should include

- **Order for medication**
- **Date and time of administration (include start/stop times for timed procedures)**
- **Medication, manufacturer, lot number, and expiration date**
- **National Drug Code, if not captured elsewhere**
- **Dose**
- **Route (eg, intramuscular) and site of administration (eg, left deltoid)**
- **Observations (eg, held by mother, no sign of adverse reaction after 5 minutes)**
- **Signature and credentials of individual administering medication**

Subcutaneous or Intramuscular Injection (Therapeutic, Prophylactic, and Diagnostic)

96372   Therapeutic, prophylactic, or diagnostic injection (specify substance or drug); subcutaneous or intramuscular

The 2022 total non-facility RVUs were 0.42.

Report code **96372** for the administration of a diagnostic, prophylactic, or therapeutic (eg, antibiotic) subcutaneous or intramuscular (IM) injection.

✖ Do not report for the administration of a purified protein derivative test.

For administration of immunizations, see discussion of codes 90460, 90461, and 90471–90474 in Chapter 8.

Example

➤ **A 2-year-old established patient presents with moderate symptoms of croup that began last evening and worsened during the night.** After obtaining history and performing an examination, the physician recommends injection of dexamethasone sodium phosphate. A 7-mg dose of dexamethasone sodium phosphate is administered by IM injection. The child is observed for reaction and released home with instructions and precautions.

ICD-10-CM	CPT
J05.0 (acute obstructive laryngitis [croup])	**99213 25** (established patient E/M with low MDM) **96372** (IM injection) **J1100** × 7 units (injection, dexamethasone sodium phosphate, 1 mg)

Teaching Point: The medication is reported with HCPCS code **J1100**, which indicates that the unit of measure for reporting is 1 mg. Because 7 mg was administered, 7 units of service are reported. Also report the appropriate 11-digit National Drug Code (NDC) and units.

The E/M service included addressing an acute, uncomplicated illness with prescription drug management, supporting code **99213**. (Although prescription drug management supports moderate MDM and code **99214**, neither the number and complexity of problems addressed nor the data to be reviewed and analyzed support this level. Two of 3 elements of MDM must meet the requirements for a level of MDM.) Modifier **25** must be appended to the E/M service code to indicate the significant, separately identifiable E/M service on the date of the injection for payers that use NCCI edits.

See Chapter 1 for more information on National Drug Codes.

Hydration and Infusions

Hydration and infusion codes are reported on the basis of the time when medication administration begins to the end of administration. Time must be documented.

When reporting multiple infusions on the same date, physicians select an initial service based on the service that is the primary reason for infusion services on that date.

Example

➤ **A patient receives infusion of a medication and a separate infusion of hydration fluid.** The physician determines whether the therapeutic infusion or the hydration was the primary service and selects the appropriate initial service code. The other service is reported with a code for sequential or subsequent administration.

Hydration

Codes **96360** (IV infusion, hydration; initial, 31 minutes to 1 hour) and **96361** (each additional hour)
- Were assigned 1.01 (**96360**) and 0.38 (**96361**) 2022 total non-facility RVUs.
- Are intended to report IV hydration infusion using prepackaged fluid and/or electrolyte solutions (eg, physiologic [normal] saline solution, D_5-0.45% physiologic saline solution with potassium). HCPCS codes and NDCs for hydration solutions may be reported in addition to the procedure codes. Note that some plans may require submission of the invoice price paid for the hydration solution and will pay up to only the amount of the invoice.
- Typically require direct physician supervision for the purpose of consent, safety oversight, or supervision of staff with little special handling for preparation or disposal of materials.
- Do not typically require advanced training of staff because there is usually little risk involved and little patient monitoring required.
- Are reported on the basis of the actual time over which the infusion is administered and do not include the time spent starting the IV and monitoring the patient after infusion.
- ✖ Are not reported when IV infusions are 30 minutes or less.

Codes 96360 and 96361 are neither used to report infusion of drugs or other substances nor reported when hydration is incidental to non-chemotherapeutic/diagnostic or chemotherapeutic services.

Medical record documentation must support the time and service reported.
- **96360** may be reported for hydration infusion lasting longer than 31 minutes and up to 1 hour.
- **96361** is reported for each additional hour of hydration infusion and for a final interval of longer than 30 minutes beyond the most recent hour reported.

Code **96361** is reported if an IV hydration infusion is provided secondary or subsequent to a therapeutic, prophylactic, or diagnostic infusion *and administered through the same IV access*.

Intra-arterial and Intravenous Push Injections

96373   Therapeutic, prophylactic, or diagnostic injection (specify substance or drug); intra-arterial

Report code **96373** for an initial intra-arterial injection. The 2022 total non-facility RVUs were 0.53.

96374   intravenous push, single or initial substance/drug

Chapter 14. Surgery, Infusion, and Sedation in the Outpatient Setting

✚**96375**   each additional sequential intravenous push of a new substance/drug

    Codes **96374** and **96375** are reported for IV push or other short infusions of less than 15 minutes. The 2022 total nonfacility RVUs were 1.16 (**96374**) and 0.47 (**96375**).

- Codes **96374** and **96375** are used only when the health care professional administering the substance or drug is in constant attendance during the administration *and* must observe the patient. The IV push must be less than 15 minutes.

> **Short infusions of less than 15 minutes are reported as a push (eg, 96374).**

- Sequential IV push of a new substance or drug is reported with add-on code **96375**.
- Each drug administered is reported separately with the appropriate infusion code.
- Code **96375** is an add-on code reported in addition to codes for IV infusion (**96365**), initial IV push (**96374**), or chemotherapy administration (**96409**, **96413**).
- Additional sequential IV push of the same substance or drug (**96376**) is not reported for services provided in the physician office (ie, is reported only by a facility).

Therapeutic, Prophylactic, and Diagnostic Infusions

96365   Intravenous infusion, for therapy, prophylaxis, or diagnosis (specify substance or drug); initial, up to 1 hour
✚**96366**   each additional hour
✚**96367**   additional sequential infusion of a new drug/substance, up to 1 hour
✚**96368**   concurrent infusion

    Table 14-3 lists primary and additional IV infusion and IV push codes. See the table notes for additional instructions on reporting multiple services.

    Codes **96365–96368**

- Are for infusions for the purpose of administering drugs or substances.
- Typically require direct physician supervision and special attention to prepare, calculate dose, and dispose of materials.
- If fluid infusions are used to administer the drug(s), they are considered incidental hydration and are not reported. Each drug administered is reported separately with the appropriate infusion code.
- Short infusions of less than 15 minutes are reported as a push (eg, **96374**).
- Only 1 initial service code (eg, **96365**) should be reported unless the protocol or patient condition requires that 2 separate IV sites must be used. A second IV site access is also reported using the initial service code with modifier **59** appended (eg, **96365, 96365 59**).
  - ✖ Do not report a second initial service on the same date caused by an IV catheter requiring a restart, an IV rate not being able to be achieved without 2 catheters, or a port of a multi-lumen catheter requiring access.
  - — If an injection or infusion is of a subsequent or concurrent nature, even if it is the first such service within that group of services, a subsequent or concurrent code from the appropriate section should be reported. For example, the first IV push given subsequent to an initial 1-hour infusion is reported by using a subsequent IV push code.
- Subcutaneous infusion is reported with codes **96369–96371** (**Table 14-3**).

    When services are performed in the physician's office, report as follows:

Initial Infusion

Report the code that best describes the key or primary reason for the service regardless of the order in which the infusions or injections occur. Only 1 initial service code (eg, **96365**) should be reported *unless the protocol or patient condition requires using 2 separate IV sites.* The difference in time and effort in providing this second IV site access is also reported by using the initial service code with modifier **59**, distinct procedural service, appended (eg, **96365, 96365 59**).

Sequential Infusion

This is an infusion or IV push of a new substance or drug following a primary or initial service. For example, if an IV push was performed through the same IV access subsequent to an IV infusion for therapy, the appropriate codes to report would be **96365** and **96375**. If an IV push was performed through a different IV access route, the services would be reported by using codes **96365** and **96374**.

    Sequential infusions are reported only 1 time for the same infusate. However, if additional hours were required for the infusion, the appropriate "each additional hour" add-on code would be reported. Different infusates can be reported by using the same code as the original sequential code. Hydration may not be reported concurrently with any other service.

● indicates a new code; ▲, revised; #, re-sequenced; ✚, add-on; ★, audiovisual technology; and ◀, synchronous interactive audio.

Table 14-3. Primary and Additional Intravenous Infusion Codesᵃ

For all services, you must specify the substance or drug administered.

Service (Select the primary reason for encounter irrespective of order of infusion services)ᵇ	IV Infusion for Therapy, Prophylaxis, or Diagnosis	Subcutaneous Infusion for Therapy or Prophylaxisᵇ	Injection IV Push for Therapy, Prophylaxis, or Diagnosis
Initial service, up to 1 h	**96365** (16 min–1 h)	**96369** (16 min–1 h)	**96374** (IV push or infusion ≤15 min)
Each additional hour (>30 min) of *same substance or drug*	✚**96366**ᶜ (List separately in addition to **96365**, **96367**.)	✚**96370** (Use **96370** in conjunction with **96369**.)	
Additional sequential infusion of *new substance or drug*	✚**96367**ᶜ	✚**96371** (additional pump setup with new subcutaneous infusion site[s])	✚**96367**
Sequential IV push of *new substance/drug*	✚**96375**		✚**96375**
Concurrent infusion	✚**96368** (Report only once per date of service.)		

Abbreviation: IV, intravenous.

ᵃ If IV infusion for hydration of >30 min is provided in addition to a therapeutic infusion service (**96365**, **96374**) through the same IV access, report ✚**96361** in addition to **96365** or **96374**.

ᵇ Includes pump setup and establishment of infusion site(s). Use **96369** and **96371** only once per encounter.

ᶜ Report **96367** only once per sequential infusion of same infusate mix. Report **96366** for each additional hour (includes final time unit of ≥31 min) beyond the first hour of the service reported with **96367**.

All sequential services require that there be a new substance or drug; only a facility may report a sequential IV push of the same drug by using **96376**.

Concurrent Infusion

This is an infusion of a new substance or drug infused at the same time as another drug or substance. This is not time based and is only reported once per day regardless of whether a new drug or substance is administered concurrently. Hydration may not be reported concurrently with any other service. A separate subsequent concurrent administration of another new drug or substance (the third substance or drug) is not reported.

Example

➤ **A 3-year-old established patient is seen with a concern of vomiting and fever for the past 24 hours.** She has refused all food and liquids and last voided 12 hours before the visit. Her diagnosis is bilateral acute suppurative otitis media with fever and dehydration. Intravenous fluids are initiated with physiologic (normal) saline solution, and IV ceftriaxone (750 mg) is infused over 30 minutes for her otitis media. After 1 hour and 45 minutes of IV hydration, she urinates, begins tolerating liquids, and is released home. The problem addressed is 1 acute illness with systemic symptoms, and the risk of morbidity from treatment is moderate, supporting moderate MDM.

ICD-10-CM	*CPT*
E86.0 (dehydration) **H66.003** (acute suppurative otitis media without spontaneous rupture of ear drum, bilateral) **R11.10** (vomiting) **R50.81** (fever in conditions classified elsewhere)	**99214 25** (established patient office E/M) **96365** (IV infusion, for therapy) **96361** (IV infusion, hydration, each additional hour) **J0696** × 3 units (ceftriaxone sodium, per 250 mg) **J7030** (infusion, normal saline solution, 1,000 cc)

Teaching Point: Link the appropriate diagnosis code to each procedure (eg, code **H66.003** is linked to code **J0696**). The NDC of the medication should be reported with the appropriate NDC units. The fluid used to administer ceftriaxone is not reported because it is considered incidental hydration.

● indicates a new code; ▲, revised; #, re-sequenced; ✚, add-on; ★, audiovisual technology; and ◀, synchronous interactive audio.

Chapter 14. Surgery, Infusion, and Sedation in the Outpatient Setting

Other Injection and Infusion Services

96523   Irrigation of implanted venous access device for drug delivery systems

Code **96523** is used to report irrigation required for implanted venous access devices for drug delivery systems when services are provided on a separate day from the injection or infusion service. Do not report **96523** in conjunction with other services.

Chemotherapy and Other Highly Complex Drug/Biologic Agent Administration

Codes **96401–96549** are reported for chemotherapy administration. *CPT* defines *chemotherapy administration* as parenteral administration of non-radionuclide antineoplastic drugs, antineoplastic agents provided for treatment of non-cancer diagnoses and to substances such as certain monoclonal antibody agents, and other biologic response modifiers.

Example

➤ **A patient with severe persistent asthma presents for a scheduled injection of omalizumab at 225 mg.** The medication is divided and injected at 2 different sites, as only 150 mg may be injected to a single site. The diagnosis code reported is **J45.50** (severe persistent asthma). Omalizumab injection is reported as a chemotherapy administration of monoclonal antibody (**96401**) with only 1 unit of service *unless prohibited by payer policy*. Omalizumab is provided in prefilled syringes of 75 mg (11-digit NDC 50242-0214-01) and 150 mg (11-digit NDC of 50242-0215-01). HCPCS code **J2357** (injection, omalizumab, 5 mg) is used to report the medication supplied by the physician practice. The following sample claim form illustrates reporting for this example:

Claim Form Sample National Drug Code										
21. Diagnosis or nature of illness or injury (Relate A–L to service line below 24E)					ICD Ind. 0					
A. J45.50	B.		C.		D.					
24. A. Dates of service	B. POS	C. EMG	D. Procedures, services or supplies *CPT/HCPCS*	Modifier	E. Diagnosis Pointer	F. Charges	G. Days or units	H. EPSDT	I. ID Qual	J. Rendering Provider No.
1/1/2023–1/1/2023	11		96401		A	$$$	1		NPI	NPI No.
N450242021401 UN1										
1/1/2023–1/1/2023	11		J2357		A	$$$	15		NPI	NPI No.
N450242021501 UN1										
1/1/2023–1/1/2023	11		J2357		A	$$$	30		NPI	NPI No.

Abbreviations: *CPT, Current Procedural Terminology*; EMG, emergency; EPSDT, Early and Periodic Screening, Diagnostic, and Treatment; HCPCS, Healthcare Common Procedure Coding System; *ICD, International Classification of Diseases*; NPI, National Provider Identifier; POS, place of service.

Teaching Point: Check payer policies before reporting administration of omalizumab and other highly complex drug/biologic agents. *CPT* instructs that administration of certain monoclonal antibody agents possibly be reported with code **96401**. However, not all payers accept code **96401** for administration of omalizumab. Some payers limit reporting to code **96372** (subcutaneous or IM injection) and/or allow only 1 administration code despite requirements to administer by 2 or more separate injections.

HCPCS codes and NDCs for the omalizumab are included on the claim with units based on the HCPCS code descriptor (eg, 75-mg dose/5-mg HCPCS unit = 15 units) and NDC quantity (shown per unit; payers may require NDC units per gram) to identify the substance administered.

Moderate Sedation

Moderate sedation codes **99151–99153** and **99155–99157** are used for reporting moderate sedation when intraservice time is 10 minutes or more. **Table 14-4** contains sedation codes and descriptors.

Codes for moderate sedation are not assigned a global period.

Moderate sedation is a drug-induced depression of consciousness.

- No interventions are required to maintain cardiovascular functions or a patent airway, and spontaneous ventilation is adequate.
- Moderate sedation provided and reported by the same physician or QHP who is performing the diagnostic or therapeutic service requires the presence of an independent trained observer.

● indicates a new code; ▲, revised; #, re-sequenced; ✚, add-on; ★, audiovisual technology; and ◀, synchronous interactive audio.

Table 14-4. Moderate Sedation		
	Intraservice Time	
Moderate Sedation	**First 15 min (10–22 min)**	**Each Additional 15 min and Last 8–22 min**
Moderate sedation services provided by the same physician or other qualified health care professional performing the diagnostic or therapeutic service that the sedation supports, requiring the presence of an independent trained observer to assist in the monitoring of the patient's level of consciousness and physiological status; initial 15 minutes of intraservice time, patient younger than 5 years of age	99151	+99153 (Report only in addition to **99151** or **99152**.)
5 years or older	99152	+99153
Moderate sedation services (other than those services described by codes **00100–01999**) provided by a physician other than the health care professional performing the diagnostic or therapeutic service that the sedation supports; younger than 5 years	99155	+99157 (Report only in addition to **99155** or **99156**.)
5 years or older	99156	+99157

✖ Do not report moderate sedation codes for medication administration for pain control, for minimal sedation (anxiolysis), or for deep sedation or monitored anesthesia care (**00100–01999**).

● Alternatively, a physician or QHP other than the person performing the diagnostic or therapeutic service may provide and report moderate sedation services.

Codes **99151–99153** are reported when

● The administration of moderate sedation is provided by the physician who is simultaneously performing a procedure (eg, fracture reduction, vessel cutdown, central catheter placement, wound repair).

● An independent trained observer is present to assist the physician in the monitoring of the patient during the procedure or diagnostic service.

An *independent trained observer* is an individual qualified to monitor the patient during the procedure but lacking other duties (eg, assisting at surgery) during the procedure.

Codes **99155–99157** are reported when

● A second physician or QHP other than the health care professional performing the diagnostic or therapeutic services provides moderate sedation.

Report codes **99153** and **99157** for each additional 15 minutes of intraservice time. The midpoint between the end of the previous 15-minute period must be passed to report an additional unit of intraservice time (ie, intraservice time must continue for at least 8 minutes beyond the last full 15 minutes of intraservice time).

● Codes are selected on the basis of intraservice time. Intraservice time
  — Begins with the administration of the sedating agent(s)
  — Ends when the procedure is completed, the patient is stable for recovery status, and the physician or other QHP providing the sedation ends personal continuous face-to-face time with the patient
  — Includes ordering and/or administering the initial and subsequent doses of sedating agents
  — Requires continuous face-to-face attendance of the physician or other QHP
  — Requires monitoring patient response to the sedating agents, including
    ▪ Periodic assessment of the patient
    ▪ Further administration of agent(s) as needed to maintain sedation
    ▪ Monitoring of oxygen saturation, heart rate, and blood pressure

✖ Do not report moderate sedation service of less than 10 minutes of intraservice time.

✖ Do not separately report the preservice work of moderate sedation services and do not include time spent in preservice work in the intraservice time. Preservice work includes
  — Assessment of the patient's past medical and surgical history with particular emphasis on cardiovascular, pulmonary, airway, or neurological conditions
  — Review of the patient's previous experiences with anesthesia and/or sedation
  — Family history of sedation complications

● indicates a new code; ▲, revised; #, re-sequenced; ✚, add-on; ★, audiovisual technology; and ◀, synchronous interactive audio.

- Summary of the patient's present medication list
- Drug allergy and intolerance history
- Focused physical examination of the patient, with emphasis on
  - Mouth, jaw, oropharynx, neck, and airway for Mallampati score assessment
  - Chest and lungs
  - Heart and circulation
  - Vital signs, including heart rate, respiratory rate, blood pressure, and oxygenation, with end-tidal carbon dioxide when indicated
- Review of any pre-sedation diagnostic tests
- Completion of a pre-sedation assessment form (with American Society of Anesthesiologists physical status classification)
- Patient informed consent
- Immediate pre-sedation assessment before first sedating doses
- Initiation of IV access and fluids to maintain patency

✖ Do not separately report or include the time of post-service work in the intraservice time. Post-service work of moderate sedation includes
- Assessment of the patient's vital signs, level of consciousness, and neurological, cardiovascular, and pulmonary stability in the post-sedation recovery period
- Assessment of the patient's readiness for discharge following the procedure
- Preparation of documentation for sedation service
- Communication with family or caregiver about sedation service

✖ Do not separately report pulse oximetry (**94760–94762**).

Documentation of moderate sedation services must include all the following items:

- **The description of the procedure**
- **Name and dosage(s) of the sedation agent(s)**
- **Route of administration of the sedation agent(s) and who administered the agent (physician or independent observer)**
- **The ongoing assessment of the child's level of consciousness and physiologic status (eg, heart rate, oxygen saturation levels) during and after the procedure**
- **The presence, name, and title of the independent observer or performing physician or other qualified health care professional**
- **Total time from administration of the sedation agent(s) (start time) until the physician's face-to-face service is no longer required (end time)**

Examples

➤ **A 3-year-old requires incision and removal of a piece of glass from a puncture wound of the right foot.** Moderate sedation is required and is performed by the Pediatric Advanced Life Support–trained physician with an independent trained observer who has been trained in pediatric basic life support. The physician supervises the administration of the sedating agent and assesses the child until an effective, safe level of sedation is achieved and continues to assess the child's level of consciousness and physiologic status while also performing the procedure. The procedure takes a total of 28 minutes from the time of administration of the agent until the physician completes the procedure and determines that the child is stable and face-to-face physician time is no longer required.

ICD-10-CM	*CPT*
S91.341A (puncture wound with foreign body, right foot) Codes for external cause, activity, and place of injury are reported when documented.	**10121** (incision and removal of foreign body, subcutaneous tissues; complex) **99151** (moderate [conscious] sedation, patient younger than 5 years, first 15 minutes) **✚99153** (moderate [conscious] sedation, each additional 15 minutes of intraservice time)

Teaching Point: If a medically necessary, significant, and separately identifiable E/M service had also been performed, an E/M visit with modifier **25** appended could have been reported. The agent itself should also be reported.

➤ **Same patient as previous example, except moderate sedation is performed by the Pediatric Advanced Life Support–trained physician while another physician performs the procedure.** The procedure, from the time of administration of the agent until the repair is complete and the child is stable and no longer requires face-to-face physician time, takes a total of 28 minutes.

ICD-10-CM	CPT
S91.341A (puncture wound with foreign body, right foot) Codes for external cause, activity, and place of injury are reported when documented.	The physician repairing the wound reports **10121** (incision and removal of foreign body, subcutaneous tissues; complex)
	The physician performing moderate sedation reports **99155** (moderate [conscious] sedation, patient younger than 5 years, first 15 minutes) **✚99157** (moderate [conscious] sedation, each additional 15 minutes of intraservice time)

Teaching Point: Each physician reports the service provided. The time of moderate sedation used in code selection is only the intraservice time.

For virtual reality dissociation services to support and optimize patient comfort and tolerance during a procedure, see codes **0771T–0774T**.

Chapter Takeaways

This chapter provides an overview of coding for procedures in the office and other outpatient settings. Following are some takeaways from this chapter:

- Many, but not all, payers use the RVUs and global periods assigned by the Medicare program. Learn how individual payers value and pay for procedural services.
- When a global service is provided, report follow-up visits during a global period with code **99024**. Append modifier **24** to codes for unrelated E/M services during a postoperative period.
- Some minor procedures are included in E/M services and not separately reported (eg, removal of non-impacted ear wax).
- All procedures include some preservice and post-service work. Only report an E/M service that is significant and separately identifiable in the documentation.

Resources

Global Periods and Relative Value Units

MPFS (www.cms.gov/medicare/medicare-fee-for-service-payment/physicianfeesched)

Online Exclusive Content at www.aap.org/cfp2023

"Office Procedures and Global Days"

Chapter 14. Surgery, Infusion, and Sedation in the Outpatient Setting

Test Your Knowledge!

1. **Which of the following services is included in the global surgical package?**
   a. Moderate sedation
   b. Local or topical anesthesia
   c. Unrelated care during the global period
   d. Any evaluation and management service within 10 days before surgery

2. **Which of the following components is included in the work of an evaluation and management service and not reported as a distinct procedural service?**
   a. Removal of impacted cerumen
   b. Removal of a foreign body from the nose
   c. Removal of foreign bodies from skin that do not require an incision
   d. Repair of a laceration by using tissue adhesive

3. **Which of the following services is reported with code 30901 for control of nasal hemorrhage?**
   a. Bleeding is controlled with manual pressure.
   b. Bleeding is controlled with placement of a nasal clamp (clip).
   c. Nasal packing is placed in the short term to administer medication.
   d. Nasal packing is placed to serve a hemostatic and/or tamponade role.

4. **Which of the following codes is used to report urinary catheterization to collect a clean-catch urine specimen?**
   a. None, this service is included in a related evaluation and management service.
   b. **51701**.
   c. **51702**.
   d. None, catheterization is included in urinalysis (eg, **81000**).

5. **Per *Current Procedural Terminology* guidance, which of the following services is reported with code 96372?**
   a. Administration of chemotherapy
   b. Administration of vaccines and toxoids
   c. Therapeutic, prophylactic, or diagnostic injections of medication other than chemotherapy
   d. Administration of a purified protein derivative test

Part 3

Primarily for Hospital Settings

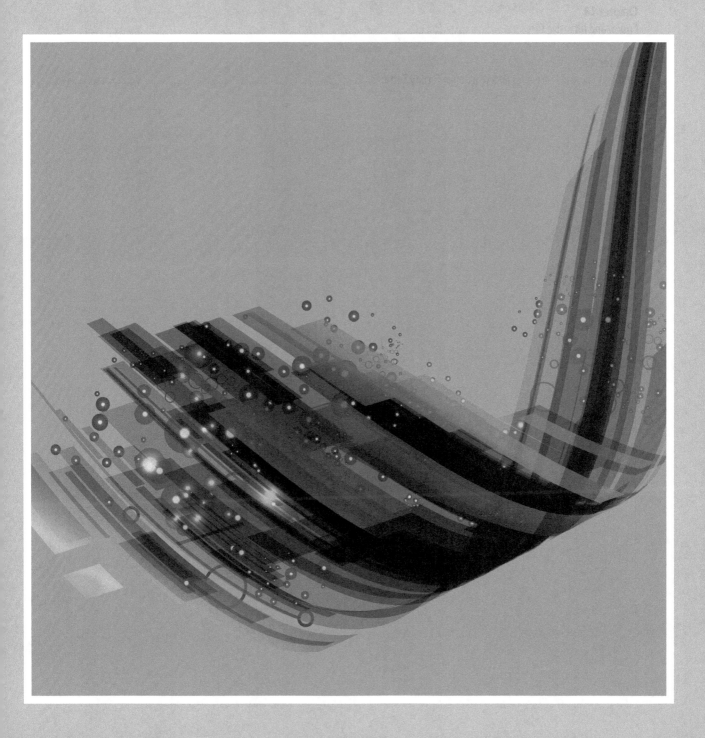

Part 3. Primarily for Hospital Settings

Emergency Department Services

CPT copyright 2022 American Medical Association. All rights reserved.

Contents

● indicates a new code; ▲, revised; #, re-sequenced; ✚, add-on; ★, audiovisual technology; and ◀, synchronous interactive audio.

Chapter Highlights

- Overview and examples of evaluation and management (E/M) code selection for emergency department (ED) services
- Documentation and coding of diagnoses for services in the ED
- Use of procedure code modifiers
- Reporting procedures in the ED
- Directing emergency medical technicians
- Reporting provision of critical care services in the ED

Emergency Department (ED) Code Updates in 2023

Significant changes to E/M codes and code selection guidelines are presented in *Current Procedural Terminology* (*CPT*®) for all services provided on and after January 1, 2023. Emergency department and other E/M services are now subject to updated guidelines that were first introduced for office and other outpatient E/M services. In particular, E/M services in the ED that were previously selected on the basis of key components (history, examination, and medical-decision-making [MDM]) are selected on the basis of MDM alone for services provided in 2023.

> Although history and examination are no longer components of code selection, documentation of pertinent history and examination is important to support the level of medical decision-making of the encounter.

Read the full discussion of the revised E/M guidelines provided in **Chapter 6** to learn the revised guidelines and definitions that apply to E/M code selection.

Using Diagnosis Codes to Support the Level of ED Visits

Emergency department physicians play critical roles in care and documentation. While multiple symptoms may be listed as the chief complaint (CC; primary concern) during the ED triage process, the physician must designate only 1 sign, symptom, disease, or injury as the CC. Hospitals depend on the physician's designation of the CC because only 1 diagnosis code may be reported for this category on the hospital claim form. This diagnosis is used to help support the urgency of the ED visit under prudent layperson guidelines. This may be different from conditions that are "present on admission" that must be tracked by hospitals.

The diagnoses on the physician's claim for professional services are equally important to support the level of ED service reported (**99281–99285**). Some health plans now compare diagnosis codes submitted on physician claims that include codes **99284** and **99285** to a predetermined list of diagnosis codes indicating conditions that typically require these levels of service. When a claim for **99284** or **99285** is submitted with diagnosis codes not included on the list, the claim may be down-coded (eg, changed to **99283**) and paid at the rate of the lesser code.

As shown in **Figure 15-1**, down-coding **99284** or **99285** to **99283** results in a significant corresponding decrease in relative value units (RVUs) and fee-for-service payment. Relative value units listed are 2022 RVUs (not geographically adjusted), as 2023 RVUs were unavailable at the time of this publication. Learn more about payment based on RVUs in **Chapter 4**.

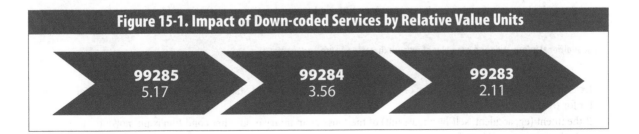

Figure 15-1. Impact of Down-coded Services by Relative Value Units

99285	99284	99283
5.17	3.56	2.11

● indicates a new code; ▲, revised; #, re-sequenced; ✚, add-on; ★, audiovisual technology; and ◀, synchronous interactive audio.

Chapter 15. Emergency Department Services

Medicaid plans also significantly limit the amount paid for any condition not included on a diagnosis list, regardless of the level of service reported. To receive the payment most appropriate under the health plan contract

- List first the diagnosis that is most responsible for the level of service provided and report the code for that diagnosis first on your claim.
- Document and report codes for all current conditions that require or affect patient care treatment or management.

Some plans consider only the first 2 diagnoses listed on the claim.

Some plans take into account all diagnoses on the claim, including

- Complicating factors (eg, **F84.0**, autism spectrum disorder)
- Social determinants of health (eg, **Z59.0**, homelessness)
- External cause of injury (eg, **W13.0XXA**, fall [on] [from] balcony)

Physicians should clearly document all diagnoses including factors that increased the level of MDM of an encounter. This documentation can help a professional coder, if used, extract the appropriate diagnosis codes. To appeal the down-coded claim, medical records supporting the higher level of service must typically be submitted to the health plan.

Reporting External Cause of Injury

States may require EDs to report codes describing the circumstances of an injury or another morbidity. These codes are referred to as *external cause* codes in *International Classification of Diseases, 10th Revision, Clinical Modification (ICD-10-CM)*. These codes capture the cause, intent, place of occurrence, activity of the patient at the time of the event, and patient status (eg, employee, military, volunteer, student). External cause codes (categories **V00–Y99**) are found in Chapter 20 of the tabular list of *ICD-10-CM*.

External cause of injury codes are found in the *International Classification of Diseases, 10th Revision, Clinical Modification* External Cause of Injuries Index. For example, under the term *struck*, sub-terms allow reporting of external causes such as a struck by baseball (W21.03-) or baseball bat (by accident [T75.0-] or assault [Y08.02-]). Combination codes allow for reporting multiple details, such as striking against an object with subsequent fall (W18.0-).

External cause codes provide information that is valuable for research on the cause and occurrence of injuries as well as evaluation of injury prevention strategies (eg, reduced reporting of head injuries because of campaigns to encourage bicycle helmet use). This is particularly important in pediatrics, as injuries remain the leading cause of death and disability. While the physician may not be required to add the specific external cause code with the discharge diagnosis, there should be sufficient documentation in the record to allow a coder to extract the proper diagnosis code.

Examples of assignment of external cause codes are provided in the ED Evaluation and Management (E/M) Codes section later in this chapter.

Key points for reporting external cause codes include

- External cause codes are never the principal or first-listed diagnosis code.
- External cause codes may be reported in conjunction with any health condition that is related to an external cause (eg, adverse effect of medical treatment).
- Report *ICD-10-CM* codes for the cause and intent of an injury or illness for the duration of treatment. The seventh character of the code indicates the nature of the encounter.
  - Initial or *active* care (**A**).
  - Subsequent care *during the healing phase* (**D**).
  - Care for *sequela* (**S**) of the injury or illness.
  - Seventh characters in some code categories provide additional details (eg, type of open fracture).

For additional information and examples of seventh characters in use, see Chapter 1.

- External cause codes indicating place of occurrence, activity, and patient status are reported only at the initial encounter for treatment.
- If the intent (eg, accident, self-harm, assault) of the cause of an injury or another condition is unknown or unspecified, code the intent as *accidental*.

● indicates a new code; ▲, revised; #, re-sequenced; ✚, add-on; ★, audiovisual technology; and ◀, synchronous interactive audio.

- No external cause code should be assigned when the cause and intent of an illness or injury are included in another reported code (eg, **T58.11XA**, initial encounter for toxic effect of carbon monoxide from utility gas, accidental).
- No external cause code should be assigned when an injury is ruled out after examination and observation (eg, **Z04.1**, encounter for examination and observation following transport accident).

Refer to the American Academy of Pediatrics *Pediatric ICD-10-CM 2023: A Manual for Provider-Based Coding* (https://shop.aap.org/pediatric-icd-10-cm-2023-8th-edition-paperback) and *International Classification of Diseases, 10th Revision, Clinical Modification* resources (www.aap.org/en/practice-management/practice-financing/coding-and-valuation/icd-10-cm-resources) for more information on codes and code selection.

Reporting Suspected or Confirmed Abuse or Other Maltreatment

ICD-10-CM includes codes for reporting suspected or confirmed neglect or abandonment; physical, sexual, or psychological abuse; forced sexual exploitation; and forced labor exploitation. These codes are selected on the basis of the type of maltreatment, whether the patient is a child or an adult, and whether the maltreatment is suspected, confirmed, or ruled out at the encounter.

Suspected (**T76.-**) or confirmed maltreatment (**T74.-**) is reported as the first-listed diagnosis when this is the reason for the encounter. Codes for associated mental health or physical injury are reported secondary to the code for suspected or confirmed abuse.

- Codes are selected on the basis of documentation. The record should clearly state whether abuse is suspected, ruled out, or confirmed.
- Codes include seventh characters **A**, **D**, and **S**.

Examples
In each example, codes for diagnosed injuries, assault, and perpetrator are reported in addition to the **T74** code.

➤ **Physical abuse is confirmed and initial active treatment is provided at an encounter.**
T74.12XA   Child physical abuse confirmed, initial encounter

➤ **Follow-up care during healing of injuries caused by confirmed physical abuse is provided at an encounter.**
T74.12XD   Child physical abuse confirmed, subsequent encounter

➤ **A child is evaluated for scar contracture that is a late effect of injuries caused by confirmed physical abuse.**
T74.12XS   Child physical abuse confirmed, sequela

- When reporting confirmed abuse (**T74.-**), also report codes for assault (**X92–Y04**; **Y08**, **Y09**) and, when known, perpetrator (**Y07.-**).

Reporting Suspected Maltreatment When Ruled Out

Report one of the following codes from category **Z04** for an encounter at which neglect, abuse, or exploitation is *suspected but ruled out* and not a code from category **T74** or **T76**:

Z04.72	Encounter for examination and observation following alleged child physical abuse
Z04.42	Encounter for examination and observation following alleged child rape
Z04.81	Encounter for examination and observation of victim following forced sexual exploitation
Z04.82	Encounter for examination and observation of victim following forced labor exploitation

ED Evaluation and Management (E/M) Codes

▲**99281**	Emergency department visit for the evaluation and management of a patient, that may not require the presence of a physician or other qualified health care professional
▲**99282**	Emergency department visit for the evaluation and management of a patient, which requires a medically appropriate history and/or examination and straightforward medical decision making
▲**99283**	Emergency department visit for the evaluation and management of a patient, which requires a medically appropriate history and/or examination and low level of medical decision making

● indicates a new code; ▲, revised; #, re-sequenced; ✚, add-on; ★, audiovisual technology; and ◀, synchronous interactive audio.

▲99284   Emergency department visit for the evaluation and management of a patient, which requires a medically appropriate history and/or examination and moderate level of medical decision making

▲99285   Emergency department visit for the evaluation and management of a patient, which requires a medically appropriate history and/or examination and high level of medical decision making

For coding purposes, an ED is defined as *an organized hospital-based facility for the provision of unscheduled episodic services to patients who present for immediate medical attention.* The facility must be available 24 hours a day, 7 days a week.

- Emergency department E/M codes **99281–99285** are reported only when care is provided to a patient who has been admitted to an ED.
  - Some states allow for freestanding EDs that are not hospital affiliated. Payers may or may not allow the use of ED codes in these circumstances.
  - Physician services provided in a freestanding hospital-affiliated ED may be subject to specific billing rules. Check payer contracts for payment and billing policies.
- Report the appropriate *CPT* office or other outpatient visit codes (**99202–99215**) and appropriate place of service code (eg, **20** for urgent care facility) for services performed in an urgent care center, a nonhospital facility, or a facility that is not open 24 hours a day. These facilities are not considered freestanding EDs.
- Append modifier **25** (significant, separately identifiable E/M service) to the ED service code (**99282–99285**) when the treating ED physician or other qualified health care professional (QHP) provides initial hospital inpatient or observation services (**99221–99223**) or same date initial hospital inpatient or observation admission and discharge (**99234–99236**) on the same date of service as the ED encounter.
  - Report codes for subsequent (**99231–99233**) or discharge (**99238**, **99239**) services for continued care on subsequent dates of service.

> **See Chapter 17 for full discussion of codes reported for hospital inpatient and observation services.**

- Payer policies may vary for reporting and payment of multiple E/M services on the same date.
- There is no differentiation between new and established patients for ED encounters.
- The level of ED codes **99282–99285** is based on the MDM. Time is not used in selection of codes **99282–99285**.
- The highest 2 of 3 elements of MDM are used to select the level of an ED E/M code.
  1. **Problem(s):** the number and complexity of presenting problems
  2. **Data:** the amount and/or complexity of data to be reviewed and analyzed
  3. **Risk:** the risk of complications and/or morbidity or mortality of patient management
- The concept of the level of MDM does not apply to **99281** because this level of service does not require a physician's or QHP's MDM.

> **Because code 99281 represents a service that does not require the presence of a physician or other qualified health care professional (QHP) and is likely performed by clinical staff employed by the facility, payment policies for the physician's or QHP's supervision may vary.**

All levels of ED service include a medically appropriate history and examination as determined by the treating physician or QHP.

Medical necessity is an overarching criterion for selecting the level of E/M service. Physicians should always consider whether the nature of the presenting problem supports the medical necessity of services rendered when selecting the level of E/M service.

Use **Table 15-1** to help you select the appropriate level of ED E/M service in the examples for each level of service that follow.

Examples

➤ **A 3-year-old presents with a splinter in his right forefoot.** The patient was playing on a wooden deck with bare feet about an hour ago and said he got a splinter. The mother wants assistance removing the splinter because the child has refused to be still for removal at home. Immunizations are up to date. The child appears well and is in no discomfort. Examination reveals a visible wood splinter that is readily grasped with tweezers and removed. Antibiotic ointment and a bandage are applied.

● indicates a new code; ▲, revised; #, re-sequenced; ✚, add-on; ★, audiovisual technology; and ◀, synchronous interactive audio.

Table 15-1. Code Selection Requirements for Emergency Department Evaluation and Management Service (Excluding 99281)

Level/Codes	Medical Decision-making (2 of 3 Required: Problems, Data,[a] Risk)		
	Problems Addressed	Data Reviewed and Analyzed[b]	Risk
Straightforward 99282	1 self-limited or minor *Examples* • Mild diaper rash • Cold or mild URTI	Minimal or none	Minimal *Examples* • Rest and plenty of fluids • Diaper ointment • Superficial wound dressing
Low 99283	Low—*Any 1 of* ≥2 self-limited or minor 1 stable chronic illness 1 acute, uncomplicated illness or injury 1 stable acute illness 1 acute, uncomplicated illness or injury requiring hospital inpatient or observation level of care *Examples* • Acute gastroenteritis • Uncomplicated hand-foot-and-mouth disease • Recheck of wound repaired at previous encounter • Resolution of URTI with continued cough	Limited (*Meet 1 of 2 categories*) <u>Category 1:</u> Tests and documents (*Any 2*)[a] • Review of prior external note(s)—each unique source • Review of the result(s) of each unique test • Ordering of each unique test <u>Category 2:</u> Assessment requiring an independent historian(s)	Low *Examples* • Over-the-counter medication(s) • Removal of sutures • Physical, language, or occupational therapy
Moderate 99284	Moderate—*Any 1 of* ≥1 chronic illness with exacerbation, progression, or side effects of treatment ≥2 stable chronic illnesses 1 undiagnosed new problem with uncertain prognosis 1 acute illness with systemic symptoms 1 acute, complicated injury *Examples* • Asthma with exacerbation but not hypoxia • Unexplained bruising • Acute gastroenteritis with dehydration • Intermittent headaches and confusion following concussion	Moderate (*Meet 1 out of 3 categories*)[a] <u>Category 1:</u> Tests and documents (*Meet any 3*) • Review of prior external note(s)—each unique source • Review of the result(s) of each unique test • Ordering each unique test • Assessment requiring an independent historian(s) <u>Category 2:</u> Independent interpretation of a test performed by another physician/other QHP[b] <u>Category 3:</u> Discussion of management or test interpretation with external physician/other QHP/appropriate source[b]	Moderate *Examples* • Prescription drug management or off-label use of over-the-counter medication • Decision about minor surgery with identified patient or procedure risk factors • Decision about elective major surgery without identified patient or procedure risk factors • Diagnosis or treatment significantly limited by social determinants of health

Continued on next page

● indicates a new code; ▲, revised; #, re-sequenced; ✚, add-on; ★, audiovisual technology; and ◄, synchronous interactive audio.

	Table 15-1 (*continued*)		
	Medical Decision-making (2 of 3 Required: Problems, Data,ª Risk)		
Level/Codes	**Problems Addressed**	**Data Reviewed and Analyzed**[b]	**Risk**
High **99285**	High—*1 of* ≥1 chronic illness with severe exacerbation, progression, or side effects of treatment 1 acute or chronic illness or injury that poses a threat to life or bodily function *Examples* • Asthma with hypoxia (status asthmaticus) • Infant with fever, tachycardia, lethargy, and dehydration • Injury or illness with shock	Extensive (*Meet 2 out of 3 categories*) Category 1: Tests and documents (*Meet any 3*)ª • Review of prior external note(s) from each unique source • Review of the result(s) of each unique test • Ordering of each unique test • Assessment requiring an independent historian(s) Category 2: Independent interpretation of a test performed by another physician/other QHP[b] Category 3: Discussion of management or test interpretation with external physician/other QHP/appropriate source[b]	High *Examples* • Drug therapy requiring intensive monitoring for toxicity • Decision about elective major surgery with identified patient or procedure risk factors • Decision about emergency major surgery • Decision about hospitalization or escalation of hospital level of care • Decision not to resuscitate or to de-escalate care because of poor prognosis • Parenteral controlled substances

Abbreviation: QHP, qualified health care professional; URTI, upper respiratory tract infection.

ª Each unique test, order, or document contributes to the combination of 2 or combination of 3 in Category 1.

[b] Do not count data review or communications reported with other codes (eg, electrocardiogram interpretation and report reported with **93010**, interprofessional consultation referral service reported with **99452**).

ICD-10-CM	*CPT*
S90.851A (superficial foreign body, right foot, initial encounter)	**99282** Straightforward MDM (problem: minimal [minor]; data: limited [independent historian]; risk: minimal)

Teaching Point: The MDM elements support code **99282**. Although the data are limited, potentially supporting low MDM, the other 2 elements support straightforward MDM. Clinically indicated history and examination are documented but do not influence code selection. Because no incision was required to remove the splinter, removal of the foreign body is not separately reported.

If the splinter removal had required an incision, a code for incision and removal of a foreign body from subcutaneous tissue would have been reported with code **10120** if simple or **10121** if complex. A separately reportable E/M service would not likely be supported (ie, would not likely be significantly beyond the typical preservice work of the procedure).

➤ **An 11-year-old patient presents with an injury to his left ankle.** The patient reports hurting his ankle by tripping during a basketball game approximately an hour earlier and is experiencing continued mild pain. He is able to bear his full weight. His parents report no prior injuries. There is discussion with the patient and family that a requested radiograph is not indicated. A compression wrap is applied, and the patient and parents are instructed on home care. They are to follow up with the patient's primary care physician. Diagnosis is sprain of the anterior talofibular ligament of the left ankle.

ICD-10-CM	*CPT*
S93.492A (sprain of other ligament of left ankle, initial encounter) **W01.0XXA** (fall on same level from slipping, tripping and stumbling without subsequent striking against object, initial encounter) **Y93.67** (activity, basketball)	**99283** Low MDM (problems: low [acute, uncomplicated injury]; data: limited [independent historian]; risk: low)

● indicates a new code; ▲, revised; #, re-sequenced; ✚, add-on; ★, audiovisual technology; and ◀, synchronous interactive audio.

Teaching Point: Low MDM supports code **99283**. All 3 elements of MDM support this level of service.

There is shared decision-making with the family regarding a lack of indication for and/or decision against testing counts toward the amount of data as if the test had been ordered. However, the number of tests, documents, and independent historian at this encounter still support a limited amount and/or complexity of data.

Codes **Y92.310** (basketball court as the place of occurrence of the external cause) and **Y99.8** (other external cause status [leisure activity]) may also be reported to add to injury information that may be necessary for determining whether another party is responsible for the patient's medical expenses (eg, school injury policy).

When a test is considered but not ordered (after discussion with the patient and/or caregivers), document that it was considered but not ordered and the reason for not ordering it (eg, not indicated, unavailable).

➤ **An 13-year-old patient presents with an injury to his left ankle.** The patient reports hurting his ankle by tripping during a basketball game approximately an hour earlier and is not able to bear full weight on his ankle. The parents detail history of a prior ankle fracture. A radiograph is ordered and images are reviewed. The ED physician chooses to speak with a radiologist about the interpretation of the radiograph. Current fracture is ruled out, and the patient and parents are provided with a walking boot and instructed on home care and follow-up with primary care physician. Diagnosis is sprain of the anterior talofibular and calcaneofibular ligaments of the left ankle.

ICD-10-CM	*CPT*
S93.412A (sprain of calcaneofibular ligament of left ankle, initial encounter) **S93.492A** (sprain of other ligament of left ankle, initial encounter) **W01.0XXA** (fall on same level from slipping, tripping and stumbling without subsequent striking against object, initial encounter) **Y93.67** (activity, basketball) **Y92.310** (basketball court as the place of occurrence of the external cause) **Y99.8** (other external cause status [leisure activity])	**99284** Moderate MDM (problems: moderate [signs or symptoms of a fracture]; data: extensive [independent visualization of images, discussion with performing physician]; risk: low)

Teaching Point: Moderate MDM is supported by the moderate complexity of the problem addressed and the extensive data analysis necessary to determine diagnosis and management. Only 2 of 3 elements are required to support the level of MDM.

The final diagnosis for a condition does not, in and of itself, determine the complexity or risk, as extensive evaluation may be required to reach the conclusion that the signs or symptoms do not represent a highly morbid condition.

➤ **An adolescent boy is brought to the ED by ambulance after a rollover automobile accident.** Emergency medical technicians relay that the patient was driving and wearing a seat belt but the older model vehicle did not have airbags. Witnesses to the accident reported that the patient lost consciousness for several minutes before arrival of the ambulance. The ED physician comprehensively examines the patient, whose Glasgow Coma Scale score is 14 because of confusion. Parenteral controlled substances are administered. Radiographs of the chest and left shoulder and a computed tomography scan of the head are ordered. The patient is found to have a closed frontal skull fracture and fractured left clavicle. Neurosurgery and orthopedic consultations are obtained, and, after discussion with the neurosurgeon and orthopedic surgeon, the patient is admitted for observation by the neurosurgeon.

Chapter 15. Emergency Department Services

ICD-10-CM	CPT
S02.0XXA (fracture of vault of skull, initial encounter for closed fracture) **S42.021A** (displaced fracture of shaft of right clavicle, initial encounter for closed fracture) **R40.2142A** (coma scale, eyes open, spontaneous, at arrival to emergency department) **R40.2242A** (coma scale, best verbal response, confused conversation, at arrival to emergency department) **R40.2362A** (coma scale, best motor response, obeys commands, at arrival to emergency department) **V48.5XXA** (car driver injured in noncollision transport accident in traffic accident, initial encounter) **Y92.413** (state road as the place of occurrence of the external cause)	**99285** (ED visit code) High MDM (problems: high [trauma with altered mental status]; data: high [3 unique tests ordered, independent historians, and discussion of management with external physicians]; risk: high [administration of parenteral controlled substances])

Teaching Point: All 3 elements of MDM support a high level of MDM in this case.

Evaluation and management services by the orthopedist would be reported with office or other outpatient consultation codes (likely **99244** or **99245**). The neurosurgeon will report an office or other consultation with modifier **25** (significant, separately identifiable E/M service) in addition to subsequent hospital inpatient or observation care (**99221–99223**). Each physician will report the diagnoses for the conditions confirmed at the conclusion of the encounter (eg, the ED physician reports what was known at the time the patient is transferred to the neurosurgeon's care).

Emergency department (ED) codes may be reported by any physician or qualified health care professional (QHP) providing unscheduled care to a patient who presents to an ED for immediate medical attention. However, if a patient is seen in the ED for the convenience of a physician or QHP, use office or other outpatient services codes (99202–99215) or other appropriate codes (eg, initial hospital inpatient or observation services) to report the E/M service.

Modifiers Used With ED Codes

Physicians need to understand when it is appropriate to report modifiers in addition to E/M or procedural service codes. Modifiers **25** (significant, separately identifiable E/M service) and **57** (decision for surgery) may be appended to ED E/M codes to indicate E/M beyond the preservice work of a procedure. Procedures performed in the ED may require reporting of modifiers such as **26** (professional component), **54** (surgical care only), or **59** (distinct procedural service) or, when accepted by the payer in lieu of modifier **59**, modifier **XE** (separate encounter), **XP** (separate practitioner), **XS** (separate structure), or **XU** (unusual nonoverlapping service). See **Chapter 2** for more detail on the use of modifiers.

Example

➤ **The ED physician is caring for a 9-year-old who has a 4-cm–long, deep laceration of the right calf and a separate 1-cm–long laceration of the right ankle from broken glass in his backyard.** The physician obtains history from the child and parents. A radiograph of the extremity is obtained and reviewed with notation of no retained radiopaque foreign bodies. The child's immunizations are current, with the last tetanus booster less than 5 years ago. The physician irrigates, carefully explores both wounds, and performs a 2-layer repair on the calf. The ankle laceration requires only single-layer closure. The child is discharged with appropriate follow-up plans.

ICD-10-CM	CPT
S81.811A (laceration without foreign body, right lower leg, initial encounter) **S91.011A** (laceration without foreign body, right ankle, initial encounter) **W25.XXXA** (contact with sharp glass, initial encounter) **Y92.007** (garden or yard of noninstitutional residence)	**99283 25** (problem: low; data: moderate; risk: low) **12032** (intermediate repair of the extremities, 2.6–7.5 cm) **12001 59** or **XS** (simple repair of the extremity, ≤2.5 cm)

Teaching Point: Modifiers are used to indicate that the laceration repairs were distinct procedures (**59**) or of a separate structure (**XS**). Append modifier **25** only when providing an E/M and other service with an E/M component (preservice and post-service work) on the same date to indicate that the E/M was significantly beyond the preservice work of the other service and distinctly documented.

See Chapter 2 for more information on these modifiers and appropriate modifier placement.

For more examples of coding for laceration repairs, see Chapter 14.

Reporting Procedures in the ED

Many procedures performed in the ED have an associated global period assigned by Medicare and other payers and/or are subject to the *CPT* surgical package. The global period affects reporting of pre- and post-procedural care. The *CPT* surgical package defines the work included in each surgical procedure. (See **Chapter 19** for the definition of the *CPT* surgical package and Medicare global period and examples of reporting procedures when follow-up care is provided by another physician.)

Modifier **54** (surgical care only) is appropriately appended to procedure codes with 10- or 90-day global periods when the patient will not return to the ED for follow-up care (eg, visits for follow-up care of a fracture). Some payers require modifier **54** only on codes assigned a 90-day global period. An example of reporting modifier **54** is included in the Fracture Care section later in this chapter.

To report an E/M service in addition to a procedure, there must be documentation of performance of a significant and separately identifiable E/M service beyond the pre- and post-procedural work typical for the procedure (eg, evaluation for a concussion and repair of wounds at 1 encounter). Post-procedural prescriptions for pain control or prophylactic antibiotics may be included in the procedure performed.

See "Emergency Department Procedures" at www.aap.org/cfp2023 for a list of procedures (with assigned Medicare global periods) commonly performed in the ED.

Any separately identifiable procedure that is personally performed by the physician may be reported, with the exception of

- Procedures that are bundled in time-based critical care codes (See **Table 18-1** for a list of services and procedures that are included in hourly critical care codes.)
- Services performed by hospital personnel because they are billed by the hospital facility (If a nurse or other clinical staff assist in part of a procedure, the ED physician may bill for the professional services if the ED physician provides the primary or key component of the procedure.)
- Hydration, infusion, and/or injection procedures (**96360–96379**) because the physician work associated with the procedures involves only confirmation of the treatment plan and not direct supervision of staff
- Procedures involving use of hospital-owned equipment (eg, pulse oximetry), unless the procedure includes both technical and professional components (If performed and documented, the professional component, such as interpretation and report of radiographic findings, may be reported with modifier **26** [professional component] appended to the procedure code.)

Fracture Care

Fracture care in the ED is typically limited to initial care. Most codes for fracture care include a 10- or 90-day period of care related to the fracture. Correct coding requires appending modifier **54** (surgical care only) to codes for fracture care when follow-up care will be provided by another physician. The physician who assumes management during the follow-up period reports the same fracture care code with modifier **55** (postoperative management only) and the same date of service. Some payers require that both physicians document the transfer of care.

Casting, splinting, or strapping may be used solely to temporarily stabilize the fracture for the comfort of a patient who will receive fracture care by an orthopedist in the next few days. When this happens, it is not considered closed fracture treatment and is reported with a code for application of casts and strapping service (**29000–29584**) in addition to any significant evaluation and management service reported with modifier **25**, when applicable.

Example

➤ **A 16-year-old patient is seen in the ED for right shoulder pain that occurred following a fall while playing soccer at a community sports field.** The patient is examined for additional injuries. Diagnosis is anterior glenohumeral dislocation of the right shoulder. The patient agrees to an attempt at reduction without analgesia, which is successful. A sling is applied. The physician refers the patient to another physician for follow-up care and documents the transfer of care.

ICD-10-CM	CPT
S43.014A (anterior dislocation of right humerus, initial encounter)	**99284 57**
W18.30XA (unspecified fall on same level, initial encounter)	**23650 54** (closed treatment of shoulder dislocation, with manipulation; without anesthesia)
Y93.66 (activity, soccer)	
Y92.322 (soccer field as place of occurrence)	

Teaching Point: The use of modifier **54** (surgical care only) alerts payers that another physician will report follow-up care for this procedure, which typically includes multiple services over a 90-day period of post-procedural care. Medical decision-making for the ED visit is moderate (assuming evaluation of body systems not directly part of the injured shoulder or independent interpretation of imaging) and moderate risk related to the decision for closed treatment of the dislocation. Modifier **57** indicates the decision for surgery during the E/M service.

See the February 2021 *AAP Pediatric Coding Newsletter* article, "Initial Fracture Care: Musculoskeletal or Evaluation and Management," for more examples of initial fracture care (https://doi.org/10.1542/pcco_book202_document005).

Nasal Fractures

Closed treatment of nasal bone fracture without manipulation is reported with an E/M code based on MDM performed and documented (ie, **99283** or **99284**). Closed treatment with manipulation is reported with codes **21315** and **21320**.

21315   Closed treatment of nasal bone fracture with manipulation; without stabilization
21320   with stabilization

Point-of-Care Ultrasound

Point-of-care ultrasound services performed by the ED physician are separately reportable in addition to the ED E/M service when *all 3 of the following conditions apply:*

- Thorough evaluation of organ(s) or anatomical region is performed.
- There is permanent image documentation (with measurements, when clinically indicated).
- A written report equivalent to that typically produced by a radiologist is documented.

Use of handheld or portable ultrasound machine that does not include all 3 of the listed elements is not separately reported.

Without all these elements, the examination is not separately reported and would be considered part of any E/M service provided. (*Exception:* Permanent image documentation is not required for ophthalmic ultrasonography for biometric measurement.)

Point-of-care ultrasound services in the ED are reported by the physician only with the professional component modifier (**26**). The technical component (eg, equipment cost, facility overhead costs) is typically reported by the facility. (Payers may limit physicians to reporting the professional component only for all facility-based services even if the physician performs the ultrasonography and/or owns the equipment used for the service. The technical component includes all associated overhead costs. Check individual payer policies for reporting.)

One use of point-of-care ultrasound services in the ED is the focused assessment with sonography for trauma (FAST) examination. This may consist of 2 distinct components: limited transthoracic echocardiography and limited abdominal ultrasonography. When 2 distinct procedures are performed, 2 codes are reported.

76705   Ultrasound, abdominal, real-time with image documentation; limited
93308   Echocardiography, transthoracic, real-time with image documentation (2D), includes M-mode recording, when performed, follow-up or limited study

Chapter 15. Emergency Department Services

Example

➤ **A child is seen in the ED for injuries sustained in a automobile accident.** The physician performs a trauma assessment, including a FAST examination. This examination may consist of 2 distinct components: limited transthoracic echocardiography and limited abdominal ultrasonography. When 2 distinct procedures are performed, 2 codes are reported.

    Teaching Point: In addition to the appropriate E/M service code, the physician reports **76705 26** and **93308 26** (see code descriptors earlier in this section). Modifier **26** signifies that the physician is reporting the professional component of each service. The facility will report the same codes with modifier **TC** to indicate reporting of the technical component of each service. When applicable and when all requirements for reporting are met, ultrasonography performed with physician-owned equipment is reported without a modifier (ie, modifiers **26** and **TC** are not applicable).

When a limited ultrasound examination of the chest is included (eg, for pneumothorax), report code **76604** (ultrasound, chest [includes mediastinum when performed], real-time with image documentation). Limited studies are defined in *CPT* as those that include examination of less than the required elements for a "complete" examination (eg, limited number of organs, limited portion of region evaluated). See your *CPT* reference for required components of complete examinations.

See the Central Venous Access section in **Chapter 19** for appropriate reporting of ultrasound guidance for vascular access (**76937**). This code is reported separately in addition to a code for primary vascular access procedure (eg, **36555**).

When ultrasound guidance is used for needle placement for procedures such as aspiration of an abscess, code **76942** is reported. Do not report code **76942** in conjunction with a service for which the code descriptor includes ultrasound guidance (eg, joint aspiration). Code **76937** (ultrasound guidance for vascular access) is not reported in conjunction with code **76942**.

Sedation

Moderate Sedation

Moderate sedation (**99151–99157**) is a drug-induced depression of consciousness during which patients may respond purposefully to verbal commands, either alone or accompanied by light tactile stimulation. Moderate sedation may be necessary for the performance of certain procedures in the ED.

99151   Moderate sedation services provided by the same physician or other qualified health care professional performing the diagnostic or therapeutic service that the sedation supports, requiring the presence of an independent trained observer to assist in the monitoring of the patient's level of consciousness and physiological status; initial 15 minutes of intraservice time, patient younger than 5 years of age

99152   initial 15 minutes of intraservice time, patient age 5 years or older

✚99153   each additional 15 minutes intraservice time (report with **99151** or **99152**)

99155   Moderate sedation services provided by a physician or other qualified health care professional other than the physician or other qualified health care professional performing the diagnostic or therapeutic service that the sedation supports; initial 15 minutes of intraservice time, patient younger than 5 years of age

99156   initial 15 minutes of intraservice time, patient age 5 years or older

✚99157   each additional 15 minutes intraservice time (report with **99155** or **99156**)

See Chapter 14 for a full discussion of coding for moderate sedation.

● Codes are selected on the basis of intraservice time. Intraservice time
  — Begins with the administration of the sedating agent(s)
  — Ends when the procedure is completed, the patient is stable for recovery status, and the physician or other QHP providing the sedation ends personal continuous face-to-face time with the patient
  — Includes ordering and/or administering the initial and subsequent doses of sedating agents
  — Requires continuous face-to-face attendance of the physician or other QHP
  — Requires monitoring patient response to the sedating agents, including
    ▪ Periodic assessment of the patient
    ▪ Further administration of agent(s) as needed to maintain sedation
    ▪ Monitoring of oxygen saturation, heart rate, and blood pressure

● Moderate sedation services of less than 10 minutes' intraservice time are not separately reported.

Example

➤ **A 5-year-old requires a procedure in the ED.** A physician other than the ED physician performs the procedure. The ED physician provides the moderate sedation and documents 25 minutes of service, beginning with administration of the sedating agent and ending when the patient is sufficiently recovered so the physician's continuous face-to-face monitoring is no longer necessary.

> **CPT**
> **99282–99285 25**
> **99156** (moderate sedation by other than physician performing procedure, first 15 minutes)
> **99157** (moderate sedation, each additional 15 minutes)

Teaching Point: The ED physician reports an E/M code as appropriate for care before the pre-sedation evaluation (eg, initial evaluation of illness or injury) and appends modifier **25** to indicate that the service was significant and is separately identifiable in the documentation. Code **99157** is reported for the final 10 minutes because the midpoint between the first and second 15-minute period was passed.

Deep Sedation

Deep sedation or analgesia is a drug-induced depression of consciousness during which patients cannot be easily aroused but respond purposefully after repeated verbal or painful stimulation (eg, purposefully pushing away the noxious stimuli). The ability to independently maintain ventilatory function may be impaired. Patients may require assistance in maintaining a patent airway, and spontaneous ventilation may be inadequate. Cardiovascular function is usually maintained. A state of deep sedation may be accompanied by partial or complete loss of protective airway reflexes.

Although ED physicians may provide deep sedation, payment for these services is limited. National Correct Coding Initiative (NCCI) edits do not allow payment of an ED visit (**99281–99285**) and deep sedation when provided by the same ED physician. No modifier will override the NCCI edits. Payers who have adopted Medicare or Medicaid NCCI edits will deny the ED visit when reported on the same date as deep sedation.

Deep sedation provided by a physician also performing the services for which the sedation is being provided is reported by appending modifier **47** (anesthesia by surgeon) to the procedure code for the service for which sedation is required. Many health plans do not pay separately for anesthesia by the physician or surgeon performing the procedure.

See **Chapter 19** for more information on deep sedation.

Directing Emergency Medical Personnel

99288   Physician or other qualified health care professional direction of emergency medical systems (EMS) emergency care, advanced life support

● Code **99288** is designated as a bundled procedure (included in the work value of other services) by Medicare. There are no relative values assigned under the Medicare Resource-Based Relative Value Scale. Check with your major payers and negotiate for coverage of this service.
● Report code **99288** (physician direction of EMS) when
  — The physician directing the services is in the hospital and in 2-way communication with EMS personnel who are in the prehospital setting providing advanced life support that requires direct or online medical control.
  — The documentation includes the times of all contacts, any orders provided, and/or directions provided to the EMS team.
● Code **99288** may be reported on the same day as ED E/M or hourly critical care services. Append modifier **25** to code **99288** to alert payers that this was a significant and separately identifiable service from ED E/M (**99282–99285**) or the critical care (**99291, 99292**) service provided.
● The supervising physician cannot report the actual procedures and interventions performed by the EMS team because they are not physically present during the transport.
● When a QHP (eg, nurse practitioner) provides critical care services during transport and those services will be reported under the QHP's National Provider Identifier or by the employing hospital, the ED physician does not report **99288**.
● See codes **99485** and **99486** in **Chapter 18** for information on supervision of inter-facility transport of a critically ill or injured patient, 24 months or younger, via direct 2-way communication with a transport team.

● indicates a new code; ▲, revised; #, re-sequenced; ✚, add-on; ★, audiovisual technology; and ◀, synchronous interactive audio.

Time-Based Critical Care in the ED

99291   Critical care, E/M of the critically ill or critically injured patient; first 30–74 minutes
✚99292   each additional 30 minutes (Use in conjunction with **99291**.)

To report **99291** and **99292**, the patient's condition must meet the specific *CPT* definition of a critically ill or injured patient. Documentation must support that the patient's condition was critical and that the services provided involved high-complexity decision-making to assess, manipulate, and support vital system function(s) to treat single or multiple vital organ system failure and/or to prevent further life-threatening deterioration of the patient's condition.

> A *critical illness* or *injury* is defined in *Current Procedural Terminology* as one that acutely impairs 1 or more vital organs such that there is a high probability of imminent or life-threatening deterioration of the patient's condition.

Guidelines for reporting critical care codes **99291** (critical care, E/M of the critically ill or injured patient; first 30–74 minutes) and **99292** (each additional 30 minutes) are described in detail in **Chapter 18**.

- Time-based critical care codes (**99291, 99292**) should be used to report the provision of critical care when performed in the ED. The global codes for pediatric or neonatal critical care should not be reported by a physician providing critical care in the ED unless that physician (eg, an intensivist) will continue to provide critical care services in the inpatient setting.
- Time spent providing critical care does not need to be continuous and includes time at the bedside as well as time in the ED reviewing data specific to the patient, discussing the patient with other physicians, and discussing the patient's management or condition with the patient's family.

> Time of any learner (eg, student, resident) involved in the patient's care may not be reported by the attending physician. Only the time specifically spent by the attending physician may be reported.

- Time reported for critical care must be devoted to the critically ill or injured patient. Therefore, the "critical care clock" stops when attention is turned to the care of another patient or the physician is not readily available in the ED.
- See **Table 18-1** for a list of services and procedures that are included in hourly critical care codes.
- Those procedures *not bundled* with codes **99291** and **99292** and personally performed by the reporting provider may be reported separately (eg, starting an intravenous line on a child aged <3 years, placing an intraosseous or central venous catheter, endotracheal intubation, cardiopulmonary resuscitation [CPR], cardioversion). Time spent performing these separately reported services must be subtracted from the critical care time calculated and reported.

Example

➤ **A 13-month-old with apparent sepsis and hypotension is brought to the ED.** The child requires placement of an intraosseous needle to achieve vascular access and subsequently receives parenteral fluids, antibiotics, and vasopressors. The child experiences cardiopulmonary arrest, prompting the ED physician to intubate the child and provide CPR. Time spent in separately reported procedures is 20 minutes. The child is in the ED for a total of 45 minutes before transfer to the critical care unit.

ICD-10-CM	CPT
I46.9 (cardiac arrest)	**99285 25**
If the physician included sepsis in the diagnosis, codes **A41.9** (sepsis, unspecified organism), **R65.21** (severe sepsis with septic shock), and **I46.8** (cardiac arrest due to other underlying condition) would be appropriate.	**92950** (CPR) **36680** (placement of intraosseous needle) **31500** (endotracheal intubation, emergency)

Teaching Point: Critical care time does not accrue during the performance of non-bundled, separately billable procedures. Because the ED physician did not spend a minimum of 30 minutes providing critical care, an ED E/M service is reported rather than critical care. Coding is based on documented elements of MDM (high-complexity problem and high risk).

> *International Classification of Diseases, 10th Revision, Clinical Modification* codes for severe sepsis (R65.20) and septic shock (R65.21) are reported secondary to the underlying infection (eg, A41.9, sepsis, unspecified organism) and followed by codes for related organ failure (eg, J96.01, acute respiratory failure with hypoxia).

Critical Care and ED E/M Services on the Same Date

Critical care and ED E/M services may both be reported on the same day when, after completion of the ED service, the condition of the patient changes and critical care services are provided. Modifier **25** should be appended to the ED E/M code when this occurs.

> Per *Current Procedural Terminology,* time-based services that are continuously provided with time continuing past midnight do not restart at midnight. For example, an episode of critical care lasting from 11:20 pm to 12:15 am is reported with 1 unit of 99291. If the same patient receives another episode of critical care beginning at 2:00 am, the first 30 to 74 minutes of service for that episode is reported with 99291.

Examples

➤ **The ED physician performs a comprehensive history and physical examination on a 13-month-old patient with severe stridor and respiratory distress believed to be secondary to croup.** Medical decision-making is highly complex. The patient's condition does not improve with nebulized epinephrine and then worsens, evidenced by progressive lethargy. The patient's capillary blood gas result shows that they have hypercapnia. Critical care is provided for 40 minutes, not including 10 minutes spent performing endotracheal intubation.

ICD-10-CM	CPT
J96.02 (acute respiratory failure with hypercapnia)	**99285 25** (ED visit code)
J05.0 (croup)	**99291 25** (critical care, first 30–74 minutes)
	31500 (endotracheal intubation, emergency)

Teaching Point: Endotracheal intubation is not bundled with critical care; therefore, time spent in the provision of the service (10 minutes for this patient) is not considered in the total critical care time. Modifier **25** is appended to codes **99285** and **99291** to indicate they were significant and separately identifiable services from each other and the endotracheal intubation.

➤ **The ED physician saw a 10-year-old for exacerbation of moderate asthma in the morning.** The child responded well to an aerosolized bronchodilator treatment and was discharged home. The child returns to the ED a few hours later with a more severe exacerbation and is seen by the same physician. The child now has respiratory failure with hypoxia. The child receives oxygen, a continuous bronchodilator nebulizer treatment, and, subsequently, a parenteral bronchodilation drug. The child improves enough to be admitted to a monitored medical ward bed with diagnosis of respiratory failure due to status asthmaticus. The ED physician spends a total of 60 minutes in patient-directed critical care.

ICD-10-CM	CPT
J96.01 (acute respiratory failure with hypoxia)	**99284 25**
J45.42 (moderate persistent asthma with status asthmaticus)	**99291**

Teaching Point: The patient received oxygen, continuous inhalation treatment, and parenteral bronchodilator in the ED. However, these services include no professional component. The facility will report the services because the cost of supplies and clinical staff time are an expense to the facility.

● indicates a new code; ▲, revised; #, re-sequenced; ✦, add-on; ★, audiovisual technology; and ◀, synchronous interactive audio.

Special Service Codes

99053 Service(s) provided between 10:00 pm and 8:00 am at 24-hour facility, in addition to basic service
99056 Service(s) typically provided in office, provided out of office at request of patient, in addition to basic service
99060 Service(s) provided on an emergency basis, out of office, which disrupts other scheduled office services, in addition to basic service

Special service codes may be used to report services that are an adjunct to the basic service provided. *CPT* guidelines do not restrict the reporting of adjunct special service codes in the ED. However, third-party payers will have specific policies for coverage and payment. Communicate with individual payers to understand their definition or interpretation of the service and coverage and payment policies.

These codes are intended to describe services that are provided outside the normal time frame and location.

Code **99053** would be reported when services are provided between the designated time limits in an ED.

CPT does not restrict reporting of any procedure or service to any specific specialty. However, it would be inappropriate for an ED physician to report code **99056** or **99060** for services provided in the ED.

If appropriate, a non-ED physician could report *CPT* code **99056** or **99060** when they provide services in the ED in addition to an outpatient office or clinic visit, ED visit, or consultation E/M code.

Continuum Model for Fever

The continuum model is a teaching tool that gives examples of how common conditions in the ED might be reported on the basis of the severity and/or complexity of the presenting problem(s). **Table 15-2** presents fever as the presenting concern across the continuum of codes **99282–99285** plus critical care.

Although the actual assignment of a code for an individual patient may vary from the examples, members of the American Academy of Pediatrics (AAP) Committee on Coding and Nomenclature generally agree that these examples provide an accurate representation of how 1 condition typically flows across the family of codes. Examples are not provided for code **99281** (typically reported for an encounter with clinical staff) because no MDM is required for services reported with this code.

Additional continuums for 3 common conditions—asthma, head injury, and laceration—are included at www.aap.org/cfp2023.

It is important to remember that 2 of 3 elements of MDM (ie, number and complexity of problems addressed, amount and/or complexity of data to be reviewed and analyzed, and risk of complications and/or morbidity or mortality of patient management) must be met to support the code selected.

Chapter 15. Emergency Department Services

Table 15-2. Continuum Model for Fever in the Emergency Department
A clinically appropriate history and examination are required for each level of service.

CPT Code Vignette	No. and Complexity of Problem(s) Addressed	Data to be Reviewed and Analyzed	Risk of Complications and/or Morbidity or Mortality of Patient Management
99282 2-year-old with temperature of 99.8°F (37.7°C), fussy before ED admission	**Minimal** 1 self-limited problem	**Limited** Required history obtained from independent historian	**Minimal** Advice for home care
99283 5-year-old with temperature of 101.0°F (38.3°C) last night and URTI symptoms	**Low:** Acute, uncomplicated illness	**Limited:** Required history obtained from independent historian	**Low:** Over-the-counter ibuprofen/acetaminophen as needed
99283 8-year-old with temperature of 101.0°F (38.3°C), cough and sore throat	**Low:** Acute, uncomplicated illness considered and ruled out after evaluation	**Limited:** 1 unique test ordered (**87636**, influenza and SARS-CoV-2 test) and required history obtained from independent historian	**Low:** Advice for home care and isolation
99284 5-year-old with temperature of 102.2°F (39.0°C)	**Low:** Acute, uncomplicated illness	**Moderate:** Complete blood count, urinalysis and urine culture, required history obtained from independent historian	**Moderate:** Antibiotic prescribed
99285 Neonate presenting with fever, not feeding well, and ill appearance	**High:** Differential diagnosis that includes neonatal sepsis	**Moderate:** CBC, CMP, blood culture, urine culture, lumbar puncture; required history obtained from independent historian	**High:** Decision regarding admission to inpatient care
99291, 99292 Febrile neonate with gray appearance	1. Patient in critically ill, unstable condition; requires >30 min of directed patient care. 2. Physician assesses, manipulates, and supports vital system function(s) to treat single or multiple vital organ system failure and/or to prevent further life-threatening deterioration of the patient's condition.		

Abbreviations: CBC, complete blood cell count; CMP, comprehensive metabolic panel; *CPT, Current Procedural Terminology;* ED, emergency department; URTI, upper respiratory tract infection.

Chapter Takeaways

In this chapter, the discussions focus on topics ranging from diagnosis coding to use of the 2023 guidelines for E/M services and reporting critical care services. Following are some takeaways from this chapter:

- The physician's designation of the CC is important because only 1 diagnosis code may be reported for this category on the hospital claim form and this diagnosis is used to help support the urgency of the ED visit under prudent layperson guidelines.
- The level of ED codes **99282–99285** is based on the highest 2 of 3 elements of MDM. Time is not used in selection of codes **99282–99285**.
- Append modifier **25** (significant, separately identifiable E/M service) to the ED service code (**99282–99285**) when the treating ED physician or QHP provides initial hospital inpatient or observation services on the same date as an ED service.
- Modifier **54** (surgical care only) is appropriately appended to procedure codes with 10- or 90-day global periods when the patient will not return to the ED for follow-up care (eg, visits for follow-up care of a fracture).

● indicates a new code; ▲, revised; #, re-sequenced; ✚, add-on; ★, audiovisual technology; and ◀, synchronous interactive audio.

Resources

AAP Coding Assistance and Education

AAP *Pediatric ICD-10-CM 2023: A Manual for Provider-Based Coding* (https://shop.aap.org/pediatric-icd-10-cm-2023-8th-edition-paperback)

ICD-10-CM resources (www.aap.org/en/practice-management/practice-financing/coding-and-valuation/icd-10-cm-resources)

AAP Pediatric Coding Newsletter™

"Initial Fracture Care: Musculoskeletal or Evaluation and Management," February 2021 (https://doi.org/10.1542/pcco_book202_document005)

"You Code It! Integumentary Repair," April 2020 (https://doi.org/10.1542/pcco_book192_document003)

Online Exclusive Content at www.aap.org/cfp2023

"Asthma, Head Injury, and Laceration: Coding Continuums"

"Emergency Department Procedures"

Test Your Knowledge!

1. **Which of the following conditions is required when selecting a code for an evaluation and management (E/M) service in the emergency department?**
   a. The meeting of 3 elements of medical decision-making (MDM)
   b. The provision of the E/M service only by an emergency medicine physician
   c. The meeting of 2 of 3 elements of MDM at the same level
   d. A diagnosis code that indicates the patient's condition posed an immediate threat to life or bodily function

2. **Which of the following statements is true for emergency department service code 99281?**
   a. This service requires at least a physician's evaluation of a minimal problem with minimal risk to the patient from management.
   b. This code has been deleted in 2023.
   c. This code is reported only by a qualified health care professional (QHP).
   d. This service does not require the presence of a physician or QHP.

3. **Which of the following seventh characters of an *International Classification of Diseases, 10th Revision, Clinical Modification* code indicates a subsequent encounter during the healing phase of an injury?**
   a. **A**
   b. **D**
   c. **S**
   d. Either **D** and **S**

4. **Which of the following statements is true of fracture care in the emergency department?**
   a. Closed treatment of nasal bone fracture without manipulation is reported with an evaluation and management code.
   b. Initial fracture care is reported with modifier **54** if another physician will provide follow-up care.
   c. Fracture care codes include care during a designated postoperative period.
   d. All of the above.

5. **Which of the following code(s) is reported when a physician provides critical care in the emergency department from 11:25 pm to 12:45 am?**
   a. **99291** × 1 unit and **99292** × 1 unit.
   b. **99291** × 1 on each date (day 1, 11:25 pm–11:59 pm, and day 2, midnight–12:40 am).
   c. Critical care is not reported for either date.
   d. **99291** × 1 unit.

● indicates a new code; ▲, revised; #, re-sequenced; ✚, add-on; ★, audiovisual technology; and ◀, synchronous interactive audio.

Hospital Care of the Newborn

CPT copyright 2022 American Medical Association. All rights reserved.

Contents

Chapter Highlights

- Neonatal period diagnoses and procedure code selection
- Codes for normal newborn and hospital inpatient care
- Codes for services throughout the course of the birth admission

Perinatal Care

This chapter focuses on coding for care of the typical newborn and newborns with conditions not requiring intensive monitoring or critical care.

The American Academy of Pediatrics (AAP) Section on Neonatal-Perinatal Medicine, in conjunction with state chapters and councils of the AAP, has developed strategies that have been successful in addressing payment concerns for neonatal care. Contact your state chapter, its pediatric council, your section district AAP Executive Committee representative, a neonatal trainer, or the AAP Committee on Coding and Nomenclature for assistance in addressing any payment inequities for neonatal services in your state.

You can also complete the AAP Hassle Factor Form (https://form.jotform.com/Subspecialty/aapcodinghotline).

Coding Definitions of the Perinatal and Neonatal Periods

For coding purposes, the *perinatal period* commences before birth and continues through the 28th day following birth. According to this definition, the *neonatal period* begins at birth and continues through *the completed 28th day after birth*, ending on the 29th calendar day after birth. The day of birth is considered day 0 (zero). Therefore, the day after birth is considered day 1. This definition is important for selection of the correct diagnosis code for conditions that originate in the perinatal period. (It is also important for selection of codes for neonatal critical care and initial intensive care.)

Expectant Parent Visits

When expectant parents request a visit to meet the pediatrician and learn about the practice, these "meet and greet" visits are not typically considered a medically necessary service. However, many pediatric practices establish policies for managing this type of visit (often at times when the practice is least busy) as a non-billable service used for marketing the practice.

> See the Consultations section later in this chapter for an example of a clinically indicated consultation provided to expectant parents at the request of another physician or other appropriate source (eg, to address risk reduction and plan newborn care in the presence of identified or suspected abnormalities). A service requested by an expectant parent is not a consultation.

Normal Newborn Care

99460	Initial hospital or birthing center care, per day, for evaluation and management of normal newborn infant
99461	Initial care, per day, for evaluation and management of normal newborn infant seen in other than hospital or birthing center
99462	Subsequent hospital care, per day, for evaluation and management of normal newborn
99463	Initial hospital or birthing center care, per day, for evaluation and management of normal newborn infant admitted and discharged on the same date
▲99238	Hospital inpatient or observation discharge day management; 30 minutes or less on the date of the encounter
▲99239	more than 30 minutes on the date of the encounter

Current Procedural Terminology (*CPT*®) codes for care of a normal newborn typically follow a pathway of daily care from initial care to subsequent care and/or discharge day management depending on the length of the newborn's hospital stay. Notable exceptions are newborns admitted and discharged on the same date (**99463**) and newborns receiving initial care in settings other than a hospital or birthing center (**99461**).

A *normal newborn* may be defined as a newborn who
- Experiences a normal transition period after birth
- May require delivery room intervention (discussed in the Attendance at Delivery section later in this chapter) but is normal after transition

Chapter 16. Hospital Care of the Newborn

- May require some testing or monitoring (eg, bilirubin, complete blood cell count [CBC], culture)
- Does not require significant intervention(s)
- May be observed for illness related to maternal pregnancy complication but is not sick
- May be born with a nonthreatening anomaly (eg, polydactyly)
- May be late preterm but requires no special care
- May be in house with sick mother/twin

> Normal newborn codes can be reported for care provided to neonates who are acting normally but recovering from fetal stress or a low Apgar score or who are being observed for a potential problem but are asymptomatic.

Codes **99460**, **99462**, **99463**, **99238**, and **99239** are used to report evaluation and management (E/M) services provided to the healthy newborn in a health care facility such as a hospital (including birthing room deliveries) or birthing center. They are reported when the neonate is cared for in the mother's room (rooming-in), a labor and delivery room, a post-partum floor, or a traditional newborn nursery and when a normal neonate is cared for after the mother is discharged (eg, awaiting foster care).

Code **99461** may be appropriate for E/M of a neonate born at home and evaluated in the physician practice soon after birth (ie, same day or next day).

> Codes **99460–99463** are not reported for telemedicine services unless specified in payer policy. These codes are not included in the *Current Procedural Terminology* listing of codes reported with modifier **95** (synchronous telemedicine service).

Guidelines for reporting include
- The neonate is considered admitted at the time of leaving the delivery room.
- Code **99463** (history and examination of the normal newborn, including discharge) should be reported when an initial history and physical examination and the discharge management are performed *on the same calendar date* for a normal newborn.
- ✖ Do not report **99463** when discharge occurs on the next calendar date even if less than 24 hours has passed since the initial newborn care.
- Code **99460** (history and examination of the normal newborn, initial service) is reported only once on the first day that the physician provides a face-to-face service in the facility. This date may not necessarily correlate with the date the patient is born or the hospital admission date.
- Code **99462** (subsequent hospital care, normal newborn) is reported once per calendar date on the date(s) subsequent to the initial normal newborn care service but *not* on the date of a discharge management service.
- Discharge management services performed on a day subsequent to initial newborn care are reported with code **99238** (hospital discharge day management; 30 minutes or less) or **99239** (hospital discharge day management; more than 30 minutes). Time must be documented when reporting **99239**.
  - Include time spent in final examination of the patient, discussion of the hospital stay, instructions to parents/care-givers for continuing care, and preparation of discharge records, prescriptions, and referral forms.

> Discharge day management codes **99238** and **99239** are valued higher than the subsequent newborn hospital care code (**99462**) to include the physician's time and work, such as reviewing and documenting the hospital stay and counseling parents about continuing care of their neonate.

- Any additional procedures (eg, circumcision) should be reported in addition to normal newborn care codes. Modifier **25** (significant, separately identifiable E/M service) should be appended to the E/M code when a procedure is performed on the same day of service.
  - When reporting an E/M service based on time (eg, discharge day management), do not include the time spent providing a separately reported service (eg, circumcision) in the time of the E/M service (eg, obtaining consent, post-procedural care instruction).

ICD-10-CM Codes for Newborn Services

International Classification of Diseases, 10th Revision, Clinical Modification (ICD-10-CM) codes from category **Z38** are used to report live-born neonates according to type of birth and are the first-listed codes for care by the attending or admitting physician during the entire birth admission. Other physicians providing care during the birth admission do not report **Z38** codes but, instead, report codes for the condition(s) they managed at each encounter. Category **Z38** codes for single and twin live-born neonates are shown in **Box 16-1**.

Box 16-1. *International Classification of Diseases, 10th Revision, Clinical Modification* **Codes for Single and Twin Live-born Neonates**	
Z38.00 (single liveborn infant, delivered vaginally)	**Z38.30** (twin liveborn infant, delivered vaginally)
Z38.01 (single liveborn infant, delivered by cesarean)	**Z38.31** (twin liveborn infant, delivered by cesarean)
Z38.1 (single liveborn infant, born outside hospital)	**Z38.4** (twin liveborn infant, born outside hospital)
Z38.2 (single liveborn infant, unspecified as to place of birth)	**Z38.5** (twin liveborn infant, unspecified as to place of birth)

See the *ICD-10-CM* manual for **Z38** codes for other multiple-birth neonates.

Report *ICD-10-CM* code **Z76.2** (encounter for health supervision and care of other healthy infant and child) when a healthy newborn continues to receive daily visits pending discharge of the mother or foster care placement or for other reasons. Code **Z76.2** is useful for indicating the reason for an extended stay of a healthy newborn. Report code **Z76.2** as secondary to the appropriate **Z38** code for services by the attending physician during the birth admission.

Examples

➤ **The physician receives a late-night call about the vaginal delivery of a healthy full-term boy.** A nurse relates that the newborn has been admitted and seems fine. The physician's standing admission orders are followed, and the physician examines the newborn the following morning. The physician reviews the record, examines the neonate, and speaks with the mother. The physician performs circumcision of the newborn (**54150**) later that day as requested by the parents. The newborn and mother remain in the hospital until the next day, when both are then discharged home. Discharge management takes 25 minutes.

ICD-10-CM	Diagnosis code for all days **Z38.00** (single liveborn, delivered vaginally)
CPT	**Day 1:** No charge (no face-to-face services provided) **Day 2: 99460 25** (initial normal newborn care) **54150** (circumcision, using clamp or other device with regional dorsal penile or ring block) **Day 3: 99238** (hospital discharge management; 30 minutes or less)

Teaching Point: Report newborn hospital care only when a face-to-face (including telemedicine) service is provided. The date of the attending physician's first evaluation of the newborn is the date of initial newborn care. When a procedure (eg, circumcision) is provided on the same date as a newborn care service, modifier **25** is appended to the code for newborn care to signify that the E/M service was significant and separately identifiable from the preservice and post-service work of the procedure in the documentation.

➤ **A baby is born vaginally in the hospital on March 3 at 4:00 pm.** The physician first sees the baby on March 4 at 7:00 am and, later the same date, determines that the newborn is ready for discharge. A history and examination of the newborn, discussion of the hospital stay with the parents, instructions for continuing care, family counseling, and preparation of the final discharge records are performed.

ICD-10-CM	**Z38.00** (single liveborn, delivered vaginally)
CPT	**99463** (initial normal newborn care and discharge on the same date)

Teaching Point: The physician's combined services are reported with **99463**.

➤ **A subsequent hospital visit is performed in the well-baby nursery on a vaginally delivered 2-day-old who is being observed for jaundice caused by hyperbilirubinemia; however, no interventions are noted, and the baby is doing well. Diagnosis is neonatal hyperbilirubinemia.**

●indicates a new code; ▲, revised; #, re-sequenced; ✚, add-on; ★, audiovisual technology; and ◄, synchronous interactive audio

ICD-10-CM	**Z38.00** (single liveborn, delivered vaginally) **P59.9** (neonatal jaundice, unspecified)
CPT	**99462** (subsequent normal newborn care)

Teaching Point: The service is normal newborn care even though the newborn is being observed for risk of jaundice. The first-listed diagnosis code is **Z38.00**. For neonatal hyperbilirubinemia, report *ICD-10-CM* code **P59.9** (neonatal jaundice, unspecified).

➤ **During a subsequent newborn care visit, the physician notes that the newborn failed the routine hearing screening.** The attending physician spends 15 minutes discussing the results with the parents and refers to an audiologist for testing to confirm or rule out hearing abnormality.

ICD-10-CM	**Z38.00** (single liveborn, delivered vaginally) **R94.120** (abnormal auditory function study)
CPT	**99462** (subsequent normal newborn care)

Teaching Point: The time spent providing the subsequent newborn care does not affect code selection, as normal newborn care services are reported per day, not per hour. Only code **Z38.00** would be reported when the result of an auditory screening is normal.

An audiologist performing confirmatory testing would report code **Z01.110** (encounter for hearing examination following failed hearing screening) and codes for any identified conditions.

Hospital Care of the Ill Newborn

Choosing Normal Newborn Care or Hospital Care

The choice between coding for normal newborn care and coding for hospital care is based on the physician's judgment and the type of symptoms demonstrated. Services to newborns that require an increased level of physician care, nursing observation, or physiologic monitoring (but not intensive care as described by codes **99477–99480**) are typically reported with hospital inpatient or observation care codes (initial, **99221–99223**; subsequent, **99231–99233**).

- A sick-newborn visit includes a manifesting problem that supports the need for diagnostic investigation or therapy. *Therapeutic intervention is typically necessary for the sick newborn.*
- The nature of the manifesting problem and extent of work required to diagnose and manage the problem should be considered when determining the appropriate procedure code.

Attendance at Delivery

99464   Attendance at delivery (when requested by the delivering physician or other qualified health care professional) and initial stabilization of newborn

Attendance at delivery (**99464**) is not reported when hospital-mandated attendance is the only basis for providing the service. When physician on-call services are mandated by the hospital (eg, attending all repeated cesarean deliveries) and not physician requested, report code **99026** (hospital-mandated on-call service; in hospital, each hour) or **99027** (hospital-mandated on-call service; out of hospital, each hour).

Attendance at delivery (**99464**)

- Service is reported only when requested by the delivering physician and indicated for a newborn who may require immediate intervention (ie, stabilization, resuscitation, or evaluation for potential problems).
- Medical record documentation must include the request for attendance at the delivery and substantiate the medical necessity of the services performed. If there is no documentation by the delivering physician for attendance at delivery, the verbal request and the reason for the request should be documented in the attendance note.
- Includes initial drying, stimulation, suctioning, blow-by oxygen, or continuous positive airway pressure or high-flow air/oxygen without positive-pressure ventilation (PPV); a cursory visual inspection of the neonate; assignment of Apgar scores; and discussion of the care of the newborn with the delivering physician and parents. A quick look into the delivery room or examination after stabilization is not sufficient to report **99464**. See the "Coding Conundrum: What

●indicates a new code; ▲, revised; #, re-sequenced; ✛, add-on; ★, audiovisual technology; and ◀, synchronous interactive audio

Service Can Be Reported When a Physician Arrives After Delivery?" box later in this chapter for more information on reporting less than full attendance at delivery services.

- May be reported in addition to initial normal newborn (**99460**), initial sick newborn (**99221–99223**), initial intensive care of the neonate (**99477**), or critical care (**99468**; **99291**, **99292**) codes.
- Is not reported in conjunction with standby service codes **99026** and **99027**.

See Chapter 17 for guidelines for standby service codes 99026 **and** 99027. **Standby services** *may be* **reported with the newborn resuscitation services** (99465) **per** *Current Procedural Terminology* **guidelines.**

Examples

➤ **A physician is called at the request of an obstetrician to attend a cesarean delivery.** The physician stands by until the neonate is delivered and provides stabilization of the neonate, who initially requires blow-by oxygen but steadily becomes more vigorous (**99464**). The same physician then provides initial normal newborn care (**99460**) on that same day.

    Teaching Point: The physician separately reports the 2 services.

➤ **A delivering physician asks a neonatologist to be present at delivery of a neonate whose mother has active infection.** The neonatologist documents stabilization, including use of continuous positive airway pressure without PPV and a comprehensive examination of the neonate, in addition to review of the maternal and fetal history and discussion with the parents and delivering physician.

    The newborn is admitted to the newborn nursery under the orders of another physician. This attending physician provides a comprehensive history and examination, orders screening tests and prophylactic interventions, and counsels the family that the neonate will be monitored closely for signs of illness. The physician also counsels about topics such as feeding, sleep, and safety. The attending physician would report code **99460** or initial hospital inpatient or observation care (**99221–99223**) if the newborn experienced an abnormal transition and required significant intervention(s) on that date.

    Teaching Point: Although a history and examination were performed, they do not equate to initial hospital care of the newborn. The neonatologist reports code **99464**.

When qualifying resuscitative efforts including PPV are provided to a neonate with respiratory or cardiac instability, report code **99465** (delivery/birthing room resuscitation, provision of PPV and/or chest compressions in the presence of acute inadequate ventilation and/or cardiac output) instead of **99464**. Do no report both **99464** and **99465** (ie, report only **99465**, when provided).

Coding Conundrum: What Service Can Be Reported When a Physician Arrives After Delivery?

There are no specific time requirements for reporting attendance at delivery. This service requires a request for attendance at delivery by the delivering physician and includes physician work as described in the Attendance at Delivery section earlier in this chapter. When a physician arrives in the delivery room after the delivery and some or all of this work has been performed, should attendance at delivery be reported? Physicians might want to consider

- When the newborn continues to require intervention or stabilization in the delivery room, reporting code **99464** (attendance at delivery) if the physician work and medical necessity are related to the initial transition or **99465** if the neonate requires resuscitative interventions
- When the work provided in the delivery room is related more to the initial hospital care (eg, neonate is examined and the physician sends the neonate to the well-baby nursery), reporting only the initial normal newborn care code (**99460**)

For example, attendance at delivery was requested by the delivering physician and the physician arrives after the delivery.

- The 1-minute Apgar score has been assigned; the neonate has been dried, stimulated, and suctioned by the nurses; and the neonate is ready to be sent to the newborn nursery by the time the pediatrician appears in the delivery room. The delivering physician acknowledges that assistance is no longer needed. The attending pediatrician reports initial normal newborn care (**99460**) after completing the initial examination of the newborn. However, if the pediatrician is not the attending pediatrician, no service can be reported.
- In the previous example, the child requires continued attendance and assistance. The pediatrician assigns the 5-minute Apgar score, performs a cursory examination, reviews the birth history, and discusses the care of the newborn with the delivering physician and parents. Code **99464** is reported because most of the basic elements of the attendance at delivery were performed and documented in the medical record.

> See Chapter 18 for more information on delivery/birthing room neonatal resuscitation and guidelines for coding intensive or critical care services.

See the "Stillborn Deliveries and Unsuccessful Resuscitation" box in **Chapter 18** for discussion of billing for services provided to a mother and/or neonate when the outcome is a stillborn neonate or unsuccessful resuscitation of an ill neonate.

Diagnosis Codes for Perinatal Conditions

There are some important guidelines for reporting conditions that originate in the perinatal period. In *ICD-10-CM*, these conditions are classified to Chapter 16 and codes **P00–P96**. Codes in this chapter are used only on the neonate's record and not that of the mother.

> Following is the order for reporting codes for neonates at the birth hospital:
>
> 1. Birth outcome (Z38-, reported only by the attending/admitting physician)
> 2. Codes from the perinatal chapter (P00–P96)
> 3. Codes from the congenital anomalies chapter (Q00–Q99)
> 4. Codes from all other chapters

Other important guidelines include that

- Perinatal condition codes are assigned for any condition that is clinically significant. In addition to clinical indications for reporting codes from other chapters, perinatal conditions are considered clinically significant if the condition has implications for future health care needs. Other clinical indications that apply to all conditions are those requiring
    - Clinical evaluation (eg, subspecialty consultation)
    - Therapeutic treatment
    - Diagnostic procedures
    - Extended hospital stay
    - Increased nursing care and/or monitoring
- Should a condition originate in the perinatal period and continue past the 28th day after birth, the perinatal code should continue to be used regardless of the patient's age.

    Typical scenarios that may require exclusive use of perinatal or neonatal codes beyond the perinatal period are those related to care of a critically ill or recovering neonate, such as necrotizing enterocolitis in newborn (**P77.-**), chronic respiratory disease arising in the perinatal period (**P27.-**), and preterm birth (**P07.-**).

> Perinatal codes are not reported for conditions with *onset after the patient is 28 days old.* For example, necrotizing enterocolitis with onset after the neonatal period is reported with codes K55.30–K55.33.

- If a newborn has a condition that could be caused by the birth process or community acquired, and documentation does not indicate which the cause is, the condition is reported as due to the birth process. Community-acquired conditions are reported with codes other than those in *ICD-10-CM* Chapter 16.
- Codes in categories **P00–P04**, newborn affected by maternal factors and by complications of pregnancy, labor, and delivery, may be reported when the conditions are suspected but have not yet been ruled out.

> If a neonate is suspected of having an abnormal condition that, after examination and observation, is ruled out, assign codes for signs and symptoms or, in the absence of signs or symptoms, a code from category Z05 (encounter for observation and evaluation of newborn for suspected diseases and conditions ruled out).

Example

➤ **A neonate was born at 36 weeks' gestation to a mother whose group B β-hemolytic streptococcal culture result was still pending at the time of delivery.** The newborn was alert with excellent Apgar scores in the delivery room and was admitted to the newborn nursery. The newborn was treated per current group B streptococcal (GBS) disease guidelines, with no indication of illness. On day 2, the mother's GBS culture result was negative. The patient was discharged home as a normal newborn.

●indicates a new code; ▲, revised; #, re-sequenced; ✚, add-on; ★, audiovisual technology; and ◀, synchronous interactive audio

| ICD-10-CM | **Day 1: Z38.00** (single liveborn, delivered vaginally), **P00.89** (newborn affected by other maternal conditions)
Day 2: Z38.00 (single liveborn, delivered vaginally), **Z05.1** (observation and evaluation of newborn for suspected infectious condition ruled out) |
| CPT | **Day 1: 99460**
Day 2: 99238 |

Teaching Point: On day 1, the patient was suspected of being affected by a localized maternal infection (**P00.89**). Normal initial newborn care is reported rather than hospital care because the neonate, although at risk for infection in this case, was not treated but observed and did not develop infection. By day 2, the condition was ruled out (**Z05.1**) and discharge day management services were performed (**99238**).

Daily Hospital Care of the Ill Newborn

Codes for hospital inpatient services 99221–99223, 99231–99233, 99234–99236, and 99238–99239 have been revised to allow code selection based on either medical decision-making or the physician's or qualified health care professional's total time directed to the patient's care on the date of service. The revised codes also include services provided to a patient in observation status. See Chapter 17 for full details.

Levels of hospital E/M services are based on all hospital care services provided on the same date by the same physician or qualified health care professional (QHP) or by multiple physicians and QHPs of the same group practice (billing under the same tax identification number) and same exact specialty.

When multiple physicians of the same specialty and same group practice provide separate initial or subsequent hospital care to a newborn on the same date, report with a single code representing the combined medical decision-making (MDM) (eg, **99223**, initial hospital inpatient or observation care with a high level of MDM) or combined total time on the date of the encounter.

Report an initial hospital or observation service when the patient has not received any professional services from the reporting physician or qualified health care professional (QHP) or another physician or QHP of the exact same specialty and subspecialty who belongs to the same group practice, during the current admission and stay.

Report a subsequent hospital or observation service when the patient has previously received professional service(s) from the physician or QHP or another physician or QHP of the exact same specialty and subspecialty who belongs to the same group practice, *during the current admission and stay.* Services provided by covering physicians are reported as if provided by the physician who is unavailable.

Initial Inpatient Hospital or Observation Care

Codes **99221–99223** are used to report the initial hospital encounter with a sick neonate who does not require intensive observation and monitoring or critical care services.

Refer to Chapter 17 and Table 17-2 for the specific coding and documentation requirements for reporting initial hospital care. Unlike with codes for office and other outpatient evaluation and management (E/M) (99202–99215), total time for hospital E/M services is described as a number of minutes that must be met or exceeded (eg, ≥55 minutes for 99222).

Examples

➤ **The pediatrician sees a newborn boy admitted to the well-baby nursery.** The baby's blood type is O+ and his Coombs test result is positive. He was born to a mother with blood type O– who has a history of 2 previous newborns with jaundice secondary to Rh incompatibility. At 8 hours of age, the neonate appears jaundiced. Total and direct bilirubin tests, CBC, and reticulocyte count are ordered; results are evaluated; the newborn's risks for kernicterus are discussed with the family; and phototherapy is started. The pediatrician performs a clinically indicated history and physical examination. The physician's total time on the date of the encounter is 50 minutes.

   ICD-10-CM: **Z38.00** (single liveborn, delivered vaginally); **P55.0** (Rh isoimmunization of newborn)

   CPT: **99222** (initial hospital inpatient or observation care with moderate level MDM or ≥55 minutes of total time)

   Level of problem addressed ⅢⅢ➡ Moderate (1 acute illness with systemic symptoms)

   Level of data reviewed and analyzed ⅢⅢ➡ Moderate (4 unique tests ordered and history required from independent historian)

   Level of risk of morbidity ⅢⅢ➡ Moderate (phototherapy)

   Teaching Point: When reporting initial hospital care based on MDM, 2 of 3 elements of MDM must be met. In this example, all 3 elements support moderate MDM.

   While code **P55.0** does not specifically mention "jaundice," the *ICD-10-CM* Index entry for newborn jaundice due to maternal/fetal Rh incompatibility directs only to code **P55.0**.

➤ **The pediatrician admits a full-term neonate, born vaginally, with Rh incompatibility (mom AB– and baby B+/Coombs test result positive).** The otherwise normal neonate is monitored for elevated bilirubin level.

ICD-10-CM	**Z38.00** (single liveborn, delivered vaginally) **P55.0** (Rh isoimmunization of newborn)
CPT	**99460** (initial newborn care)

   Teaching Point: The neonate is being observed but not treated, supporting **99460**.

Subsequent Hospital Care

Subsequent hospital care codes (**99231–99233**) are reported for each day of service subsequent to initial encounter for the newborn who continues to be sick (ie, not a typical neonate but not in critical condition and not requiring intensive observation and interventions).

> Refer to Chapter 17 and Table 17-2 for detailed coding and documentation requirements for codes **99231–99233**.

- When a neonate is not treated but only observed for the potential development of illness, normal newborn codes would be reported.
- Report the appropriate code for the highest acuity on each date of service. On subsequent dates when a previously sick neonate is improved and requires no more care than a normal newborn, the subsequent normal newborn care code (**99462**) should be reported.

Example

➤ **On day 2 of the birth admission, the attending pediatrician provides subsequent hospital care to a full-term neonate, born vaginally, with ABO incompatibility (mom O+/antibody test negative and baby B+/Coombs test result negative).** The total serum bilirubin level is elevated. The pediatrician orders phototherapy and follow-up laboratory tests. Clinically indicated history, obtained from the parents, and examination are documented.

   ICD-10-CM: **Z38.00** (single liveborn, delivered vaginally); **P55.1** (ABO incompatibility)

   CPT: **99232** (subsequent hospital inpatient or observation care with moderate level MDM or ≥35 minutes of total time)

   Level of problem addressed ⅢⅢ➡ Moderate (1 acute illness with systemic symptoms)

> *Level of data reviewed and analyzed* ▯▯▯➡ Limited or moderate (1 test reviewed, at least 1 test ordered [eg, follow-up bilirubin], and history required from independent historian)
> *Level of risk of morbidity* ▯▯▯➡ Moderate (phototherapy)
> **Teaching Point:** On day 2, the neonate continues to require therapeutic management, supporting subsequent hospital care.

Discharge Management

Dependent on total time involved in the discharge, either code **99238** or **99239** (hospital discharge management) is reported when discharge occurs on a day separate from the initial hospital care.

- A newborn who dies on the date of birth is not discharged from the hospital. The attending physician should report a code for the level of hospital care provided (ie, initial hospital sick care, intensive care, or critical care) as appropriate. Codes for discharge services are not reported.
- When a neonate is transferred to another facility, the physician providing care before transfer reports the appropriate code for the type of care provided on that date (eg, hourly critical care **99291** and, when appropriate, **99292**) before the transfer, but not the discharge management.
- Time must be documented to support code **99239** (ie, time of >30 minutes).

> Chapter 17 includes more information on discharge management codes **99238** and **99239**.

Example

➤ **The physician performs a follow-up visit for a neonate who will be discharged with a home apnea monitor.** The parents are counseled on their neonate's condition and given instructions for home care and follow-up. Forty-five minutes was spent on the floor reviewing the hospital course and expected follow-up and counseling the parents.
▲**99239** (discharge management, more than 30 minutes)
Teaching Point: Time (45 minutes unit/floor time dedicated to the patient) is the key controlling factor. If time spent in discharge day management is not documented, code **99238** must be reported.

Consultations

A consultation is reported when a physician, other QHP, or other appropriate source (eg, attorney, nonclinical social worker) requests an opinion and/or advice from another physician or QHP. This request must be in writing or given verbally by the requester and documented in the consultation record. The consulting physician evaluates the patient, renders advice, records it, and returns a report to the requesting physician or appropriate source (either in a shared electronic health record [EHR] or by separate written communication).

99251 has been deleted in 2023. Codes **99252–99255** are reported for newborn care when the following circumstances are true:

- The encounter meets the definition of a consultation.
- The encounter is the first face-to-face professional service provided to the patient by the consulting physician or QHP (or another physician or QHP of the same exact specialty and same group practice) during the admission/stay.

A consulting physician's follow-up visits with a newborn (newly requested consultation or continuing care) are reported as subsequent hospital care (**99231–99233**) unless the service meets the requirements for reporting hourly critical care (see **Chapter 18** for requirements of critical care).

> Chapter 17 details the specific reporting, documentation, and coding requirements for inpatient consultations.

Examples

➤ **At the request of a primary care physician, a neonatologist evaluates a full-term gestation neonate with moderate tachypnea after birth.** A detailed history is obtained from the mother, noting that she had a positive GBS screening result. Review of labor and delivery records reveals that she received 1 dose of intravenous ampicillin 2 hours before delivery. Because of fetal tachycardia and a non-reassuring fetal heart rate pattern, a cesarean delivery was performed. After birth, the newborn had Apgar scores of 7 and 9 but was noted to have tachypnea with mild substernal retractions. The neonatologist recommends obtaining blood cultures and beginning antibiotics pending the results of the cultures, as well as a follow-up CBC at 12 hours. The neonatologist counsels the baby's parents, writes a detailed medical record note, and discusses her recommendations with the attending physician by phone. The attending physician does not want the neonatologist to assume responsibility for all the patient's care but requests follow-up of the possible infection.

At a follow-up visit later that day, the 12-hour CBC and C-reactive protein test results are reassuring, the blood culture result has remained negative, and the tachypnea has resolved. The neonatologist recommends continuing the antibiotics until culture results are negative at 48 hours but otherwise signs off on the case, remaining available for further questions. The neonatologist's total time on the date of the encounter is 75 minutes.

ICD-10-CM: **P00.82** (newborn affected by [positive] maternal group B streptococcus [GBS] colonization)

CPT: **99254** (hospital inpatient or observation consultation, with moderate level MDM or total time ≥60 minutes)

Level of problem addressed ⅢⅢ➡ Moderate (1 undiagnosed problem with uncertain prognosis)

Level of data reviewed and analyzed ⅢⅢ➡ Moderate (3 tests reviewed and/or ordered and history required from independent historian)

Level of risk of morbidity ⅢⅢ➡ Moderate (intravenous antibiotics)

Teaching Point: Both the level of MDM and total time on the date of the encounter support code **99254**. If the payer policy does not allow payment for consultation codes, the 75 minutes of service supports initial hospital or observation care code **99223**.

➤ **At the request of an obstetrician, a pediatric urologist provides a consultation to a family whose male fetus (single gestation) has an enlarged bladder and bilateral dilated ureters in the second trimester of pregnancy based on prenatal ultrasound.** The request for consultation is documented by the obstetrician and the urologist. The urologist spends 10 minutes reviewing records of this new patient provided by the obstetrician, including ultrasounds of the fetus before the consultation on the same date. The consultation with the family takes place via a secure, real-time audiovisual connection with the physician in an outpatient clinic and the patient at home. The service includes discussing how the mother's treatment will be affected (eg, follow-up testing and delivery will occur at a facility with resources that may be required to care for the neonate). The time spent in consultation with the family is 34 minutes. The urologist documents the time spent and a summary of the discussion. Additionally, the urologist discusses ongoing patient management and delivery with the obstetrician via secure messaging. A written report is also produced and sent to the requesting obstetrician with a copy maintained in the patient's record. The urologist's total time on the date of the encounter is 65 minutes.

ICD-10-CM: **O35.8XX0** (maternal care for other [suspected] fetal abnormality and damage)

CPT: **99245 95** (outpatient consultation with moderate MDM or total time ≥55 minutes, by telemedicine)

Teaching Point: The patient in this example is not a newborn but, rather, the expectant mother. The physician's total time supports code **99245**. Modifier **95** (synchronous telemedicine service rendered via a real-time interactive audio and video telecommunications system) is appended to indicate that the service met the requirements of a telemedicine service. If the consultation took place in person while the mother was hospitalized, code **99254** (inpatient or observation consultation with moderate level MDM or total time ≥60 minutes) would be reported.

Prolonged E/M Service on the Date of a Hospital Encounter

#★✚●**99418** Prolonged inpatient or observation evaluation and management service(s) time with or without direct patient contact beyond the required time of the primary service when the primary service level has been selected using total time, each 15 minutes of total time

Code **99418** is reported in addition to a code for a face-to-face E/M service in a facility setting under the following circumstances:

- Only in conjunction with hospital inpatient or observation services (**99223, 99233, 99236, 99255**) or nursing facility services (**99306, 99310**)
- Only when the code for the primary E/M service was selected on the basis of the physician's or QHP's total time on the date of the encounter
- Only when the total time required for the highest level of service in a code category (eg, **99223** for initial hospital or observation care) has been exceeded by at least 15 minutes

See **Table 17-7** for illustration of required total time to report **99418** in conjunction with inpatient and observation E/M services.

Do not report **99418**

✖ When the total time on the date of the encounter exceeds the required time of the primary service by less than 15 minutes

✖ For any time spent providing a separately reported service (eg, a procedure or interpretation and report of a diagnostic test)

✖ For any increment of less than 15 minutes beyond the required time of the primary service or the most recent unit of prolonged service

✖ For prolonged services on a date other than the date of a face-to-face E/M service (See **99358–99359**, discussed in the Prolonged E/M on a Date Before or After a Direct Service section later in this chapter.)

Example

➤ **A physician reports code 99223 on the basis of the required total time of 75 or more minutes.** The physician's total time on the date of the encounter is 95 minutes. The physician reports **99223** and **99418** × 1 unit.

Teaching Point: The physician's total time of 95 minutes exceeds the required time of 75 minutes or more for code **99223** by more than 15 minutes. Only 1 unit of code **99418** is reported because the initial unit of service for **99418** includes 15 to 29 minutes beyond the total time of the related service.

At the time of publication, a separate Healthcare Common Procedure Coding System code for prolonged inpatient service has been proposed for the Medicare program in 2023. Verify individual payer's policy for prolonged E/M services to identify payable codes and time requirements.

Prolonged E/M on a Date Before or After a Direct Service

99358   Prolonged evaluation and management service before and/or after direct patient care; first hour (minimum 30 minutes)

✚99359   each additional 30 minutes (minimum 15 minutes)

Prolonged service without direct patient contact (**99358**, **99359**) may be reported only in relation to an E/M service *when it occurs on a date other than the date of a face-to-face E/M service.* Report **99358** and **99359**

● For non–face-to-face E/M services of 30 or more minutes' total duration on a single date of service

● For prolonged services in relation to any E/M service *regardless of whether time was used to select the level of the face-to-face service*

● When the prolonged E/M service is related to a service during or patient for which (face-to-face) patient care has occurred or will occur and relates to ongoing patient management

Do not report **99358** and **99359** when

✖ An E/M service that is selected on the basis of total time (eg, in-person or telemedicine E/M service) is provided on the same date.

✖ Less than 30 minutes of time is directed to the individual patient on the date of service.

✖ The same time is attributed to another service (eg, medical team conference or interprofessional telephone/internet/EHR consultation).

Example

➤ **An infant will be transferred from a Level III neonatal intensive care unit (NICU), following a 30-day hospital stay, to a community Level II unit to complete recovery before home discharge.** The receiving physician spends 1 hour 20 minutes reviewing the extensive transfer records on the evening before the patient arrives at the receiving facility.

99358 (prolonged non–face-to-face services; first hour)

99359 × 1 (each additional 30 minutes)

Teaching Point: This service included 80 minutes of prolonged service time on a date when no direct E/M service was provided. Code **99358** represents the first 60 minutes. Code **99359** is reported for the final 20 minutes of prolonged service. If less than 75 minutes of prolonged services were provided, code **99359** would not be reported because this code is reported for time that lasts at least 15 minutes beyond the first hour or final 30 minutes.

●indicates a new code; ▲, revised; #, re-sequenced; ✚, add-on; ★, audiovisual technology; and ◀, synchronous interactive audio

Coding for Transitions to Different Levels of Neonatal Care

During a hospital stay, a newly born or readmitted neonate may require multiple levels of care. A normal newborn may end up becoming sick, becoming intensively ill, or requiring critical care during the same hospital stay. As they improve, recovering neonates require lower levels of care (eg, normal neonatal care) before home discharge.

It is important to remember that

- When a patient initially qualifies after birth for normal newborn care and, at a subsequent encounter on the same day, becomes ill and requires a higher service level, normal newborn care (**99460** or **99462**) may be reported in addition to the following codes on the same day:
  — Initial intensive care (**99477**)
  — Initial critical care (**99468**)
  — Time-based critical care (**99291**, **99292**)
- *CPT* instructs to report the appropriate E/M code with modifier **25** for these services in addition to the normal newborn code.
- ✖ Do not report both hospital care (**99221–99223**, **99231–99233**) and initial newborn care (**99460**, **99462**) on the same date.

> It may be beneficial to document the time spent providing normal newborn care to a neonate who is being observed for illness because this time may be added to the time of hospital care provided later on the same date and used in selecting the level of initial or subsequent hospital care.

Examples

➤ **A physician admits a full-term neonate, born vaginally, with Rh incompatibility (mom AB– and baby B+/Coombs test result positive).** The mother had not received RhoGAM injection during her pregnancy. A complete examination of the neonate is normal in findings, with no hydrops or hepatosplenomegaly. The initial hemoglobin test result is borderline, and the reticulocyte count is elevated. The parents are counseled, and the initial plan is to monitor the bilirubin and hemoglobin levels every 4 hours. The physician documents 30 minutes spent providing normal newborn care. The physician is notified of a rise in the bilirubin level to 10 mg/mL and returns to the hospital. The child's progress and feeding history are obtained from nurses and parents, and the examination is documented, noting the dermal progression of the jaundice while eliminating any other clinical change. The parents are counseled that the child will require a few days of continued hospital care and phototherapy, which is initiated at the visit. All the parents' questions are answered. The physician's total time on the date of the encounter is 75 minutes.

ICD-10-CM	**Z38.00** (single liveborn, delivered vaginally) **P55.0** (Rh isoimmunization of newborn)
CPT	**99223** (initial hospital care requiring high MDM or total time meeting or exceeding 75 minutes)

Teaching Point: The neonate was initially being observed but not treated, supporting **99460** (assigned 2.75 total relative value units [RVUs] and 1.92 work RVUs). However, the neonate required hospital care for illness on the same date, so only one of the daily hospital care codes is reported (ie, normal newborn or hospital care). The physician may select the initial hospital care code based on MDM or total time directed to care of the individual patient on the date of service. The documented total time of 75 minutes supports **99223** (assigned 5.73 total RVUs and 3.86 work RVUs).

➤ **A neonate who was initially normal becomes ill several hours after Physician A provided normal newborn care and the neonate moved to a higher level of care.** Physician B of another group practice assumes management of the newborn's care and provides an initial hospital care service with moderate-level MDM.

Physician A reports **99460**	Physician B reports **99222**

> **Teaching Point:** No modifier is required because the physicians are not of the same group practice, although they may each be general pediatricians (eg, a community physician provides normal newborn care, whereas a hospitalist/neonatologist assumes care of an ill newborn).

- Once an initial-day care code for a higher service level has been reported, an *initial* code for a lower service level within the same hospital stay will not be reported.
  - If an ill neonate has required intensive care (**99477–99480**) but no longer qualifies for intensive care and is transferred to the care of a physician of a different specialty or different group practice, the receiving physician will report subsequent hospital care (**99231–99233**) based on the level of service provided.
  - The receiving physician *will not report* initial hospital care (**99221–99223**) for the first encounter after the transfer. If the neonate is no longer ill but requires continued hospital observation, the receiving physician will report subsequent normal newborn care (**99462**). If the neonate is still ill but no longer requires intensive observation, the subsequent hospital care codes (**99231–99233**) will be reported.
  - The transferring physician may report initial neonatal intensive care (**99477**) if provided earlier on the date of transfer. However, when the ill neonate improves and is transferred on a date after the initial day of intensive care, a transferring physician will report subsequent hospital care (**99231–99233**) and not subsequent neonatal intensive care (**99478–99480**). The level of care determines the code, not the location of the newborn. Care provided in the NICU does not automatically support intensive care.

Example

➤ **A neonate (2,600 g) is transferred from neonatal intensive care by Dr A to Dr B, who is of a different specialty (eg, pediatrician, hospitalist), to complete recovery before home discharge.** On the day of transfer, Dr A determines that the ill but recovering neonate no longer requires intensive care and documents 25 minutes spent on the unit/floor arranging the transfer. Dr B provides a face-to-face E/M service to the neonate, documenting 75 minutes of time directed to the patient.

Dr A reports	Dr B reports
99231 (subsequent hospital care, 25 minutes)	**99233** (subsequent hospital care, typical time 50 minutes)
	99418 × 1 (direct prolonged services, first 15 minutes)

> **Teaching Point:** Dr B may not report initial hospital care for services to the patient who has received prior initial hospital services (eg, initial neonatal intensive care) in the same facility. The typical time of code **99233** was exceeded by 25 minutes, supporting code **99418**.

The AAP *Newborn Coding Decision Tool 2023* (https://shop.aap.org/newborn-coding-decision-tool-2023) provides a quick reference to help determine appropriate codes for transitions in care.

Other Newborn Hospital Care

Circumcision

54150 Circumcision, using clamp or other device with regional dorsal penile or ring block

- If the circumcision using a clamp or other device is performed without dorsal penile or ring block, append modifier **52** (reduced services) to **54150**.
- Medicare has a global period of 0 (zero) assigned to code **54150**.
- When performing a circumcision and a separately identifiable E/M service on the same day (eg, **99462**, subsequent normal newborn care; **99238**, discharge services <30 minutes), append modifier **25** to the E/M code. Link the appropriate *ICD-10-CM* code (eg, **Z38.00**) to the E/M service and to the circumcision code.
- The American Hospital Association *Coding Clinic* instructs that code **Z41.2** (encounter for routine and ritual male circumcision) *is not assigned* during the birth admission, as circumcision is a routine part of the newborn's hospital care.

54160 Circumcision, surgical excision other than clamp, device, or dorsal slit; neonate (28 days of age or less)
54161   older than 28 days

Unlike with code **54150**, Medicare has a global period of 10 days assigned to codes **54160** and **54161**. A physician who performs a procedure with a 10-day global period must append modifier **24** (unrelated E/M service by the same physician or other qualified health care professional during a postoperative period) to the E/M code for subsequent newborn or hospital care or discharge management (eg, **99238 24**) provided in the 10-day period following the procedure for general care of the newborn unrelated to the procedure.

> **See Chapter 12 for information on coding for circumcisions performed in the office.**

Frenotomy

40806	Incision of labial frenum (frenotomy)
41010	Incision of lingual frenum (frenotomy)

Occasionally, a newborn experiences issues with latching on or sucking effectively because of a tight frenulum. If these issues are severe enough to warrant intervention by incision of the frenulum, report code **41010** for lingual frenotomy or **40806** for labial frenotomy. This may be completed in the hospital before discharge. Link *ICD-10-CM* codes **P92.5** (neonatal difficulty in feeding at the breast) and **Q38.1** (ankyloglossia) to the procedure code on the claim.

● If the physician performing the incision is also performing newborn care on the same date, be sure to append modifier **25** to the hospital care service also being reported. Link this service to the appropriate **Z38** code followed by **P92.5** and **Q38.1**.

✖ Do not report *CPT* code **41115** (excision of lingual frenum [frenectomy]) when the frenulum is only incised or clipped.

Car Safety Seat Testing

Codes **94780** and **94781** (car seat testing) are reported when determining whether *an infant through 12 months of age* may be safely transported upright in a car seat or must be transported by lying down in a car bed.

● Car seat testing codes may be reported in addition to the subsequent hospital or discharge day management codes when performed and documented. *Note:* These codes cannot be reported in addition to critical or intensive care services.

● Time spent in car seat testing is not counted as time spent in discharge day management.

● Car seat testing may also be provided to an infant in an outpatient setting to determine if the infant can safely move from car bed to car seat transportation.

> **See Chapter 18 for more information on car seat testing.**

To test your knowledge of the information presented in this chapter, complete the quiz found at the end of it, after the resources. Answers to each quiz are found in **Appendix IV**.

Chapter Takeaways

This chapter addresses coding for services provided during the course of a newborn's birth admission. Following are some takeaways from this chapter:

● The *neonatal period* begins at birth and continues through *the completed 28th day after birth,* ending on the 29th calendar day after birth. The day of birth is considered day 0 (zero).

● *ICD-10-CM* codes from category **Z38** are used to report live-born neonates according to type of birth and are the first listed for care by the attending or admitting physician during the entire birth admission.

● The choice between coding for normal newborn care and coding for hospital care is based on the physician's judgment and the type of symptoms demonstrated.

● *CPT* codes for care of a normal newborn typically follow a pathway of daily care from initial care to subsequent care and/or discharge day management.

Resource

AAP Coding Assistance and Education

AAP *Newborn Coding Decision Tool 2023* (https://shop.aap.org/newborn-coding-decision-tool-2023)

Test Your Knowledge!

1. **A neonate is born on the evening of January 1. Which of the following codes is reported by an attending physician who provides initial normal newborn and discharge management services at separate encounters on January 2?**
   a. **99460**
   b. **99461**
   c. **99462**
   d. **99463**

2. **Which of the following codes is not reported in addition to attendance at delivery (99464)?**
   a. **99465**
   b. **99461**
   c. **99221**
   d. None of the above

3. **Which of the following codes or code pairs is reported when an attending physician provides subsequent newborn care to a neonate who was previously suspected to be affected by a maternal streptococcal infection but is determined to be normal on this date of service?**
   a. **P00.82** (newborn affected by [positive] maternal group B streptococcus [GBS] colonization)
   b. A category **Z38** code (liveborn infant) and **P00.82**
   c. **Z05.42** (observation and evaluation of newborn for suspected infectious condition ruled out)
   d. A category **Z38** code (liveborn infant) and **Z05.42**

4. **Which of the following reporting takes place when a physician provides discharge management services to a normal newborn with a total time of 20 minutes?**
   a. Subsequent normal newborn care (**99462**) is reported for discharge of a normal newborn.
   b. Discharge management services of less than 30 minutes are not reported.
   c. **99238** is reported.
   d. **99462** and **99238** are reported.

5. **Which of the following codes or code series is reported for a follow-up evaluation and management service provided to an ill newborn (not requiring critical care) by a physician who provided a consultation earlier in the admission?**
   a. **99231–99233** (subsequent hospital or observation care)
   b. **99252–99255** (inpatient or observation consultation)
   c. **99221–99223** (initial hospital care)
   d. Either a consultation or an initial hospital care code as determined by payer policy

Chapter 16. Hospital Care of the Newborn

CHAPTER 17

Noncritical Hospital Evaluation and Management Services

CPT copyright 2022 American Medical Association. All rights reserved.

Contents

Chapter 17. Noncritical Hospital Evaluation and Management Services

Chapter Highlights

- Changes to the guidelines and descriptors for codes used to report services provided in hospital patient and observation settings
- How 2 of 3 elements of medical decision-making (MDM) are used to select a level of MDM
- Changes to code selection based on time

Following are significant changes to reporting hospital evaluation and management (E/M) services in 2023:
- Observation E/M codes **99217**, **99218–99220**, and **99224–99226** have been deleted.
- Codes **99221–99223**, **99231–99233**, and **99238** and **99239** have been revised to describe E/M services to patients in either hospital inpatient or observation status.
- Codes **99234–99236** are revised to mirror the code descriptor language now applicable to all inpatient or observation E/M services.
- Consultation code **99251** has been deleted, and codes **99252–99255** have been revised.
- Prolonged service codes **99354–99357** have also been deleted and replaced with code **99418**.
- Codes previously selected on the basis of 3 key components or typical unit/floor time are now selected on the basis of either
  — The level of MDM
  — The total time directed to care of the individual patient by a physician and/or qualified health care professional (QHP) on the date of service (includes time on and off the unit/floor) regardless of the amount of time spent in counseling and/or coordination of care

Coding for Noncritical Hospital Evaluation and Management (E/M) Services

This chapter discusses codes and guidelines for all E/M services that are provided in a hospital inpatient or observation setting except critical care services. (See **Chapter 18** for discussion of critical care services.) Hospital inpatient or observation care codes are used to report partial hospitalization services in addition to inpatient and observation services.

Codes for reporting hospital inpatient and observation services (other than consultations reported with **99252–99255**) are shown in **Table 17-1**. For a separate discussion of consultation codes, see the Consultation Guidelines section later in this chapter.

> All levels of initial and subsequent hospital or observation care include a medically appropriate history and/or examination, but neither is a component of code selection for services provided in 2023.

Table 17-1. Hospital Inpatient and Observation Evaluation and Management Codes
Except for 99238 and 99239, codes are selected on the basis of either MDM or meeting or exceeding the listed total time on the date of the encounter. (Consultation codes not included here. See Table 17-6.)

Category of Service	Straightforward or Low MDM	Moderate MDM	High MDM
Admit/discharge on the same date	▲99234 Total time: ≥45 min	▲99235 Total time: ≥70 min	▲99236 Total time: ≥85 min
Initial inpatient or observation	▲99221 Total time: ≥40 min	▲99222 Total time: ≥55 min	▲99223 Total time: ≥75 min
Subsequent inpatient or observation care	▲99231 Total time: ≥25 min	▲99232 Total time: ≥35 min	▲99233 Total time: ≥50 min
Inpatient or observation discharge management	▲99238 ≤30 min ▲99239 >30 min		

Abbreviations: E/M, evaluation and management; MDM, medical decision-making.

See E/M guidelines (discussed in **Chapter 6**) for selecting a level of MDM and determining total time.

● indicates a new code; ▲, revised; #, re-sequenced; ✚, add-on; ★, audiovisual technology; and ◀, synchronous interactive audio.

See **Chapter 6** for specific documentation requirements. See also the American Academy of Pediatrics (AAP) *Pediatric Evaluation and Management: Coding Quick Reference Card 2023* (https://shop.aap.org/pediatric-evaluation-and-management-coding-quick-reference-card-2023) or the *Pediatric Inpatient Evaluation and Management Pocket Card 2023* (https://shop.aap.org/pediatric-inpatient-evaluation-and-management-pocket-card-2023).

> Although evaluation and management codes for hospital inpatient and observation care are combined, admission orders should distinctly designate the patient's admission status, as this may be important for payer coverage and payment rates. When a patient transitions from observation to inpatient status, an order for inpatient admission should be clearly documented in the patient record.

Guidelines for Inpatient and Observation Services

Following are basic guidelines for reporting hospital inpatient or observation E/M services with the codes in **Table 17-1**:
- There are no distinctions between new and established patients. However, most codes differentiate initial from subsequent hospital or observation care.
    — Report an initial hospital or observation service when the patient has not received any professional services from the reporting physician or QHP or another physician or QHP of the exact same specialty and subspecialty who belongs to the same group practice (ie, has the same tax identification number or group National Provider Identifier [NPI]) during the current admission and stay.
    — Report a subsequent hospital or observation service when the patient has received professional service(s) from the physician or QHP or another physician or QHP of the exact same specialty and subspecialty who belongs to the same group practice, on a prior date during the current admission and stay.

> *Current Procedural Terminology* no longer states that initial hospital inpatient or observation care codes are for reporting by the admitting physician. When initial inpatient or observation care is provided by physicians of a different specialty or group practice from the admitting physician, report initial hospital inpatient or observation services (except when conditions for reporting an inpatient or observation consultation are met).

    — When physicians and QHPs are working together, they are considered to be in the same specialty and subspecialty (eg, neonatology, hospital medicine).
    — A physician or QHP who is covering for another physician or QHP reports a service as if it were provided by the physician or QHP who is unavailable.
    — A hospital stay that includes a transition between observation and inpatient is a single stay.

Examples

➤ **A neonate was born by cesarian delivery on Monday and received normal newborn care from Dr A of Pediatric Hospitalists, Inc, on Monday and Tuesday.** On Wednesday, the neonate is evaluated by Dr B (also an employee of Pediatric Hospitalists, Inc, and of the same exact specialty as Dr A) and found to have developed hyperbilirubinemia requiring initiation of phototherapy. Dr B's service includes clinically indicated history and examination with moderate MDM. The diagnosis is jaundice caused by ABO incompatibility.
  ICD-10-CM: **Z38.01** (single liveborn infant, delivered by cesarean)
  P55.1 (ABO isoimmunization of newborn)
  CPT: **99232** (subsequent hospital inpatient or observation with moderate MDM)
  Teaching Point: The neonate's service by Dr B is a subsequent encounter because Dr A of the same group practice and same specialty has provided E/M services during this stay.

➤ **A neonate was born by cesarian delivery late on Monday and received normal newborn care from Dr A of Pediatric Hospitalists, Inc, on that date.** On Tuesday, Dr A requests that Dr B, a specialist, evaluate the neonate, who may have risk factors for an infection that was diagnosed in the mother. Dr B and no other physician or QHP of the same specialty and same group practice has provided a professional service to the neonate during this stay.
  Teaching Point: The neonate's service by Dr B is an initial service. If all requirements for reporting a consultation are met, codes **99252–99255** are reported. However, if the service does not meet the requirements of a consultation or the payer does not pay for services reported with consultation codes, Dr B reports initial hospital inpatient or observation services.

● indicates a new code; ▲, revised; #, re-sequenced; ✛, add-on; ★, audiovisual technology; and ◀, synchronous interactive audio.

- Codes are reported on the basis of the cumulative inpatient or observation services (*MDM or total time on the date of service*) provided by 1 or more physicians or other QHPs
  - Of the same exact specialty
  - With the same tax identification number (or group NPI)
  - *On a single calendar date*
- Services may be performed and reported by any physician of any specialty (eg, hospitalist, primary care physician, specialist) or other QHPs.
- Any professional service (eg, procedure, interpretation and report) with a *Current Procedural Terminology* (*CPT*) code may be reported separately when performed by the reporting provider or group and documented.
  - Do not include the time spent performing separately reported procedures in the time of the E/M service.
- Evaluation and management services may be provided by the same physician or QHP in an outpatient (eg, office, emergency department [ED]) or other facility (eg, nursing facility) setting before admission to observation or inpatient status on the same date. Under new *CPT* guidelines, these services *are separately reportable* with modifier **25** appended to the E/M code for the initial encounter on that date. Individual payer policies for more than 1 E/M service provided on the same date may vary.

Example

➤ **A physician provides an E/M service to a patient in an outpatient clinic and determines that admission to observation care is indicated.** Later that day, a QHP, who is of the exact same specialty and same group practice, visits the patient in the hospital and provides initial observation care. Despite management, the patient's condition continues to deteriorate and the physician orders admission to inpatient status.

　　Teaching Point: The physician may report the outpatient E/M service with modifier **25** appended to the appropriate E/M code (eg, **99214 25**) and the QHP reports an initial hospital inpatient or observation E/M service code (without a modifier).

Multiple Sites of Evaluation and Management Services

If a physician or qualified health care professional (or individuals of the same specialty and same group practice) provides care to a patient in an encounter in another site of service (eg, emergency department, office, nursing facility) on the same date before admission and also initial hospital or observation care on that same date, the code for the initial evaluation and management (E/M) service is separately reported with modifier **25** (significant, separately identifiable E/M service) appended.

For separate discussion of consultations provided before admission to inpatient or observation status, see the Consultation Guidelines section later in this chapter. Note that some payer policies may not align with *Current Procedural Terminology* guidance for reporting of more than 1 E/M service on a single date of service.

General E/M Code Selection Guidelines

As detailed in **Chapter 6**, code selection for E/M services that were previously based on key components or unit/floor time are now selected on the basis of MDM alone or total time on the date of the encounter (regardless of the amount of time spent in counseling and/or coordination of care). The following sections provide some key points about using either MDM or total time on the date of service to select codes.

　　An overarching key point is that any initial or subsequent hospital inpatient or observation care service code *may be selected on the basis of either MDM or total time.* The reported code is determined by using whichever method most benefits the reporting physician or QHP.

Medical Decision-making

Code selection based on MDM always requires that 2 of 3 elements be met at the level reported. As a reminder, the 3 elements of MDM are

1. Number and complexity of *problems addressed* (problems addressed)
2. Amount and/or complexity of *data to be reviewed and analyzed* (data)
3. Risk of complications and/or morbidity or mortality *of patient management* (risk)

　　Do not select a code on the basis of 1 element of MDM (eg, high risk alone does not support high MDM).

Chapter 17. Noncritical Hospital Evaluation and Management Services

---

Problems Addressed

For subsequent hospital inpatient and observation care services, the problem addressed is the problem status on the date of the encounter, which may significantly differ from that on admission. It is the problem(s) addressed by the reporting physician or QHP on the date of the encounter and not necessarily the problem(s) that prompted admission (eg, a physician addresses a new problem that manifested after admission, or a consultant is asked to evaluate a problem that was not the problem that prompted admission).

> A problem is addressed or managed when evaluated or treated at the encounter by the reporting physician or qualified health care professional. Do not count problems that are not evaluated and/or do not affect medical decision-making at the current encounter.

Determining the highest-complexity problem(s) addressed is key to selecting the number and complexity of problems addressed. Addressing multiple problems of the same complexity affects only the level of problems addressed when addressing either 2 or more self-limited or minor problems or 2 or more stable chronic illnesses.

Examples

➤ **A patient is admitted with diagnosis of type 1 diabetic ketoacidosis without coma (E10.10).** The number and complexity of problems addressed for the initial encounter is high because of addressing 1 or more chronic illnesses with severe exacerbation, progression, or side effects of treatment.

On the next date, the patient is improved but is receiving follow-up care for the uncontrolled (or new) diagnosis of type 1 diabetes mellitus with hyperglycemia (**E10.65**). The problem addressed is 1 or more chronic illnesses with exacerbation, progression, or side effects of treatment supporting a moderate number and complexity of problems addressed.

Teaching Point: The problem addressed is the problem status on the date of the encounter, which may significantly differ from that on admission. It is the problem being managed or comanaged by the reporting physician or QHP, and not necessarily the cause of the admission or continued stay, that is to be coded on the encounter date.

➤ **A patient with cerebral palsy was admitted as an inpatient for orthopedic surgery and, during the hospital stay, developed a urinary tract infection (UTI).** A hospitalist who has been managing the patient's conditions unrelated to the surgery provides a subsequent hospital inpatient or observation service to address the UTI.

Teaching Point: The problem addressed by the hospitalist, UTI, was not the reason for the admission. The hospitalist's code selection, when based on MDM, will include selecting the number and complexity of the problem addressed (ie, the UTI and any other problem addressed at the encounter).

The underlying chronic condition, cerebral palsy, may influence the level of MDM when addressed and results in an increased amount and/or complexity of data to be reviewed and analyzed or an increased risk of complications and/or morbidity or mortality of patient management. An *International Classification of Diseases, Tenth Revision, Clinical Modification (ICD-10-CM)* diagnosis code for cerebral palsy will be reported in addition to the code for the UTI when the cerebral palsy influences MDM.

Data

Following are important guidelines for determining the amount and/or complexity of data to be reviewed and analyzed:
- The data counted toward the level of MDM are data that are analyzed (ie, used as part of the MDM) at the current encounter.
- Review of tests ordered by the same physician or QHP (or individuals covering for or of the same specialty and group practice) at a prior encounter are not counted toward the data analyzed at the current encounter.

> Each unique test is counted once toward the amount and/or complexity of data. Do not count both the order for and the review of the same unique test.
>
> When a test with multiple components can be reported with a single code (eg, test panel or a test that is described as bilateral or with a specific number of images), count the test once for the purpose of data to be reviewed and analyzed.

- Any test for which the reporting individual or another individual of the same specialty and same group practice will separately report a code for interpretation and report is not counted toward the data analyzed at the encounter.

Example

➤ **A cardiologist who provides subsequent hospital care to a patient also reports the interpretation and report of an electrocardiogram (ECG).**

Teaching Point: The cardiologist does not include the order for or review of the ECG in the amount and/or complexity of data to be reviewed and analyzed because the interpretation and report of test results are separately reported.

Risk

Determine the level of risk of management decisions made at each individual encounter. Following are a few key points regarding selection of the level of risk:

- The element of risk of MDM is the *risk of management* and not the risk of the problem itself. For example, the risk of treating a child with a parenteral controlled substance is higher than the risk of other prescription drug management.
- Risk may be increased by a decision against a management option (testing, treatment, or hospitalization) that was *considered but not selected.*
- The risk associated with a decision for surgery is not determined by the global period assigned to the procedure but, rather, by how trained clinicians would commonly classify the risks of the procedure, also considering the patient-specific risk factors. For example, an orthopedic heel-cord release would be a low-risk procedure, but that risk would be significantly increased if the patient had cerebral palsy with respiratory and neurological disease.
- A decision regarding escalation of the level of service (eg, a decision to transfer to intensive or critical care) indicates a higher level of risk in the patient's management.

For examples in the discussion of initial, subsequent, and same date hospital or observation admission and discharge services, see the Selecting Hospital Inpatient or Observation Care Codes section later in this chapter, which further expands on the elements of MDM.

Time-Based Code Selection

It is important to understand the different use of time in selecting codes for hospital services in 2023. The time used for code selection is the physician's and/or QHP's total time directed to the individual patient's care on the date of the encounter. See **Chapter 6** for a full discussion of activities that may contribute to the total time.

Inpatient hospital or observation care code descriptors include a *minimum amount of time that must be met or exceeded.*

Following are some key points regarding total time of service:

- Total time is not limited to time spent on the unit/floor. Count all time in activities necessary for care of the individual patient.
- Time may be the basis for code selection regardless of the amount of the unit/floor time that was spent in counseling and/or coordination of care.
- When time is used as the controlling factor in the selection of the code, *the total time spent on the date of the encounter must be documented in the medical record.*
- Continuous service time that crosses midnight is counted as a single service on a single date. When there is no continuous episode of care crossing midnight, separately report the services provided on each calendar date.

Do not count time spent on

✖ The performance of other services that are reported separately (eg, bedside procedure)

✖ Travel

✖ Teaching that is general for any patient admitted to the hospital and not specific to the management of the patient's problem(s) presently being addressed

✖ Time spent in activities normally performed by clinical staff (eg, assisting the patient to the bathroom or changing a diaper)

For examples in the discussion of initial, subsequent, and same date hospital or observation admission and discharge services, see the Selecting Hospital Inpatient or Observation Care Codes section later in this chapter, which further expands on time-based code selection.

Hospital or Observation Services by Multiple Physicians and QHPs

Concurrent Care

Concurrent care is defined by *CPT* as the provision of similar services to the same patient by more than one physician on the same day. Concurrent care may be provided by physicians from different practices or physicians from the same practice but different specialties. When concurrent care is provided, the diagnosis code(s) reported by each physician should reflect the medical necessity for the provision of services by more than one physician on the same date of service. Although it is easier to justify concurrent care when each treating physician reports different diagnoses, if the diagnosis code is reported for the same condition, it does not prevent billing for the services.

Example

➤ **The attending physician wants the consultant to provide ongoing management of 1 problem (eg, heart failure) while the attending physician provides ongoing management for other active problems (eg, pneumonia with respiratory distress).**

   Teaching Point: Both physicians would report subsequent hospital care codes and link the *CPT* codes to the appropriate diagnosis codes.

   See **Chapter 1**, **Figure 1-1**, for an example of linking diagnoses to procedure codes on a claim.

Reporting Services Split or Shared by a Physician and a QHP

In general, a split or shared E/M service is one in which a physician and a QHP from the same specialty and group practice, who could otherwise independently report an E/M service, each personally perform a medically necessary portion of 1 or more face-to-face E/M services on the same date. Split/shared billing may allow a physician to report the combined work and receive payment at a higher fee schedule rate than would be paid if reported by the QHP. (Some health plans pay <100% of the plan's physician fee schedule [eg, 85%] for services reported by QHPs.)

   Split/shared billing policy may not apply when a payer does not allow direct billing by a QHP. In this event, follow the payer's policy for reporting (eg, always bill for the combined work under the physician's NPI).

> Split or shared billing differs from incident-to billing, which is allowed only in a non-facility setting. See Chapter 7 for information on incident-to billing.

CPT® Guidelines for Split/Shared Services

CPT defines a "shared or split visit" as a visit in which a physician and QHP(s) jointly provide the face-to-face and non–face-to-face work related to a visit. The *CPT* guidelines for split/shared services address use of time for code selection as follows:

● When time is used to select the appropriate level of hospital or observation service, the time personally spent by the physician and QHP(s) assessing and treating the patient and/or counseling, educating, or communicating results to the patient or family/caregiver on the date of the encounter is summed to define total time.
● When 2 or more individuals of the same specialty and same group practice jointly meet with or discuss the patient, only the time of one individual should be counted.

   CPT does not designate circumstances under which a split/shared visit must be reported by the QHP in lieu of the physician.

Medicare Guidelines for Split/Shared Services

The Medicare program applies the split/shared billing policy only to services provided in a facility setting. Other payers may differ in their policies or may not distinctly address split/shared services.

   The following requirements apply to all split/shared services when Medicare guidelines are applied:

● *When reporting based on total time, the provider with the highest total time on the date of the encounter reports the service under their NPI.* Medicare policy for reporting based on history, examination, or MDM was not finalized at the time of this publication.

> This instruction is based on Medicare policy for 2023 as published in 2021 and early 2022. Please check for updates to policies of Medicare and other payers before billing for split or shared services.

- When reporting based on time, documentation must support the total time of the combined service.
- The reporting physician or QHP must authenticate/sign the documentation of the service per Medicare policy. Each individual should independently document their work and time spent on the date of the encounter.
- A physician cannot merely sign off on the documentation of the work by the QHP.
- Shared services are generally not permitted if the QHP is a hospital employee. (Exceptions may apply under value-based care payment arrangements.)

Under Medicare policy, a split/shared service must be reported with modifier **FS** (split or shared E/M visit) appended to the code reported for the split/shared encounter.

Examples

➤ **A QHP provides initial hospital care and documents 35 minutes spent providing the service.** Later that day, a physician from the same specialty and same group practice is called to see the patient, who is exhibiting new symptoms, and to review new laboratory test results. The physician spends 40 minutes reassessing the patient, entering new orders, and documenting the service. When accounting for both services, which have been individually documented and signed, an initial hospital inpatient service with total time of service of 75 minutes is reported.

   Teaching Point: Because both health care professionals are from the same group practice and have signed off on their individually provided services, the services may be shared and billed under the physician as code **99223** (initial hospital care with a minimum total time of 75 minutes). The service is reported by the physician who provided most of the total time spent on the date of the service. If required by the payer, modifier **FS** is appended to code **99223**.

➤ **A QHP provides initial hospital care and documents 45 minutes spent providing the service.** Later that day, a physician from the same specialty and same group practice is called to see the patient to answer questions from a parent who was not present at the QHP's service. The physician spends a total of 20 minutes reviewing the patient's medical record, briefly reassessing the patient, and discussing the anticipated hospital course with the patient's parents. When accounting for both services, which have been individually documented and signed, an initial hospital inpatient service with total time of service of 65 minutes is reported.

   Teaching Point: The total time of the combined services supports code **99222** (initial hospital care with a minimum total time of 55 minutes). If the payer follows Medicare guidelines for split/shared services, the QHP must report the service because the greater portion of the total time was spent by the QHP and **99222 FS** would be reported.

Selecting Hospital Inpatient or Observation Care Codes

The following section provides an overview of each category of hospital inpatient or observation E/M service with time and MDM reporting criteria and examples of each level of service. Following are key points to remember in code selection:

- Examples given are not clinical recommendations, and levels of service supported may vary on the basis of documentation and patient age and presentation (eg, ill appearance beyond what is typical for concern).
- Select a code based on either total physician/QHP time on the date of service or MDM.
- Report an initial service when the patient has not received any professional services from the physician or QHP (or another physician or QHP of the exact same specialty and subspecialty who belongs to the same group practice) during the current hospital or observation stay.

Table 17-2 provides guidance for selecting a code based on the level of MDM supported by 2 of 3 elements of MDM or based on total time on the date of the encounter. This table is useful when reviewing examples of services provided in discussions of each category of hospital inpatient or observation E/M service.

Chapter 17. Noncritical Hospital Evaluation and Management Services

---

● indicates a new code; ▲, revised; #, re-sequenced; ✚, add-on; ★, audiovisual technology; and ◀, synchronous interactive audio.

Table 17-2. Hospital or Observation Evaluation and Management Services: Code Selection Requirements (also included at www.aap.org/cfp2023)

Level/Codes/Total Time (min)[a]	Medical Decision-making (2 of 3 Required: Data,[b,c] Problems, Risk)		
	Problems Addressed	Data Reviewed and Analyzed[b]	Risk
Straightforward *Same date admission and discharge* ▲99234 (≥45) *Initial service* ▲99221 (≥40) *Subsequent service* ▲99231 (≥25) *Consultation* ▲99252 (≥35)	1 self-limited or minor	Minimal or none	Minimal
Low *Same date admission and discharge* ▲99234 (≥45) *Initial service* ▲99221 (≥40) *Subsequent service* ▲99231 (≥25) *Consultation* ▲99253 (≥45)	Low—*Any 1 of* • ≥2 self-limited or minor • 1 stable chronic illness • 1 acute, uncomplicated illness or injury • 1 stable acute illness • 1 acute, uncomplicated illness or injury requiring hospital inpatient or observation level of care	Limited (*Meet 1 of 2 categories*) <u>Category 1:</u> Tests and documents (*Any 2*) • Review of prior external note(s)—each unique source • Review of the result(s) of each unique test • Ordering of each unique test <u>Category 2:</u> Assessment requiring an independent historian(s)	Low *Examples* • Over-the-counter medication(s) • Removal of sutures • Physical, language, or occupational therapy
Moderate *Same date admission and discharge* ▲99235 (≥70) *Initial service* ▲99222 (≥55) *Subsequent service* ▲99232 (≥35) *Consultation* ▲99254 (≥60)	Moderate—*Any 1 of* ≥1 chronic illness with exacerbation, progression, or side effects of treatment ≥2 stable chronic illnesses 1 undiagnosed new problem with uncertain prognosis 1 acute illness with systemic symptoms 1 acute, complicated injury	Moderate (*Meet 1 out of 3 categories*) <u>Category 1:</u> Tests and documents (*Meet any 3*) • Review of prior external note(s)—each unique source • Review of the result(s) of each unique test • Ordering each unique test • Assessment requiring an independent historian(s) <u>Category 2:</u> Independent interpretation of a test performed by another physician/other QHP[c] <u>Category 3:</u> Discussion of management or test interpretation with external physician/other QHP/appropriate source	Moderate *Examples* • Prescription drug management or off-label use of over-the-counter medication • Decision about minor surgery with identified patient or procedure risk factors • Decision about elective major surgery without identified patient or procedure risk factors • Diagnosis or treatment significantly limited by social determinants of health

● indicates a new code; ▲, revised; #, re-sequenced; ✚, add-on; ★, audiovisual technology; and ◀, synchronous interactive audio.

Level/Codes/Total Time (min)ᵃ	Medical Decision-making (2 of 3 Required: Data,ᵇ,ᶜ Problems, Risk)		
	Problems Addressed	**Data Reviewed and Analyzedᵇ**	**Risk**
High *Same date admission and discharge* ▲**99236** (≥85) *Initial service* ▲**99223** (≥75) *Subsequent service* ▲**99233** (≥50) *Consultation* ▲**99255** (≥80)	High—*1 of* ≥1 chronic illness with severe exacerbation, progression, or side effects of treatment 1 acute or chronic illness or injury that poses a threat to life or bodily function	Extensive (*Meet 2 out of 3 categories listed in the previous row*)	High *Examples* • Drug therapy requiring intensive monitoring for toxicity • Decision about hospitalization or escalation of hospital level of care • Decision about elective major surgery with identified patient or procedure risk factors • Decision about emergency major surgery • Decision not to resuscitate or to de-escalate care because of poor prognosis • Parenteral controlled substances

Abbreviation: QHP, qualified health care professional.

ᵃ Include only time personally spent by physicians and QHPs of the same specialty and same group practice directed to the individual patient's care on the date of the encounter.

ᵇ Each unique test, order, or document contributes to the combination of 2 or combination of 3 in Category 1.

ᶜ Do not count data review or communications reported with other codes (eg, test interpretation, interprofessional consultation).

Same Date Admission and Discharge Services

▲**99234**   Hospital inpatient or observation care, for the evaluation and management of a patient including admission and discharge on the same date, which requires a medically appropriate history and/or examination and straightforward or low level of medical decision making.

When using total time on the date of the encounter for code selection, 45 minutes must be met or exceeded.

▲**99235**   Hospital inpatient or observation care, for the evaluation and management of a patient including admission and discharge on the same date, which requires a medically appropriate history and/or examination and moderate level of medical decision making.

When using total time on the date of the encounter for code selection, 70 minutes must be met or exceeded.

▲**99236**   Hospital inpatient or observation care, for the evaluation and management of a patient including admission and discharge on the same date, which requires a medically appropriate history and/or examination and high level of medical decision making.

When using total time on the date of the encounter for code selection, 85 minutes must be met or exceeded.

(For services ≥100 minutes, see discussion of prolonged service add-on code **99418** in the Prolonged Service on the Date of an E/M Service section later in this chapter.)

> Prolonged service may be reported only in addition to the highest-level code in the category of evaluation and management service (eg, code **99418** is reported in addition to code **99236** but not codes **99234** and **99235**) and only when code selection is based on total time.

Codes **99234–99236** are reported when a physician or QHP provides a hospital inpatient or observation admission service and, *after reevaluation later on the same date,* provides discharge management services.

● Two or more encounters are required *on the same calendar date.* Report **99234–99236** only when 1 encounter consists of an initial admission service and another consists of a discharge management.

● For a patient admitted and discharged at a single face-to-face encounter, report only initial hospital inpatient or observation service codes **99221–99223**.

● indicates a new code; ▲, revised; #, re-sequenced; ✚, add-on; ★, audiovisual technology; and ◀, synchronous interactive audio.

— Do not report discharge management codes **99238** and **99239** in conjunction with **99221–99223** for admission and discharge services performed on the same calendar date.

> **Report 99463** for admission and discharge services provided to normal newborns on the same calendar date.

Code selection is based on *either MDM or total time* on the date of the encounter.

- Include the combined MDM or total time provided by the same physician or physicians of the same specialty and same group practice provided on a single date of service.
- Except where payer guidance specifies otherwise, reporting of initial observation or inpatient care is based on the date of the face-to-face assessment and not the date of admission or designation of a status by a facility (eg, when changed on physician order).

> **When Payers Use Medicare Policy**
>
> Medicaid and private payers may adopt a Medicare policy that limits reporting of hospital inpatient and observation services to encounters during which a patient is admitted to observation or inpatient status for at least *8 hours and not more than 24 hours*. Under this policy, when a patient is admitted to inpatient or observation care for less than 8 hours on the same calendar date, only the initial hospital inpatient or observation service (99221–99223) is reported. A separate code for discharge services is not reported.
>
> Medicare also requires that there must be a medical observation record for the patient that contains dated and timed physician's orders for the inpatient or observation services the patient is to receive, nursing notes, and progress notes prepared by the physician indicating physical presence and personal performance of services. This record must be in addition to (and not a copy and paste of) any record prepared as a result of an emergency department or outpatient clinic encounter before the admission.

Use **tables 17-2** and **17-3** to assign codes for the services based on MDM or total time on the date of the encounter that follow.

> For ease of reference, a printable version of Table 17-2 is included at www.aap.org/cfp2023.

Table 17-3. Codes for Admission and Discharge on the Same Date			
Medical Decision-making	**Straightforward or Low**	**Moderate**	**High**
Code/Total Time	▲99234 Total time: ≥45 min	▲99235 Total time: ≥70 min	▲99236 Total time: ≥85 min

Examples

➤ **6:00 am: An 8-year-old girl is admitted from the ED to observation for generalized abdominal pain.** The physician orders monitoring of vital signs and small amounts of clear fluids pending test results. Nursing staff monitors the patient periodically. The physician adds an order for a stool softener and suppository, which produce stooling, and symptoms are slowly resolved. Decision for discharge to home is made at 11:00 am. Diagnosis is abdominal pain due to fecal impaction. The physician's total time on the date of the encounter is 55 minutes, including all face-to-face and non–face-to-face time spent in review and documentation of the patient's health information and in discussions directly related to care of this patient.

ICD-10-CM: **K56.41** (fecal impaction)

CPT: **99234** (same date admission and discharge service with 45 minutes met or exceeded)

Teaching Point: Per *CPT* guidance, a code from the **99234–99236** series would be reported because observation admission and discharge services were provided by the same physician on the same date, including 2 distinct face-to-face services.

Alternatively, if the payer requires an observation stay of 8 hours to report **99234–99236**, an initial inpatient or observation care code (**99221–99223**) is reported for this 5-hour stay. Code **99222** (55 minutes met or exceeded) is supported.

● indicates a new code; ▲, revised; #, re-sequenced; ✚, add-on; ★, audiovisual technology; and ◀, synchronous interactive audio.

➤ **A 14-year-old patient with an acute exacerbation of asthma is admitted to an observation stay.** The attending physician performs the initial history and physical examination at 4:00 am and orders continued fluids, inhalation treatments, and continued close monitoring. Another physician from the attending physician's same specialty and group practice returns to the hospital at 5:00 pm that same day and, after evaluation of the child, discharges the patient home with new prescriptions for asthma control and emergency-use medications.

    ICD-10-CM: **J45.41** (moderate persistent asthma with exacerbation)

    CPT: **99235** (initial inpatient E/M service with moderate MDM)

    Level of problem addressed |||➡ Moderate (an exacerbated chronic condition)

    Level of data reviewed and analyzed |||➡ Minimal or none

    Level of risk of morbidity |||➡ Moderate (prescription drug management)

    Teaching Point: Because the physicians of the same specialty and same group practice provided inpatient admission and discharge services on the same date, code **99235** is reported by one of the physicians. Determination of who reports the service may be based on the attending physician of record or practice policy.

Initial Inpatient Hospital Care

▲**99221**   Initial hospital inpatient or observation care, per day, for the evaluation and management of a patient, which requires a medically appropriate history and/or examination and straightforward or low level medical decision making.

         When using total time on the date of the encounter for code selection, 40 minutes must be met or exceeded.

▲**99222**   Initial hospital inpatient or observation care, per day, for the evaluation and management of a patient, which requires a medically appropriate history and/or examination and moderate level medical decision making.

         When using total time on the date of the encounter for code selection, 55 minutes must be met or exceeded.

▲**99223**   Initial hospital inpatient or observation care, per day, for the evaluation and management of a patient, which requires a medically appropriate history and/or examination and high level medical decision making.

         When using total time on the date of the encounter for code selection, 75 minutes must be met or exceeded.

(For services ≥90 minutes, see discussion of prolonged service add-on code **99418** in the Prolonged Service on the Date of an E/M Service section later in this chapter.)

- Initial hospital inpatient or observation service codes are used to report initial face-to-face services provided to a patient admitted as a hospital inpatient or in observation status.
- Initial hospital encounters may be reported by more than one physician. For discussion of consultations in hospital inpatient or observation settings, see the Consultation Guidelines section later in this chapter.
- The code is reported on the first day that a face-to-face (physician-patient) service is provided.
- The date of initial hospital inpatient or observation care that the physician reports does not need to correlate with the facility's date of admission.
- Only one initial hospital inpatient or observation care code is reported per stay. A transition from observation to inpatient does not constitute a new stay.

    Use **tables 17-2** and **17-4** to review the requirements used to select level of service in the examples that follow.

Table 17-4. Codes for Initial Hospital Inpatient or Observation Services			
Medical Decision-making	**Straightforward or Low**	**Moderate**	**High**
Code/Total Time	▲99221 Total time: ≥40 min	▲99222 Total time: ≥55 min	▲99223 Total time: ≥75 min

Examples

➤ **A 5-year-old patient is admitted to observation from the ED for treatment of diarrhea with moderate dehydration. At 5:00 am, a hospitalist provides the initial observation encounter on the patient's unit.** The hospitalist orders include a time-based oral rehydration plan by using an electrolyte solution. The patient is reevaluated by the hospitalist at 7:00 am and again at 10:00 am and determined to be sufficiently recovered for discharge to home at the 10:00 am encounter. The hospitalist orders the discharge and documents all the services, including 50 minutes of total time spent directed to the care of the patient. Diagnosis is viral gastroenteritis with mild dehydration.

ICD-10-CM: **A08.4** (viral intestinal infection, unspecified), **E86.0** (dehydration)

CPT: The patient's health benefit plan requires reporting initial hospital or observation care, in lieu of same date admission and discharge services, for the 5-hour stay. Code **99221** (straightforward to low MDM, ≥40 minutes) is reported in lieu of **99234** (same date admission and discharge with straightforward to low MDM, ≥45 minutes).

Teaching Point: The hospitalist's service is reported as directed by the benefit plan policy, although the service provided supports same date admission and discharge (ie, the patient was evaluated at more than one encounter, and both an admission and a discharge management service were provided on the same date).

➤ **An 60-day-old girl is admitted from the ED to Dr A's service.** The patient's mother reported that the infant seemed warm to the touch, seemed irritable, breast fed much less than normal, and mother had noticed fewer wet diapers and 1 normal stool in the past 24 hours.

Laboratory evaluation: complete blood cell count (CBC) with white blood cells at 12,000/mcL, no left shift on differential count, normal absolute neutrophil count (ANC); urinalysis results normal or negative with pH of 7.0, specific gravity of 1.020. Urine and blood culture results pending. The C-Reactive Protein was normal (less than 3.1). The comprehensive metabolic panel was normal except for CO_2 of 16 mEq/L. COVID-19 test was negative. Because of patient's age and continued symptoms, concern for sepsis or undetected bacterial infection; doubt pyelonephritis given normal urinalysis; less likely meningitis given mild clinical findings; doubt bronchiolitis given lack of viral symptoms.

Assessment: 8-week-old with fever, mild dehydration, and lethargy.

Plan: Admit for intravenous (IV) antibiotics and IV fluids. Will closely observe for sepsis and pyelonephritis but normal exam, CBC, UA, and CRP results. Will follow blood and urine cultures. Continue breastfeeding ad lib. Discussed current diagnostic and treatment plans with parents and advised that a QHP from the same group practice visit later today to reevaluate the patient and plan for any needed overnight changes in management or for home discharge.

ICD-10-CM: **R50.9** (fever, unspecified), **E86.0** (dehydration), **R53.83** (lethargy), **E87.21** (acute metabolic acidosis)

CPT: **99222** (moderate MDM)

Level of problem addressed ⅢⅢ➡ Moderate (undiagnosed new problem with uncertain prognosis)

Level of data reviewed and analyzed ⅢⅢ➡ Moderate (3 tests reviewed and independent historian [Category 1 data])

Level of risk of morbidity ⅢⅢ➡ Moderate (prescription drug management)

Teaching Point: Moderate MDM and code **99222** are supported by all 3 elements of MDM.

➤ **Later that same calendar day, a QHP of the same specialty and of the same group practice reexamines the infant.** The QHP spends 25 minutes in care of the patient, including time reviewing records, examination of the infant (who shows signs of improvement), discussion with parents and clinical staff, and documenting the service.

Plan: Reevaluate tomorrow; continue IV antibiotics pending result of cultures.

The total time of service for the 2 separate encounters is 70 minutes (45 + 25 = 70).

ICD-10-CM: **R50.9** (fever, unspecified), **E86.0** (dehydration), **R53.83** (lethargy), **E87.21** (acute metabolic acidosis)

CPT: **99222** (moderate MDM, ≥55 minutes). Modifier **FS** (split/shared service) is appended if required by the payer.

Teaching Point: The hospital E/M services provided on this date include the total time spent by the 2 individuals of the same specialty and same group practice. Dr A, who spent most of the total time of service and ordered the tests reviewed by the QHP, submits the bill for the calendar day's service. In this scenario, both the physician's total time and level of MDM were higher than that of the QHP as the problem was improving at the time of the QHP's visit, review of test results was included in the order by a physician of the same group and specialty, and the risk of management is unchanged.

Had the combined total time of service met or exceeded 75 minutes, code **99223** would have been reported.

➤ **A 14-year-old patient is admitted to inpatient status from the ED at 8:00 pm on Tuesday with status asthmaticus.** The admitting physician's documentation includes notes of a discussion with an ED physician and decision for general pediatric unit admission rather than intensive care unit. She reviews the results of 3 unique tests (eg, BMP, CBC, spirometry, and/or blood gas analysis). The admitting diagnosis is status asthmaticus, stable on albuterol inhalation treatments and IV methylprednisolone. *Plan:* Continue albuterol inhalation therapy and IV methylprednisolone. Monitor peak expiratory flow rate, serum electrolyte levels, and glucose level.

ICD-10-CM: **J45.42** (moderate persistent asthma with status asthmaticus)

CPT: **99223** (initial inpatient E/M service with high MDM)

Teaching Point: The high-level MDM in this example is supported by all 3 elements of MDM.

Level of problem addressed |||➡ High complexity (severe exacerbation of a chronic condition)

Level of data reviewed and analyzed |||➡ Extensive because of 2 of 3 categories of data: Category 1 (order or review of ≥3 tests) and Category 3 (discussion with an external physician [physician of another specialty])

Level of risk of morbidity |||➡ High (decision to admit to a unit/floor)

Subsequent Hospital Care

★▲**99231**   Subsequent hospital inpatient or observation care, per day, for the evaluation and management of a patient, which requires a medically appropriate history and/or examination and straightforward or low level of medical decision making.

   When using total time on the date of the encounter for code selection, 25 minutes must be met or exceeded.

★▲**99232**   Subsequent hospital inpatient or observation care, per day, for the evaluation and management of a patient, which requires a medically appropriate history and/or examination and moderate level of medical decision making.

   When using total time on the date of the encounter for code selection, 35 minutes must be met or exceeded.

★▲**99233**   Subsequent hospital inpatient or observation care, per day, for the evaluation and management of a patient, which requires a medically appropriate history and/or examination and high level of medical decision making.

   When using total time on the date of the encounter for code selection, 50 minutes must be met or exceeded.

(For services ≥65 minutes, see discussion of prolonged service add-on code **99418** in the Prolonged Service on the Date of an E/M Service section later in this chapter.)

● Codes include all E/M services by a physician or QHP of the same specialty and same group practice provided on a subsequent day of inpatient or observation service. The level of service reported will be dependent on the total services provided and documented.

● Codes **99231–99233** are also reported by consulting physicians when reporting an inpatient or observation consultation code is inappropriate (eg, when an outpatient consultation was provided before admission on the same date). For additional discussion of consultations, see the Consultation Guidelines section later in this chapter.

● Selection of the code is based on either MDM or total time on the date of the encounter.

Use **tables 17-2** and **17-5** to help select the appropriate codes in the examples that follow.

Table 17-5. Codes for Subsequent Hospital Inpatient or Observation Services			
Medical Decision-making	**Straightforward or Low**	**Moderate**	**High**
Code/Total Time	▲**99231** Total time: ≥25 min	▲**99232** Total time: ≥35 min	▲**99233** Total time: ≥50 min

Examples

➤ **A physician reevaluates an 8-week-old who has fever, dehydration, and lethargy and received initial hospital care from a physician of the same specialty and same group practice on the prior day.** *Progress note:* "No new reported problems overnight; breastfeeding has improved but patient continues to have low-grade fever (38.2°C [100.8°F] maximum temperature) overnight; no reported apnea or cyanosis; no respiratory distress. Drinking better, more wet diapers, more alert, less irritable, and more active."

Laboratory: No growth in blood or urine cultures at less than 24 hours. Glucose level normal.

● indicates a new code; ▲, revised; #, re-sequenced; ✚, add-on; ★, audiovisual technology; and ◀, synchronous interactive audio.

Assessment/plan: Continued fever. Continued concern for sepsis; suspect viral etiology given negative workup so far for common serious bacterial infections, such as pyelonephritis, pneumonia, meningitis, and bacteremia. Continue IV antibiotics until culture results are negative for 48 hours; continue breastfeeding ad lib. Spoke with mother and reviewed overnight events, morning laboratory results, current plan, and possible discharge to home tomorrow.

ICD-10-CM: **R50.9** (fever, unspecified)

CPT: **99232** (moderate MDM, ≥35 minutes)

Teaching Point: In this example, the MDM is moderate (3 of 3 elements support moderate, although only 2 of 3 are required).

Level of problem addressed ||||➡ Moderate (undiagnosed with uncertain prognosis)

Level of data reviewed and analyzed ||||➡ Limited (if tests were ordered by the physician of the same specialty and same group practice) or moderate (if the 3 unique test results reviewed were ordered by a physician of another group practice or other specialty)

Level of risk of morbidity ||||➡ Moderate (managing IV antibiotics)

Time cannot be used as the controlling factor in selection of the code because the documentation does not indicate the total time spent on the date of the encounter. It is strongly recommended that all admission and progress notes document the time of the total encounter. If a colleague must see the patient later in the day, the total time for the day may allow a higher level of care.

Tests are counted toward the level of data for the encounter at which the tests are ordered because review of results is included in the order. However, when a physician or QHP reviews results of tests ordered by a physician or QHP of another specialty or other group practice, the review is counted toward the amount and/or complexity of data for that visit.

➤ **A physician reevaluates a 14-year-old who was seen in consultation late on the prior evening following admission to observation for a first-time tonic-clonic seizure.** The physician obtains additional history from the patient and parents, completes a focused examination, reviews new laboratory test results, and explains a suspected diagnosis of juvenile generalized epilepsy. Additional testing is planned for early the next morning. The physician's total time devoted to the patient's care on this date is 45 minutes.

ICD-10-CM: **R56.9** (unspecified convulsions)

CPT: **99232** (≥35 minutes)

Teaching Point: The physician's total time supports code **99232**. Fifty minutes or more is required to report **99233** on the basis of total time.

Hospital Inpatient or Observation Discharge Management

▲**99238**   Hospital inpatient or observation discharge day management; 30 minutes or less on the date of the encounter
▲**99239**   more than 30 minutes on the date of the encounter

Codes **99238** (≤30 minutes) and **99239** (>30 minutes) are reported for discharge management services by the physician or QHP who is responsible for discharge services (the attending physician). Services by other physicians or QHPs who may have interacted with the patient/family and who provided additional instructions to the patient/family and coordinated post-discharge services may be reported with subsequent care codes **99231–99233**.

Same date admission and discharge services, performed at 2 distinct encounters, are reported with codes **99234–99236**. For admission and discharge services provided at 1 encounter (1 patient visit), report **99221–99223**.

Reporting is based on the total time (does not have to be continuous) spent performing all final discharge services, including, *as appropriate,* examination of the patient, discussion of the hospital stay, patient and/or family counseling, instructions for continuing care to all relevant caregivers, and preparation of referral forms, prescriptions, and medical records.

> If the total time spent in performing discharge management is not documented in the medical record, code 99239 cannot be supported.

- Although time is the total time spent in discharge management on the date of the encounter (eg, time of documentation), a face-to-face physician-patient encounter in the hospital is required.
- Only the physician's total time spent on the date of the discharge management is reported with codes **99238** and **99239**. Do not include time spent documenting discharge on a date after the service was rendered.

● indicates a new code; ▲, revised; #, re-sequenced; ✚, add-on; ★, audiovisual technology; and ◀, synchronous interactive audio.

- Time spent on the day of discharge performing separately reported services (eg, newborn circumcision) is not included in the discharge management time.
- Report discharge management services **99238** or **99239** provided to patients who die during their hospital stay *when the service is provided on the date of death.* An exception is a neonate who dies on the date of birth; report only the appropriate level of hospital care (ie, initial hospital care, intensive care, or critical care) in this instance.
  — Codes **99238** and **99239** are not reported for completion of a death certificate or for completion of records *on a date after the date of death.*

> **Most health plans do not pay for services provided after the date of the patient's death (ie, the date that the patient's coverage ended).**

Discharge codes are not reported

✖ When a patient is transferred to another physician or another unit in the same facility or for transitions between observation and inpatient status.

✖ When a patient is transferred to another hospital and receives care from the same physician or a physician of the same group and specialty. Report subsequent hospital care in lieu of discharge management (and initial hospital care).

Examples

➤ **An attending physician provides a final inpatient visit to an adolescent boy who was admitted on a prior date.** The physician explains to the patient that he will need outpatient care after discharge. The emancipated minor left foster care a year ago and has been working, but his health plan has high out-of-pocket costs that he cannot afford. The patient also shares a concern that he may be evicted from the motel where he lives because of inability to pay the weekly rent. The physician orders a consultation with a hospital social worker to connect the patient with his financial assistance before discharge. The physician also meets with a utilization management nurse regarding the need to connect the patient with a source of continued care after discharge, preferably with a clinic that offers a fee schedule based on the patient's ability to pay. The physician's documented total time on the date of the encounter is 70 minutes. The patient goes home the next morning after follow-up care has been arranged. If the physician provides a face-to-face service on that date, it is reported with a code for subsequent hospital care (**99231–99233**).

    Teaching Point: Time would be used as the controlling factor in selection of the code because the total time of service supports code **99239**. The date of discharge management may or may not coincide with the date that the patient leaves the facility.

    Reporting *ICD-10-CM* codes for the social determinants of health that affected patient management (eg, **Z59.86**, financial insecurity; **Z59.01**, sheltered homelessness; **Z59.7**, insufficient social insurance and welfare support) can help demonstrate the complexity of the service (ie, reason for time spent) and alert a payer that a patient may require care coordination and other benefits as available under health plan policy.

➤ **An attending physician is notified by phone of the death of a patient who was an inpatient.** The physician comes into the facility the next morning and completes documentation.

    Teaching Point: Discharge management services (**99238**, **99239**) are not reported when no face-to-face encounter (eg, pronouncement of death or hospital discussion with family) is provided by the attending physician.

Inpatient or Observation Consultations

Consultation Guidelines

> **Code 99251 has been deleted. See code 99252 to report a hospital consultation with straightforward medical decision-making.**

    CPT defines consultations as *initial encounters* provided by a physician or QHP at the request of another physician, QHP, or appropriate source (eg, nonclinical social worker, educator, lawyer, insurance company) to recommend care for a specific condition or problem. Codes **99252–99255** represent consultations provided to hospital inpatients, observation-level patients, nursing facility residents, or partial hospital setting patients.

Services requested by patients or by parents or other caregivers are not reported as consultations.

Consultation codes should not be reported by the physician who has agreed to accept transfer of care before an initial evaluation. Consultation codes are appropriate to report if the decision to accept transfer of care is not made until after the consultant's initial evaluation, regardless of site of service.

- When the role of attending physician is transferred to the consultant after the initial encounter, report subsequent hospital care codes (**99231–99233**) to indicate the level of service provided until the day of discharge management (**99238, 99239**).

> Codes 99252–99255 are not reported when the patient has received any face-to-face professional services from the consultant or another physician or qualified health care professional of the exact same specialty and subspecialty who belongs to the same group practice during the stay.

Consultation Following a Related E/M Service

If a consultation is performed in anticipation of, or related to, an admission by another physician or QHP and then the same consultant performs an encounter after the patient is admitted, report the consultant's inpatient or observation encounter with the appropriate subsequent care code (**99231–99233**). This instruction applies whether the consultation occurred on the date of the admission or a date previous to the admission. It also applies for consultations reported with any appropriate code (eg, office or other outpatient visit or office or other outpatient consultation).

- Report subsequent care codes (**99231–99233**) for follow-up visits provided by the same physician or QHP (or individuals of the same group practice and same exact specialty). Examples of a follow-up visit might be to complete the initial consultation when test results become available or to respond to a change in the patient's status.
- When a consultant has provided an outpatient E/M service to a patient before performing an inpatient or observation consultation on the same date, the consultant reports the outpatient E/M service with modifier **25** appended (eg, **99245 25** for outpatient consultation) and a subsequent hospital inpatient or observation care code **99231–99233** for the second service on the same date.

Examples

➤ **Dr A consulted with Dr B, requesting clearance for surgery for a patient who has cystic fibrosis and may benefit from gastrostomy and enteral feeding.** Dr B sees the patient in his office and recommends that the patient undergo the procedure as an inpatient with Dr B's medical management. Dr A admits the patient a few days later and consults Dr B for medical management.

Teaching Point: Dr B reports the outpatient consultation (eg, **99244** or, if the payer does not allow payment for consultation codes, **99214**) for the initial date of service and an applicable subsequent hospital inpatient or observation code (**99231–99233**) for the initial encounter in the hospital setting.

➤ **Dr A consulted Dr B, requesting Dr B's advice on treating a patient who has cystic fibrosis and is having increasingly poor pulmonary function.** After evaluating the patient, Dr B calls Dr A by phone and recommends hospital admission. Dr A, who does not provide hospital care, agrees with admission under the care of a hospitalist, who will consult Dr B for pulmonary E/M. Dr B provides an initial inpatient E/M service on the same date as the outpatient consultation.

Teaching Point: Dr B reports the outpatient consultation (eg, **99244 25** or, if the payer does not accept consultation code, **99214 25**) and an applicable subsequent hospital inpatient or observation code (**99231–99233**) for the initial encounter in the hospital setting on the same date of service.

Medicare Consultation Guidelines

Medicare does not recognize consultation codes but pays for the services by using codes for other E/M services. Detailed information on the *CPT* and Centers for Medicare & Medicaid Services (CMS) Medicare guidelines for reporting consultations for office and outpatient consultations is provided in **Chapter 7**. Please review those guidelines carefully as general guidelines that apply for all consultations.

Payers that adopt Medicare guidelines require that initial consultations provided to patients in observation or inpatient hospital status are reported by using hospital inpatient or observation care codes (eg, **99221–99223**). The admitting physician must report the initial hospital care services with modifier **AI** (principal physician of record) appended to the

● indicates a new code; ▲, revised; #, re-sequenced; ✚, add-on; ★, audiovisual technology; and ◀, synchronous interactive audio.

appropriate code to distinguish the services from the consulting physician. Subsequent face-to-face services, including new consultations within the same admission, are reported with subsequent inpatient or observation care codes **99231–99233** (see **Table 17-5**). Modifier **AI** is not required when reporting subsequent care codes.

Check with your commercial payers to learn if they follow Medicare consultation guidelines or have otherwise adopted consultation guidelines that differ from *CPT.*

Inpatient and Observation Consultations

99252 Inpatient or observation consultation for a new or established patient, which requires a medically appropriate history and/or examination and straightforward medical decision making.

When using total time on the date of the encounter for code selection, 35 minutes must be met or exceeded.

99253 Inpatient or observation consultation for a new or established patient, which requires a medically appropriate history and/or examination and low level of medical decision making.

When using total time on the date of the encounter for code selection, 45 minutes must be met or exceeded.

99254 Inpatient or observation consultation for a new or established patient, which requires a medically appropriate history and/or examination and moderate level of medical decision making.

When using total time on the date of the encounter for code selection, 60 minutes must be met or exceeded.

99255 Inpatient or observation consultation for a new or established patient, which requires a medically appropriate history and/or examination and high level of medical decision making.

When using total time on the date of the encounter for code selection, 80 minutes must be met or exceeded.

(For services ≥95 minutes, see discussion of prolonged services add-on code **99418** in the Prolonged Service on the Date of an E/M Service section later in this chapter.)

Codes **99252–99255** are reported only for an initial encounter, as defined previously in this chapter, per hospital inpatient or observation admission. There are no specific guidelines for the length of stay.

● Procedures performed by the consultant will be separately reported, although the time spent performing the procedure is not added to the total time of the E/M service.

Use **tables 17-2** and **17-6** to help select the appropriate codes in the example that follows.

Table 17-6. Codes for Hospital Inpatient or Observation Consultation Services				
Medical Decision-making	**Straightforward**	**Low**	**Moderate**	**High**
Code/Total Time	▲99252 ≥35 min	▲99253 ≥45 min	▲99254 ≥60 min	▲99255 ≥80 min

Example

➤ **A 10-year-old patient who was admitted to inpatient status from the ED for vomiting and general abdominal pain is under the care of a hospitalist, Dr A.** Dr A consults Dr B, a pediatric surgeon, regarding a diagnosis of acute appendicitis and a recommendation for appendectomy versus continued antibiotic therapy. Dr B's service on this day is an initial encounter (ie, the first encounter by Dr B or another individual in the same exact specialty and same group practice). Dr B evaluates the patient, discusses options with the patient's parents, and recommends surgery the next day because of the patient's risk of rupture. Dr B documents a written report in the medical record, including an independent interpretation of a sonogram and a discussion with Dr A about the recommended procedure. Dr B's total time of service is 45 minutes.

ICD-10-CM: **K35.80** (unspecified acute appendicitis)

CPT: **99255 57** (inpatient or observation consultation)

Teaching Point: Dr B's service is a consultation based on Dr A's request to recommend care for the patient's specific problem. The level of MDM supported is high because of the extensive review of data, including independent interpretation of a sonogram and discussion of management with Dr A and a decision for emergent surgery. Modifier **57**

indicates that a decision for surgery was made at the encounter and may prevent bundling of the initial hospital care with the preservice work of the procedure.

If the patient's health plan did not pay for services reported with consultation codes, Dr B would report initial hospital or observation care **99223 57** because of the high MDM.

Interprofessional Telephone/Internet/Electronic Health Record Consultation

A consultation request by a patient's physician or QHP soliciting opinion and/or treatment advice by telephone, internet, or electronic health record from a physician with specialty expertise (consultant) is reported by the consultant with interprofessional consultation codes **99446–99451**. Codes are selected on the basis of the minutes of medical consultative discussion and review.

- When reporting codes **99446–99449** (consultation with verbal and written report), the consultant must spend at least 5 minutes, with more than 50% of the time reported as interprofessional consultation spent in medical consultative verbal or internet discussion rather than review of data (eg, medical records, test results).
- The service time for code **99451** (consultation with written report only) is based on total review and interprofessional communication time. No face-to-face contact between the patient and consultant is required. The patient may be in the inpatient or outpatient setting.

Code **99452** may be reported by a requesting physician who spends 16 to 30 minutes on the date of service preparing for the referral and/or communicating with the consultant.

For full code descriptors and a detailed discussion of interprofessional consultation, see **Chapter 9**.

Prolonged Hospital E/M Services

Prolonged Service on the Date of an E/M Service

#★✚●**99418** Prolonged inpatient or observation evaluation and management service(s) time with or without direct patient contact beyond the required time of the primary service when the primary service level has been selected using total time, each 15 minutes of total time

(List separately in addition to the code for the primary E/M service.)

Code **99418** is used to report prolonged total time provided by the physician or QHP on the date of an inpatient or observation service (or nursing facility service). Report **99418** only when

- The code for the primary E/M service was selected on the basis of the physician's or QHP's total time on the date of the encounter.
- The total time exceeds the minimum total time of the highest level of service in the code category (ie, **99223**, **99233**, **99236**, **99255**, **99306**, **99310**) *by no less than 15 minutes.*
- Time spent performing other separately reported services (eg, procedures, interpretation and report of test results) is not included in the total time of the E/M service.

Table 17-7 provides time ranges for reporting **99418** in conjunction with each applicable code.

Table 17-7. Direct Prolonged Service Codes for Inpatient and Observation Care	
Primary Service Code (min)	**Time Range (min) = Codes × Unit(s)**
99223 (≥75)	90–104 = **99223, 99418** × 1. 105–119 = **99223, 99418** × 2.
99233 (≥50)	65–79 = **99233, 99418** × 1. 80–94 = **99233, 99418** × 2.
99236 (≥85)	100–114 = **99236, 99418** × 1. 115–129 = **99236, 99418** × 2.
99255 (≥80)	95–109 = **99255, 99418** × 1. 110–124 = **99255, 99418** × 2.

● indicates a new code; ▲, revised; #, re-sequenced; ✚, add-on; ★, audiovisual technology; and ◀, synchronous interactive audio.

Do not report **99418**

✖ For any unit of less than 15 minutes beyond the required time of the primary E/M service or prior unit of prolonged service

✖ On the same date of service as psychotherapy services (eg, **90833**, **90836**, **90838**)

✖ On the same date as prolonged service on a date when no E/M service is provided (**99358**, **99359**) or when reporting prolonged clinical staff time (**99415**, **99416**)

Examples

➤ **Dr A spends a total of 140 minutes reviewing extensive medical records and providing initial hospital care to a patient whose condition required multiple episodes of care throughout the day.**

Teaching Point: Codes **99223** (≥75) and **99418** × 4 units are reported. Each additional unit of **99418** is supported by at least 15 minutes beyond the prior unit.

➤ **Dr A spends 40 minutes reviewing extensive medical records in addition to an initial inpatient E/M service reported on same date.** The code for the initial inpatient E/M service (**99223**) was selected on the basis of high MDM and is not supported by the physician's total time.

Teaching Point: Code **99418** would not be reported. Prolonged service is not reported when the code for the related E/M service is not selected on the basis of total time. Because Dr A provided a face-to-face E/M service on this date, codes **99358** and **99359** are not reported.

Prolonged Service on Date Other Than the Face-to-face E/M Service Without Direct Patient Contact

99358   Prolonged evaluation and management service before and/or after direct patient care; first hour

99359   each additional 30 minutes (Use code **99359** in conjunction with code **99358**.)

Report **99358** and **99359** only when a prolonged service is *provided on a date other than the date of a face-to face E/M encounter* with the patient and/or family/caregiver. Services are indirect but related to care of a single patient (eg, reviewing medical records, imaging, and/or developing and coordinating a patient management plan).

Codes **99358** and **99359**

● Represent the total time spent by a physician or QHP (ie, not by clinical staff) on a single date of service.

● Must relate to a face-to-face professional service provided or planned to be provided by a physician or QHP and must be relevant to ongoing care.

● Are always provided and reported on a different date than the related E/M service. The related primary service may be any E/M service whether or not time was used to select the level of the face-to-face service.

● Are not reported for a physician's or QHP's time attributed to other services such as care plan oversight (CPO; **99374–99380**), chronic care management by a physician or QHP (**99491**, **99437**), or principal care management by a physician or QHP (**99424**, **99425**).

Prolonged service of less than 30 minutes' total duration on a given date is not separately reported. **Table 17-8** shows the required time for reporting code **99358** (30–74 minutes) and **99359** (1 unit for each 30 minutes beyond the 1st hour and each additional 30 minutes). Code **99359** may be reported for the last 15 to 30 minutes of service beyond the prior reported unit of service. Do not add times of services *provided on different dates* to meet the time requirements for codes **99358** and **99359**.

Table 17-8. Indirect Prolonged Service Codes and Time Units	
Time of Service (min)	**Code(s) × Unit(s)**
<30	Not reported separately
30–74	**99358** (always reported with 1 unit of service)
75–104	**99358**, **99359** × 1
≥105	**99358**, **99359** × ≥2 (have an additional unit added for each 15–30 min beyond the prior unit)

● indicates a new code; ▲, revised; #, re-sequenced; ✚, add-on; ★, audiovisual technology; and ◄, synchronous interactive audio.

Examples

➤ **Dr A spends 40 minutes reviewing extensive medical records on the evening before an initial encounter with an inpatient whose admitting physician has requested a consultation.**

    Teaching Point: Code **99358** would be reported. Prolonged service of less than 30 minutes' total duration would not be separately reported.

➤ **Dr A spends 40 minutes reviewing extensive medical records before an initial inpatient consultation provided later on the same date.**

    Teaching Point: Code **99358** would not be reported. The time spent reviewing the medical records is included in the total time on the date of the encounter when selecting a code for the consultation service.

At the time of this publication, the CMS has proposed creation of a Healthcare Common Procedure Coding System **G** code for reporting prolonged service in conjunction with inpatient and observation services. See individual payer policy for reporting prolonged service to verify payable codes and time requirements.

Hospital-Mandated On-Call Services

99026	Hospital mandated on-call service; in-hospital, each hour
99027	out of hospital, each hour

- Codes **99026** and **99027** describe services provided by a physician who is on call per hospital mandate as a condition of medical staff privileges.
- Used to report on-call time spent by the physician when they are not providing other services.
- Time spent performing separately reportable services should not be included in time reported as mandated on-call services.
- Most payers do not cover these services because they consider this a contract issue between the hospital and physician. However, these codes may be used either for tracking purposes or for credit in larger groups by assigning the code a relative value unit (RVU) when determining annual bonuses based on individual RVU production.

Continuing Care After Hospitalization

Prevention of readmittance and/or ED visits following hospitalization is a key goal of many quality improvement programs. In recent years, *CPT* and payers have recognized a need for codes to capture services related to care coordination and management of chronic and episodic conditions that may lead to unnecessary emergency and inpatient care. For physicians continuing patient care after hospital discharge, services such as transitional care management, principal (ie, single serious disease) care management, or chronic (ie, multiple chronic illnesses) care management offer opportunities to provide and be compensated for care aimed at reducing the risk of decline, exacerbation, and/or functional decline.

See **Chapter 10** for more information on care management services and other indirect services such as medical team conferences, CPO, and advance care planning.

The AAP *Pediatric Evaluation and Management: Coding Quick Reference Card 2023* (https://shop.aap.org/pediatric-evaluation-and-management-coding-quick-reference-card-2023) is an easy-to-use card that will help users navigate the steps to ensure proper code-level reporting for many E/M services (eg, it provides tables showing key component and time requirements for each type of code).

Chapter Takeaways

This chapter informs on many aspects of code selection for services provided to patients in hospital inpatient or observation status.

- *CPT* no longer includes separate codes for differentiating E/M services provided to patients in observation status. The retained codes are used to report initial, subsequent, and discharge management services in either inpatient or observation status.
- **99234–99236** are now reported only when 2 distinct encounters are provided for admission and discharge on the same date of service.
- **99252–99255** are reported only when the service qualifies as a consultation, is the initial encounter during the hospital stay, and does not relate to another E/M service by the same physician or QHP provided to the patient on the same or different date.
- Prolonged service in a facility setting is reported with code **99418** when the required time of the associated E/M service, which was selected on the basis of time, has been exceeded by at least 15 minutes.
- Prolonged service codes **99358** and **99359** are not reported on the same date as a face-to-face E/M service that may be reported on the basis of the total time on the date of the encounter.

Resources

AAP Coding Assistance and Education

AAP *Pediatric Evaluation and Management: Coding Quick Reference Card 2023* (https://shop.aap.org/pediatric-evaluation-and-management-coding-quick-reference-card-2023)

Online Exclusive Content at www.aap.org/cfp2023

"Hospital or Observation Evaluation and Management Services: Code Selection Requirements" (**Table 17-2**, printable version)

Chapter 17. Noncritical Hospital Evaluation and Management Services

Chapter 17. Noncritical Hospital Evaluation and Management Services

Test Your Knowledge!

1. **When can a physician select a code for an initial hospital care service based on time?**
   a. When the physician has documented the total time spent on the date of the encounter.
   b. Physicians cannot select initial hospital care codes based on time.
   c. Only when more than 50% of the total unit/floor time was spent in counseling and/or coordinating care.
   d. Only when the unit/floor time of the highest level of initial hospital care has been met.

2. **Under Medicare split or shared guidelines, which determines who (ie, the treating physician or qualified health care professional) reports a split/shared hospital care service reported based on total time?**
   a. The physician must always report the service.
   b. Split/shared guidelines do not determine who reports the service.
   c. The individual who spent the greater portion of the combined time reports the service.
   d. Total time cannot be used in code selection for a split/shared service.

3. **True or false? An outpatient evaluation and management (E/M) service provided on the same date may by separately reported in addition to an initial inpatient or observation E/M service.**
   a. True
   b. False

4. **Which of the following services is reported when an attending physician provides both an initial face-to-face hospital service and discharge management at 1 encounter?**
   a. Same date admission and discharge service (**99234–99236**)
   b. Initial hospital or observation service (**99221–99223**)
   c. Subsequent hospital or observation service (**99231–99233**)
   d. Discharge management (**99238, 99239**)

5. **Which of the following codes is reported when a physician documents 90 minutes spent providing initial hospital care with documentation of moderate medical decision-making?**
   a. **99222, 99418** × 2
   b. **99223**
   c. **99222, 99418** × 1
   d. **99223, 99418** × 1

Critical and Intensive Care

CPT copyright 2022 American Medical Association. All rights reserved.

Contents

● indicates a new code; ▲, revised; #, re-sequenced; ✚, add-on; ★, audiovisual technology; and ◀, synchronous interactive audio.

Chapter Highlights

- This chapter focuses on correctly coding critical and intensive care services, including
  - Attendance at delivery
  - Neonatal resuscitation
  - Hourly critical care
  - Critical care of the neonate, infant, and child younger than 6 years
  - Intensive care of the recovering or low birth weight neonate and infant
- Services commonly reported before and after intensive or critical care services, such as care during emergency transport, are also included.

Evaluation and management (E/M) of the child who no longer requires intensive or critical care is discussed in **Chapter 17**.

Defining Critical Care

- A *critical illness or injury* is defined by *Current Procedural Terminology* (*CPT*®) as one that acutely impairs 1 or more vital organs such that there is a high probability of imminent or life-threatening deterioration of the patient's condition.
- Services qualify as critical care *only if both* the injury or illness *and* the treatment being delivered meet the following criteria:
  - The illness or injury acutely impairs 1 or more vital organs as defined previously.
  - The treatment delivered involves high-complexity medical decision-making (MDM) to prevent life-threatening deterioration of the patient's condition.
- Critical care involves high-complexity MDM to assess, manipulate, and support vital organ system function(s); treat single or multiple organ system failure; and/or prevent further life-threatening deterioration of the patient's condition.
- Immaturity alone, or any of the specific procedures, equipment, or therapies associated with care of the immature neonate, does not define critical care.
- Coding critical care is not determined by the location in which the care is delivered but by the nature of the care being delivered and the condition of the patient requiring care.
- Critical care is not limited to an inpatient setting or a critical care area, and a physician of any specialty can provide these services. Services must be provided directly by the physician or other qualified health care professional (QHP).
- Many typically performed procedures are included (bundled) in the work valuation of each critical care code and cannot be reported separately (**Table 18-1**). (See also the Procedures *Not* Bundled With Critical/Intensive Care Services section later in this chapter for commonly provided services not bundled with hourly and/or neonatal and pediatric critical care service.)

Table 18-1. Critical Care Bundled Services			
CPT Code and Procedure	**Hourly Critical Care** 99291, 99292	**Pediatric Transport** 99466, 99467	**Neonatal/Pediatric Critical and Intensive Care** 99468–99476, 99477–99480
Interpretation and Monitoring			
71045 X-ray, chest; single view **71046** X-ray, chest; 2 views	X	X	X
✛93598 Cardiac output measurement(s), thermodilution or other indicator dilution method, performed during cardiac catheterization for the evaluation of congenital heart defects	X	X	X
94760 Pulse oximetry; single determination **94761** multiple determinations (eg, during exercise) **94762** by continuous overnight monitoring	X	X	X

Continued on next page

• indicates a new code; ▲, revised; #, re-sequenced; ✛, add-on; ★, audiovisual technology; and ◄, synchronous interactive audio.

Table 18-1 (*continued*)

CPT Code and Procedure	Hourly Critical Care 99291, 99292	Pediatric Transport 99466, 99467	Neonatal/Pediatric Critical and Intensive Care 99468–99476, 99477–99480
Vascular Access Procedures			
36000 Introduction of needle or intracatheter, vein	X	X	X
36140 Catheterization extremity artery			X
36400 Venipuncture, <3 years, requiring physician or QHP skill; femoral or jugular vein **36405** scalp vein **36406** other vein		X	X
36410 Venipuncture, ≥3 years, requiring physician or QHP skill	X		X
36415 Collection of venous blood by venipuncture	X	X	X
36420 Venipuncture, cutdown; younger than age 1 year			X
36430 Transfusion, blood or blood components **36440** Push transfusion, blood, 2 years or younger			X
36510 Catheterization of umbilical vein, newborn			X
36555 Insertion of non-tunneled CICC; <5 years of age			X
36591 Collection blood from venous access device	X	X	X
36600 Arterial puncture, withdrawal of blood for diagnosis	X	X	X
36620 Arterial catheterization, percutaneous **36660** Catheterization, umbilical artery, newborn			X
Other Procedures			
31500 Endotracheal intubation, emergency			X
43752 Nasogastric or orogastric intubation, fluoroscopic guidance	X	X	X
43753 Gastric intubation including lavage if performed	X	X	X
51100 Aspiration of bladder; by needle			X
51701 Insertion of non-indwelling bladder catheter **51702** Temporary indwelling bladder catheter; simple			X
62270 Spinal puncture, lumbar, diagnostic			X
92953 Temporary transcutaneous pacing	X	X	X
94002 Ventilation initiation; inpatient/observation, initial day **94003** each subsequent day	X	X	X
94004 Ventilation initiation; nursing facility, per day	X		X
94375 Respiratory flow volume loop			X
94610 Intrapulmonary surfactant administration			X
94660 CPAP, initiation and management **94662** CNP, initiation and management	X	X	X
94780 Car seat/bed testing, infants through 12 months; 60 minutes **94781** each additional full 30 minutes			X

Abbreviations: CICC, centrally inserted central venous catheter; CNP, continuous negative pressure; CPAP, continuous positive airway pressure; *CPT, Current Procedural Terminology;* QHP, qualified health care professional.

● indicates a new code; ▲, revised; #, re-sequenced; ✚, add-on; ★, audiovisual technology; and ◄, synchronous interactive audio.

Procedures *Not* Bundled With Critical/Intensive Care Services

When reporting hourly critical or neonatal and pediatric critical and intensive care services, many services commonly performed in the provision of critical care are not bundled into the intensive or critical care services. However, claim edits may require appending a modifier to indicate that the services were distinct. Examples (not all inclusive) of procedures that are not bundled with critical care services include

- Thoracentesis (**32554, 32555**) (via needle or pigtail catheter)
- Percutaneous pleural drainage with insertion of indwelling catheter (**32556, 32557**)
- Complete (double volume) exchange transfusion (**36450**, newborn; **36455**, other)
- Partial exchange transfusion (**36456**)
- Abdominal paracentesis (**49082, 49083**)
- Bone marrow aspiration (**38220**)
- Circumcision (**54150**)
- Cardioversion (**92960**)
- Cardiopulmonary resuscitation (**92950**)
- Extracorporeal membrane oxygenation (ECMO) (**33946–33949**)
- Peripherally inserted central catheter (**36568–36573**)
- Insertion of non-tunneled centrally inserted central venous catheter, older than 5 years (**36556**)
- Replacement (rewire) of non-tunneled centrally inserted central venous catheter (**36580**)
- Therapeutic apheresis (**36511–36514**)
- Insertion of cannula for hemodialysis, other purpose (separate procedure); vein to vein (**36800**)
- Placement of needle for intraosseous infusion (**36680**)
- Initiation of selective head or total body hypothermia in the critically ill neonate (**99184**)

Example

➤ **In addition to providing 45 minutes of critical care in the emergency department (ED), a physician places a needle for intraosseous infusion.**

99291 (critical care, first 30–74 minutes)

36680 (needle placement for intraosseous infusion)

Critical care service time is documented and distinctly identifiable in the patient record from time spent performing the separately reportable needle placement (ie, the total time or the start and stop times of the procedure are documented).

National Correct Coding Initiative (NCCI) edits do not bundle **36680** and **99291**; however, individual payer edits may require appending modifier **25** to code **99291** to indicate that the critical care service was significant and separately identifiable from the separately reported procedure.

> Emergency cardiac defibrillation is included in cardiopulmonary resuscitation (CPR; 92950). Per the Medicaid National Correct Coding Initiative manual, if emergency cardiac defibrillation without CPR is performed in the emergency department or critical/intensive care unit, the cardiac defibrillation service is not separately reportable. Report code 92960 only for elective cardioversion.

Many practice management and billing systems include claim scrubbers providing an alert that claim edits apply and a modifier may be appropriate on the basis of clinical circumstances. Payers may also offer online tools for determining when code pair edits apply.

Hourly Critical Care

99291   Critical care, E/M of the critically ill or critically injured patient; first 30–74 minutes

✛99292   each additional 30 minutes (Use in conjunction with **99291**.)

Guidelines for reporting codes **99291** and **99292**

- Report only when critical care is provided for 30 minutes or more
  - In the outpatient setting (eg, ED, office, clinic) *regardless of age*
  - To an inpatient 6 years or older (Daily critical care of a child younger than 6 years is discussed in the Neonatal and Pediatric Daily Critical Care Codes section later in this chapter.)

● indicates a new code; ▲, revised; #, re-sequenced; ✛, add-on; ★, audiovisual technology; and ◄, synchronous interactive audio.

 Chapter 18. Critical and Intensive Care

- Concurrently by a second physician from a different specialty to a critically ill or injured patient, regardless of age
- To an inpatient 5 years or younger when the patient is being transferred to another facility where a receiving physician of the same specialty but different medical group will be reporting the daily inpatient critical care service codes (**99468** and **99469**, **99471** and **99472**, **99475** and **99476**)
- By the physician physically transporting a critically ill child older than 2 years or when payer policy does not recognize codes **99466** and **99467** (face-to-face transport care of the critically ill or injured patient 24 months or younger [discussed in the Face-to-face Pediatric Critical Care Patient Transport section later in this chapter])
- Review **Table 18-1** and the Procedures *Not* Bundled With Critical/Intensive Care Services section, presented earlier in this chapter, to determine which services are bundled (ie, included in the value assigned to critical care services) and which ones are separately reported (eg, lumbar puncture, endotracheal intubation, thoracentesis).

> The reported time of critical care cannot include any time spent performing procedures or services that are reported separately.

- Report **99291** and, when appropriate, **99292** when another physician or QHP of a *different specialty* (from either the same or a different group practice) provides neonatal or pediatric critical care services (**99468–99476**) on the same date.
- A teaching physician may report time-based critical care services only they were present for the entire period for which the claim is submitted and that time is supported in documentation of the service.
- When inpatient and outpatient critical care services are provided to a neonate, infant, or child younger than 6 years on the same date by the same physician (or physician of the same group and specialty), only the daily *inpatient* critical care codes are reported (**99468–99476**). For exceptions, see the Neonatal and Pediatric Daily Critical Care Codes and Emergency Medical Services Supervision and Patient Transport sections later in this chapter.
- Other significant, separately identifiable E/M services (eg, **99282–99285** for ED E/M services) can be reported in addition to time-based critical care services as appropriate. Do not count time spent in separately reported E/M services in critical care time.

> Payer policies for same date/same physician critical care and other evaluation and management (E/M) services may vary. Medicare policy limits payment of emergency department services 99281–99285 and other E/M services on the same date as critical care services to when all the following circumstances are true:
>
> 1. The other E/M visit was provided before the critical care services at a time when the patient did not require critical care.
> 2. The services were medically necessary.
> 3. The services were separate and distinct, with no duplicative elements from the critical care services provided later in the day.
>
> Modifier 25 (significant, separately identifiable E/M service) is appended to the code for the noncritical care service.

Time Units of Hourly Critical Care

For codes **99291** and **99292**, reporting is time based. **Table 18-2** lists times and billing units. The total floor or unit time devoted to the patient in the provision of critical care is used in code selection.

Critical care time is counted *when the physician or QHP is immediately available to the patient,* including face-to-face time spent between the physician and patient and other time spent directly related to the patient's care (eg, reviewing test results, discussing care with other medical staff or family, documenting services in the medical record).

Table 18-2. Reporting Hourly Critical Care Services

Do not report services of <30 min as critical care; report the appropriate E/M service for the site where service is provided.

Duration of Face-to-face Critical Care	30–74 min	75–104 min	105–134 min	135–164 min	165–194 min
CPT Codes and Units of Service	99291	99291 × 1, 99292 × 1	99291 × 1, 99292 × 2	99291 × 1, 99292 × 3	99291 × 1, 99292 × 4

Abbreviations: *CPT, Current Procedural Terminology;* E/M, evaluation and management.

- Time spent in the provision of critical care does not need to be continuous. The cumulative time of critical care provided on a single date of service is used to calculate the units of service provided.

When a *continuous period* of critical care occurs before and after midnight, report the total time on the date that the period of care was initiated. Do not report a second initial hour of critical care for the continuous period beginning at midnight.

- Code **99291** is reported once on a given date of service when 30 to 74 minutes of critical care is performed. If less than 30 minutes of critical care is provided, an appropriate E/M service (eg, **99202–99215**, **99282–99285** for ED services) is reported.
- Code **99292** is reported with 1 unit for each additional period up to 30 minutes beyond the previous period. Time spent providing critical care services must be documented in the medical record.

Unless otherwise indicated in payer policy, services of physicians and QHPs of the same group practice and exact same specialty are typically considered to be provided by a single physician or QHP.

- Code **99291** is reported once for 30 to 74 minutes of critical care performed by 1 or more physicians or QHPs of the same group practice and same exact specialty.
- When the combined times of physicians and QHPs in the same group practice and specialty support reporting of code **99292**, follow payer guidelines regarding reporting by each individual physician or QHP (eg, the same physician reports **99291** and **99292**, or the first physician reports **99291** and the other physician reports **99292**, as indicated).

Medicare's Assignment of a Qualified Health Care Professional's Specialty

When qualified health care professionals (QHPs) work with physicians, *Current Procedural Terminology* considers the QHPs to be working in the exact same specialty and exact same subspecialties as the physician. This guideline is not consistent with Medicare policy. Under Medicare policy, distinct specialty codes are assigned to QHPs such as nurse practitioners (50), physician assistants (97), and clinical nurse specialists (89). This assignment affects how critical care is reported to Medicare, and plans that follow Medicare policy, when provided in part by a physician and in part by a QHP.

See the Split or Shared Critical Care Services section later in this chapter to learn how Medicare policy allows for a combination of a physician's and a QHP's time spent in providing critical care on the same date of service.

Medicare Guidelines for Critical Care Services

Medicare policy is often adopted by other payers (eg, Medicaid plans, group health plans). For this reason, it is good to be aware of Medicare policies that may affect how services are reported.

Hourly Critical Care Services by Physicians of the Same Specialty and Same Group Practice

When 2 physicians of the same specialty and same group practice or 2 QHPs of the same group practice provide hourly critical care services on the same date, Medicare policy allows reporting based on the combined times of each physician or each QHP.

See the Split or Shared Critical Care Services section later in this chapter for Medicare payment policy that may apply to critical care services provided by a physician and QHP in the same group practice on the same date of service.

Under the Medicare policy for reporting critical care services provided by 2 or more individuals of the same specialty and same group practice,

- The time of critical care services by 2 physicians or by 2 QHPs may be combined to support code **99291**.
- A second physician cannot report **99291** when the initial 30 to 74 minutes of critical care services on the same date were provided by another physician of the same specialty and same group practice. The physician who provided the initial period of critical care services reports **99291**. If the requirements for reporting **99292** are met by the combined critical care service times of the 2 physicians, the second physician may report **99292**.

All the time attributed to critical care services must be medically necessary, and each visit must meet the definition of critical care to combine the times for the purpose of code selection.

Examples

➤ **Dr A spends 20 minutes providing initial critical care services to the child and orders a transfer to another facility.** Dr B, a physician of the same specialty and same group practice, assumes management and provides 45 minutes of critical care to the child during transport to the receiving facility.

Dr A or Dr B reports **99291** × 1 (critical care, first 30–74 minutes).

● indicates a new code; ▲, revised; #, re-sequenced; ✚, add-on; ★, audiovisual technology; and ◀, synchronous interactive audio.

Teaching Point: Dr A's time does not support **99291**. However, because Dr B is in the same group practice and same specialty, the time spent by each physician is combined (20 + 45 = 65) to support **99291**. Medicare does not designate which physician reports the service.

➤ **A 13-year-old adolescent is admitted to the intensive care unit in respiratory distress.** Nurse practitioner A, who specializes in pulmonology, spends 50 minutes providing initial critical care services. Later, on the same date, Nurse practitioner B, of the same group practice and who specializes in infectious disease, provides 40 minutes of critical care.

Nurse practitioner A reports **99291** (critical care, first 30–74 minutes).

Nurse practitioner B reports **99292** × 1 (additional 30 minutes).

Teaching Point: The nurse practitioners are considered by Medicare policy to be of the same specialty, so only the first period of critical care services is reported with code **99291**.

Split or Shared Critical Care Services

Because Medicare does not consider QHPs to be working in the same specialty as physicians, a policy known as split or shared (split/shared) services is applied by Medicare policy when physicians and QHPs, not hospital employees, jointly provide E/M services in a facility setting. (In an office setting, incident-to policy [discussed in **Chapter 7**] applies, rather than split/shared.)

Under the split/shared policy, hourly critical care services (ie, the service times of a physician and QHP of the same group practice) can be combined and reported as a single service. However, the policy requires that the service be reported by *the individual who spent the greater amount of time providing critical care services.*

● Modifier **FS** (split or shared E/M visit) must be appended to the critical care code(s) on the claim (ie, **99291 FS** and, when applicable, **99292 FS**).

● When 2 or more physicians and QHPs spend time jointly meeting with or discussing the patient as part of a critical care service, the time can be counted only once for the purpose of reporting the split (or shared) critical care visit.

● The physician and the QHP must document their personally performed services, but the reporting individual (the one who spent the greater portion of time) is responsible for authenticating and dating the record.

Example

➤ **A 4-year-old arrives to the ED in critical condition.** The ED physician provides 50 minutes of critical care before the child's condition is stabilized so they may be transferred to another facility. Pending transfer, a QHP of the same group practice assumes treatment of the patient in now-stable condition. The patient's condition deteriorates, and the QHP provides another 30 minutes of critical care before a team arrives to accept treatment of the patient during transport.

The ED physician reports **99291 FS** and **99292 FS** × 1 (additional 30 minutes).

Teaching Point: The ED physician who provided the substantive or greater amount (ie, 50 of 80 minutes) of the total time reports the critical care services with modifier **FS** appended to indicate that the services were split/shared. The physician and the QHP each document the individually provided services and time spent. Under Medicare policy, the individual reporting the service must authenticate/sign and date the record of the split/shared services reported.

Neonatal and Pediatric Daily Critical Care

Defining the Neonatal Period

For coding purposes, the neonatal period begins at birth and continues through the completed 28th day after birth, ending on the 29th calendar day after birth. The day of birth is considered day 0 (zero). Therefore, the day after birth is considered day 1.

This definition is important in selecting the initial- and subsequent-day neonatal critical care codes **99468** and **99469** as well as code **99477** for the initial hospital care of the neonate, 28 days or younger, who requires intensive observation, frequent interventions, and other intensive care services.

ICD-10-CM Guidelines and Neonatal Critical Care

It is important to correctly assign *International Classification of Diseases, 10th Revision, Clinical Modification* (ICD-10-CM) codes that reflect the diagnoses for which critical care services were required. Assign codes for neonatal conditions that require treatment or further investigation, prolong the length of stay, or require resource utilization as well as codes for conditions that have implications for future health care needs.

> When care is provided by the attending physician during the birth admission, report first a code from category Z38 (liveborn infants according to place of birth and type of delivery). Codes for abnormal conditions are reported as secondary to the code for live birth. When a neonate is transferred to another facility after birth, the admission to the receiving facility is not a birth admission and Z38 codes are not reported.

- ICD-10-CM contains codes (**P00–P96**) for conditions originating in the perinatal period. These codes are reported for conditions described as having their origin in the fetal or perinatal period (before birth through the first 28 days after birth) even if morbidity occurs later. Again, this period includes the completed 28th day after birth with the day of birth being counted as day 0 (zero).
  — These codes are to be reported only when the condition originates in this time, but they can be reported beyond the perinatal period if the condition(s) causes morbidity or is the primary reason for or contributing to the reason the patient is receiving health care.
  — The perinatal code should continue to be used regardless of the patient's age if a condition originates in the perinatal period and continues throughout the patient's life.

Example

➤ **A 30-day-old who was a 26-weeks' gestation preterm neonate continues to require critical or intensive care due to a condition originating in the perinatal period.**
    Teaching Point: The *ICD-10-CM* code that is linked to the critical or intensive care service is the appropriate perinatal code (**P00–P96**) for the condition(s) managed or treated.

- Any condition *originating* after the perinatal period (29th calendar day after birth and beyond) is not reported with codes for perinatal conditions.
- A diagnosis of prematurity must be documented to support reporting a code for prematurity. Coders cannot assign codes for prematurity based solely on documented gestational age.
- Codes in category **P05** are reported for the newborn affected by fetal growth restriction or slow intrauterine growth.
  — Codes in subcategory **P05.0** are used to report that the neonate is light for gestational age but not small (weight below but length above the 10th percentile). These neonates have often been said to exhibit *asymmetrical growth restriction.*
  — Codes in subcategory **P05.1** are used to report that the neonate is small and light (both weight and length below the 10th percentile) for gestational age. These newborns have often been said to exhibit *symmetrical growth restriction* or *intrauterine growth restriction.*
- Code **P05.2** is provided for reporting fetal (intrauterine) malnutrition affecting a newborn whose weight is not below the 10th percentile and has a significant disparity between weight and length percentiles.

> Learn more about reporting codes in category P05 in the December 2020 *AAP Pediatric Coding Newsletter* article, "Coding for Abnormalities in Fetal Growth" (https://doi.org/10.1542/pcco_book200_document002).

- Codes from category **P07** (disorders of newborn related to short gestation and low birth weight [not due to fetal malnutrition]) are reported on the basis of the recorded birth weight (*not less than the 10th percentile*) and estimated gestational age to indicate that these conditions are the cause of morbidity or reason for additional care of the newborn.
  — When both are documented, weight is sequenced before age.
  — These codes may be reported for a child as well as for an adult who was preterm or had a low birth weight as a newborn and this is affecting the patient's current health status.

  Codes in subcategory **P07.3-** (preterm newborn) should be reported for neonates born at 36 weeks' gestation who stay in the newborn nursery or who are cared for in the neonatal intensive care unit (NICU).

Chapter 18. Critical and Intensive Care

Do not report codes in subcategory **P07.0-** (extremely low birth weight newborn) and **P07.1-** (other low birth weight newborn) in conjunction with codes in category **P05** (disorders of the newborn due to slow fetal growth and fetal malnutrition). However, subcategory **P07.2-** (extreme immaturity of newborn) and **P07.3-** (preterm newborn) may be reported in addition to category **P05**.

Attendance at Delivery and Neonatal Resuscitation

Attendance at Delivery

99464   Attendance at delivery (when requested by the delivering physician or other qualified health care professional) and initial stabilization of newborn

Attendance at delivery (**99464**) is reported only when the physical presence of the provider is requested by the delivering physician and indicated for a newborn who may require immediate intervention (ie, stabilization, resuscitation, or evaluation for potential problems).

● Includes initial drying, stimulation, suctioning, blow-by oxygen, or continuous positive airway pressure (CPAP) without positive-pressure ventilation (PPV); a cursory visual inspection of the neonate; assignment of Apgar scores; and discussion of the care of the newborn with the delivering physician and parents. A quick look in the delivery room or examination after stabilization is not sufficient to support reporting of **99464**.

    — When qualifying resuscitative efforts are provided, code **99465** (delivery/birthing room resuscitation) is reported instead. Codes **99464** and **99465** cannot be reported on the same day of service.

See **Chapter 16** for further discussion and coding examples for code **99464**.

Neonatal Resuscitation

99465   Delivery/birthing room resuscitation, provision of positive pressure ventilation and/or chest compressions in the presence of acute inadequate ventilation and/or cardiac output

Attendance at delivery with neonatal resuscitation (**99465**)

● Requires PPV delivered by any means (resuscitation bag or T-piece resuscitator) and/or cardiac compressions.

✖ Do not report when T-piece resuscitator is used to provide CPAP only. If the neonate responds to provision of CPAP with an adequate respiratory effort, code **99464** should be reported.

● May be reported in addition to any initial care service, including initial daily inpatient critical care (**99468**), hourly critical care (**99291**, **99292**), initial neonatal intensive care (**99477**), or normal newborn care (**99460**) if the resuscitation results in a stable full-term neonate.

Payers may require modifier **25** (significant, separately identifiable evaluation and management [E/M] service) appended to the code for E/M services reported in addition to code **99464** or **99465**. However, National Correct Coding Initiative edits do not bundle these services.

● Medically necessary procedures (eg, **31500**, intubation, endotracheal, emergency procedure; **31515**, laryngoscopy, direct, for aspiration; **36510**, catheterization of umbilical vein for diagnosis or therapy, newborn; **94610**, surfactant administration) essential to successful resuscitation that are performed in the delivery room before admission may also be reported in addition to codes **99465** and **99468** or **99477** (initial daily inpatient neonatal critical or intensive care).

    — Do not separately report services performed as a convenience before admission to the NICU.

    — Medical record documentation must clearly support that the services are provided as a required measure for emergency resuscitation and not as part of an admission protocol.

Documentation of neonatal resuscitation should explicitly state that the neonate demonstrated respiratory and/or cardiac instability requiring intervention, including apnea or inadequate respiratory effort to support gas exchange; that the provider instituted positive-pressure ventilation (PPV); and the neonate's response to the PPV.

See the "Stillborn Deliveries and Unsuccessful Resuscitation" box later in this chapter for discussion of billing for services provided to a mother and/or neonate when the outcome is a stillborn neonate or unsuccessful resuscitation of an ill neonate.

Example

➤ **A neonatologist attends an emergency cesarean delivery of a 34-weeks' gestation neonate whose mother has known, poorly controlled diabetes mellitus and a history of drug misuse. The neonate is born limp and cyanotic with no spontaneous respiratory activity.** The resuscitation includes PPV, intubation, and placement of an umbilical vein catheter with physiologic (normal) saline bolus (solution). The newborn, who is continuously bradycardic and pale, is admitted to the NICU where the neonatologist administers surfactant and initiates red blood cell transfusion.

The intubation and umbilical vein catheterization are separately reported procedures provided as part of the resuscitation and not as a convenience to the physician before admission.	**CPT** **99465** (delivery/birthing room resuscitation) **31500** (endotracheal intubation, emergency) **36510** (catheterization of umbilical vein for diagnosis or therapy, newborn) **99468 25** (initial daily neonatal critical care) **36450** (exchange transfusion, blood; newborn)

Teaching Point: Modifier **25** is appended to code **99468** to signify a significant, separately identifiable E/M service provided in addition to codes **31500** and **36510** because these services are bundled by NCCI edits. Codes **99465** and **99468** are not bundled by NCCI edits, but individual payers may require modifier **25** to designate separately identifiable critical care services on the same date. The surfactant administration is not separately reported when performed in conjunction with neonatal critical care. However, the red blood cell transfusion is separately reported.

Stillborn Deliveries and Unsuccessful Resuscitation

Questions arise on documentation, coding, and billing for services provided to a baby who is stillborn or is thought to be viable (eg, showing fetal distress before delivery) but who, shortly after birth, despite resuscitative efforts, never shows active signs of a heartbeat.

If a baby is delivered but is known to have expired in utero, a separate medical record will not be created. Therefore, any services performed by a pediatrician or neonatologist will be documented in the maternal record. The physician could be called on to perform an examination and/or discuss any known or discovered fetal anomalies. In this circumstance, the physician could charge an initial hospital inpatient or observation encounter (with the mother as the patient) only with counseling, by using time to determine the code level (99221–99223), which includes the physician's total time devoted to this service on the date of the encounter. In practice, many physicians may not charge for this service.

As with a known intrauterine fetal demise, a neonate who was felt to be viable may be born without evidence of a heart rate or respiratory effort. Resuscitative efforts may be started and then stopped after a determined amount of time. Although neonatal resuscitation (99465) could be coded and billed for, a separate medical record may not be created for the neonate. The service may be billed by using the mother as the patient; however, medical records would likely have to accompany the claim. Most payers will deny this claim, so an appeal would be required. It would be best to create a record for the baby so the services can be documented for both the physician and nursing staff. Again, in practice, many physicians do not charge for this service.

For a live-born neonate who experiences distress and dies in the delivery room, an individual medical record should be created to document the care. This service will be reported as neonatal resuscitation services (99465) with the deceased neonate as the recipient of care. Remember to also document and report any other separately billable services (eg, surfactant administration), when performed.

Although all services and procedures performed must be clearly documented in the maternal or neonatal medical record (if one is created), billing for the services will be up to the individual physician.

Neonatal Critical and Intensive Care Supervision Requirements

CPT states that codes **99468**, **99469**, and **99471–99476** are used to report services provided by a single individual "directing the inpatient care" of a critically ill neonate, infant, or child through 5 years of age. Constant in-house attendance by the supervising physician or QHP is not a requirement of neonatal critical and intensive care. However, the codes' values were established under the assumption that the reporting individual is physically present and participating directly in the patient's care for a significant portion of the reported service.

● Documentation in the patient's medical record should reflect this active participation, including documentation of hands-on care, such as a personal physical examination, and of the patient's condition that requires critical or intensive care.

Chapter 18. Critical and Intensive Care

- Supervision of all the care from a distance without face-to-face care is not reported as critical or intensive care.
- Medical record documentation must support the need for and meet the definition of critical care (eg, complex MDM, high probability of imminent or life-threatening deterioration, organ system failure).
- Care must be provided by the reporting individual, but it includes the services provided by the health care team functioning under the direct supervision of the physician *or a QHP (eg, neonatal nurse practitioner [NNP]) who is not employed by the hospital* when allowed under state licensure requirements.
- Typically, a neonate or an infant is evaluated during numerous intervals throughout a calendar day, depending on the clinical needs of the patient. The extent of the reporting individual's personal service (eg, overnight in-house care) and presence is determined by the complexity of the total population of neonates cared for in a nursery or the changes in a specific neonate's or infant's condition that cannot be adequately assessed or managed over the telephone.

For more information, refer to "Global Per Diem Critical Care Codes: Direct Supervision and Reporting Guidelines" at www.aap.org/cfp2023.

Coding Conundrum: Selecting the Appropriate Code

Many diagnoses or conditions, such as respiratory distress, infection, seizures, mild to moderate hypoxic-ischemic encephalopathy, and metabolic disorders, can be reported with codes **99468**, **99477**, or **99221–99223**. The patient's clinical status, required level of monitoring and observation, and present body weight determine which of these code series is chosen. Selection of the service must be justified by medical record documentation.

Neonatal and Pediatric Daily Critical Care Codes

Codes are
- Reported for critical care of children younger than 6 years in the inpatient setting.
- Global. They encompass all E/M services by an attending physician or QHP (including individuals of the exact same specialty in the same group practice) *on 1 calendar date.* (For exceptions [eg, critical care transport], see the Guidelines for Reporting Neonatal or Pediatric Inpatient Critical Care section later in this chapter.)

Only the attending or principal physician or qualified health care professional (QHP) reports daily critical or intensive care services. Other physicians and QHPs providing concurrent critical care must report hourly critical care code 99291 or 99292.

- Bundled. They have commonly performed procedures included in the E/M codes. See **Table 18-1** for services and procedures that are included with neonatal critical care codes.
- Not time based. Prolonged services *may not* be reported in conjunction with neonatal or pediatric critical care services.
- Not based on typical E/M rules as applied to services for which codes are selected on the basis of a level of MDM or total time on the date of an encounter.
- Reported on the basis of postnatal age (see Defining the Neonatal Period at the beginning of the Neonatal and Pediatric Daily Critical Care section earlier in this chapter) and initial or subsequent care (**Table 18-3**).

Table 18-3. Neonatal and Pediatric Daily (Global) Critical Care

Daily (Global) Critical Care	28 Days or Younger	29 Days Through 24 Months of Age	2 Through 5 Years of Age
Initial daily critical care	99468	99471	99475
Subsequent daily critical care	99469	99472	99476

Guidelines for Reporting Neonatal or Pediatric Inpatient Critical Care

- The physician or NNP (subject to state regulations, scope of practice, and hospital privilege credentials) primarily responsible for the patient on the date of service should report the neonatal or pediatric critical care codes. When both the physician and the NNP provide critical care services to a patient, only one may report the code.
- If critical care is provided in both the outpatient and inpatient settings by the same physician or a physician of the same specialty and group, only the inpatient code is reported.

● indicates a new code; ▲, revised; #, re-sequenced; ✚, add-on; ★, audiovisual technology; and ◀, synchronous interactive audio.

- Daily critical care codes are reported only once per day, per patient.
- When the same physician or physicians of the same specialty and group practice provide pediatric critical care during transport of a child 24 months or younger (**99466**, **99467**, **99485**, **99486**) and critical care after admission to the receiving facility, both services are reported and modifier **25** is appended to the transport code.
- Initial daily inpatient critical care codes (**99468**, **99471**, **99475**) are reported only once per calendar day and *once per hospital stay* for a given patient. For a second episode of critical care during the same hospital stay, report a subsequent critical care code (**99469**, **99472**, **99476**).
- Subsequent critical care may be reported on multiple days even if there is no change in the patient's condition if the patient continues to meet the critical care definition and documentation supports this level of service.
- Care may be provided on any unit of a hospital facility.

Subsequent-day intensive care codes (**99478–99480**, discussed in the Initial and Continuing Intensive Care section later in this chapter) are reported when critical care is no longer required and the neonate or infant who weighs 5,000 g or less on the day of service requires more intensive care than what is typically provided under routine subsequent hospital care (**99231–99233**). Once a neonate weighing at least 5,001 g no longer requires critical care services, report an appropriate level of subsequent-day inpatient hospital care codes (**99231–99233**).

Neonatal Critical Care

99468   Initial inpatient neonatal critical care, per day, for the evaluation and management of a critically ill neonate, 28 days of age or younger

99469   Subsequent inpatient neonatal critical care, per day, for the evaluation and management of a critically ill neonate, 28 days of age or younger

Selection of the appropriate code will depend on the patient's condition and the intensity of the service provided and documented on a particular day of service.

- Report **99468** and, when appropriate, **99469** in addition to normal newborn care (**99460**, **99462**) or neonatal consultation (**99252–99255**) when these services are provided on the same date that the patient later requires a separate encounter for critical care. Each service should be reported with the appropriate diagnosis code to support the service (eg, diagnosis codes for well newborn and the critical illness). However, a neonatologist would report only critical or intensive care services if a transfer of care occurs at the initial consultation.

> National Correct Coding Initiative edits bundle normal newborn care to neonatal critical care, but you may use modifier **25** (significant, separately identifiable evaluation and management service) to override the edit under appropriate circumstances (eg, separate encounters).

- If the neonate or infant becomes critically ill on a day when initial or subsequent intensive care services (**99477–99480**) have been provided and the same physician(s) or QHP(s) from the same group practice provide critical care services, report only initial or subsequent critical care (**99468–99476**) on the basis of the patient's age and whether this is the first or subsequent admission for critical care during the same hospital stay.

Coding Conundrum: Applying the Critical Care Definition

While immaturity commonly leads to many levels of organ dysfunction that will increase the risk of a critical illness in a newborn, neither immaturity alone nor any of the specific procedures or therapies associated with care of the immature neonate or infant qualifies alone for reporting critical care. The physician must use their experience and judgment in assigning the *Current Procedural Terminology* definition of critical care. In summary, these are patients presently at clear risk of death or serious morbidity, requiring close observation and frequent interventions and assessments, and high-level medical decision-making (MDM) is apparent in the medical record documentation. No single criterion places or excludes a patient from this category, and the patient is not required to demonstrate all the characteristics listed in this chapter. The most convincing way to demonstrate the appropriate application of a critical care code is to clearly document the neonate's condition in the medical record, noting the risks to the patient, frequency of needed assessments and interventions, degree and type of organ failure(s) the patient is presently experiencing, and level of the MDM.

● indicates a new code; ▲, revised; #, re-sequenced; ✚, add-on; ★, audiovisual technology; and ◀, synchronous interactive audio.

Chapter 18. Critical and Intensive Care

Examples

➤ **A full-term 3,500-g neonate is born cyanotic following a vaginal delivery.** He has minimal respiratory distress and appears otherwise vigorous. He is brought to the NICU, where a chest radiograph shows dramatic cardiomegaly and a marked increase in pulmonary markings. The attending neonatologist inserts an umbilical artery catheter and umbilical vein catheter to determine blood gas pressures. Electrocardiography is performed, and a pediatric cardiologist is consulted to obtain an emergency echocardiogram.

   Teaching Points: It is important to remember that respiratory support (ie, mechanical ventilation) is not required to report critical care services. In this case, serious cyanosis and clear evidence of cardiac decompensation qualify as critical care. Code **99468** would be reported for the neonatologist's initial date of neonatal critical care services. The umbilical vessel catheterizations are bundled with **99468**.

   Depending on the findings on the echocardiogram and a need for cardiac intensive care, the cardiologist may report critical care services (**99291**, **99292**), consultative services (**99252–99255**), or, if the payer does not accept consultation codes, initial hospital care (**99221–99223**) on the basis of the level of service provided. (See **Chapter 17** for more information on reporting consultations and reporting to payers who do not recognize consultation codes.)

➤ **Same patient as prior example.** The neonate is transferred to a cardiac center by the neonatologist.

   Teaching Point: The neonatologist would report time-based critical care codes (**99291**, **99292**) for the care provided before the transfer rather than **99468**. The receiving physician in the cardiac center would report code **99468** for the initial date of critical care.

> Only 1 individual reports daily critical care services for each patient per date of service. Other physicians and qualified health care professionals of different specialties and/or different group practices report critical care services by using **99291** and, when appropriate, **99292**.

➤ **A 6-day-old born at 31 weeks' gestation with unstable apnea is weaned off the ventilator to CPAP.** She is continued on caffeine, partial parenteral nutrition by central vein, and intravenous (IV) antibiotics.

   Code **99469** is reported because the medical record continues to document the neonate's instability and the continued need for critical care services.

Coding Conundrum: Apnea in Neonates

Apnea in neonates may be an expected component of preterm birth and may be effectively managed by manual stimulation, pharmacological stimulation, high-flow nasal oxygen, or continuous positive airway pressure. At other times, this symptom is associated with a serious underlying problem(s) and reflects the instability of a critically ill neonate. When this is the case, 1 or more of the same interventions will be required. The physician must employ their best clinical judgment and clearly document the factors that make the patient's present condition critical (or require intensive care). The same requirements for organ failure, risk of imminent deterioration, and complex medical decision-making apply. With apnea and many other conditions, the following information drives correct code selection: the total picture of the neonate with the diagnosis, clinical presentation, and immediate threat to life; the amount of hands-on and supervisory care provided by the physician; and the level of intervention needed to manage that neonate's conditions on a given day. When critical care codes are reported, the documentation must support the physician's judgment that the patient is critically ill and services provided are commensurate with the condition on that day of service on which critical care codes are reported.

Pediatric Critical Care

99471	Initial inpatient pediatric critical care, per day, for the evaluation and management of a critically ill infant or young child, 29 days through 24 months of age
99472	Subsequent inpatient pediatric critical care, per day, for the evaluation and management of a critically ill infant or young child, 29 days through 24 months of age
99475	Initial inpatient pediatric critical care, per day, for the evaluation and management of a critically ill infant or young child, 2 through 5 years of age
99476	Subsequent inpatient pediatric critical care, per day, for the evaluation and management of a critically ill infant or young child, 2 through 5 years of age

Services are provided to patients who are at least 29 days of age (postnatal age with day of birth being 0 [zero]) until the child reaches 6 years of age. Time-based critical care services (**99291**, **99292**) are reported for critical care services provided to children who are 6 years or older on the date of service.

Initial pediatric critical care codes (**99471**, **99475**) are reported by a single physician or QHP only once *per hospital stay* for a given patient. If the patient is stepped down from critical care to continued hospital care and then requires a subsequent episode of critical care during the same hospital stay, report a subsequent critical care code (**99472**, **99476**) for services on each date the child's condition remains critical.

Examples

➤ **A 22-month-old girl with status epilepticus is initially treated by the ED physician (1 hour of critical care).** Although seizures were initially controlled, pharmacological management led to irregular respiratory activity, lethargy, and hypotension. The patient was admitted to the pediatric intensive care unit at 11:00 pm that evening by the critical care attending physician, who intubated her, placed her on a ventilator, began fluid expansion, used dobutamine to control her blood pressure, and made arrangements for a bedside electroencephalogram (EEG).

> **Teaching Point:** The ED physician would report 1 hour of critical care (**99291**). The pediatrician or intensivist would report initial inpatient pediatric critical care code (**99471**) for that calendar day, even though only 1 hour of care was provided. One hour later, after midnight, a new date of service would begin. The intubation is bundled with **99471** and cannot be separately billed.

➤ **A hospitalist admits a 5-year-old to observe for exacerbation of asthma that initially improved with treatment.** Later the same day, the patient is found to be in respiratory failure and the hospitalist provides 35 minutes of critical care services before transferring the patient's care to a pediatric intensivist. The pediatric intensivist assumes management of the critically ill patient at 10:00 pm.

> **Teaching Point:** The hospitalist reports initial hospital inpatient or observation care (**99221–99223**) on the basis of the level of service provided and appends modifier **25** to indicate that this service is significant and separately identifiable from critical care services reported with code **99291**. The intensivist reports code **99475** (initial inpatient pediatric critical care, per day, for the E/M of a critically ill infant or young child, 2 through 5 years of age). The intensivist will report code **99476** for each subsequent calendar day on which critical care services are provided.
>
> Daily critical care codes do not apply to children 6 years or older. If the child in this example were 6 years old, the intensivist would report codes **99291** and **99292** for the amount of time spent providing critical care services on each date that the child remained critically ill. If less than 30 minutes of critical care were provided on any date, hospital inpatient or observation care codes would be reported (initial, **99221–99223**; subsequent, **99231–99233**).

Patients Critically Ill After Surgery

Postoperative care of a surgical patient is included in the surgeon's global surgical package. For some neonatal surgical care, critical care days are included in the work values assigned to surgical procedures (eg, **39503** [repair of diaphragmatic hernia], **43314** [esophagoplasty, thoracic approach; with repair of tracheoesophageal fistula], **49605** [repair of large omphalocele or gastroschisis; with or without prosthesis]).

However,

- If a second physician (eg, intensivist, hospitalist) provides routine postoperative care for the patient, the surgeon must append modifier **54** (surgical care only) to the surgical code. (A formal transfer of care should be documented.)

> Under Medicare policy, the intensivist accepting a transfer of care from a surgeon during a postoperative period reports modifier **55** (postoperative management only) and, if the condition managed is unrelated to the surgical procedure, modifier **FT** (unrelated E/M visit during a postoperative period). The diagnosis code(s) reported should reflect the problem(s) addressed and may differ from the diagnosis for which the patient underwent surgery.

Example

➤ **A 1-month-old underwent bowel resection for volvulus and was recovering well 8 days after surgery.** On day 9, the patient's temperature is 38.4°C (101.1°F). The incision area is swollen and erythematous. Sepsis evaluation is initiated and antibiotics are started. Within hours the patient becomes hypotensive, requiring vasopressors. The surgeon requests a transfer of care to an intensivist, who accepts the transfer and provides critical care to the critically ill patient.

Teaching Point: The intensivist reports code **99471** (initial inpatient pediatric critical care, per day, for the E/M of a critically ill infant or young child, 29 days through 24 months of age). The intensivist will report **99472** for each subsequent calendar day on which critical care services are provided. The surgeon's postoperative care, other than a return to the operating/procedure room, is included in the global period of the surgery.

Initial and Continuing Intensive Care

99477	Initial hospital care, per day, for the evaluation and management of the neonate, 28 days of age or younger, who requires intensive observation, frequent interventions, and other intensive care services
99478	Subsequent intensive care, per day, for the evaluation and management of the recovering very low birth weight infant (present body weight less than 1500 grams)
99479	Subsequent intensive care, per day, for the evaluation and management of the recovering low birth weight infant (present body weight of 1500–2500 grams)
99480	Subsequent intensive care, per day, for the evaluation and management of the recovering infant (present body weight of 2501–5000 grams)

> Continuing intensive care services provided to an infant weighing more than 5,000 g (approximately 11.02 lb) are reported with subsequent hospital care codes (99231–99233). Codes 99231–99233 are reported on the basis of the documented level of medical decision-making or the physician's or qualified health care professional's total time directed to the individual patient's care on the date of service.

Neonatal and pediatric intensive care codes (**99477–99480**) may be used to report daily care of neonates or infants who are not critically ill but have a need for intensive monitoring, observation, and frequent assessments by the health care team and supervision by the physician or QHP. This includes

● Neonates who require intensive but not critical care services from birth
● Neonates who are no longer critically ill but require intensive physician and health care team observation and interventions
● Recovering low birth weight infants who require a higher level of care than that defined by other hospital care services

These neonates or infants often have a continued need for oxygen, parenteral or gavage enteral nutrition, treatment of apnea of prematurity, and thermoregulation from an Isolette or radiant warmer, and may be recovering from cardiac or surgical care. The intensive services described by these codes include intensive cardiac and respiratory monitoring, continuous and/or frequent vital sign monitoring, heat maintenance, enteral and/or parenteral nutritional adjustments, and laboratory and oxygen saturation monitoring when provided. Patients are under constant observation by the health care team, which is under direct supervision by a physician or QHP.

● **Table 18-4** illustrates codes for initial- and subsequent-day neonatal and pediatric intensive care services (**99477–99480**) by age and present body weight.

Table 18-4. Neonatal and Pediatric Intensive Care

Description	Present Weight <1,500 g	Present Weight 1,500–2,500 g	Present Weight 2,501–5,000 g	Present Weight ≥5,001 g
Initial intensive care of a neonate (28 days or less)	99477			99221–99223
Initial intensive care of an infant (29 days or older)	99221–99223			
Subsequent intensive care	99478	99479	99480	99231–99233

● These are bundled services and include the same procedures that are bundled with neonatal and pediatric critical care services (**99468–99476**). See **Table 18-1** for a list of all the services and procedures that are included.

Code **99477** is used to report the more intensive services that an ill but not critically ill neonate (28 days or younger) requires on the day of admission to inpatient care. Code **99477** includes all E/M services on that date, excluding

● Attendance at delivery (**99464**) or newborn resuscitation (**99465**), which may be reported in addition to code **99477**, when performed.
● Normal newborn care (**99460–99462**), when performed.

Append modifier **25** to code **99477** when reporting on the same date as **99460–99462**, **99464**, or **99465**.

> Payers that have adopted the Medicare National Correct Coding Initiative (NCCI) edits will not allow payment of codes 99460–99462 and 99477 for services by the same physician or physicians of the same specialty and group practice on the same date. Only code 99477 is reported under these circumstances. For more about NCCI edits, see Chapter 2.

- If the infant is older than 28 days at admission but weighs less than 5,000 g, codes **99221–99223** should be used for intensive care on the date of hospital admission (typically **99223**, under the assumption that documentation of high-level MDM or total time is ≥75 minutes).
- Services are typically (but not required to be) provided in a NICU or special care unit and require a higher intensity of care than would be reported with codes **99221–99223** (initial hospital care of sick patient).
- ✖ Do not report code **99477** twice in the same hospital admission. If a patient requires a new episode of intensive care during the same hospital stay, report subsequent intensive care services (**99478–99480**) for the first and each successive day that the patient requires intensive care services.
- Codes **99478–99480** depend on the *present* body weight of the infant, not the infant's age, on the date of service. Therefore, code selection may change from one day to the next depending on the infant's present body weight and condition.
- Codes **99478–99480** are typically used for subsequent days, as long as the neonate or infant continues to require intensive care, and include all the attending physician's or QHP's E/M services (and bundled procedures) provided to the patient on each date of service.
- Once the baby's weight exceeds 5,000 g, subsequent hospital care codes (**99231–99233**) are reported until the date of discharge (**99238**, **99239**).

Examples

In these examples, the neonate is not critically ill but continues to require intensive monitoring and constant observation by the health care team under direct supervision by the reporting physician or QHP.

➤ **A 1,500-g neonate has mild respiratory distress on the initial date of hospital care.** She is on 30% oxygen by nasal cannula, a cardiorespiratory monitor, and continuous pulse oximetry. Laboratory tests and radiographs are ordered, and IV fluids and antibiotics are started. Frequent monitoring and observation are required and ordered.

Code **99477** (initial hospital care for the ill neonate, 28 days of age or less, who requires intensive observation and monitoring) is reported by the attending physician or QHP.

➤ **A 1,250-g infant, now 40 days old, is stable on 1.5 L oxygen by nasal cannula with fraction of inspired oxygen of 30%. The patient is on caffeine for apnea of prematurity, tolerates orogastric feeds, and requires use of an Isolette for temperature stability.**

Code **99478** is reported because the infant weighs less than 1,500 g.

➤ **A 15-day-old, 1,600-g neonate remains in an Isolette for thermoregulation and is on methylxanthines for intermittent apnea and bradycardia, for which the neonate requires continuous cardiorespiratory and pulse oximetry monitoring.** The physician adjusts the neonate's continuous gavage feeds on the basis of tolerance and weight.

Code **99479** is reported for the infant whose present body weight is 1,500 to 2,500 g.

➤ **A baby requires intensive care and weighs 2,500 g on Monday.** The following day, she continues to require intensive care and her weight is 2,504 g.

Code **99479** is reported for the care provided on Monday. Code **99480** is reported for the continuing intensive care provided the following day.

Coding for Transitions to Different Levels of Neonatal Care

During a hospital stay, a newborn or readmitted neonate may require different levels of care. A normal newborn may end up becoming sick, intensively ill, or critical during the same hospital stay. Neonates who were initially sick may also improve to require lower levels of care (eg, normal neonatal care).

● indicates a new code; ▲, revised; #, re-sequenced; ✚ add-on; ★, audiovisual technology; and ◀, synchronous interactive audio.

An initial-day critical or intensive care code (eg, **99468**, **99477**) is reported only once per hospital stay. If the patient recovers and is later stepped up again to that higher level of care, only the subsequent-level codes (**99469**, **99478–99480**) are reported.

Refer to the American Academy of Pediatrics (AAP) *Newborn Coding Decision Tool 2023* (https://shop.aap.org/newborn-coding-decision-tool-2023) for numerous scenarios of coding for newborn care throughout admissions and transfers of care.

Emergency Medical Services Supervision and Patient Transport

Pediatric Critical Care Patient Transport

Face-to-face Pediatric Critical Care Patient Transport

99466   Critical care face-to-face services, during an interfacility transport of critically ill or critically injured pediatric patient, 24 months of age or younger; first 30–74 minutes of hands-on care during transport

99467   each additional 30 minutes (List separately in addition to code **99466**)

Codes **99466** and **99467** are used to report the physical attendance and direct face-to-face care provided by a physician or QHP during the inter-facility transport of a critically ill or injured patient aged 24 months or younger.

- The patient's condition must meet the *CPT* definition for critical care.
- Face-to-face time begins when the physician or other QHP assumes primary responsibility for the patient at the referring hospital or facility and ends when the receiving hospital or facility accepts responsibility for the patient's care. Only the time the physician spends in direct face-to-face contact with the patient during transport should be reported.
  - Less than 30 minutes of face-to-face time cannot be reported.
  - Time must be documented.
  - Code **99467** is used to report each additional 30 minutes of physician face-to-face time of critical care provided on the same day of service beyond the first 74 minutes.
- Codes include the bundled services listed in **Table 18-1**. Codes **99466** and **99467** may be reported separately from any other procedures or services that are not bundled and performed on the date of transfer. The time involved in performing any procedures that are not bundled and are reported separately should not be included in the face-to-face transport time.
- Procedures or services that are performed by other members of the transport team with the physical presence, participation, and supervision of the accompanying physician may be reported by the physician. Documentation must support the physician's participation.
- Medical record documentation must include the total face-to-face time spent with the patient, the critical nature of the patient's condition, and any performed procedures that are not bundled.
- The pediatric critical care transport codes are preadmission codes and may be reported in addition to neonatal (**99468**) or pediatric (**99471**) initial-day critical care codes. For payers that have adopted NCCI edits, modifier **25** is required to indicate the significant and separately identifiable E/M services. Append modifier **25** to code **99466** when reporting in conjunction with daily critical care codes.
- Face-to-face critical care services provided during an inter-facility transport of a child older than 24 months are reported with hourly critical care codes (**99291** and **99292**).
- If an NNP employed by the neonatal group is on the transport team, the NNP may report codes **99466** and **99467** if independent billing by an NNP is allowed by the state and the activities are covered in the scope of practice. The neonatologist from that same group would not report codes **99485** and **99486** (physician direction of pediatric critical care transport) or **99288** (physician direction of emergency medical systems emergency care). The facility (hospital) could also report these services if the NNPs are employed by the hospital. In this case, the neonatologist would report codes **99485** and **99486** for supervision of inter-facility transport because the NNP is not of the same group practice.
- *CPT* does not include specific codes for face-to-face transport of a patient when criteria for critical care are not met. When face-to-face care during transport of a patient is medically necessary but critical care is not, report code **99499** (unlisted E/M service).

Example

➤ **A 4-week-old with tetralogy of Fallot is brought to the local ED with concerns of feeding intolerance, blue lips, labored breathing, and crying.** Transport is dispatched form the regional neonatal center. On arrival, the transport neonatologist finds a cyanotic neonate, with low oxygen saturation despite receiving supplemental oxygen. The

● indicates a new code; ▲, revised; #, re-sequenced; ✚, add-on; ★, audiovisual technology; and ◀, synchronous interactive audio.

neonatologist intubates the patient and administers morphine, which, over time, improves oxygen saturation. A peripheral IV line is placed and fluids are initiated. The neonatologist spends 50 minutes face-to-face evaluating and stabilizing the newborn at the transferring facility followed by 45 minutes during transport to the receiving nursery. Frequent assessments of vital signs and ventilator settings are performed on the transport back. The neonatologist spent a total of 95 minutes of face-to-face critical care time with the neonate; 10 minutes are subtracted for the performance of non-bundled procedures. The time spent in critical care during the transport is 85 minutes. The neonatologist continues care of the newborn in the NICU.

99466 25	(first 74 minutes)
99467 25 × 1 unit	(final 11 minutes)
31500	(endotracheal intubation, emergency)
99468 25	(initial daily inpatient neonatal critical care)

Modifier **25** is appended to each of the services to designate a significant and separately identifiable E/M service provided by the same physician on the same date of service. Endotracheal intubation is bundled with daily neonatal critical care but is separately reported when provided during transport of the critically ill or injured neonate.

Non–face-to-face Pediatric Critical Care Patient Transport

#99485   Supervision by a control physician of interfacility transport care of the critically ill or critically injured pediatric patient, 24 months of age or younger, includes two-way communication with transport team before transport, at the referring facility and during the transport, including data interpretation and report; first 30 minutes

#99486   each additional 30 minutes (List separately in addition to code **99485**)

Code **99485** is used to report the first 16 to 45 minutes of a control physician's documented non–face-to-face supervision of inter-facility critical care transport of a patient 24 months or younger, which includes all 2-way communication between the control physician and the specialized transport team before transport, at the referring facility, and during transport to the receiving facility.

Each additional 30-minute period of communication is reported with add-on code **99486**.

- The patient's condition must meet the *CPT* definition of critical care.
- Only report for patients 24 months or younger who are critically ill or injured.
- The control physician does not report any services provided by the specialized transport team.
- The control physician reports only cumulative time spent communicating with the specialty transport team members during an inter-facility transport. Communication between the control physician and the referring facility before or following patient transport *is not* counted.
- Reportable time begins with the initial discussions with the transport team, including discussions of the best mode of transport and strategies for therapy on arrival. Time ends when the patient's care is handed over to the receiving facility team.
- ✖ Do not report **99485** or **99486** for services of 15 minutes or less or for any time spent in supervision of a QHP from the same group who is reporting **99466** or **99467**.
- Time spent with the individual patient's transport team and reviewing data submissions should be recorded. Time spent discussing the patient with the referring physician or facility is not counted.
- Total communication time of 15 minutes or less is not reported with code **99485**. Code **99288** (discussed in the Direction of Emergency Medical Services section later in this chapter) may be reported when requirements for code **99485** are not met.
- Codes **99485** and **99486** represent preadmission services and may be reported by the same or different individual(s) of the same specialty and same group when neonatal or pediatric critical care services (**99468–99476**) are reported for the same patient on the same day.

Example

➤ **An ED physician requests transfer of an infant with possible sepsis and respiratory distress.** The pediatric intensivist dispatches the transport team, consisting of a hospital-employed transport nurse and a respiratory therapist. On the trip to the referring hospital, the intensivist converses by telephone for 10 minutes with the team, explaining the infant's condition and formulating an initial treatment plan. After arrival, the nurse evaluates the infant and telephones the intensivist to discuss the findings. The decision is made to transport the patient. Because of the critical nature of the infant, the intensivist elects to remain on the telephone until transport is in motion and the patient is critical but stable (15 minutes). On the return trip, another telephone contact lasting 10 minutes is made to receive additional guidance from the intensivist on the infant's worsening respiratory status. The transport is completed and the infant is admitted.

The intensivist spent a total of 35 minutes in direct 2-way telephone communication with the team in 3 discrete episodes. The intensivist carefully documents the time spent in communication with the transport team, the nature of the infant's critical illness, and what decisions were made during each contact in the medical record. Code **99485** is used to report this service.

Direction of Emergency Medical Services

99288   Physician or other qualified health care professional direction of emergency medical systems (EMS) emergency care, advanced life support

See the Non–face-to-face Pediatric Critical Care Patient Transport section earlier in this chapter for discussion of physician non–face-to-face supervision of inter-facility transport of a critically ill or injured pediatric patient 24 months or younger (**99485**, **99486**).

Code **99288**

- May be reported by any physician of any specialty or QHP when advanced life support services are provided via 2-way voice communications (eg, cardiac and/or pulmonary resuscitation; administration of IV fluids, antibiotics, or surfactant).
- This code reflects all the services provided by the directing physician and is not based on any time requirements. Code **99288** may be reported when less than 16 minutes is spent in physician non–face-to-face supervision of inter-facility transport of a critically ill or injured pediatric patient (ie, requirements for reporting **99485** are not met).
- The directing physician should maintain documentation of the times of all contacts, orders, and/or directions for treatment or management of the patient.
- Services or procedures performed by emergency medical services (EMS) personnel are not reported by the physician because they were not physically present.
- When an advance practice professional provides and reports face-to-face services during transport, the physician will not report **99288**.
- The appropriate diagnoses are linked to the service.

If, after directing EMS personnel, the physician performs the initial critical care, the appropriate critical care code (eg, **99468**, initial daily inpatient neonatal critical care) would also be reported with modifier **25** appended to indicate that 2 separate and distinct E/M services were provided by the same physician on the same day of service.

There is no assigned Medicare relative value unit to this service, so it is carrier priced and payments will vary by payer.

Medicare considers code **99288** a bundled service and does not pay separately for the service. Check with your Medicaid program and other payers to determine their coverage policy.

Total Body Systemic and Selective Head Hypothermia

99184   Initiation of selective head or total body hypothermia in the critically ill neonate, includes appropriate patient selection by review of clinical, imaging and laboratory data, confirmation of esophageal temperature probe location, evaluation of amplitude EEG, supervision of controlled hypothermia, and assessment of patient tolerance of cooling

        (Do not report **99184** more than once per hospital stay)

Examples

➤ **A full-term neonate born with evidence of hypoxic-ischemic encephalopathy is admitted to the NICU and receives critical care services.** Laboratory, EEG, blood gas, and imaging studies confirm that the neonate meets objective criteria for *total body cooling*. Continuous total body cooling is undertaken.

Code **99184** is reported for total body systemic hypothermia in addition to **99468**, initial day of neonatal critical care.

● indicates a new code; ▲, revised; #, re-sequenced; ✚, add-on; ★, audiovisual technology; and ◀, synchronous interactive audio.

➤ **A full-term neonate born with evidence of hypoxic-ischemic encephalopathy is admitted to the NICU and receives critical care services.** Laboratory, EEG, blood gas, and imaging studies confirm that the neonate meets objective criteria for *selective head cooling*. Continuous selective head cooling is undertaken.

　　Code **99184** is reported for selective head hypothermia in addition to **99468**, initial day of neonatal critical care.

When total body systemic or selective head hypothermia is used in treatment of a critically ill neonate, code **99184** represents the work of initiating the service.

Documentation for use of total body systemic hypothermia and selective head hypothermia should include the neonatal criteria that support initiating this service.

- During either cooling approach, monitoring includes
  - Radiographic confirmation of core temperature probe
  - Continuous core temperature assessment and adjustment
  - Repeated assessment of skin integrity
  - Recurrent objective evaluation of evolving neurological changes (eg, Sarnat stage), which may also include assessment of continuous amplitude EEG monitoring
- In addition, cooling-related laboratory evaluations are required to monitor for cooling-specific complications, including metabolic and coagulation alterations.

Extracorporeal Membrane Oxygenation (ECMO) or Extracorporeal Life Support (ECLS) Services

Prolonged ECMO and extracorporeal life support (ECLS) services commonly involve multiple physicians and supporting health care personnel to manage each patient. ECMO and ECLS codes differentiate components of initiation and daily management of ECMO and ECLS from daily management of a patient's overall medical condition.

　　These services include cannula insertion (**33951–33956**), ECMO or ECLS initiation (**33946, 33947**), daily ECMO or ECLS management (**33948, 33949**), repositioning of the ECMO or ECLS cannula(e) (**33957–33964**), and cannula removal (**33965–33986**).

ECMO/ECLS Cannula Insertion, Repositioning, and Removal

Codes for insertion, repositioning, and removal of ECMO and ECLS are reported on the basis of the patient's age, with separate codes for procedures performed on newborns through 5 years of age and on patients 6 years and older. Codes for these services are shown in **Table 18-5**. While typically only performed by surgeons, other pediatric providers may perform them as well.

- Do not separately report repositioning of the ECMO or ECLS cannula(e) (**33957–33964**) at the same session as insertion (**33951–33956**).
- Report replacement of ECMO or ECLS cannula(e) in the same vessel by using only the insertion code (**33951–33956**).
- If a cannula(e) is removed from one vessel and a new cannula(e) is placed in a different vessel, report the appropriate cannula(e) removal (**33965–33986**) and insertion (**33951–33956**) codes.
- Fluoroscopic guidance used for cannula(e) repositioning (**33957–33964**) is included in the procedure when performed and should not be separately reported.
- Extensive repair or replacement of an artery may be additionally reported (eg, **35226, 35286, 35371, 35665**).
- Direct anastomosis of a prosthetic graft to the artery sidewall to facilitate arterial perfusion for ECMO or ECLS is separately reported with code **33987** in addition to codes **33953–33956**.

+33987　　Arterial exposure with creation of graft conduit (eg, chimney graft) to facilitate arterial perfusion for ECMO/ECLS (List separately in addition to code for primary procedure)

　　　　Do not report **33987** in conjunction with **34833** (open iliac artery exposure with creation of conduit for delivery of aortic or iliac endovascular prosthesis, by abdominal or retroperitoneal incision, unilateral).

ECMO/ECLS Initiation and Daily Management

33946　　Extracorporeal membrane oxygenation (ECMO)/extracorporeal life support (ECLS) provided by physician; initiation, venovenous

33947　　　　initiation, venoarterial

33948　　　　daily management, each day, venovenous

33949　　　　daily management, each day, venoarterial

Table 18-5. Extracorporeal Membrane Oxygenation or Extracorporeal Life Support Cannula(e) Procedures

Approach	Birth Through 5 Years of Age	6 Years and Older	Do Not Report With
Insertion			
Percutaneous peripheral (arterial/venous) cannula(e)[a]	33951	33952	33957–33964
Open peripheral (arterial/venous) cannula(e)	33953	33954	33957–33964, 34812, 34820, 34834
Central cannula(e) by sternotomy or thoracotomy	33955	33956	33957–33964, 32100, 39010
Reposition[b]			
Percutaneous, reposition peripheral (arterial and/or venous) cannula(e)[a]	33957	33958	33946, 33947, 34812, 34820, 34834
Open, reposition peripheral (arterial and/or venous) cannula(e)[a]	33959	33962	33946, 33947, 34812, 34820, 34834
Central cannula(e) reposition by sternotomy or thoracotomy[a]	33963	33964	33946, 33947, 32100, 39010
Removal[c]			
Removal of peripheral (arterial and/or venous) cannula(e), percutaneous	33965	33966	Not applicable
Removal of peripheral (arterial and/or venous) cannula(e), open	33969	33984	34812, 34820, 34834, 35201, 35206, 35211, 35216, 35226
Removal of central cannula(e) by sternotomy or thoracotomy	33985	33986	35201, 35206, 35211, 35216, 35226

[a] Includes fluoroscopic guidance when performed.
[b] Repositioning of cannula(e) at the same session, as insertion is not separately reported.
[c] Report only the insertion when cannula(e) is replaced in the same vessel.

Initiation of the ECMO or ECLS circuit and setting parameters (**33946, 33947**) involves determining the necessary ECMO or ECLS device components, blood flow, gas exchange, and other necessary parameters to manage the circuit.

Daily care for a patient on ECMO or ECLS includes managing the ECMO or ECLS circuit and related patient issues. These services may be performed by one physician while another physician manages the overall patient medical condition and underlying disorders, but a single physician may provide both services. Regardless of the patient's condition, the basic management of ECMO and ECLS is similar. Documentation for each service should be distinct in the medical record.

✖ Do not report modifier **63** (procedure performed on infants <4 kg) when reporting codes **33946–33949**.

● The physician reporting daily ECMO or ECLS oversees the interaction of the circuit with the patient, management of blood flow, oxygenation, carbon dioxide clearance by the membrane lung, systemic response, anticoagulation and treatment of bleeding, cannula positioning, alarms and safety, and weaning the patient from the ECMO or ECLS circuit when heart and/or lung function has sufficiently recovered.

● Daily management of the patient may be separately reported by using the relevant hospital observation services, hospital inpatient services, or critical care E/M codes (**99221–99223, 99231–99233, 99234–99236, 99291, 99292, 99468–99480**).

● Daily management (**33948, 33949**) or cannula repositioning (**33957–33959, 33962–33964**) may not be reported on the same date as initiation (**33946, 33947**) by the same or different physician.

Each physician providing part of the ECMO/ECLS services may report the services they provide except when prohibited by *CPT* instruction (eg, cannula repositioning is not reported by the same or another physician on the same date as initiation of ECMO/ECLS).

Example

➤ **Venoarterial ECMO is initiated for a patient with cardiac and respiratory failure.** Physician A inserts the cannulae. Physician B manages the initial transition to ECMO, including the work with Physician A, ECMO specialists, and others to initiate an ongoing assessment of anticoagulation, venous return, cannula positioning, and optimal flow.

Chapter 18. Critical and Intensive Care

Physician B also provides daily management of the patient's overall care. When ECMO is discontinued, Physician A returns and removes the cannulae.

Physician A will report codes for insertion and later removal of the ECMO cannulae (eg, **33952** and **33966**) with the appropriate dates of each service. Physician B will report the code for initiation of venoarterial ECMO (**33947**), the appropriate hospital and/or critical care codes for overall treatment of the patient for each day provided (eg, **99468–99476**; **99291**, **99292**; or **99231–99233**), and the code for daily management of ECMO (**33949**) for each day provided.

Sedation

Refer to **Chapter 19** for specific guidelines for reporting sedation services, including moderate (conscious) sedation (**99151–99157**) and deep sedation.

Car Seat/Bed Testing

94780   Car seat/bed testing for airway integrity, for infants through 12 months of age, with continual clinical staff observation and continuous recording of pulse oximetry, heart rate and respiratory rate, with interpretation and report; 60 minutes

✚94781   each additional full 30 minutes (List separately in addition to **94780**.)

Neonates who required critical care during their initial hospital stay are most often those patients who require monitoring to determine if they may be safely transported in a car seat or must be transported in a car bed. While these codes are bundled under neonatal and pediatric critical and intensive care codes (**99468–99472**, **99477–99480**), the services most often take place when a neonate is about to go home and, therefore, can be reported if hospital care services (**99231–99233**) or hospital discharge services (**99238**, **99239**) are being reported instead.

Report codes **94780** and **94781** when the following conditions are met:

- The patient must be an infant (ie, aged ≤12 months). Assessment after the patient is 29 days or older may be necessary.
- Continual clinical staff observation with continuous recording of pulse oximetry, heart rate, and respiratory rate is required.
- Inpatient or office-based services are reported.
- Vital signs and observations must be reviewed and interpreted and a written report generated by the physician.
- Codes are reported on the basis of the total observation time spent and documented.
- If less than 60 minutes is spent in the procedure, code **94780** may not be reported.
- Each additional full 30 minutes (ie, not <90 minutes) is reported with code **94781**.
- ✖ Do not include the time of car seat/bed testing in time attributed to discharge day management services (**99238**, **99239**).
- These codes may be reported with discharge day management (**99238**, **99239**), normal newborn care services (**99460**, **99462**, **99463**), or subsequent hospital care codes (**99231–99233**).

Examples

➤ **A neonate born at 26 weeks' gestation requires a car seat test on the date of discharge from the hospital.**
    Code **94780** is reported in addition to hospital discharge management code **99238** or **99239**.

➤ **A neonate born at 26 weeks' gestation requires a car seat test before discharge from the hospital.** The newborn has received 60 minutes of testing reported with **94780** and now receives an additional 30 minutes.
    Codes **94780** and **94781** are reported.

Values and Payment

Although not exact or applicable for every patient, the preservice, intraservice, and post-service times assigned to codes for neonatal and pediatric critical and intensive care services provide a point of reference for differentiation of the services. Relative value units for each code also allow for comparison of the work and time included in each service. "Times and Values for Pediatric Critical Care/Intensive Care Services" is included at www.aap.org/cfp2023.

● indicates a new code; ▲, revised; #, re-sequenced; ✚, add-on; ★, audiovisual technology; and ◀, synchronous interactive audio.

Payment Advocacy

The AAP encourages chapter development of pediatric councils as forums to discuss pediatric issues with payers. Pediatric councils have the potential to facilitate better working relationships between pediatricians and health insurance plans and to improve quality of care for children. Learn more about AAP pediatric councils at www.aap.org/en/practice-management/practice-financing/payer-contracting-advocacy-and-other-resources/aap-payer-advocacy/aap-pediatric-councils.

The AAP Section on Neonatal-Perinatal Medicine, in conjunction with state chapters and councils of the AAP, has developed strategies that have been successful in addressing payment concerns for neonatal care. Contact your state chapter, its pediatric council, your section district AAP Executive Committee representative, a neonatal trainer, or the AAP Committee on Coding and Nomenclature for assistance in addressing any payment inequities for neonatal services in your state.

Chapter Takeaways

This chapter reviews the definitions of critical care and neonatal intensive care and code assignment for many services often provided to a critically ill or injured patient. Following are some takeaways from this chapter:

- A *critical illness or injury* is defined by *CPT* as one that acutely impairs 1 or more vital organs such that there is a high probability of imminent or life-threatening deterioration of the patient's condition.
- Physicians should be aware of services that are included in the critical and intensive care services and those that can be reported separately in addition to codes for critical or intensive care services.
- When multiple physicians and QHPs provide critical or intensive care services on the same date, it is important to report the correct codes for the service provided (eg, daily critical or intensive care by the attending physician vs concurrent time-based critical care or hospital care by consulting physicians or QHPs).
- Payer guidelines, state regulations, and other factors, such as employment status, affect how services provided by QHPs are reported in conjunction with a physician's services on the same date. Neonatal nurse practitioners, who are not employed by a facility, may be able to independently report services.

Resources

AAP Coding Assistance and Education

AAP Section on Neonatal-Perinatal Medicine coding trainers are available to provide coding education through local educational seminars and continuing education events. Contact section manager Jim Couto (jcouto@aap.org) for additional information about these valuable services.

AAP *Newborn Coding Decision Tool 2023* (https://shop.aap.org/newborn-coding-decision-tool-2023)

AAP pediatric councils (www.aap.org/en/practice-management/practice-financing/payer-contracting-advocacy-and-other-resources/aap-payer-advocacy/aap-pediatric-councils)

AAP Pediatric Coding Newsletter™

"Coding for Abnormalities in Fetal Growth," December 2020 (https://doi.org/10.1542/pcco_book200_document002)

Online Exclusive Content at www.aap.org/cfp2023

"Global Per Diem Critical Care Codes: Direct Supervision and Reporting Guidelines"

"RUC Times and Values for Pediatric Critical Care/Intensive Care Services"

"Times and Values for Pediatric Critical Care/Intensive Care Services"

Chapter 18. Critical and Intensive Care

Test Your Knowledge!

1. **Which of the following codes is separately reportable in conjunction with neonatal critical care services (99468, 99469)?**
   a. Initiation of selective head or total body hypothermia (**99184**)
   b. Oral or nasogastric tube placement (**43752**)
   c. Catheterization of umbilical vein, newborn (**36510**)
   d. Intrapulmonary surfactant administration (**94610**)

2. **To which of the following critical care services may Medicare's split or shared service policy apply when care is provided to the same patient on a single date?**
   a. 2 physicians of the same specialty and same group practice provide critical care.
   b. 2 physicians of different specialties but the same group practice provide critical care.
   c. A physician and a qualified health care professional (QHP) of the same group practice provide critical care services.
   d. A physician and a hospital-employed QHP provide critical care services.

3. **Which of the following code pairs or series is reported by a receiving physician for services provided to a sick neonate who no longer requires intensive or critical care?**
   a. Initial hospital inpatient or observation care (**99221–99223**)
   b. Subsequent hospital inpatient or observation care (**99231–99233**)
   c. Hourly critical care (**99291, 99292**)
   d. Subsequent intensive care, per day (**99478–99480**)

4. **Which of the following codes or code pairs is reported when a consulting physician (ie, a physician other than the attending physician) provides an initial critical care service to a critically ill neonate?**
   a. Critical care face-to-face services, during an interfacility transport (**99466, 99467**)
   b. Supervision by a control physician of interfacility transport care of the critically ill or critically injured pediatric patient (**99485, 99486**)
   c. Initial daily inpatient neonatal critical care (**99468**)
   d. Hourly critical care services (**99291, 99292**)

5. **Which of the following codes or code series is reported when a physician accepts a transfer of a 15-day-old, 1,600-g neonate in a step-down from critical care to intensive care services (same admission)?**
   a. Initial intensive care of a neonate (**99477**)
   b. Subsequent hospital inpatient or observation care (**99223**)
   c. Subsequent intensive care, infant weighing 1500–5000 grams (**99479**)
   d. Hospital inpatient or observation consultation (**99252–99255**)

● indicates a new code; ▲, revised; #, re-sequenced; ✚, add-on; ★, audiovisual technology; and ◀, synchronous interactive audio.

Common Surgical Procedures and Sedation in Facility Settings

CPT copyright 2022 American Medical Association. All rights reserved.

Contents

Chapter 19. Common Surgical Procedures and Sedation in Facility Settings

● indicates a new code; ▲, revised; #, re-sequenced; ✚, add-on; ★, audiovisual technology; and ◀, synchronous interactive audio.

Chapter 19. Common Surgical Procedures and Sedation in Facility Settings

Chapter Highlights

- Work reported with surgical codes
- Reporting special circumstances (eg, partial procedures, work of an assistant surgeon)
- Teaching physician guidelines for reporting surgical procedures
- Anesthesia and sedation

Surgical Package Rules

This chapter discusses coding for surgery and related services in a facility setting. *Current Procedural Terminology* (*CPT*®) surgical codes (**10004–69990**) are packaged or global codes including all the necessary services normally furnished by a surgeon before, during, and after a procedure. *CPT* defines only a surgical package, whereas the Centers for Medicare & Medicaid Services (CMS) defines the surgical package in terms of global periods based on the preoperative, intraoperative, and postoperative work values assigned to each procedure.

- Most Medicaid programs follow the CMS definition.
- Each commercial insurance company will have its own policy for billing and payment of global surgical care, and most will designate a specific number of follow-up days for surgical procedures.

  Both *CPT* and the CMS agree:
- Surgical codes include local infiltration, metacarpal/metatarsal/digital block, or topical anesthesia by the physician performing the procedure.
- Preoperative care
  - Includes evaluation and management (E/M) service(s) *subsequent to the decision for surgery* (eg, assessing the site and condition, explaining the procedure, obtaining informed consent) on the day before and/or on the date of the procedure (including history and physical examination).
  - When the initial decision to perform surgery is made on the day before or on the day of surgery, the appropriate-level E/M visit may be reported separately with modifier **57** (decision for surgery) appended. This modifier shows the payer that the E/M service was necessary to make the decision for surgery (ie, not the routine preoperative evaluation).
  - When an E/M service performed on the day of the procedure is unrelated to the decision to perform surgery and is significant and distinct from the usual preoperative care associated with the procedure, it may be reported with modifier **25** (significant, separately identifiable E/M service by the same physician on the same day of the procedure or other service) appended.
  - Medical record documentation must support that the service was significant, separately identifiable, and medically necessary. An E/M service performed before the decision to perform the procedure is separately reportable.
  - Different diagnoses are not required when reporting an E/M visit and procedure.

Medicare Policy Addresses Preoperative Care Differently for Minor and Major Procedures

When a payer adopts Medicare policy, the evaluation and management (E/M) visit on the date of a minor procedure (ie, procedure assigned a 0- or 10-day global period or endoscopy) is considered a routine part of the procedure regardless of whether it is prior or subsequent to the decision for surgery. In these cases, modifier **57** is not recognized.

An E/M code may be reported on the same day as a minor surgical procedure only when a significant, separately identifiable E/M service is performed; modifier **25** is appended to the E/M code.

When the initial decision to perform a major surgical procedure (ie, procedure assigned a 90-day global period) is made on the day before or on the day of a procedure, the E/M service may be reported with modifier **57** appended. Medical record documentation should support that the decision for surgery was made during the encounter and that time was spent in performing counseling of the risks, benefits, and outcomes.

- Postoperative care
  - Includes all associated typical postoperative care (eg, dictating progress notes; counseling with the patient, family, and/or other physicians; writing orders; evaluating the patient in the postanesthesia recovery area).
  - Care for therapeutic surgical procedures includes only the care that is usually part of the surgical service.

● indicates a new code; ▲, revised; #, re-sequenced; ✛, add-on; ★, audiovisual technology; and ◀, synchronous interactive audio.

— Care for diagnostic procedures (eg, endoscopies, arthroscopies, injection procedures for radiography) includes only the care that is related to the recovery from the diagnostic procedure.

— Care resulting from complications of surgery.

— Any complications, exacerbations, recurrence, treatment of unrelated diseases or injuries, or the presence of other diseases or injuries that require additional services may be reported separately.

Medicare Policy for Reporting Postoperative Medical or Surgical Services

- **All additional medical or surgical services required of the surgeon during the postoperative period of the surgery because of complications *that do not require additional trips to the operating/procedure room* are included in the global package (not separately reported).**
- **Does not include treatment of the underlying condition or an added course of treatment that is not part of normal recovery from surgery. (For discussion of modifiers 24, 58, and 79, see the Global Periods and Modifiers for Reporting Postoperative Care section that follows.)**

Global Periods and Modifiers for Reporting Postoperative Care

The CMS-designated global periods for each *CPT* procedure code can be found on the Resource-Based Relative Value Scale of the Medicare Physician Fee Schedule (MPFS) at www.cms.gov/medicare/medicare-fee-for-service-payment/physicianfeesched.

- It designates specific postoperative periods for certain procedure codes (ie, 0, 10, or 90 days). When determining the postoperative period, the day after surgery is day 1 of a 10- or 90-day period.
- In addition to the *CPT* code, physicians use modifier **78** for return to the operating/procedure room (OR) for a related procedure during a postoperative period. This includes return to the OR for treatment of complications of the first procedure.
- For return to the OR for staged or more extensive procedures and therapeutic procedures following a diagnostic procedure, append modifier **58**.
- Report procedures during the postoperative period that are unrelated and not caused by complications of the original procedure with modifier **79** and unrelated E/M services with modifier **24** (documentation is typically required before payment).
- Other codes are designated YYY, which means the postoperative period is set by the carrier. There are no associated postoperative days included in the payment for codes assigned with status codes XXX (the global concept does not apply) or ZZZ (assigned to an add-on code for a service that is always related to another service to which the global period is assigned).

Reporting Postoperative Care

- Report *CPT* code **99024** (postoperative follow-up visit) for follow-up care provided by the physician who performed a procedure (or the covering physician or other qualified health care professional [QHP]) during the global surgery period.
  - Reporting of inpatient or observation follow-up visits is typically not required.
  - Reporting code **99024** allows a practice to track the number of visits performed by individuals during the postoperative period of specific procedures, calculate office overhead expenses (eg, supplies, staff, physician time) associated with the procedure, and potentially use the data to negotiate higher payment rates.

Payers track the postoperative care provided. If a physician is not providing or reporting the postoperative care (99024) typically performed for a procedure, payers may reduce payment for the surgical service because payment includes postoperative care as part of the procedure.

- Append modifier **24** (unrelated E/M service by the same physician during a postoperative period) to the code for an unrelated E/M service provided by the physician who performed a procedure during the postoperative period.
- When physicians from different practices perform part of a surgical package, the procedure should be reported with one of the following modifiers:
  - **54** (surgical care only)
  - **55** (postoperative management only)
  - **56** (preoperative management only)

● indicates a new code; ▲, revised; #, re-sequenced; ✛, add-on; ★, audiovisual technology; and ◀, synchronous interactive audio.

> See Chapter 2 for a more detailed description of modifiers. For critical care following surgery, see the Patients Critically Ill After Surgery section in Chapter 18.

These situations require communication among the surgeon, the physician providing preoperative or postoperative care, and each physician's respective billing personnel to ensure accurate reporting and payment.

- No modifier is required when a physician (different specialty or group practice) other than the surgeon provides unrelated services to a patient during the postoperative period.

Despite the use of different National Provider Identifiers and diagnosis codes, some payers with assigned global surgical periods will deny the service. The claim should be appealed for payment with a letter advising the payer that the service was unrelated to any surgery.

Removal of Sutures and Staples

> New in 2023! *Current Procedural Terminology* code 15850 (removal of sutures under anesthesia [other than local], same surgeon) has been deleted, and code 15851 (removal of sutures under anesthesia [other than local], other surgeon) has been revised. Additionally, codes 15853 and 15854 are added for reporting removal of sutures and/or staples not requiring anesthesia.

▲**15851**   Removal of sutures or staples requiring anesthesia (ie, general anesthesia, moderate sedation)

Code **15851** is reported only when the patient requires general anesthesia or moderate sedation during suture or staple removal.

\#✚●**15853**   Removal of sutures or staples not requiring anesthesia

\#✚●**15854**   Removal of sutures and staples not requiring anesthesia

Codes **15853** and **15854** are reported on the basis of whether sutures *or* staples or sutures *and* staples are removed. These codes represent the practice expense associated with removal of sutures and/or staples following a procedure that does not include a postoperative period (eg, 0-day global procedure).

Multiple Procedures on the Same Date

Often, multiple, separately reportable services are provided in one session or on one date of service. However, it is important to recognize which surgical services are considered a component of another procedure and which are separately reported.

- It is not appropriate to report multiple Healthcare Common Procedure Coding System (HCPCS)/*CPT* codes when a single, comprehensive HCPCS/*CPT* code describes the procedures performed.

Example

➤ **Code 42820 describes tonsillectomy and adenoidectomy in a patient younger than 12 years.** It would not be appropriate to separately report **42825** (tonsillectomy) and **42830** (adenoidectomy).

- Surgical access (eg, laparotomy) is integral to more comprehensive procedures (eg, appendectomy) and not separately reported.
- When the surgical approach fails, report only the code for the approach that resulted in the completed procedure. For example, if laparoscopy fails and an open approach is used to complete the procedure, report only the open procedure.
- It is advisable to adopt a process for checking the National Correct Coding Initiative (NCCI) edits or payer-specific edit tools before submitting multiple procedure codes for services on the same date. Code edit tools may be provided through a provider portal.
- For Medicaid, the NCCI manual is also informative regarding correct reporting and use of modifiers to override NCCI edits.

> See Chapter 2 for more information on the National Correct Coding Initiative.

- When more than one procedure/service is performed on the same date, during the same session, or during a post-operative period, several *CPT* modifiers may apply. Documentation must support the reason for applying a modifier (eg, indicate a separate incision).
  - Modifier **59** (distinct procedural service) is often appended to surgical procedure codes to override payer edits that would otherwise not allow payment for services that may be components of other services.
  - It is important to carefully consider whether other modifiers are more appropriate (eg, **50**, bilateral service; an anatomical modifier such as **E4**, lower right eyelid) to indicate a distinct service.

Separate Procedure Designation

One designation in *CPT* helps identify procedures that are commonly performed as an integral component of another procedure. The parenthetical comment "(separate procedure)" follows the code descriptor for these services.

- Services designated as a separate procedure should not be reported in addition to the code for the total procedure or service of which they are considered an integral component.
- A procedure or service that is designated as a separate procedure may be
  - Carried out independently and be the only code reported
  - Considered to be unrelated or distinct from other procedures/services provided at that time and reported in addition to other procedures/services by appending modifier **59** (distinct procedural service)

Increased or Decreased Procedural Services

Increased Procedural Service

Modifier **22** (increased procedural service) may be appended to the code for a surgical procedure when the work required to provide the service was *significantly greater* than typically required for that procedure. To substantiate modifier **22**, documentation must support that the procedure was more difficult due to 1 or more of the following conditions:

- Increased intensity or time
- Technical difficulty
- The severity of the patient's condition
- Significantly increased physical and mental effort

Example

➤ **A child undergoes surgery for acute appendicitis with rupture.** The procedure takes 45 minutes longer than typical due to subhepatic location and rupture of the appendix. The surgeon documents the increased work and time of the procedure and reports

    44970 22   Laparoscopy, surgical, appendectomy

    Teaching Point: Because the work of the procedure was significantly increased by the location and rupture of the appendix, modifier **22** is appropriately appended.

See Chapter 2 for discussion of other surgical modifiers (eg, **62**, 2 surgeons; **66**, surgical team) and general information on modifiers.

Reporting Terminated or Partial Procedures

- When a procedure is started but cannot be completed due to extenuating circumstances, physicians should consider the individual situation, including the reason for termination of the procedure and the amount of work that was performed, when determining how to report the service rendered.
- When a procedure was performed but not entirely successful (eg, portion of foreign body removed), it may be appropriate to report the procedure code that represents the work performed without modification.
- Only report reduced services (modifier **52**) or discontinued procedure (modifier **53**) when the service was significantly reduced from the typical service and as instructed in *CPT*.

Example

➤ *CPT* instructs to append modifier **52** (reduced service) to codes **36572**, **36573**, or **36584** with modifier **52** when insertion or replacement of a peripherally inserted central venous catheter (PICC) is performed without confirmation of catheter tip location (eg, via radiography or ultrasonography).

- If the work performed before discontinuation was insignificant, it may be appropriate to not report the procedure.
- When not reporting the procedure, consider whether the level of a related E/M service was increased because of the level of medical decision-making (MDM) associated with the attempted procedure, any complicating factors, and the revised management or treatment plan.
- *CPT* includes specific instructions for reporting certain services when reduced or discontinued (eg, endoscopy). Be sure to verify *CPT* instructions before reporting reduced or terminated services.

Know Payer Policies for Modifiers 52 (Reduced Service) and 53 (Discontinued Procedure)

Individual payer policies may specify allowed uses and reporting requirements for reduced or discontinued services. Pediatricians should be aware that some payer policies automatically reduce payment to 25% to 50% of the fee schedule amount for the service reported with modifier **52** or **53**.

When indicated, modifier **52** or **53** should always be reported. Documentation should support the reason for reduced or discontinued service and the extent of the service performed. Payers may audit the patient's medical record or, for facility-based services, use electronic processes to compare a physician's claim to a facility claim for the same service that was reported with modifier **73** or **74** (outpatient hospital/ambulatory surgical center discontinued service). If modifier **52** or **53** was indicated but not reported, a payer may demand return of previous payments.

For more information on reporting discontinued or incomplete procedures, see the May 2021 *AAP Pediatric Coding Newsletter* article, "Discontinued or Reduced Services: Modifier 52 or 53" (https://doi.org/10.1542/pcco_book205_document003).

Reporting by Assistant Surgeon

An assistant surgeon is a physician or other QHP who provides active assistance in the performance of a procedure when clinically indicated (eg, technically complex procedure).

- See the Assistant Surgeon in a Teaching Facility section later in this chapter for guidance on reporting assistant surgeon services by a physician in a teaching facility.
- Global rules do not apply to services performed by an assistant surgeon. Payment is based on a percentage of the fee schedule amount allowed for the procedure performed (eg, Medicare allows 16%).
- Modifiers are appended to the code(s) for the procedure on the assistant's claim. See **Box 19-1** for modifiers for reporting services by an assistant surgeon.
- Reductions for multiple procedures on the same date may apply.
- See individual payer policies for assistant at surgery, as many limit payment to only specific procedures and/or may require documentation substantiating the need for assistance.

Box 19-1. Modifiers for Reporting Assistant Surgeon Services	
80	Assistant surgeon (Use for doctor of medicine or osteopathy.)
81	Minimum assistant surgeon
82	Assistant surgeon (when qualified resident surgeon not available)

Procedures Performed on Infants Less Than 4 kg

Modifier **63** is used to identify procedures performed on neonates and infants with present body weight of up to 4 kg. This modifier signals significantly increased complexity and physician or other QHP work commonly associated with these patients.

- Append modifier **63** to codes for procedures performed on these infants only when there is no instruction prohibiting reporting.

Chapter 19. Common Surgical Procedures and Sedation in Facility Settings

- Services that cannot be reported with modifier **63** are those that have been valued on the basis of the intensity of the service in patients weighing less than 4 kg. See "Summary of *CPT* Codes Exempt from Modifier **63**" in your *CPT* reference for a list of codes exempt from modifier **63**.
- Unless otherwise designated, this modifier may be appended only to procedures or services listed in the **20100–69999** code series and codes **92920**, **92928**, **92953**, **92960**, **92986**, **92987**, **92990**, **92997**, **92998**, **93312–93318**, **93452**, **93505**, **93593–93598**, **93563**, **93564**, **93568**, **93569**, **93573–93575**, **93580–93582**, **93590–93592**, **93615**, and **93616**. Modifier **63** is not appended to codes from the E/M, anesthesia, radiology, or pathology/laboratory section of *CPT*.
- Use of modifier **63** may require submission of an operative note with the claim. The operative note should include the patient's weight. It is also beneficial to report the patient's weight on the claim.
- Payer acceptance of modifier **63** may be limited to specific procedures and increased payment allowance (above the payment for the same procedure in a patient weighing >4 kg) varies. Verify policies of individual health plans for reporting this modifier.

Examples

➤ **A 13-day-old weighing 2.4 kg requires peripheral cannulae insertion for extracorporeal membrane oxygenation (ECMO).** The physician reports

33951 63   Extracorporeal membrane oxygenation (ECMO)/extracorporeal life support (ECLS) provided by physician; insertion of peripheral (arterial and/or venous) cannula(e), percutaneous, birth through 5 years of age (includes fluoroscopic guidance, when performed)

Teaching Point: The patient weighed less than 4 kg, and the procedure is not listed as modifier **63** exempt. Therefore, modifier **63** is appropriately appended to indicate the increased intensity and/or work of performing the procedure on the neonate. Note that modifier **63** cannot be appended to codes for initiation or daily management of ECMO/ECLS (**33646–33949**).

➤ **An infant weighing 3 kg undergoes diagnostic laryngoscopy.** The physician reports

31520   Laryngoscopy, direct, with or without tracheoscopy; diagnostic newborn

Teaching Point: The parenthetical instruction below code **31520** ("Do not report modifier **63** in conjunction with **31520**") prohibits reporting modifier **63**, including when this procedure is performed on an infant weighing less than 4 kg.

Physicians at Teaching Hospitals Guidelines for Billing Procedures

The CMS established and maintains guidelines for documentation and billing by teaching physicians. Physicians at Teaching Hospitals guidelines for billing procedures are less complex than those for billing E/M services. Guidelines specify that

- When a procedure is performed by a resident, teaching physician attendance and participation are required and must be documented. For examples of appropriate documentation, see **Table 19-1**.
- The level of participation required by the teaching physician depends on the type of procedure being performed.
- A resident, nurse, or teaching physician may document the teaching physician's attendance.

To obtain the rules for supervising physicians in teaching settings, see Chapter 100 of the *Medicare Claims Processing Manual* at https://cms.hhs.gov/manuals/downloads/clm104c12.pdf.

> **Modifier GC must be appended to procedure codes for services performed by a resident under the direction of a teaching physician.**

Minor Procedures

- The CMS defines a minor procedure as one taking *5 minutes or less* to complete with relatively little decision-making once the need for the procedure is determined.
- Minor procedures are usually assigned a 0- to 10-day global period.
- Teaching physicians may bill for a minor procedure when they personally perform the service or when a resident performs the service and they are present for the entire procedure.
- The resident may document the procedure but must attest to the teaching physician's presence.

● indicates a new code; ▲, revised; #, re-sequenced; ✚, add-on; ★, audiovisual technology; and ◀, synchronous interactive audio.

Table 19-1. Examples of Appropriate Documentation of Teaching Physician Presence

Presence	Documentation
Minor procedure	*"Dr Teaching Physician was present during the entire procedure."* —Nurse *"Dr Teaching Physician observed me as I performed this procedure."* —Dr Resident
Interpretation of diagnostic radiological findings and other diagnostic test results	*"I personally reviewed the MRI with Dr Resident and agree with his findings."* —Dr Teaching Physician *"I personally reviewed the CT scan with Dr Resident. Findings indicate [cite specifics]."* —Dr Teaching Physician
Endoscopy	*"I was present during the entire viewing of this endoscopy."* —Dr Teaching Physician
Surgery other than minor procedure	*"Dr Teaching Physician was present during the entire surgery."* —Dr Resident *"I was present during and observed Dr Resident perform the key portion of this procedure."* —Dr Teaching Physician
Complex or high-risk surgery or procedure	*"I was physically present during this entire procedure exception for the [opening and/or closing], as that overlapped with the key portion of another case."* —Dr Teaching Physician *"Dr Y was immediately available during the overlapping portions of this case, which included [cite specifics]."* —Dr Teaching Physician

Abbreviations: CT, computed tomography; MRI, magnetic resonance image.

Interpretation of Diagnostic Radiology and Other Diagnostic Tests

- The teaching physician may bill for interpretation of the diagnostic service if they interpret tests or review findings with the resident.
- Documentation must support a personal interpretation or a review of the resident's notes with indication of agreement with the resident's interpretation.
- Changes to the resident's interpretation must be documented.

Endoscopy

- The teaching physician must be present for the entire viewing starting at the time of insertion and ending at the time of removal of the endoscope.
- Viewing the procedure through a monitor located in another room does not meet the requirements for billing.
- The presence of the teaching physician must be documented in the medical record. The teaching physician's presence must be stated.

Complex or High-risk Surgery or Procedure

- A complex procedure or surgery (eg, cardiac catheterization) requires the direct or personal supervision of a physician as specified in Medicare or local policy or in the *CPT* description.
- A teaching physician must be present with a resident for the entire procedure when billing for a service identified by the CMS or local policy as complex and requiring personal supervision by a physician.
- Documentation must support that the teaching physician was present.

Surgery Other Than Minor, Complex, or High-risk Procedure

- The teaching physician must assume the responsibility of preoperative, operative, and postoperative care of the patient. They must be present during all critical and key portions (as determined by the teaching physician) of the procedure. For example, if opening or closing is not considered to be key or critical, the teaching physician does not need to be present.

- The teaching physician must be immediately available to furnish services during the entire procedure.
- If circumstances prevent the physician from being immediately available, arrangements must be made with another qualified surgeon to be immediately available to assist with the procedure.
- The physician's presence for single surgical procedures may be demonstrated in notes made by the teaching physician, resident, or nurse.
- When the teaching physician is present for the entire procedure, only the written attestation of their presence is required.
- If the teaching physician is present during only the key or critical portions of the surgery, documentation must indicate their presence at those portions of the procedure (the resident may still document the operative report).
- When billing for 2 overlapping (concurrent) surgical procedures, the teaching physician must be present for the key or critical portions of both procedures and must personally document their presence. The surgeon cannot be involved in a second case until all key or critical portions in the first case have been completed.
- Arrangements may be made with another qualified surgeon to be present at one of the surgical procedures. The name of the other surgeon who was immediately available during overlapping surgical procedures must be documented.

Postoperative Care

- The teaching physician determines which postoperative visits are considered key or critical and require their presence.
- If the teaching physician is not providing postoperative care included in the global surgery package, they will report the procedure(s) with modifiers **54** (surgical care only) and **56** (preoperative management only).
- Postoperative care is reported by another physician with the same surgical procedure code with modifier **55** (post-operative management only).
- The surgeon and physician providing postoperative care must keep a copy of a written transfer agreement in the patient's medical record.

Assistant Surgeon in a Teaching Facility

Medicare will not pay for the services of assistants at surgery furnished in a teaching hospital that has a training program related to the medical specialty required for the surgical procedure and has a qualified resident available to perform the service. This policy may be applied by Medicaid and other payers.

- When the MPFS allows payment for an assistant surgeon and a physician assists a teaching physician because no qualified resident was available, modifier **82** (assistant surgeon [when qualified resident surgeon not available]) is appended to the code for the procedure performed on the assistant surgeon's claim.
- The unavailability of a qualified resident surgeon is a prerequisite for use of modifier **82**. Documentation must specify that no qualified resident was available or that there was no residency program related to the medical specialty required for the surgical procedure.
- This modifier is used only in teaching hospitals and only if there is no approved training program related to the medical specialty required for the surgical procedure or no qualified resident was available.

Burn Care

CPT code **16000** (initial treatment, first-degree burn, where no more than local treatment is required) is reported when initial treatment is performed for the symptomatic relief of a first-degree burn that is characterized by erythema and tenderness.

16020	Dressings and/or debridement of partial-thickness burns, initial or subsequent; small or less than 5% total body (eg, finger)
16025	medium or 5%–10% total body surface area (eg, whole face or whole extremity)
16030	large or greater than 10% total body surface area (eg, more than 1 extremity)
16035	Escharotomy; initial incision
+16036	each additional incision

Codes **16020–16030**

- Are used to report treatment of burns with dressings and/or debridement of small to large partial-thickness burns (second degree), whether initial or subsequent.
- Are reported on the basis of the percentage of total body surface area (TBSA) affected.
- The percentage of TBSA involved must be calculated and documented when reporting care of second- or third-degree burns.

● indicates a new code; ▲, revised; #, re-sequenced; ✚, add-on; ★, audiovisual technology; and ◄, synchronous interactive audio.

Pediatric physicians often use the Lund-Browder classification method for estimating the TBSA based on patient age. (The Lund-Browder diagram and classification method table are in *CPT 2023 Professional Edition*.)

- An E/M visit (critical care, emergency department [ED] services, inpatient or outpatient E/M) may be provided for evaluation of the patient's injuries and management of complications such as dehydration, shock, infection, multiple organ dysfunction syndrome, electrolyte imbalance, cardiac arrhythmias, and respiratory distress.
  - Report the E/M code appropriate to the setting and care provided with modifier **25** appended to indicate that the significant, separately identifiable E/M service is medically indicated, performed, and documented in addition to the burn care.
- Codes **16000–16036** do not include other services such as pulmonary testing/therapy or procedures such as hyperbaric oxygenation, grafting, or tracheotomy. Separately report other services provided on the same date as burn care.
- Codes **16020–16030** include dressing application (whether initial or subsequent) and any associated debridement or curettement.
- It is advisable to use *International Classification of Diseases, 10th Revision, Clinical Modification* (ICD-10-CM) category **T31**, burns classified according to extent of body surface involved, as an additional code for reporting purposes when there is mention of a third-degree burn involving 20% or more of the body surface.
- Codes **16020–16030** include the application of materials (eg, dressings) not described in codes **15100–15278** (skin grafts and substitutes).

  Codes **16035** and **16036**

- Are reported per incision of eschar (dead tissue cast off from the surface of the skin in full-thickness burns).
- Are not reported on the basis of anatomical site; report with 1 unit of code **16035** only for the first incision and 1 unit of code **16036** for each additional incision regardless of body area.

Surgical Preparation and Skin Grafting

Surgical Preparation

15002	Surgical preparation or creation of recipient site by excision of open wounds, burn eschar, or scar (including subcutaneous tissues), or incisional release of scar contracture, trunk, arms, legs; first 100 sq cm or 1% of body area of infants and children
+15003	each additional 100 sq cm, or part thereof, or each additional 1% of body area of infants and children
15004	Surgical preparation or creation of recipient site by excision of open wounds, burn eschar, or scar (including subcutaneous tissues), or incisional release of scar contracture, face, scalp, eyelids, mouth, neck, ears, orbits, genitalia, hands, feet and/or multiple digits; first 100 sq cm or 1% of body area of infants and children
+15005	each additional 100 sq cm, or part thereof, or each additional 1% of body area of infants and children

Surgical preparation codes **15002–15005** for skin replacement surgery describe removal of nonviable tissue to treat a burn, traumatic wound, or necrotizing infection.

Report codes **15002–15005** for preparation of a clean and viable wound surface for placement of an autograft, flap, or skin substitute graft or for negative pressure wound therapy (NPWT).

> An incisional release of scar contracture may also be used to create a clean wound bed.

- Code selection for surgical preparation codes is based on the location and size of the defect. Measurements apply to the recipient area.
  - Adults and children 10 years and older: 100 cm^2
  - Infants and children younger than 10 years: each percentage of body surface area
- Codes **15002–15005** are always preparation for healing by primary intention. Do not report codes **15002–15005** for chronic wounds left to heal by secondary intention.
- Report the appropriate codes when closure is achieved by adjacent tissue transfer (codes **14000–14061**) or a complex repair (codes **13100–13153**) rather than skin grafts or substitutes.

Example

➤ **An 8-year-old patient undergoes surgical preparation for skin grafting of face, front of right arm, and right hand.** The body areas are measured as face, 4% of body area; right arm, 4%; and right hand, 1%.

ICD-10-CM	CPT
Appropriate codes for burns by depth and body area	**15004** (first 1% of body areas of face and hand) **15005** × 4 (each additional 1%) **15002 59** (first 1% body area of arm) **15003** × 3 (each additional 1%)

Teaching Point: Because the face and hand are both included in the descriptor for codes **15004** and **15005**, the percentages of body areas are combined. Because the preparation of an area on the arm is described by codes **15002** and **15003**, the body area of the arm is not added to that of the face and hand. Modifier **59** indicates that the procedure reported with code **15002** was performed on distinct body areas not described by code **15004**.

Skin Grafts and Skin Graft Substitutes

A chart of codes for skin grafts of infants and children is included at www.aap.org/cfp2023.

- When burn wounds are treated and subsequently require skin grafting at the same session, report the burn code along with the appropriate skin graft code.
- A skin graft procedure may be a staged procedure (delayed) with the preparation of the recipient site and the graft procedure being performed on different dates. In these cases, modifier **58** (staged procedure) is appended to the grafting procedure code performed during the global period.
- The appropriate code for harvesting cultured skin autograft is **15040** (harvest of skin for tissue cultured skin autograft, 100 sq cm or less).
- Debridement is considered a separate procedure only when
  — Gross contamination requires prolonged cleansing.
  — Appreciable amounts of devitalized or contaminated tissue are removed.
  — Debridement is carried out separately without immediate primary closure.
- Measurements apply to the recipient area.
  — For patients 10 years and older, report 1 unit per 100 sq cm.
  — Report 1 unit per 1% of body area of children 9 years and younger.
- Procedures involving the wrist and/or ankle are reported with codes that include "arm" or "leg" in the descriptor.
- The physician should select the skin substitute graft application code based on the actual size of the wound, after wound preparation has been performed, and not the amount of the skin graft substitute used.
- The party supplying skin substitute graft products reports HCPCS codes for the products.

Musculoskeletal Procedures

> An object intentionally placed by a physician or other qualified health care professional for any purpose (eg, diagnostic, therapeutic) is considered an implant. If an implant (or part thereof) has moved from its original position, or is structurally broken and no longer serves its intended purpose or presents a hazard to the patient, it qualifies as a foreign body for coding purposes, unless *Current Procedural Terminology* (*CPT*) coding instructions direct otherwise or a specific *CPT* code exists to describe the removal of that broken/moved implant.

Fracture and Dislocation Care Codes

Codes for fracture/dislocation care

- Are listed by anatomical location.
- Are provided (in most cases) for closed or open treatment, with or without manipulation and with or without internal fixation.
- Typically include a 90-day period of follow-up care under the Medicare global package. Append modifier **57** (decision for surgery) to an E/M code when the decision for the procedure is made during a visit on the day before or day of the procedure.
- Are appended with modifier **54** to the usual procedure code if you provide initial fracture care (with or without manipulation) but transfer to another physician for follow-up care (applies to procedures with a 10- or 90-day global period). The transfer of care should be documented (eg, patient to see Dr X for continuing fracture care Monday morning).

> Do not report a fracture care code when stabilization (eg, temporary cast/splint/strap) is performed to protect an injury and provide comfort to the patient until another physician performs initial fracture or dislocation care. Instead, report an evaluation and management service and the application of a cast, splint, or strapping (29000–29584), as indicated.

The physician providing follow-up care will report the same date of service and procedure code appended with modifier **55**. The claim will also denote the date of the transfer of care, which should be documented by both physicians.

- Include the initial casting, splinting, or strapping, but do not include radiographs.
- Routine follow-up visits during the global period are reported with no charge with code **99024** (post-op follow-up visit related to the original procedure).
- Only the first cast is included in the code for fracture care. It is appropriate to append modifier **58** (staged or related procedure during the postoperative period) to the fracture care code when reporting a cast change (**29000–29799 58**). However, payer guidance on use of modifier **58** may vary.
- Are appended with modifier **76** to the usual procedure code to indicate repeated procedure or service by the same physician or other QHP for re-reduction of a fracture and/or dislocation.

Examples

➤ **An orthopedic surgeon is consulted to evaluate a child in the ED for an injury to the left elbow following a fall caused by overturning her bicycle on the sidewalk of her apartment complex.** The orthopedic surgeon evaluates the child and diagnoses a displaced supracondylar humerus fracture. A decision is made to proceed with closed reduction and pinning. The surgeon's total time spent in provision and documentation of the E/M service is 40 minutes. The procedure takes place on the same date. The orthopedic surgeon provided consultation in the ED and a surgical procedure requiring an inpatient admission on the same date.

ICD-10-CM	CPT
S42.412A (displaced simple supracondylar fracture without intercondylar fracture of left humerus, initial encounter for closed fracture) **V18.0XXA** (pedal cycle driver injured in noncollision transport accident in nontraffic accident, initial encounter) **Y92.480** (sidewalk as the place of occurrence of the external cause)	**99244 57** (outpatient consultation with moderate MDM or ≥40 minutes) or, if the payer does not pay consultation codes, **99215 57** (office or other outpatient E/M service with high MDM or 40–54 minutes) **24538** (percutaneous skeletal fixation of supracondylar or transcondylar humeral fracture, with or without intercondylar extension)

Teaching Point: Because code **24538** is assigned a 90-day global period in the MPFS, modifier **57** (decision for surgery) is appended to the E/M code reported for the same date of service. Individual payers may have different policies. The postoperative care in the hospital is not separately reported. Follow-up visits in the office should be reported with code **99024** (postoperative follow-up visit).

➤ **An orthopedic surgeon sees a child for follow-up care after percutaneous skeletal fixation of a supracondylar fracture.** The surgeon replaces a splint that was applied at the time of the procedure with a long-arm cast.

ICD-10-CM	CPT
S42.412D (displaced simple supracondylar fracture without intercondylar fracture of left humerus, subsequent encounter for fracture with routine healing) **V18.0XXD** (pedal cycle driver injured in noncollision transport accident in nontraffic accident, subsequent encounter) **Y92.480** (sidewalk as the place of occurrence of the external cause)	**29065 58** (application cast; shoulder to hand)

Teaching Point: Because the cast is not part of the initial fracture care, it is separately reported. Cast removal on a later date will not be separately reported.

Chapter 19. Common Surgical Procedures and Sedation in Facility Settings

See the February 2021 *AAP Pediatric Coding Newsletter* article, "Initial Fracture Care: Musculoskeletal or Evaluation and Management," for additional examples of coding for fracture care (https://doi.org/10.1542/pcco_book202_document005).

Removal of Musculoskeletal Hardware

20665	Removal of tongs or halo applied by another individual
20670	Removal of implant; superficial (eg, buried wire, pin or rod) (separate procedure)
20680	deep (eg, buried wire, pin, screw, metal band, nail, rod or plate)

Removal of a halo or tongs is included in the placement procedure. However, removal of a halo or tongs by another physician is separately reported with code **20665**. (*Note:* Physicians of the same specialty and same group practice are typically considered as the same physician for billing purposes.)

Codes **20670** and **20680** may be reported for removal of orthopedic hardware. If it is necessary to remove an implant within the global period (eg, due to breakage), report the appropriate removal code with modifier **78** (unplanned return to the operating/procedure room by the same physician or other QHP following initial procedure for a related procedure during the postoperative period.)

Respiratory

Intubation and Airway Management

31500	Intubation, endotracheal, emergency

- Moderate sedation (**99151–99157**) may be reported in addition to the intubation if used to sedate the patient before and during the intubation procedure (eg, in rapid sequence intubation) and reporting criteria are met. See the Sedation section later in this chapter for more on moderate sedation.
- Endotracheal intubation is included in the neonatal and pediatric critical care services reported with **99468–99476** and intensive care services reported with **99477–99480**. Code **31500** is separately reported for endotracheal intubation performed as part of neonatal resuscitation in the delivery room (ie, before admission).

31502	Tracheostomy tube change prior to establishment of fistula tract

Report code **31502** only when an indwelling tracheostomy tube is replaced before establishment of a fistula tract.

Routine changing of a tracheostomy tube after a fistula tract has been established is included in a related evaluation and management service. Code 31575 (laryngoscopy, flexible; diagnostic) may be reported when performed to check tracheostomy tube placement.

31505–31520 Indirect laryngoscopy

Report code **31505** for indirect diagnostic laryngoscopy. If, while performing this procedure, a foreign body is removed, report code **31511** (laryngoscopy with removal of foreign body).

31515	Direct laryngoscopy with or without tracheoscopy

Code **31515** is reported when laryngoscopy is performed for aspiration.

When diagnostic direct laryngoscopy, with or without tracheoscopy, is performed on a newborn, report code **31520**. Do not report modifier **63** (procedure performed on infant <4 kg) in conjunction with code **31520**.

31525	Laryngoscopy, direct, with or without tracheoscopy; diagnostic except newborn

Thoracostomy, Thoracentesis, and Pleural Drainage

32551	Tube thoracostomy, includes connection to drainage system (eg, water seal), when performed, open (separate procedure)
32554	Thoracentesis, needle or catheter, aspiration of the pleural space; without imaging guidance
32555	with imaging guidance
32556	Pleural drainage, percutaneous, with insertion of indwelling catheter; without imaging guidance
32557	with imaging guidance

- Thoracostomy (**32551**) represents an open procedure involving incision into a rib interspace with dissection extending through the chest wall muscles and pleura. Thoracentesis and percutaneous pleural drainage may be more commonly performed in pediatrics with the exception of neonatal and pediatric critical care.

● indicates a new code; ▲, revised; #, re-sequenced; ✛, add-on; ★, audiovisual technology; and ◀, synchronous interactive audio.

— Percutaneous image guidance cannot be reported in conjunction with code **32551**, which represents an open procedure.

— Diagnostic ultrasonography performed before thoracostomy to localize a collection in the pleural space is separately reportable only when the complete ultrasound study of the chest (**76604**) is performed with permanent recording of images.

● Thoracentesis codes **32554** and **32555** represent a procedure in which the surgical technique is puncture of the pleural space to remove fluid or air. Although a catheter (eg, pigtail catheter) may be used, it is not left in place at the end of the procedure.

● Percutaneous pleural drainage codes **32556** and **32557** represent procedures in which an indwelling catheter is inserted into the pleural space and remains at the end of the procedure. The catheter is secured in place and connected to a suction drainage system.

● Removal of chest tubes and non-tunneled indwelling pleural catheters is included in a related E/M service and not a separately reportable procedure.

● For insertion of a tunneled pleural catheter with cuff, see code **32550**. For removal of a tunneled pleural catheter with cuff, see **32552**.

Cardiovascular Procedures

New in 2023! Codes 93569 and 93573–93575 have been added for reporting selective pulmonary angiography in addition to codes for reporting certain primary procedures. Codes 33900–33904 are added for reporting percutaneous pulmonary artery revascularization by stent placement.

Selective Pulmonary Angiography

Add-on codes **93569** and **93573–93575** have been added for reporting selective pulmonary angiography in addition to codes for reporting certain primary procedures. Each code is described as an injection procedure during cardiac catheterization including imaging supervision, interpretation, and report for specified vessels as follows:

✚●**93569**   for selective pulmonary arterial angiography, unilateral

✚●**93573**   for selective pulmonary arterial angiography, bilateral

✚●**93574**   for selective pulmonary venous angiography of each distinct pulmonary vein during cardiac catheterization.

✚●**93575**   for selective pulmonary angiography of major aortopulmonary collateral arteries (MAPCAs) arising off the aorta or its systemic branches, during cardiac catheterization for congenital heart defects, each distinct vessel

For nonselective pulmonary arterial angiography, use ▲93568.

Add-on codes **93569** and **93573–93575** are used for reporting selective pulmonary angiography in addition to codes for reporting certain primary procedures, including shunting procedures to create effective intracardiac blood flow in patients with congenital heart defects (**33741**, **33745**), transcatheter interventions for revascularization or repair for coarctation of the aorta (**33894**, **33895**), endovascular repair of pulmonary artery stenosis by stent placement (**33900–33904**), cardiac catheterization other than for congenital heart defect (**93451–93453**; **93456**, **93457**; **93460**, **93461**), percutaneous transcatheter repair of structural heart defect (**93580–93583**), and cardiac catheterization for congenital heart disease (**93593–93598**). See your *CPT* reference for a full listing of codes to which **93569** and **93573–93575** are additionally reported.

● **93569** and **93573–93575** include the selective introduction and positioning of the angiographic catheter, injection, and radiological supervision and interpretation.

● **93574** and **93575** are reported for evaluation of each distinct named vessel (eg, right upper pulmonary vein or MAPCA vessel 1 from the underside of the aortic arch). Documentation must clearly identify each vessel evaluated.

Echocardiography

✚**93319**   3D echocardiographic imaging and postprocessing during transesophageal echocardiography, or during transthoracic echocardiography for congenital cardiac anomalies, for the assessment of cardiac structure(s) (eg, cardiac chambers and valves, left atrial appendage, interatrial septum, interventricular septum) and function, when performed (List separately in addition to code for echocardiographic imaging)

● indicates a new code; ▲, revised; #, re-sequenced; ✚, add-on; ★, audiovisual technology; and ◀, synchronous interactive audio.

Chapter 19. Common Surgical Procedures and Sedation in Facility Settings

> Three-dimensional echocardiographic imaging and postprocessing is reported when performed during transesophageal echocardiography in patients with or without congenital cardiac anomalies. When 3-dimensional echocardiographic imaging and postprocessing are performed during transthoracic echocardiography, report code 93319 only if the patient has congenital cardiac anomalies.

When performed, report code **93319** in conjunction with transthoracic echocardiography for congenital cardiac anomalies (complete [**93303**] or follow-up/limited [**93304**] study); echocardiography, transesophageal, real time with image documentation (**93312, 93314**); or transesophageal echocardiography for congenital cardiac anomalies (**93315, 93317**).

✖ Do not report **93319** in conjunction with 3D rendering with interpretation and reporting (**76376, 76377**), Doppler echocardiography color flow velocity mapping (**93325**), or echocardiography, transesophageal, for guidance of a transcatheter intracardiac or great vessel(s) structural intervention(s) (**93355**).

Cardiac Catheterization for Congenital Heart Defects

Codes **93593–93598** are reported *only when cardiac catheterization is performed for evaluation of congenital cardiac defects.*

See "Cardiac Catheterization for Congenital Heart Defect: Code Chart" at www.aap.org/cfp2023 for a quick reference to codes for cardiac catheterization for congenital anomalies, with codes included for many services that are separately reported when performed during the catheterization.

> Diagnostic heart catheterization in a patient without congenital defect (eg, any acquired heart disease, such as dilated cardiomyopathy secondary to viral myocarditis, coronary artery diagnosis, or intervention in Kawasaki disease) is reported with codes 93451–93456, 93460, and 93461.

There is no age limit for services reported with codes **93593–93598**. As long as there is evaluation of congenital cardiac defects, it is appropriate to report these codes. These codes take into account

- The added technical difficulty presented when structures may be in abnormal positions and locations and access is through abnormal native connections.
- Additional preservice time in both discussing the procedure with parents and reviewing noninvasive data, previous cardiac catheterizations, and previous surgical procedures.
- Procedures may be more time consuming due to small vessels, multiple measurements that must be made, hemodynamic instability of patients, frequency of multiple sites of arterial-venous admixture, and performance of other required interventions.

Heart catheterization includes ultrasound guidance of vascular access, generalized fluoroscopy to guide catheter manipulation, and any limited echocardiographic guidance when performed by the proceduralist. Echocardiography by another cardiologist during the same session is separately reported.

93593 Right heart catheterization for congenital heart defect(s) including imaging guidance by the proceduralist to advance the catheter to the target zone; normal native connections

93594   abnormal native connections

> For reporting purposes, when the morphologic left ventricle or left atrium is in a subpulmonic position due to congenital heart disease (eg, transposition of the great arteries), catheter placement in either of these structures is considered part of right-sided heart catheterization and does not constitute left-sided heart catheterization.

93595 Left heart catheterization for congenital heart defect(s) including imaging guidance by the proceduralist to advance the catheter to the target zone, normal or abnormal native connections

93596 Right and left heart catheterization for congenital heart defect(s) including imaging guidance by the proceduralist to advance the catheter to the target zone(s); normal native connections

93597   abnormal native connections

> Report the appropriate code for right- and left-sided heart catheterization if catheter placement with hemodynamic assessment of the double outlet ventricle *is performed during the right-sided heart catheterization and separately from the arterial approach.* Catheter placement with hemodynamic assessment of the morphologic left ventricle during right-sided heart catheterization alone (ie, not separately from the arterial approach) is considered part of that procedure.

● indicates a new code; ▲, revised; #, re-sequenced; ✚, add-on; ★, audiovisual technology; and ◀, synchronous interactive audio.

✛93598   Cardiac output measurement(s), thermodilution or other indicator dilution method, performed during cardiac catheterization for the evaluation of congenital heart defects (List separately in addition to code for primary procedure)

> **Thermodilution cardiac output assessment is not typically included in right-sided heart catheterization for congenital heart defects. Report code 93598 in addition to the code for diagnostic cardiac catheterization, when performed.**

- Codes for right-sided heart or right- and left-sided heart catheterization for congenital defects are determined on the basis of access through normal or abnormal native connections.
  - Normal native connections exist when blood flow follows the expected course (ie, superior vena cava/inferior vena cava to right atrium, then right ventricle, then pulmonary arteries, for the right side of the heart; left atrium to left ventricle, then aorta, for the left side of the heart). Examples of congenital heart defects with normal connections would include acyanotic defects such as isolated atrial septal defect, ventricular septal defect, or patent ductus arteriosus.
  - Abnormal native connections exist when there are alternative connections for the pathway of blood flow through the heart and great vessels. Abnormal connections are typically present in patients with cyanotic congenital heart defects, any variation of single ventricle anatomy (eg, hypoplastic right or left side of the heart, double outlet right ventricle), unbalanced atrioventricular canal (endocardial cushion) defect, transposition of the great arteries, valvular atresia, tetralogy of Fallot with or without MAPCAs, total anomalous pulmonary veins, truncus arteriosus, and any lesions with heterotaxia and/or dextrocardia.
- The work of imaging guidance, including fluoroscopy and ultrasound guidance for vascular access and catheter placement for hemodynamic evaluation, is included in the cardiac catheterization for congenital heart defects codes, when performed by the same operator.
- Procedures such as percutaneous transcatheter closure of patent ductus arteriosus (**93582**) include right- and left-sided heart catheterization for congenital cardiac anomalies. Be sure to read the *CPT* instructions for procedures performed in conjunction with congenital cardiac catheterization to determine if the catheterization is separately reportable.

Related Procedures

Codes **93462–93464** are reported in conjunction with many services, including cardiac catheterization for congenital heart defects, when applicable.

✛93462   Left heart catheterization by transseptal puncture through intact septum or by transapical puncture

   Report code **93462** in conjunction with **33741, 33745, 33477, 93452, 93453, 93458–93461, 93595–93597, 93582, 93653,** and **93654**.

- Also report code **93462** with **93581** for transseptal or transapical puncture performed for percutaneous transcatheter closure of ventricular septal defect.
- For *transapical puncture* performed for left-sided heart catheterization and percutaneous transcatheter closure of paravalvular leak, report code **93462** in conjunction with **93590** and **93591**. However, do not report **93462** in conjunction with **93590** for *transeptal puncture* through intact septum performed for left-sided heart catheterization and percutaneous transcatheter closure of paravalvular leak.

✛93463   Pharmacologic agent administration (eg, inhaled nitric oxide, intravenous infusion of nitroprusside, dobutamine, milrinone, or other agent) including assessing hemodynamic measurements before, during, after and repeat pharmacologic agent administration, when performed (List separately in addition to code for primary procedure)

   Report code **93463** in conjunction with **33477, 93451–93453, 93456–93461, 93593–93597,** or **93580–93582**.

✛93464   Physiologic exercise study (eg, bicycle or arm ergometry) including assessing hemodynamic measurements before and after

   Report code **93464** in conjunction with **33477, 93451–93453, 93456–93461,** and **93593–93597**.

Pericardiocentesis and Pericardial Drainage

33016	Pericardiocentesis, including imaging guidance, when performed
33017	Pericardial drainage with insertion of indwelling catheter, percutaneous, including fluoroscopy and/or ultrasound guidance, when performed; 6 years and older without congenital cardiac anomaly
33018	birth through 5 years of age or any age with congenital cardiac anomaly

---

● indicates a new code; ▲, revised; #, re-sequenced; ✛, add-on; ★, audiovisual technology; and ◀, synchronous interactive audio.

33019   Pericardial drainage with insertion of indwelling catheter, percutaneous, including CT guidance

- Codes **33016–33019** include imaging guidance when performed. Do not separately report imaging guidance (eg, **75989**, **76942, 77002, 77012, 77021**) with codes **33016–33019**.

    For thoracoscopic (video assisted) pericardial procedures, see code **32601, 32604, 32658, 32659**, or **32661**.

- Echocardiography, when performed solely for the purpose of pericardiocentesis guidance, is not separately reported in addition to codes **33016–33018**.
- For the purpose of reporting percutaneous pericardial drainage with insertion of indwelling catheter (**33017–33019**), congenital cardiac anomaly is defined as
    — Abnormal situs (heterotaxy, dextrocardia, mesocardia)
    — Single ventricle anomaly/physiology
    — Any patient in the first 90-day postoperative period after repair of a congenital cardiac anomaly defect
- Report **33017–33019** only when the catheter remains in place when the procedure is completed and not when a catheter is placed to aspirate fluid and then removed at the conclusion of the procedure.

Atrial Septostomy

33741   Transcatheter atrial septostomy (TAS) for congenital cardiac anomalies to create effective atrial flow, including all imaging guidance by the proceduralist, when performed, any method (eg, Rashkind, Sang-Park, balloon, cutting balloon, blade)

33745   Transcatheter intracardiac shunt (TIS) creation by stent placement for congenital cardiac anomalies to establish effective intracardiac flow, all imaging guidance by the proceduralist when performed, left and right heart diagnostic cardiac catheterization for congenital cardiac anomalies, and target zone angioplasty, when performed (eg, atrial septum, Fontan fenestration, right ventricular outflow tract, Mustard/Senning/Warden baffles); initial intracardiac shunt

+33746   each additional intracardiac shunt location (List separately in addition to code for primary procedure)

Codes **33741–33746** are typically used to report creation of effective intracardiac blood flow in the setting of congenital heart defects.

Code 33741

- Involves the percutaneous creation of improved atrial blood flow (eg, balloon/blade method), typically in infants weighing 4 kg or less with congenital heart disease. Do not append modifier **63** (procedures performed on infants <4 kg) to **33741**.
- Ultrasound guidance for vascular access and fluoroscopic guidance for the intervention is included, when performed. Intracardiac echocardiography including imaging supervision and interpretation is separately reported with code **93662**, when performed.
- Use **93462** to report transseptal puncture performed in conjunction with **33741**.
- Diagnostic cardiac catheterization is not typically performed at the same session as code **33741**; separately report each service when performed. See instructions in *CPT* addressing when it is appropriate to separately report cardiac catheterization. Do not separately report cardiac catheterization that is fluoroscopic guidance for the intervention or limited hemodynamic and angiographic data used solely for the purpose of accomplishing the intervention.

Codes 33745 and 33746

- Include intracardiac stent placement, target zone angioplasty preceding or after stent implantation, and *complete diagnostic right- and left-sided heart catheterization* (not separately reported), when performed.
    — Ultrasound guidance for vascular access and fluoroscopic guidance for the intervention is included, when performed. Intracardiac echocardiography including imaging supervision and interpretation is separately reported with code **93662**, when performed.
    — Includes all balloon angioplasties performed in the target lesion, including any pre-dilation or post-dilation following stent placement, or use of larger/smaller balloon to achieve therapeutic result.
    — Angioplasty in a separate and distinct intracardiac lesion may be reported separately with modifier **59** (distinct procedural service) appended to the angioplasty code.
- Although diagnostic angiography (**93563, 93565–93568, 93569, 93573–93575**) is typically performed during **33745**, target vessels and chambers are highly variable and, *when performed for an evaluation separate and distinct from the stent delivery,* may be reported separately.

Append modifier **59** to codes for diagnostic angiography performed at the same session for angiographic evaluation separate and distinct from the shunt creation.

- When additional, different intracardiac locations are treated in the same session, code **33746** may be reported for each additional intracardiac shunt creation by stent placement at a separate location.

> **Multiple stents placed in a single location may be reported only with a single code and not a first or additional unit of** 33746.

Valvuloplasty

33390 Valvuloplasty, aortic valve, open, with cardiopulmonary bypass; simple (ie, valvotomy, debridement, debulking, and/or simple commissural resuspension)

33391 complex (eg, leaflet extension, leaflet resection, leaflet reconstruction, or annuloplasty)

Do not report code **33391** in conjunction with code **33390**.

Codes for open valvuloplasty of the aortic valve

- Are descriptive of currently performed valvuloplasty procedures
  - Code **33390** is specifically for reporting valvotomy, debridement, debulking, and/or simple commissural resuspension.
  - Code **33391** represents more complex procedures not limited to the examples in the code descriptor.
- May be reported in conjunction with the code for transmyocardial revascularization (**33141**), operative tissue ablation and reconstruction of atria (**33255–33259**), and reoperation, valve procedure, more than 1 month after original operation (**33530**), when appropriate

Open procedures for aortic valve replacement are reported with codes **33405**, **33406**, and **33410** on the basis of the type of replacement valve (ie, prosthetic, homograft, or stentless).

Transcatheter Pulmonary Valve Implantation

33477 Transcatheter pulmonary valve implantation, percutaneous approach, including pre-stenting of the valve delivery site, when performed

The key instructions for reporting code **33477** are that it

- Should be reported only once per session
- Includes, when performed,
  - Percutaneous access, placement of the access sheath, advancement of the repair device delivery system into position, repositioning of the device as needed and deployment of the device(s), angiography, all cardiac catheterization(s) for hemodynamic measurements, intraprocedural contrast injections, radiological supervision, and interpretation performed to guide transcatheter pulmonary valve implantation.

    Do not separately report diagnostic angiography (**93563**, **93566–93568**, **93569**, **93573**) or right-sided heart catheterization (**93451–93461**; **93593**, **93594**; **93596–93598**) that is intrinsic to the procedure.
  - Percutaneous balloon angioplasty of the conduit or treatment zone, valvuloplasty of the pulmonary valve conduit, and stent deployment within the pulmonary conduit or an existing bioprosthetic pulmonary valve.

Diagnostic angiography and right-sided heart catheterization may be separately reported (append modifier **59**) only when one of the following circumstances is true:

- No prior study is available and a full diagnostic study is performed.
- A prior study is available, but, as documented in the medical record, one of the following circumstances applies:
  - There is inadequate visualization of the anatomy and/or pathology.
  - The patient's condition with respect to the clinical indication has changed since the prior study.
  - There is a clinical change during the procedure that requires new evaluation.

Other cardiac catheterization services may be reported separately when performed for diagnostic purposes not intrinsic to transcatheter pulmonary valve implantation.

- **Does not include** (Report separately, when performed.)
  - Codes **92997** and **92998** when pulmonary artery angioplasty is performed at a site separate from the prosthetic valve delivery site
  - Codes **37236** and **37237** when pulmonary artery stenting is performed at a site separate from the prosthetic valve delivery site
  - Same-session/same-day *diagnostic* cardiac catheterization services (See your *CPT* reference for further instruction and append catheterization code with modifier **59**.)
  - Diagnostic coronary angiography performed at a separate session from an interventional procedure
  - Percutaneous coronary interventional procedures

● indicates a new code; ▲, revised; #, re-sequenced; ✚, add-on; ★, audiovisual technology; and ◀, synchronous interactive audio.

Chapter 19. Common Surgical Procedures and Sedation in Facility Settings

— Percutaneous pulmonary artery branch interventions
— Percutaneous ventricular assist device procedure codes (**33990–33993**), ECMO/ECLS procedure codes (**33946–33989**), or balloon pump insertion codes (**33967, 33970, 33973**)
— Percutaneous peripheral bypass (**33367**), open peripheral bypass (**33368**), or central bypass (**33369**)

Transcatheter Interventions for Revascularization/Repair for Coarctation of the Aorta

33894   Endovascular stent repair of coarctation of the ascending, transverse, or descending thoracic or abdominal aorta, involving stent placement; across major side branches
33895   not crossing major side branches
33897   Percutaneous transluminal angioplasty of native or recurrent coarctation of the aorta

Codes **33894, 33895,** and **33897** include all fluoroscopic guidance of the intervention, diagnostic congenital left-sided heart catheterization, all catheter and wire introductions and manipulation, and angiography of the target lesion. For additional diagnostic right-sided heart catheterization in the same setting as **33894** and **33895,** see codes **93593** and **93594.**

Code **33897** may be reported in addition to **33894** or **33895** for balloon angioplasty of an additional coarctation of the aorta in a segment *separate from the treatment zone* for the coarctation stent. However, balloon angioplasty *within the target treatment zone,* either before or after stent deployment, is not separately reportable in conjunction with **33894** or **33895.** For angioplasty and other transcatheter revascularization interventions *of additional upper or lower extremity vessels* in the same setting as **33897,** use the appropriate code from the Surgery/Cardiovascular System section of *CPT.*

✖ Do not report **33897** in conjunction with open or percutaneous transluminal angioplasty (**37246**) or with transcatheter stent placement for occlusive disease (**37236**).

Codes **33894** and **33895** include stent introduction, manipulation, positioning, and deployment as well as any additional stent delivery in tandem with the initial stent for extension purposes.

● Codes **33894** and **33895** are differentiated by whether or not stent placement crosses major side branches of the aorta. Major side branches include
— Thoracic aorta: brachiocephalic, carotid, and subclavian arteries
— Abdominal aorta: celiac, superior mesenteric, inferior mesenteric, and renal arteries

✖ Do not separately report the following services when reporting codes **33894, 33895,** and **33897:**
— Insertion of a temporary pacemaker (**33210**) to facilitate stent positioning, when performed
— Introduction, positioning, and deployment of an endograft for treatment of abdominal aortic pathology (**34701–34706**)
— Introduction of catheter, aorta (**36200**)
— Thoracic or abdominal aortography (**75600, 75605, 75625**)
— Left heart catheterization for congenital heart defect(s) (**93595**)
— Right and left heart catheterization for congenital heart defect(s) for normal or abnormal native connections (**93596, 93597**)

✖ Do not separately report balloon angioplasty of the aorta *within the coarctation treatment zone* (transluminal angioplasty, **37246**; open or percutaneous angioplasty with transcatheter stent placement for occlusive disease, **37236**; or **33897**) when reporting **33894** and **33895.**

● The following services may be separately reported when performed before or after coarctation stent deployment during endovascular repair of coarctation of the aorta (**33894, 33895**):
— Balloon angioplasty or stenting of the innominate, carotid, subclavian, visceral, iliac, or pulmonary artery
— Arterial or venous embolization
— Additional atrial, ventricular, pulmonary, or coronary or bypass graph angiography with injection procedure during cardiac catheterization (**93563–93568**)

For angiography of other vascular structures, use the appropriate code from the Radiology/Diagnostic Radiology section of *CPT.*

Percutaneous Pulmonary Artery Revascularization

●**33900**   Percutaneous pulmonary artery revascularization by stent placement, initial; normal native connections, unilateral
●**33901**   normal native connections, bilateral
●**33902**   abnormal connections, unilateral
●**33903**   abnormal connections, bilateral
✚●**33904**   Percutaneous pulmonary artery revascularization by stent placement, each additional vessel or separate lesion; normal or abnormal connections

● indicates a new code; ▲, revised; #, re-sequenced; ✚, add-on; ★, audiovisual technology; and ◀, synchronous interactive audio.

Endovascular repair of pulmonary artery stenosis by stent placement is reported on the basis of normal native or abnormal connections and unilateral or bilateral procedures.

- Stent placement within the pulmonary arteries via normal native connections (**33900**, **33901**) is reported when the pathway to stent placement is through the superior vena cava/inferior vena cava to right atrium, then right ventricle, then pulmonary arteries.
- Stent placement via abnormal connections with codes **33902** and **33903** includes placement within the pulmonary arteries, the ductus arteriosus, or a surgical shunt; via abnormal connections; or through postsurgical shunts (eg, Blalock-Taussig shunt, Sano shunt, or post Glenn operation or Fontan procedure).
- Code **33904** is an add-on code that describes placement of stent(s) in additional vessels or lesions beyond the primary vessel or lesion treated regardless of whether access occurs via normal or abnormal connections.
- Codes **33900–33904** include vascular access and all catheter and guidewire manipulation; fluoroscopy to guide the intervention; any post-diagnostic angiography for the purpose of road mapping; post-implant evaluation; stent positioning, and balloon inflation for stent delivery; and radiological supervision and interpretation of the intervention.
- Report only **33904** in conjunction with **33900–33903**.

> Diagnostic right- and left-sided heart catheterization, diagnostic coronary angiography, and diagnostic angiography may be separately reported only in conjunction with **33900–33904** when the services are separate and distinct from pulmonary artery revascularization. Be sure to read the *CPT* instructions to determine whether the catheterization is separately reportable.

✖ **Do not report diagnostic cardiac catheterization and diagnostic angiography codes (93451–93568, 93593–93598) in conjunction with 33900–33904 for any of the following procedures:**
— Contrast injections, angiography, road mapping, and/or fluoroscopic guidance for the stent placement
— Pulmonary conduit angiography for guidance
— Right-sided heart catheterization for hemodynamic measurements before, during, and after stent placement

✖ **Do not report balloon angioplasty within the same target lesion as the stent implant, either before or after stent deployment.** Balloon angioplasty for a distinct lesion or in a different artery may be separately reported with **92997** and **92998** when performed at the same session.

Percutaneous Transcatheter Closure of Patent Ductus Arteriosus

93582   Percutaneous transcatheter closure of patent ductus arteriosus

- Includes, when performed (do not separately report)
  — Introduction of catheter, right heart or main pulmonary artery (**36013**)
  — Selective catheter placement, left or right pulmonary artery (**36014**)
  — Introduction of catheter, aorta (**36200**)
  — Aortography, thoracic, without serialography, radiological supervision and interpretation (**75600**)
  — Aortography, thoracic, by serialography, radiological supervision and interpretation (**75605**)
  — Heart catheterization or catheter placement for coronary angiography (**93451–94361**)
  — Heart catheterization for congenital cardiac anomalies (**93593–93598**)
  — Injection procedure during cardiac catheterization including imaging supervision, interpretation, and report; for supravalvular aortography (**93567**)
- Separately report when performed at the time of transcatheter patent ductus arteriosus closure
  — Pharmacologic agent administration (**93463**)
  — Intracardiac echocardiography during therapeutic/diagnostic intervention, including imaging supervision and interpretation (**93662**)
  — Add-on codes for injection procedures during cardiac catheterization, including imaging supervision, with interpretation and report, for
    ▪ Selective coronary angiography during congenital heart catheterization (**93563**)
    ▪ Selective opacification of aortocoronary venous or arterial bypass graft(s) to 1 or more coronary arteries and in situ arterial conduits, whether native or used for bypass to 1 or more coronary arteries during congenital heart catheterization, when performed (**93564**)
    ▪ Selective left ventricular or left atrial angiography (**93565**)
    ▪ Selective right ventricular or right atrial angiography (**93566**)
    ▪ Nonselective pulmonary arterial angiography (**93568**) or selective pulmonary angiography (**93569**, **93573–93575**) performed during congenital heart catheterization

> Modifier **63** may be appended to code **93582** when the procedure is performed on an infant weighing less than 4 kg.

Vascular Access

Many vascular access procedures are included in the services reported with critical or intensive care codes. Please see **Chapter 18** for a list of procedures that are not separately reported by a physician or QHP who is reporting critical care services on the same date.

Central Venous Access

There is no distinction between venous access achieved percutaneously or via cutdown. Report the venous access code appropriate to the

- Type of insertion (ie, centrally inserted or peripherally inserted)
- Type of catheter (eg, non-tunneled vs tunneled)
- Device (eg, with or without port)
- Age of child

   In non-facility settings, code **96522** may be reported for refilling and maintenance of an implantable pump or reservoir for systemic (intravenous, intra-arterial) drug delivery.

   Irrigation of an implanted venous access device for drug delivery (**96523**) is reported only in non-facility settings and when no other service is reported by the same individual on the same date.

- Codes for refilling and maintenance and/or irrigation are not reported by physicians in facility settings.

> If an existing central venous access device is removed and a new one *placed via a separate venous access site,* appropriate codes for both procedures (removal of old, if code exists, and insertion of new device) should be reported. See replacement codes for removal with replacement *via the same venous access site.*

Insertion or Replacement of Centrally Inserted Central Venous Access Device

See "Centrally Inserted Central Venous Catheter: Codes for Insertion and Replacement" at www.aap.org/cfp2023 for a comparison of codes by procedure and the patient's age.

- Codes **36555–36558** and **36560** and **36561** are selected on the basis of the patient's age on the date of the procedure to insert the catheter.
- Codes for insertion of a tunneled centrally inserted central venous catheter (**36563–36566**) are not selected on the basis of the patient's age.
- To qualify as a centrally inserted central venous access device, both the following circumstances must be true:
  - The entry site must be the *jugular, subclavian, or femoral vein or the inferior vena cava.*
  - The tip of the catheter must terminate in the *subclavian, brachiocephalic (innominate), or iliac veins; the superior or inferior vena cava; or the right atrium.*
- Moderate sedation services are separately reportable with codes **99151–99157**. For more information on reporting moderate sedation, see the Sedation section later in this chapter.
- Report imaging guidance for gaining access to venous entry site or manipulating the catheter into final central position (in addition to codes **36555–36558**) with either of the following codes:
  - **76937** (ultrasound guidance for vascular access requiring ultrasound evaluation of potential access sites, documentation of selected vessel patency, concurrent real-time ultrasound visualization of vascular needle entry, with permanent recording and reporting)
  - **77001** (fluoroscopic guidance for central venous access device placement, replacement [catheter only or complete], or removal [includes fluoroscopic guidance for vascular access and catheter manipulation, any necessary contrast injections through access site or catheter with related venography radiologic supervision and interpretation, and radiographic documentation of final catheter position])
- ✖ *Do not separately report ultrasonography only for vessel identification.*
- Report replacement of the catheter only with **36578**, or report complete replacement with **36578–36583**.

Insertion of Peripherally Inserted Central Venous Access Device

Midline catheters terminate in the peripheral venous system. Midline catheter insertion is not reported as a peripherally inserted central venous catheter insertion. See codes 36400, 36406, and 36410 for midline catheter insertion.

See "Peripherally Inserted Central Venous Catheter: Codes" at www.aap.org/cfp2023 for comparison of codes for PICC insertion procedures and codes for PICC replacement procedures.

- To qualify as a PICC, both the following circumstances must be true:
  - The entry site must be a peripheral vein (eg, axillary, basilic, or cephalic).
  - The tip of the catheter must terminate in the subclavian, brachiocephalic (innominate), or iliac veins; the superior or inferior vena cava; or the right atrium.
- Codes **36568** and **36569** are reported for PICC insertion without a subcutaneous port *and without imaging guidance* on the basis of the patient's age. This includes placement by using magnetic guidance or any guidance modality that does not include imaging with image documentation.
- ✖ Do not report imaging guidance (**76937**, **77001**) in conjunction with codes **36568** and **36569**.
- If imaging guidance is used in PICC insertion, see codes **36572**, **36573**, and **36584**. Imaging guidance is included in the placement (**36572**, **36573**) or complete replacement (**36584**) of a PICC without subcutaneous port or pump.
- ✖ Do not report chest radiographs (**71045**–**71048**) for the purpose of documenting the final catheter position by the same physician on the same day of service as the PICC insertion (**36572**, **36573**, or **36584**). If PICC insertion is performed without confirmation of the catheter tip location, append modifier **52** (reduced service) to the code for catheter insertion (**36572**, **36573**, or **36584**).
- Documentation of services includes
  - Images from all modalities used (eg, ultrasonography, fluoroscopy) stored to the patient record
  - Associated supervision and interpretation
  - Venography performed through the same venous puncture
  - The final central position of the catheter with imaging
- Report PICC insertion *with a subcutaneous port* with codes **36570** and **36571**.
  - Ultrasound (**76937**) or fluoroscopic guidance (**77001**) may be separately reported when performed and documented.
  - Documentation of ultrasound guidance for PICC placement should include evaluation of the potential puncture sites, patency of the entry vein, and real-time ultrasound visualization of needle entry into the vein.

Repair of Central Venous Catheters

36575	Repair of tunneled or non-tunneled central venous access catheter, without subcutaneous port or pump, central or peripheral insertion site
36576	Repair of central venous access device, with subcutaneous port or pump, central or peripheral insertion site
36593	Declotting by thrombolytic agent of implanted vascular access device or catheter
36595	Mechanical removal of pericatheter obstructive material (eg, fibrin sheath) from central venous device via separate venous access

For radiological supervision and interpretation of mechanical removal of pericatheter obstructive material from a central venous device via separate venous access, report 75901.

36596	Mechanical removal of intraluminal (intracatheter) obstructive material from central venous device through device lumen
36598	Contrast injection(s) for radiologic evaluation of existing central venous access device, including fluoroscopy, image documentation and report

Repair of a central venous catheter includes fixing the device without replacement of the catheter or port/pump.

- For the repair of a multi-catheter device, with or without subcutaneous ports or pumps, use the appropriate code describing the service with 2 units of service.
- Repair of any central venous access catheter *without a port or pump* is reported with code **36575**.
- Repair of any central venous catheter *with a port or pump* is reported with code **36576**.
- Code **36593** is reported for declotting of an implanted vascular device or catheter *by thrombolysis*.
- Code **36593** *is not reported* for declotting of a pleural catheter. Use unlisted procedure code **32999** for declotting of a pleural catheter.

- Code **36595** and **36596** are reported for a procedure with *mechanical removal* of pericatheter or intraluminal obstructive material.
  - Radiological supervision and interpretation are separately reported with code **75901**.
  - Do not report code **36595** or **36596** in conjunction with code **36593** or **36598**.
- When the patency of a central catheter is evaluated under fluoroscopy, code **36598** is reported for the contrast injection, image documentation, and report.
  - Fluoroscopy (**76000**) is not separately reported.
  - See codes **75820–75827** for complete venography studies.

Removal of Central Venous Catheters

36589   Removal of tunneled central venous catheter, without subcutaneous port or pump

36590   Removal of tunneled central venous access device, with subcutaneous port or pump, central or peripheral insertion

Removal codes are reported for removal of the entire device. See replacement codes for partial replacement (catheter only) or complete exchange *in the same venous access site* of central venous access devices.

- For removal of both catheters (placed from separate venous access sites) of a multi-catheter device, with or without subcutaneous ports/pumps, use the appropriate code describing the service with 2 units of service.
- When removal of an existing central venous access device is performed in conjunction with placement of new device *via a separate venous access site*, report both procedures.

Arterial Access

36600   Arterial puncture, withdrawal of blood for diagnosis

36620   Arterial catheterization or cannulation for sampling, monitoring or transfusion (separate procedure); percutaneous

36625   cutdown

- An arterial puncture for diagnosis is reported with code **36600**.
- Code **36620** is reported when a percutaneous peripheral arterial catheterization is performed. Code **36625** is reported when a cutdown is performed.

Transfusions

36430   Transfusion, blood or blood components

36440   Push transfusion; blood, 2 years or younger

> **Push transfusion (36440) is used only for patients younger than 2 years.**

36450   Exchange transfusion, blood, newborn

36455   other than newborn

36456   Partial exchange transfusion, blood, plasma, or crystalloid necessitating the skill of a physician or other qualified health care professional; newborn

> **The placement of catheters to support exchange transfusions may be reported separately with the appropriate vascular access codes.**

- Transfusion (**36430**) or push transfusion (**36440**) should be used only if the physician personally infuses the substance and not if the blood is administered by nursing personnel and allowed to enter the vessel via gravity or meter flow. Codes **36430** and **36440** are not separately reported when the same physician or physicians of the same specialty and same group practice are reporting neonatal or pediatric critical care (**99468–99472, 99475, 99476**).
- Complete exchange transfusions (double volume) performed during the neonatal period are reported by using code **36450**; exchange transfusions for all other age-groups are reported by using code **36455**.
  - The assumption is that the exchange for the neonate is performed via the umbilical vein, while an exchange for an older child or adult is performed via a peripheral vessel.
  - The actual placement of catheters to support the exchange transfusion may be reported separately with the appropriate vascular access codes.

● indicates a new code; ▲, revised; #, re-sequenced; ✚, add-on; ★, audiovisual technology; and ◀, synchronous interactive audio.

- Partial exchange transfusions (eg, for hyperviscosity syndrome in the neonate) should be reported using code **36456**.
- ✖ Do not report other transfusion codes (**36430**, **36440**, or **36450**) with **36456**.
- ✖ Do not append modifier **63** (procedure performed on infants <4 kg) when reporting code **36450** or **36456**.

> See Chapter 14 for information on coding for hydration and intravenous infusion services.
>
> These services *are not reported by a physician or other qualified health care professional when performed in a facility setting* because the physician work associated with these procedures involves only affirmation of the treatment plan and direct supervision of the staff performing the services. These codes may be reported by the facility.

Ear, Nose, and Throat Procedures

69421   Myringotomy including aspiration and/or eustachian tube inflation requiring general anesthesia
69436   Tympanostomy (requiring insertion of ventilating tube), general anesthesia

- For bilateral procedure, report code **69436** with modifier **50**.
- Insertion of ventilation tube(s) is not separately reported when performed in conjunction with another middle ear procedure (eg, tympanoplasty) without significant increase in work.
- Cleaning debris from the lateral drum, including a pars flaccida retraction pocket, is inclusive to the tube placement code.
- Use of an operating microscope is included in the procedure described by **69436**.

> Code 69436 may be reported without a modifier (eg, 52, reduced service) when a ventilating tube is replaced under general anesthesia. See 69433 (tympanostomy requiring insertion of a ventilation tube) for replacement by using local or topical anesthetic in the office.

92511   Nasopharyngoscopy with endoscope (separate procedure)

   Code **92511** is designated as a "separate procedure" and should not be reported in addition to the code for the total procedure or service of which it is considered an integral component.

- When carried out independently, report code **92511**.
- When considered to be unrelated or distinct from other procedures or services provided at that time, report code **92511 59** in addition to other procedures or services.

Laryngoplasty

#31551   Laryngoplasty; for laryngeal stenosis, with graft, without indwelling stent placement, younger than 12 years of age
#31552   age 12 years or older
#31553   Laryngoplasty; for laryngeal stenosis, with graft, with indwelling stent placement, younger than 12 years of age
#31554   age 12 years or older
31580   Laryngoplasty; for laryngeal web, with indwelling keel or stent insertion
31584   Laryngoplasty; with open reduction and fixation of (eg, plating) fracture, includes tracheostomy, if performed

- ✖ Do not report graft separately if harvested through the laryngoplasty incision (eg, thyroid cartilage graft).
- Report only one of the following codes for a single operative session: **31551–31554** or **31580**.
- Codes for treatment of laryngeal stenosis by laryngoplasty with graft are selected on the basis of whether or not the procedure includes indwelling stent placement and by the age of the patient (<12 years or ≥12 years).
- Open treatment of a hyoid fracture is reported with code **31584** (repair procedure on the larynx).
- To report tracheostomy, see code **31600**, **31601**, **31603**, **31605**, or **31610**.
- Report laryngoplasty, not otherwise specified or for removal of a keel or stent, with code **31599**.

Adenoidectomy and Tonsillectomy

42820   Tonsillectomy and adenoidectomy; younger than age 12
42821   age 12 or over
42825   Tonsillectomy, primary or secondary; younger than age 12
42826   age 12 or over

● indicates a new code; ▲, revised; #, re-sequenced; ✚, add-on; ★, audiovisual technology; and ◄, synchronous interactive audio.

42830	Adenoidectomy, primary; younger than age 12
42831	age 12 or over
42835	Adenoidectomy, secondary; younger than age 12
42836	age 12 or over

For partial ablation of tonsils with laser, report the appropriate code from **42820** or **42821**, or **42825** or **42826**, with modifier **52** (reduced service).

For control of hemorrhage following tonsillectomy or adenoidectomy, see codes **42960–42972**.

✹ Do not append modifier **52** (reduced service) when intracapsular tonsillectomy is performed. Report the procedure (tonsillectomy or tonsillectomy with adenoidectomy) by using the appropriate code without a modifier, as the work of the procedure and outcome are unchanged.

Digestive System Procedures

Gastric Intubation and Aspiration

| 43752 | Naso- or orogastric tube placement, requiring physician's skill and fluoroscopic guidance (includes fluoroscopy, image documentation and report) |
| 43753 | Gastric intubation and aspiration(s), therapeutic (eg, for ingested poisons), including lavage if performed |

Do not report code **43752** or **43753** in conjunction with critical or intensive care services (**99291, 99292; 99466–99469; 99471–99476;** or **99477–99480**). Append modifier **25** to codes for other significant, separately identifiable E/M services (eg, hospital care, consultation).

Note that code **43752** is reported when a physician's skill is required for placement of a nasogastric or orogastric tube using fluoroscopic guidance.

● This service is not separately reported when a physician's skill is not required or placement is performed without fluoroscopic guidance.

● Replacement of a nasogastric tube requiring physician's skill and fluoroscopic guidance may also be reported with code **43752**.

✹ Do not separately report **43752** for tube placement to insufflate the stomach before percutaneous gastrointestinal tube placement.

Examples

➤ **A 10-year-old is brought to the ED after having ingested drugs.** Gastric intubation and lavage are performed.
Code **43753** would be reported in addition to the appropriate E/M service (eg, ED services **99281–99285**).

➤ **A patient requires placement of a nasogastric tube.** Attempts by nursing staff are unsuccessful, so placement by the physician is required. The physician places the tube by using fluoroscopic guidance.
Code **43752** would be reported in addition to the appropriate E/M service but is not reported when the service is performed by the physician out of convenience rather than necessity for a physician's skill. Use of fluoroscopic guidance is required and must be documented (ie, image documentation and report).

Appendectomy

44950	Appendectomy
+44955	when done for indicated purpose at time of other major procedure
44960	for ruptured appendix with abscess or generalized peritonitis
44970	Laparoscopy, surgical, appendectomy
44979	Unlisted laparoscopy procedure, appendix

As a sole procedure, appendectomy coding is fairly straightforward, with 3 code choices: **44950**, **44960**, and **44970**.

CPT instructs that incidental appendectomy (ie, not due to disease or symptom) during intra-abdominal surgery does not usually warrant reporting a code for the appendectomy procedure.

● If it is necessary to report an incidental appendectomy performed during another intra-abdominal procedure, append modifier **52** (reduced service).

● indicates a new code; ▲, revised; #, re-sequenced; ✚, add-on; ★, audiovisual technology; and ◀, synchronous interactive audio.

- The Medicaid NCCI manual also instructs that incidental removal of a normal appendix during another abdominal surgery is not separately reportable. This instruction is likely followed by other payers.

  Appendectomy performed for an indicated purpose (ie, problem with the appendix) in conjunction with another procedure is separately reported.

- Report add-on code **44955** in addition the code for the primary procedure when open appendectomy is performed (due to clinical indication) in conjunction with another procedure.
- For a laparoscopic appendectomy when done for an indicated purpose at the time of another major procedure, report code **44979**.
- A separate diagnosis code (distinct from the diagnoses for which other intra-abdominal procedures were performed) should be linked to the appendectomy procedure code to indicate the medical necessity of the procedure.

Hernia Repair

49491	Repair, initial inguinal hernia, preterm infant (younger than 37 weeks gestation at birth), performed from birth up to 50 weeks postconception age, with or without hydrocelectomy; reducible
49492	incarcerated or strangulated
49495	Repair, initial inguinal hernia, full term infant younger than age 6 months, or preterm infant older than 50 weeks postconception age and younger than age 6 months at the time of surgery, with or without hydrocelectomy; reducible
49496	incarcerated or strangulated
49500	Repair initial inguinal hernia, age 6 months to younger than 5 years, with or without hydrocelectomy; reducible
49501	incarcerated or strangulated
49505	Repair initial inguinal hernia, age 5 years or older; reducible
49507	incarcerated or strangulated
49520	Repair recurrent inguinal hernia, any age; reducible
49521	incarcerated or strangulated

- For the purpose of reporting inguinal hernia repair, postconception age equals gestational age at birth plus age of newborn/infant in weeks at the time of the hernia repair.
- Initial inguinal hernia repair performed on preterm newborns and infants who are older than 50 weeks' postconception age and younger than 6 months at the time of surgery should be reported by using codes **49495** and **49496**.
- ✖ Do not append modifier **63** (procedure performed on infants <4 kg) to code **49491**, **49492**, **49495**, or **49496**.
- Separately report inguinal hernia repair (**49495–49525**) performed in conjunction with inguinal orchiopexy (**54640**).

> See Appendix II for new codes for reporting anterior abdominal hernia(s) (ie, epigastric, incisional, ventral, umbilical, spigelian), by any approach (**49591–49618**) and for reporting repair of parastomal hernia (**49621, 49622**).

Genitourinary System Procedures

Anogenital Examination

99170	Anogenital examination, magnified, in childhood for suspected trauma including image recording when performed

Moderate sedation of 10 minutes or more may be separately reported when performed by the same physician performing the anogenital examination.

Example

➤ **A child is brought to the ED for concern of sexual molestation after blood was found in the child's underpants.**
The physician performs a comprehensive history and physical examination. Because of the findings on general examination, the physician elects to further examine the child's genitalia with magnification to document findings that may be consistent with abuse or trauma.

Chapter 19. Common Surgical Procedures and Sedation in Facility Settings

ICD-10-CM	CPT
Report confirmed abuse with all the following codes: **T74.22XA** (child sexual abuse, confirmed, initial encounter) An appropriate injury code (eg, **S39.848A**, other specified injuries of external genitals, initial encounter) A code from categories **X92–Y06** or **Y08** for assault A code from category **Y07** to identify the perpetrator of assault If abuse is suspected but not confirmed, report **T76.22XA** (child sexual abuse, suspected, initial encounter) and a code for injury. If there are no findings, report **Z04.42** (encounter for examination and observation following alleged child rape or sexual abuse).	**99285** (comprehensive ED examination) **99170** (anogenital examination) If the same physician performs moderate (conscious) sedation, also report code **99152**. For more on moderate sedation, see the Sedation section later in this chapter.

Lysis/Excision of Labial or Penile Adhesions

Lysis of labial or penile adhesions performed by the application of manual pressure without the use of an instrument to cut the adhesions is considered part of the evaluation and management visit and not reported separately.

54162   Lysis or excision of penile post-circumcision adhesions

Code **54162** is reported only when lysis is performed under general anesthesia or regional block, with an instrument, and under sterile conditions.

- This code has a 2022 total relative value of 5.87 when performed in a facility setting and a Medicare 10-day global surgery period, which payers may or may not use.
- If post-circumcision adhesions are manually broken during the postoperative period by the physician or physician of the same group and specialty who performed the procedure, it would be considered part of the global surgical package. Code **99024** is reported for the service.

An integumentary repair performed in conjunction with lysis or excision of penile post-circumcision adhesion is not reported in addition to code **54162**.

- Report the service with *ICD-10-CM* code **N47.0**, adherent prepuce in a newborn, or **N47.5**, adhesions of prepuce and glans penis (patients aged >28 days).

For repair of incomplete circumcision with removal of excessive residual foreskin, see code **54163**.

56441   Lysis of labial adhesions

Code **56441** is performed by using a blunt instrument or scissors under general or local anesthesia.
- The 2022 total relative value units for this procedure in a facility setting are 4.61, and the procedure is assigned a Medicare 10-day global surgery period, which may or may not be used by payers.
- *ICD-10-CM* code **Q52.5** (fusion of labia) would be reported with *CPT* code **56441**.
- When provided without anesthesia, modifier **52** may be appended to indicate reduced services. Payer guidance may vary with regard to use of modifier **52**.

Correction of Chordee and Hypospadias

54300   Plastic operation of penis for straightening of chordee (eg, hypospadias), with or without mobilization of urethra

54304   Plastic operation on penis for correction of chordee or for first stage hypospadias repair with or without transplantation of prepuce and/or skin flaps

---

● indicates a new code; ▲, revised; #, re-sequenced; ✚, add-on; ★, audiovisual technology; and ◀, synchronous interactive audio.

▲54340   Repair of hypospadias complication(s) (ie, fistula, stricture, diverticula); by closure, incision, or excision, simple

▲54344   requiring mobilization of skin flaps and urethroplasty with flap or patch graft

▲54348   requiring extensive dissection, and urethroplasty with flap, patch or tubed graft (including urinary diversion, when performed)

▲54352   Revision of prior hypospadias repair requiring extensive dissection and excision of previously constructed structures including re-release of chordee and reconstruction of urethra and penis by use of local skin as grafts and island flaps and skin brought in as flaps or grafts

Code **54300** is appropriately reported for *straightening* of the chordee to correct congenital concealed penis (**Q55.64**). This procedure may also be performed to correct an entrapped penis after newborn circumcision (eg, release of concealed penis with coverage of deficient penile ventral skin by using penile skin-raised Byars flaps and re-circumcision).

Codes **54304–54336** describe procedures performed to *correct* hypospadias in either single-stage or multiple-stage procedures.

✖ Do not separately report codes **54300**, **54304**, or **54360** (plastic operation on penis to correct angulation) when reporting single-stage repair of hypospadias.

   Correction of penile chordee or penile curvature is included in all single-stage repairs of hypospadias.

● For more detailed information on reporting procedures to repair hypospadias, see the American Urological Association policy and advocacy brief, "Pediatric Hypospadias Repair: A New Consensus Document on Coding," at www.auanet.org/Documents/practices-resources/coding-tips/Pediatric-Hypospadias-Repair.pdf; download required.

● Repair or revision of hypospadias complication is reported with codes **54340–54352**.

✖ Do not separately report the following procedures when reporting code **54352**: application of skin substitute graft (**15275**); formation of direct or tubed pedicle (**15574**); island pedicle flap (**15740**); excision of urethral diverticulum (**53235**); one-stage urethroplasty of anterior urethra (**53410**); repair of hypospadias or hypospadias correction described by codes **54300**, **54336**, **54340**, **54344**, and **54348**; or plastic operation to correct penile angulation (**54360**).

Negative Pressure Wound Therapy

97605   Negative pressure wound therapy (eg, vacuum assisted drainage collection), utilizing durable medical equipment (DME), including topical application(s), wound assessment, and instruction(s) for ongoing care, per session; total wound(s) surface area less than or equal to 50 square centimeters

97606   total wound(s) surface area greater than 50 square centimeters

97607   Negative pressure wound therapy (eg, vacuum assisted drainage collection), utilizing disposable, non-durable medical equipment including provision of exudate management collection system, topical application(s), wound assessment, and instructions for ongoing care, per session; total wound(s) surface area less than or equal to 50 square centimeters

97608   total wound(s) surface area greater than 50 square centimeters

   Negative pressure wound therapy

● Requires direct (one-on-one) physician or QHP contact with the patient

● May be initiated in a hospital or surgical center setting and continued in the home setting after discharge

● Includes application of dressings

● Is separately reported when performed in conjunction with surgical debridement (**11042–11047**)

● Includes documentation of current wound assessment, including
  — Quantitative measurements of wound characteristics (eg, site, surface area and depth)
  — Any previous treatment regimens
  — Debridement (when performed)
  — Prescribed length of treatment
  — Dressing types and frequency of changes
  — Other concerns that affect healing

● Includes documentation of progress of healing and changes in the wound, including measurement, amount of exudate, and presence of granulation or necrotic tissue at encounters for ongoing NPWT

   Codes **97605** and **97606** represent NPWT provided via a system that includes a *non-disposable* suction pump and drainage collection device. Supplies, including dressings, are reportable with HCPCS codes (eg, **A6550**, wound care set, for NPWT electrical pump, includes all supplies and accessories).

● Codes **97607** and **97608**
  — Report NPWT that uses a *disposable* suction pump and collection system
  — Are not reported in conjunction with codes **97605** and **97606**

● indicates a new code; ▲, revised; #, re-sequenced; ✚, add-on; ★, audiovisual technology; and ◀, synchronous interactive audio.

Chapter 19. Common Surgical Procedures and Sedation in Facility Settings

— Require verification of coverage policy of the patient's health plan before provision of services, as services may be subject to payer policies limiting to care of specific types of wounds that require NPWT to improve granulation tissue formation and to certain types of NPWT equipment

Supplies for a disposable system are reported with code **A9272**, which also includes all dressings and accessories.

Sedation

Moderate Sedation

Moderate sedation is reported with codes **99151–99153** (provided by the same physician or QHP performing the diagnostic or therapeutic service) and **99155–99157** (provided by a different physician or QHP who is not performing the diagnostic or therapeutic service). See **Chapter 14**, **Table 14-4**, for full code descriptors and time requirements.

Moderate sedation codes are not used to report administration of medications for pain control, minimal sedation (anxiolysis), deep sedation, or monitored anesthesia care (**00100–01999**).

Moderate sedation is discussed in more detail in **Chapter 14**.

Deep Sedation/Anesthesia Services

Deep sedation/analgesia is a drug-induced depression of consciousness during which patients cannot be easily aroused but respond purposefully after repeated verbal or painful stimulation (eg, purposefully pushing away the noxious stimuli). A state of deep sedation may be accompanied by partial or complete loss of protective airway reflexes. Cardiovascular function is usually maintained.

CPT codes for reporting anesthesia services, including deep sedation, monitored anesthesia care, or general anesthesia, are **00100–01999**. These codes are not as specific as codes for other services and generally identify a body area or type of procedure.

00102	Anesthesia for procedures involving plastic repair of cleft lip
01820	Anesthesia for all closed procedures on radius, ulna, wrist, or hand bones

Anesthesia services include
- Preoperative evaluation of the patient
- Administration of anesthetic, other medications, blood, and fluids
- Monitoring of physiologic parameters
- Other supportive services
- Postoperative E/M related to the surgery (Ongoing critical care services by an anesthesiologist may be separately reportable.)

Pediatricians who provide deep sedation services for procedures performed outside the operating suite should follow the same anesthesia policies and coding instructions as other providers of anesthesia services.

> If surgery is canceled, subsequent to the preoperative evaluation, payment may be allowed to the anesthesiologist for an evaluation and management (E/M) service and the appropriate E/M code (eg, consultation) may be reported. See Chapter 17 for information on reporting these services.

Add-on codes may be reported to identify special circumstances that increase the complexity of providing anesthesia care, including

+99100	Patient under 1 year or older than 70 years (not reported in conjunction with codes **00326**, **00561**, **00834**, or **00836**)
+99116	Anesthesia complicated by total body hypothermia
+99135	Anesthesia complicated by controlled hypotension
+99140	Emergency conditions

Emergency is defined by *CPT* as a situation in which delay in treatment of the patient would lead to a significant increase in the threat to life or body part.

Modifiers are reported in addition to anesthesia codes to indicate the physical status of the patient. The American Society of Anesthesiologists (ASA) classification of the patient's physical status is represented by the following HCPCS modifiers:

P1	Normal healthy patient
P2	Patient with mild systemic disease

● indicates a new code; ▲, revised; #, re-sequenced; ✚, add-on; ★, audiovisual technology; and ◄, synchronous interactive audio.

P3	Patient with severe systemic disease
P4	Patient with severe systemic disease that is a constant threat to life
P5	Moribund patient who is not expected to survive without the operation
P6	Declared brain-dead patient whose organs are being removed for donor purposes

Base units for anesthesia services are published in the ASA *Relative Value Guide* and by the CMS for each anesthesia procedure code. Payers do not typically require reporting of base units on the claim for services.

- Many private payers will allow additional base units for physical status modifiers **P3** (1 unit), **P4** (2 units), and **P5** (3 units).
- Anesthesia time is reported in minutes unless a payer directs to report units (1 unit per 15 minutes). Start and stop times must be documented, including multiple start and stop times when anesthesia services are discontinuous.

Other modifiers that may be required by payers for anesthesia services by pediatric physicians are those identifying the type of anesthesia or anesthesia provider.

AA	Anesthesia services performed personally by anesthesiologist

> Payers may require this modifier for services personally rendered by physicians other than anesthesiologists. This signifies that services were not rendered by a nonphysician provider, such as a certified registered nurse anesthetist.

GC	This service has been performed in part by a resident under the direction of a teaching physician
G8	Monitored anesthesia care for deep complex, complicated, or markedly invasive surgical procedure
G9	Monitored anesthesia care for patient who has history of severe cardiopulmonary condition
QS	Monitored anesthesia care service

> Medicare considers deep sedation equivalent to monitored anesthesia care. Private payers may vary.

Postoperative Pain Management

Generally, the surgeon is responsible for postoperative pain management. However, a surgeon may request assistance with postoperative pain management (eg, epidural or peripheral nerve block).

- Payers may require a written request by the surgeon for postoperative pain management by the anesthesia provider.
- When a catheter is placed as the mode of anesthesia (eg, epidural catheter) and retained for use in postoperative pain management, this is not separately reported.
- When separately reporting postoperative pain management, append modifier **59** (distinct procedural service) to indicate the separate service and document this service distinctly (and preferably separately) from the anesthesia record.
- When an epidural catheter is used for postoperative pain management, code **01996** (daily management of epidural) may be reported on days subsequent to the day of surgery. Daily management of other postoperative pain management devices may be reported with subsequent hospital care codes (**99231–99233**).

Example

➤ **An orthopedic surgeon requests preanesthetic insertion of a catheter to provide a continuous infusion of the femoral nerve for postoperative pain relief for a patient undergoing an arthroscopy of the knee with lateral meniscectomy.** The anesthesiologist uses ultrasound guidance to insert a catheter for continuous infusion before inducing general anesthesia for the surgical procedure.

ICD-10-CM	CPT
Appropriate diagnosis code	**01400** (anesthesia for open or surgical arthroscopic procedures on knee joint; not otherwise specified) **64448 59** (injection, anesthetic agent[s] and/or steroid; femoral nerve, continuous infusion by catheter [including catheter placement])

Teaching Point: Because the anesthetist provided a distinct service separate from the anesthesia for the procedure, the catheter insertion is separately reported with modifier **59**. Had the procedure been performed under an epidural block and the epidural catheter left in place for postoperative pain management, no additional code would be reported.

To test your knowledge of the information presented in this chapter, complete the quiz found at the end of it, after the resources.

Chapter Takeaways

This chapter discusses many aspects of coding for surgical care in a facility setting. Following are some takeaways from this chapter:

- Surgical services are packaged to include all the necessary services normally furnished by a surgeon before, during, and after a procedure.
- Payers may assign a global period (eg, 0, 10, or 90 days) based on the periods published in the MPFS or assign other global periods. It is important to identify the global periods when contracting with payers.
- Report code **99024** (postoperative follow-up visit) for follow-up care during the global surgery period.
- It is important to recognize which surgical services are considered a component of another procedure and which are separately reported. Append a modifier, when appropriate, to indicate that a service was distinct from another service provided on the same date.

Resources

AAP Pediatric Coding Newsletter™

"Discontinued or Reduced Services: Modifier **52** or **53**," May 2021 (https://doi.org/10.1542/pcco_book205_document003)

"Initial Fracture Care: Musculoskeletal or Evaluation and Management," February 2021 (https://doi.org/10.1542/pcco_book202_document005)

Online Exclusive Content at www.aap.org/cfp2023

"Cardiac Catheterization for Congenital Heart Defect: Code Chart"

"Centrally Inserted Central Venous Catheter: Codes for Insertion and Replacement"

"Peripherally Inserted Central Venous Catheter: Codes"

"Skin Grafts of Infants and Children: Codes"

Surgery

CMS-designated global periods, Medicare Resource-Based Relative Value Scale Physician Fee Schedule (www.cms.gov/Medicare/Medicare-Fee-for-Service-Payment/PhysicianFeeSched/PFS-Relative-Value-Files.html; see column O)

American Urological Association policy and advocacy brief, "Pediatric Hypospadias Repair: A New Consensus Document on Coding" (www.auanet.org/Documents/practices-resources/coding-tips/Pediatric-Hypospadias-Repair.pdf; download required)

Teaching Physician

Medicare Claims Processing Manual, Chapter 100 (https://cms.hhs.gov/manuals/downloads/clm104c12.pdf)

● indicates a new code; ▲, revised; #, re-sequenced; ✚, add-on; ★, audiovisual technology; and ◀, synchronous interactive audio.

Test Your Knowledge!

1. **Which of the following indications calls for appending modifier 78?**
   a. A patient requires removal of sutures or staples.
   b. A patient requires insertion of a central catheter unrelated to follow-up during the postoperative period of a hernia repair.
   c. A patient is returned to the operating/procedure room for control of postoperative bleeding.
   d. The patient's condition required staged procedures.

2. **When should a reduced service (modifier 52) or discontinued procedure (modifier 53) be reported?**
   a. When required by *Current Procedural Terminology* instruction
   b. When a procedure is canceled before the patient enters the operating/procedure room
   c. When a procedure performed was significantly less than the typical service
   d. Both a and c

3. **Which of the following statements is true of teaching physician rules for surgery other than minor, complex, or high-risk procedures?**
   a. The teaching physician must be personally present for the entire procedure.
   b. The teaching physician must be immediately available to furnish services during the entire procedure.
   c. The teaching physician must personally perform the entire procedure.
   d. The teaching physician must personally perform the key or critical portions of the procedure.

4. **Which of the following cardiac catheterization procedures does not include code selection based on the presence of normal or abnormal connections?**
   a. Right-sided heart catheterization for congenital heart defect.
   b. Left-sided heart catheterization for congenital heart defect.
   c. Right- and left-sided heart catheterization for congenital heart defect.
   d. All cardiac catheterization codes are selected on the basis of normal or abnormal connections.

5. **Which of the following codes or services would be reported when post-circumcision adhesions are manually broken during the postoperative period by the physician who performed the procedure?**
   a. **99024**.
   b. **54162** (lysis or excision of penile post-circumcision adhesions).
   c. Subsequent hospital care is reported.
   d. This service is not reported.

Chapter 19. Common Surgical Procedures and Sedation in Facility Settings

● indicates a new code; ▲, revised; #, re-sequenced; ✚, add-on; ★, audiovisual technology; and ◀, synchronous interactive audio.

Part 4
Digital Medicine Services

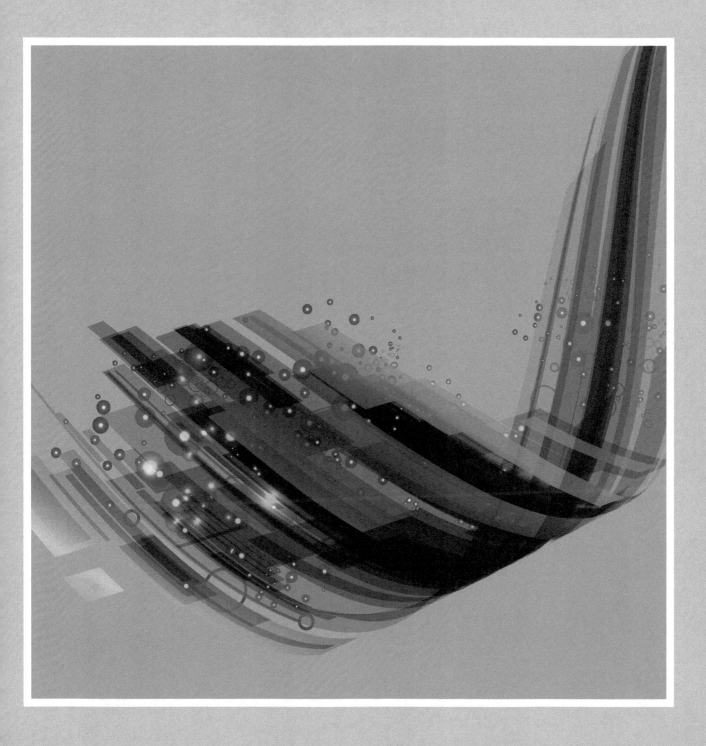

Part 4. Digital Medicine Services

Telemedicine Services

CPT copyright 2022 American Medical Association. All rights reserved.

Contents

Chapter Highlights

- Definitions of telemedicine services
- Identification of codes, modifiers, and places of service (POSs) for telemedicine services
- Differentiation of telemedicine services from telephone or online digital evaluation and management (E/M) services

Telemedicine Services

This chapter provides information on coding for services provided via telemedicine. Put simply, telemedicine allows a physician or other qualified health care professional (QHP) in a distant location to provide medical services to a patient without the need for either party to physically travel. Provision of and payment for telemedicine services has expanded greatly since 2020, when telemedicine became an important method for providing medical care during the COVID-19 public health emergency (PHE).

Telemedicine in *Current Procedural Terminology* (*CPT®*)

Telemedicine is the term used by *Current Procedural Terminology* (*CPT*) to describe synchronous (real-time) provision of medical services via telecommunications. Telemedicine may also be referred to as *telehealth;* definitions for each term vary by state and payer, but *telehealth* is more commonly used to reference any health service provided via telecommunications (eg, collection and interpretation of digitally stored and/or transmitted physiologic data [for a discussion of this data, see **Chapter 21**]).

    CPT describes and provides for reporting of 2 types of telemedicine services.

1. Synchronous telemedicine service rendered via a real-time interactive audio and video telecommunications system
2. Synchronous telemedicine service rendered via telephone or other real-time interactive audio-only telecommunications system

---

Telemedicine Terminology

Key terms in differentiating telemedicine services from other digital services are *synchronous* and *asynchronous*. Telemedicine services (other than a special Medicare demonstration project) always include synchronous communication.

- **Synchronous telemedicine services include simultaneous interaction between a physician or other qualified health care professional and a patient who is located at a distant site.**
- **Asynchronous communication does not require simultaneous interaction from both parties. Examples of asynchronous communication are email and data and/or images transferred for review and subsequent response.**

    CPT does not limit telemedicine services to services reported only by physicians and QHPs whose scope of practice includes E/M services. Many of the services that may be reported as telemedicine are reported by nonphysician QHPs such as psychologists, licensed clinical social workers, dietitians, and speech pathologists.

    Before providing telemedicine or any digital medicine service, understand local and state laws, ensure that communications will be Health Insurance Portability and Accountability Act (HIPAA) of 1996 compliant, establish written guidelines and procedures, educate payers and negotiate for payment, and educate patients. Note that many popular communication platforms, such as FaceTime, Google Talk, and Skype, are not HIPAA compliant and should not be used for health care communications (except when specifically allowed by an emergency use authorization declared by state and federal authorities).

The COVID-19 public health emergency (PHE) prompted some permanent and temporary Medicare payment policy changes that extend to at least December 31, 2023. Changes to state regulations during and as an outcome of the PHE may more directly affect pediatric practice when addressing the location of the patient receiving care via telemedicine (eg, home, non-rural locale), payment parity with in-person services, and practice across state lines. Be sure that your practice is monitoring payment policies and is aware of end dates for temporary policies.

● indicates a new code; ▲, revised; #, re-sequenced; ✛, add-on; ★, audiovisual technology; and ◀, synchronous interactive audio.

Chapter 20. Telemedicine Services

Payer Coverage

Payment for telemedicine services may be affected by state and federal regulations in addition to payer policy. Review the payment policies of health plans and payers such as Medicaid before initiating telemedicine services, as coverage and payment policies may vary.

Although state regulations may require that health plans originating in the state cover and pay equitably for telemedicine services, plans subject to other regulations (eg, self-funded health plans governed by the Employee Retirement Income Security Act of 1974) may be exempt from these state regulations.

When contracting with payers, be aware of plans that include virtual-first or other restrictions of patient access to telemedicine services by community physicians. Virtual-first plans require or encourage patients to use one select telehealth agency for initial health care services and receive a referral before receiving services from a physician or QHP in the patient's community. (This process does not typically apply to services such as recommended preventive services that require in-person examination.) The patient may have access to the plan's virtual care network without out-of-pocket costs versus application of a co-payment and/or deductible to services by other physicians and QHPs.

Medicare has published a list of codes covered when provided via telemedicine (www.cms.gov/Medicare/Medicare-General-Information/Telehealth/Telehealth-Codes), but this list may be more restrictive than the lists used by Medicaid plans and other payers. Private payers may limit telemedicine services to those described by specific codes with benefit policy based on state telemedicine or telehealth regulations. It is important to verify the services and sites of service that are covered by each patient's health plan.

Many health plans develop policies that designate covered and non-covered telemedicine services. Services that are most often not reportable as a telemedicine service include

- A service provided on the same day as an in-person visit, when performed by the same provider and for the same condition

> Typically, the work of 2 evaluation and management (E/M) services provided by the same physician (or physicians of the same group practice and same specialty) addressing the same problem at different times on the same date may be combined and reported as a single E/M service. If reporting 2 E/M services by the same physician addressing different problems, the services may be separately reported with modifier 25 (significant and separately identifiable E/M service) appended to the code for the second E/M service.

- A service that is incidental to an E/M service and limited to clinical staff communication of test results, scheduling additional services, or providing educational resources
- Any service that is not a covered benefit, such as travel vaccines or travel counseling
- Any service that is not separately paid because the service is included in the postoperative work of a procedure (eg, E/M services within 90 days of a major surgery)

Medicaid Payment

For purposes of Medicaid, telemedicine is a service that includes 2-way, real-time interactive communication between the patient and the physician or QHP including, at a minimum, audio and video technology. Although exceptions were made during the PHE, Medicaid plans may limit telemedicine services to those provided to patients who are located in an originating site that is a physician office or other health care facility at the time of service (ie, exclude services to patients in their home).

State telehealth laws often include mandates for coverage of telemedicine services, and some include parity of payment (ie, equal to in-person services). Medicaid payment policies often align with state regulations. Policies vary widely by state and may vary between Medicaid managed care plans (eg, a specific plan may allow more than is required by standard Medicaid policy or regulation).

> **Medicare and Medicaid Telemedicine Terminology**
>
> *Originating site:* location of the patient at the time of service
> *Distant site:* location of the physician or other qualified health care professional at the time of service

Medicaid plans may pay the physician or other QHP at the distant site for each service rendered via telemedicine and pay a facility fee to the originating site (eg, hospital), when applicable. States can also pay any additional costs, such as technical support, transmission charges, and equipment. These add-on costs can be incorporated into the fee-for-service rates or separately paid as an administrative cost by the state. If they are separately billed and paid, the costs must be linked to a covered Medicaid service.

● indicates a new code; ▲, revised; #, re-sequenced; ✚, add-on; ★, audiovisual technology; and ◀, synchronous interactive audio.

States may also choose to pay for services delivered with technology that does not meet the definition of telemedicine services (eg, telephones, facsimile machines, email systems, remote patient monitoring).

> **See Chapter 21 for information on remote patient monitoring services.**

States may cover telemedicine services reported with a variety of *CPT* and Healthcare Common Procedure Coding System (HCPCS) codes. Plans may also pay **T1014** (telehealth transmission, per minute) to originating sites (other than patient's home) or **Q3014** (telehealth originating site facility fee). Modifiers are often required to designate a telemedicine service. For further discussion, see the Telemedicine Modifiers section later in this chapter.

Reporting Telemedicine Services

From a *CPT* coding perspective, telemedicine services are synchronous services provided via audiovisual communication technology (or telephone, for a limited number of services) and reported with the same E/M codes that would be appropriate for in-person encounters.

Synchronous telemedicine service is defined by *CPT* as a real-time interaction between a physician or QHP and a patient who is located at a separate site. The total communication between the physician or QHP and the patient during the course of the synchronous telemedicine service must be of an amount and nature that would be sufficient to meet the requirements of the same service when rendered via a face-to-face interaction.

- *CPT* codes for services that are typically performed face-to-face but may be rendered via a synchronous interactive audio and video telecommunications system are preceded by a star (★) and listed in Appendix P of the *CPT* manual.
- *CPT* codes for telemedicine services that may be delivered by technology including at least synchronous interactive audio communication, in lieu of audiovisual technology, are preceded by an audio symbol (◀) and listed in Appendix T of the *CPT* manual.

> **See Chapter 9 for information on coding for evaluation and management services provided via telephone or online digital communication technology (eg, secure email, patient portal). *Current Procedural Terminology* does not include these services in the listing of telemedicine services for the purpose of code assignment.**

Documentation of Services

Documentation of telemedicine services should be like that of services provided in traditional patient care settings, such as the following documentation:

- The reason for the visit and the requesting party (eg, patient, another physician or QHP)
- Relevant history and physical examination (if there is one)
- Assessment and plan of care and/or recommendations

Documentation must support the service reported (eg, it must describe a critical illness and time spent in remote critical care services). For most E/M services, this requirement means that documentation supports reporting services based on the required medical decision-making (MDM) or total time spent by the physician or QHP directed to care of the individual patient on the date of service.

> **See Chapter 6 for more information on documentation of evaluation and management services and instructions for reporting based on time.**

In addition, some plans require documentation of the patient's and/or caregiver's consent to receive services via telemedicine. Other documentation elements include

- Patient's or family's consent to receive a service via telemedicine.
- Platform or modality by which the service is occurring. It must be HIPAA compliant.
- Patient's location and physician's location.
- Any other individuals present with the patient, including, when offered, identification of and contributions from a tele-presenter (ie, a health care professional who is present with the patient to facilitate the service).
- Start and end times for the telemedicine encounter.

> **Document any technology (eg, digital examination camera, digital stethoscope) used during a telemedicine encounter.**

Place of Service Codes

Use of the correct POS code on claims for telemedicine services is important for appropriate payment. There are 2 POS codes that identify that a service was provided to a patient in a place other than their home or to a patient in their home.

02   Telehealth provided other than in patient's home

10   Telehealth provided in patient's home

Payment may be affected by the POS code, as some services include payment for a physician's or QHP's practice expense for services provided in a non-facility setting (eg, office) versus a facility setting (eg, hospital or hospital-based clinic). Place of service code **02** typically triggers payment at a lower facility-based rate, when applicable.

Some payers accept the POS code for the location where the physician or QHP would provide the service if performed in person (eg, **11**, office) in addition to appending modifier **95** (discussed later in this chapter) to the procedure code to indicate that the service was delivered via telemedicine.

> **See Chapter 4 for more information on place of service codes.**

See an individual payer's telemedicine policy to determine if there are reporting requirements for the specific site of service (eg, physical location from which services were rendered or received).

Field 32 of the 1500 paper claim form and its electronic equivalent is used to report the site of service (eg, hospital name, address, National Provider Identifier). This is typically the physical location of the physician or other provider of service at the time of service when payment is influenced by geographic location.

Telemedicine Modifiers

Modifiers are used to indicate that a service was somehow modified from what is typical (ie, reduced or increased service). *CPT* and HCPCS include modifiers for indicating that a service was provided by telemedicine. It is important to append an indicated modifier as directed by *CPT* or, when applicable, in compliance with an individual health plan's payment policy.

93—Synchronous Telemedicine Service Rendered via Telephone or Other Real-time Interactive Audio-Only Telecommunications System

Modifier **93** has limited utility for physicians and QHPs. Modifier **93** is appended only to services preceded by an audio symbol (◀) and included in *CPT* Appendix T. Some services included in Appendix T include

- Individual behavior change interventions (**99406–99409**)
- Advance care planning (**99497, 99498**)
- Psychiatric services (**90791, 90792; 90832–90840; 90845; 90846, 90847;** and **90785**).
- Health risk assessment (**96160, 96161**)
- Developmental screening (**96110**)

Do not report modifier **93** in conjunction with codes not included in Appendix T (eg, office or other outpatient services **99202–99205** or **99212–99215**).

See modifier **FQ**, discussed later in this chapter, when payer policy requires use of modifier **FQ** (eg, when reporting of follow-up mental health and substance use disorder treatment services provided via audio-only technology).

95—Synchronous Telemedicine Service Rendered via a Real-time Interactive Audio and Video Telecommunications System

Modifier **95** may be appended only to the codes preceded by a star (★) and included in *CPT* Appendix P. Appending modifier **95** to the appropriate procedure code identifies to the payer that telemedicine services were rendered via real-time interactive audio and video telecommunications. This modifier is not applied if the communication is not real-time interactive audio and video.

Appendix P codes that may be of particular interest to pediatricians include

- New and established patient office or other outpatient E/M services (**99202–99205, 99212–99215, 99417**)
- Subsequent hospital inpatient or observation care (**99231–99233**)
- Inpatient or observation (**99252–99255**) and outpatient (**99242–99245**) consultations

---

● indicates a new code; ▲, revised; #, re-sequenced; ✚, add-on; ★, audiovisual technology; and ◀, synchronous interactive audio.

- Administration of patient-focused health risk assessment instrument (eg, health hazard appraisal) with scoring and documentation, per standardized instrument (**96160**)
- Administration of caregiver-focused health risk assessment instrument (eg, depression inventory) for the benefit of the patient, with scoring and documentation, per standardized instrument (**96161**)
- Individual behavior change interventions (**99406–99409**)
- Transitional care management services (**99495**, **99496**)

Appendix P also includes codes for services such as psychotherapy, health and behavior assessment and intervention, medical nutrition therapy, and education and training for patient self-management, allowing for telemedicine services provided by certain qualified nonphysician health care professionals in addition to subspecialty physicians.

> When providing services via telemedicine, it is important to note whether each service may be reported with a telemedicine modifier. While many evaluation and management codes are included in Appendix P of the *CPT* manual, related services may not be included. For instance, use of a structured screening instrument to assess mental or behavioral health (96127) is not included in Appendix P. Individual payers may provide unique lists of codes that may be reported when provided via telehealth with either *Current Procedural Terminology* or Healthcare Common Procedure Coding System modifiers.

Healthcare Common Procedure Coding System (HCPCS) Modifiers

FQ—The Service Was Furnished Using Audio-Only Communication Technology

Modifier **FQ** is used specifically for reporting *telehealth for mental health and substance use disorder treatment services* furnished to a patient in their home by using audio-only communications technology. This modifier is not reported in conjunction with codes for other services unless specified as such in payer policy. See **Chapter 2** for additional information.

Modifier **FQ** may apply to either E/M services or psychiatric services when the reason for the service is continuing management of a diagnosed mental health or substance use disorder.

GQ—Via Asynchronous Telecommunications System

The application of **GQ** is limited to services provided via asynchronous technology (eg, store-and-forward of digital images for interpretation and report).

GT—Via Interactive Audio and Video Telecommunication Systems

Some payers accept modifier **GT** in lieu of modifier **95**. Critical access hospitals billing under Method II report modifier **GT** (via interactive audio and video telecommunication systems) because no POS code is reported on Method II claims to identify telemedicine services. Some health plans may also require modifier **GT,** although this modifier is no longer accepted by Medicare on claims for physician services.

Medicaid plans may also use modifiers **U1–UD** (as defined by the state) to identify, track, and pay for telemedicine services.

HCPCS Telehealth Codes

While *CPT* codes are accepted by most plans covering telemedicine services, payers may require HCPCS codes that are used in the Medicare/Medicaid programs for consultations and other services with specific coverage policies (eg, telehealth critical care consultation).

- HCPCS codes are used for telemedicine consultations with Medicare beneficiaries because *CPT* consultation codes are not payable under the Medicare Physician Fee Schedule.

G0406	Follow-up inpatient consultation, limited, physicians typically spend 15 minutes communicating with the patient via telehealth
G0407	intermediate, physicians typically spend 25 minutes communicating with the patient via telehealth
G0408	complex, physicians typically spend 35 minutes communicating with the patient via telehealth
G0425	Telehealth consultation, emergency department or initial inpatient, typically 30 minutes communicating with the patient via telehealth
G0426	typically 50 minutes communicating with the patient via telehealth
G0427	typically 70 minutes or more communicating with the patient via telehealth
G0459	Inpatient telehealth pharmacologic management, including prescription, use, and review of medication with no more than minimal medical psychotherapy

● indicates a new code; ▲, revised; #, re-sequenced; ✚, add-on; ★, audiovisual technology; and ◀, synchronous interactive audio.

G0508   Telehealth consultation, critical care, physicians typically spend 60 minutes communicating with the patient via telehealth (initial)

G0509   Telehealth consultation, critical care, physicians typically spend 50 minutes communicating with the patient via telehealth (subsequent)

> For further discussion of critical care provided via telemedicine, see the Critical Care via Telemedicine section later in this chapter.

Individual plans vary in their payment policies for telemedicine and HCPCS and *CPT* codes and modifiers used to report telemedicine services. Managers and billing staff must maintain an awareness of these policies to receive appropriate payment.

When payer policies include payment to an originating site for the cost of telehealth transmission and/or a site facility fee, report **T1014** (telehealth transmission, per minute) to originating sites (other than the patient's home) and/or **Q3014** (telehealth originating site facility fee).

Examples of Coding for Telemedicine Services (*CPT*, HCPCS)

The following examples are solely for the purpose of demonstrating coding and are not clinical guidelines. Additionally, code assignment depends on the nature of the service provided as documented in the patient record.

For each example, assume that health plan benefits for telemedicine services have been verified before the encounter.

Example: Hospital Consultation

➤ **A consultation is requested of a physician at a children's hospital for an inpatient in a rural hospital, 75 mi away.** Through real-time interactive technology, the physician performs a consultation, including moderate MDM. The total time of the interactive communication is 30 minutes. A written report to the requesting physician is transmitted via secure electronic health information exchange. The physician's total time, including pre-consultation review of records, documentation, and report to the requesting physician, is 50 minutes.

MDM: Moderate *History:* Comprehensive *Physical examination:* Comprehensive	**CPT** **99254 95** (initial inpatient consultation, which requires moderate MDM or total time of ≥60 minutes) or, if payer requires HCPCS codes, **G0425** (telehealth consultation, emergency department [ED] or initial inpatient, typically 30 minutes communicating with the patient via telehealth)

Teaching Point: Although the physician's total time was less than 60 minutes, the moderate level of MDM supports code **99254**. A payer that does not accept consultation codes may require that the physician report a code for initial hospital inpatient or observation care (**99222 95**, which requires moderate MDM or total time ≥55 minutes) in lieu of the previous codes.

If payer policy allows payment for overhead expenses related to telemedicine services, also report **T1014**, telehealth transmission, per minute, professional services bill separately. Because this is billed per minute, 30 units are reported. The rural hospital, as the originating facility, may also report **Q3014**, telehealth originating site facility fee.

Example: Telemedicine With Prolonged Service

➤ **A parent requests an established patient telemedicine appointment with her 6-year-old son's physician for evaluation of increased asthma symptoms.** The physician obtains history from the patient and his mother via a secure audiovisual connection. The parent reports that the child, who has a history of intermittent asthma, has had nighttime cough and increased awakenings despite daily control medication. The child is asymptomatic at the time of the telemedicine visit. The patient's asthma symptom log is reviewed, and his asthma action plan is updated. A new control medication is prescribed, and approval is obtained from the patient's pharmacy benefit management company. The physician's total time directed to the patient's care is 30 minutes, including the physician's time to document the service.

● indicates a new code; ▲, revised; #, re-sequenced; ✚, add-on; ★, audiovisual technology; and ◀, synchronous interactive audio.

On the evening of the same date, the physician receives a request for an additional telemedicine service because the child is coughing and wheezing. The second evaluation results in referral to the ED because of increasing symptoms despite multiple inhalation treatments. The physician's total time directed to the care of this patient on the date of the encounter is 65 minutes, including both encounters, time spent speaking with a physician in the ED to advise on referral for treatment, and documenting the service.

ICD-10-CM	CPT
J45.22 (mild intermittent asthma with status asthmaticus)	**99215 95** (office or other outpatient visit for an established patient, high level MDM or total time of 40–54 minutes) **99417 95** × 1 unit (prolonged outpatient E/M service[s] time with or without direct patient contact beyond the required time of the primary service when the primary service level has been selected using total time, each 15 minutes)

Teaching Point: The physician's total time of 65 minutes supports code **99215** and one 15-minute period of prolonged outpatient service, **99417**. Both E/M codes are reported with modifier **95** because the service was provided via synchronous audiovisual telemedicine.

When an audiovisual connection cannot be achieved or maintained, some payers advise that the service be reported on the basis of the method by which most of the service was provided. For instance, if a real-time audiovisual encounter is scheduled but the service must be changed to an audio-only (eg, telephone) service because of lack of connectivity, a telephone evaluation and management service should be reported rather than a service provided via real-time audiovisual communication. Payer instructions on these circumstances may vary.

Example: Audio-Only Telemedicine

➤ **A parent requests that her 16-year-old son's scheduled telemedicine appointment for reevaluation of anxiety be changed to a telephone service.** The patient has previously received synchronous audiovisual services, but the parent's internet service has been discontinued because of inability to pay increased rates. The patient's health plan covers audio-only health follow-up services for mental health conditions when provided to patients in their homes. Clinical staff spend 5 minutes before the telephone service obtaining the patient's responses to a structured instrument for evaluation of anxiety and scoring the instrument. At the appointment, the physician spends 30 minutes communicating with the patient and his mother by telephone and recommends a medication change and an in-person follow-up visit in 4 weeks. After the telephone service, the physician spends another 10 minutes ordering a different medication that requires prior authorization by the patient's health plan and documenting the service.

ICD-10-CM	CPT
F41.9 (anxiety)	**99215 FQ** (office or other outpatient visit for an established patient, high level MDM or total time of 40–54 minutes) **96127** (brief emotional/behavioral assessment, with scoring and documentation, per standardized instrument)

Teaching Point: The physician's total time on the date of the encounter (40 minutes) supports code **99215**. Clinical staff time is not included in the time of the E/M service. Modifier **FQ** is reported in lieu of modifier **93**, as code **99215** is not included in the list of codes reported in conjunction with modifier **93** (ie, is not listed in *CPT* Appendix T).

Code **96127** is reported for the collection and scoring of the standardized instrument used in assessment of the patient's anxiety.

Payer policies for telemedicine services are changing frequently because of changes in state regulations, changes in code sets, and availability of communication technology. It is important that practice and billing managers maintain an awareness of state regulations for telemedicine and individual payer policies that may specify allowable codes and required modifiers.

Example: Telemedicine Converted to Digital Evaluation and Management

➤ **A parent requests an established patient telemedicine appointment with her 6-year-old's physician for evaluation of chronic idiopathic urticaria.** At the appointment, the physician attempts to establish a secure audiovisual connection with the parent. However, the connection could not be established. Instead, the physician and parent connect via messaging on the practice's patient portal and the parent sends digital photographs of the rash for the physician's evaluation. Owing to the history and severity of the rash, the physician prescribes steroids and long-acting antihistamines. The patient will be seen in follow-up in 10 days. The physician spends a total of 20 minutes directed to the patient's care, including time spent in electronic communication with the patient's mother, review of the digital images, and generation of prescriptions. The portal messages and images received from the parent are automatically saved to the patient's record. No other E/M service is provided within the next 7 days.

ICD-10-CM	CPT
L50.1 (idiopathic urticaria)	**99422** (online digital evaluation and management service, for an established patient, for up to 7 days, cumulative time during the 7 days; 11–20 minutes of medical consultative discussion and review)

Teaching Point: Online digital E/M services are not considered telemedicine because a telemedicine encounter must include real-time (synchronous) communication. Online digital E/M service codes (**99421–99423**) are selected on the basis of the reporting physician's or QHP's cumulative time devoted to the service during a 7-day period. No modifier is required because the service was provided as described by code **99422**.

Codes **99421–99423** are assigned lower relative value units than telemedicine services provided via synchronous telephone or audiovisual technology.

Learn more about evaluation and management services provided by telephone or online digital communication in Chapter 9.

Critical Care via Telemedicine

CPT codes for critical and intensive care services are not included in *CPT* Appendix P. *CPT* instructs to report unlisted E/M service code **99499** for critical care provided via telemedicine. (Payers may instruct to append modifier **95** when reporting **99499**.) Alternatively, payers may include HCPCS codes **G0508** and **G0509** as covered critical care consultation services when provided via telemedicine.

Example

➤ **A pediatric intensivist is contacted via live audiovisual telecommunications to provide remote critical care to an infant who presented with fever, lethargy, and suspected sepsis.** The intensivist views radiographs and other data from monitoring devices in addition to performing visual and audio examination of the infant. The attending physician at the hospital where the infant is an inpatient performs necessary procedures as advised by the intensivist (eg, lumbar puncture). The infant remains at the same hospital under the care of the pediatrician. A total of 65 minutes of remote critical care service is provided.

The consulting physician reports	**G0508** (telehealth consultation, critical care, physicians typically spend 60 minutes communicating with the patient via telehealth [initial]) or, if a payer does not accept this code, **99499 95** (unlisted E/M service) (Enter description of service on claim or attachment.)
The attending physician reports	*CPT* codes for services personally performed (eg, initial hospital care, intubation, lumbar puncture)

Teaching Point: Code **G0508** is reported only once per date of service per patient. Alternatively, the pediatric intensivist may report an inpatient consultation (**99252–99255**) as allowed under the specific payer's policy for telemedicine.

A payer may require modifier **GT** (via interactive audio and video telecommunication systems) appended to code **G0508**.

● indicates a new code; ▲, revised; #, re-sequenced; ✚, add-on; ★, audiovisual technology; and ◀, synchronous interactive audio.

Continuing Changes in Telemedicine Services

Payer policies and legislation that affect provision of and payment for telemedicine services continue to evolve. It is important that physician practices monitor local and regional payer policies for opportunities to provide medical care via telemedicine, when appropriate, and get paid for the physician work and practice expense of providing these services.

To test your knowledge of the information presented in this chapter, complete the quiz found at the end of it, after the resources. Answers to each quiz are found in **Appendix IV**.

Chapter Takeaways

Telemedicine is an evolving practice resulting in frequent changes to codes, modifiers, guidelines, and payer policies. Following are some takeaways from this chapter:

- From a coding perspective, telemedicine describes synchronous (real-time) provision of medical services via telecommunications.
- Telemedicine services typically require real-time audiovisual communication, but certain services may be reported with modifier **93** or **FQ** when provided via audio-only communication technology.
- State regulations and payer policies for coverage of and payment for telemedicine services vary. Practices must monitor and adapt to these changes to support provision and payment for telemedicine services.

Resources

CPT Telemedicine Code List

CPT list of codes that may be reported with modifier **93** and **95** (See appendixes P and T of your *CPT* coding reference.)

Medicare Telehealth Policies and Service List

Medicare list of codes covered when provided via telemedicine (www.cms.gov/Medicare/Medicare-General-Information/Telehealth/Telehealth-Codes)

Telemedicine Originating Site Eligibility Analyzer

Health Resources and Services Administration Medicare Telehealth Payment Eligibility Analyzer for originating site payment (https://data.hrsa.gov/tools/medicare/telehealth)

● indicates a new code; ▲, revised; #, re-sequenced; ✚, add-on; ★, audiovisual technology; and ◀, synchronous interactive audio.

Test Your Knowledge!

1. **Per *Current Procedural Terminology*, which of the following services is required to append modifier 95?**
   a. Collection and interpretation of digitally transmitted physiologic data
   b. Any non–face-to-face service
   c. Store-and-forward telehealth service
   d. Synchronous telemedicine service

2. **Which of the following services is signified by modifier 93?**
   a. Clinical staff contacted a patient by telephone to relay test results.
   b. A service was provided via synchronous audiovisual technology.
   c. A service was provided via synchronous audio-only technology.
   d. A service was provided via asynchronous audio-only technology.

3. **Which of the following Medicaid terms describes the location of the physician or qualified health care professional delivering a telemedicine service?**
   a. *Distant site*
   b. *Place of service code*
   c. *Originating site*
   d. *Modifier*

4. **What differentiates modifier 93 from modifier FQ?**
   a. Any service represented by a *Current Procedural Terminology* (*CPT*) code may be reported with modifier **93**.
   b. Only modifier **93** can be appended to a *CPT* code.
   c. Modifier **FQ** is used only when reporting services to manage mental health or substance use disorders.
   d. Modifier **FQ** is reported only when the service is synchronous.

5. **True or false? Code selection for telemedicine services is based solely on the time spent in direct communication with the patient and/or caregiver.**
   a. True
   b. False

● indicates a new code; ▲, revised; #, re-sequenced; ✚, add-on; ★, audiovisual technology; and ◀, synchronous interactive audio.

Remote Data Collection and Monitoring Services

CPT copyright 2022 American Medical Association. All rights reserved.

Contents

This chapter reviews codes for reporting services that include collection of data over time with submission/transmission of data for review and report at the conclusion of the service period and for reporting remote monitoring of patient data with concurrent treatment management services.

Codes included describe the following related services:
- Device supply and data capture/transfer services
- Patient education/training and device calibration

Chapter Highlights
- General documentation elements for remote data collection and monitoring services
- Identification and differentiation of codes for specific types of remote data collection and monitoring or management services

Getting Paid for Remote Data Monitoring

Although some remote data collection and monitoring services have been available for decades, increased access to and advances in technology have expanded the types of data that may be collected, monitored, and used in patient management. According to the Center for Connected Health Policy, as of September 2021, Medicaid plans in 27 states offer some form of payment for remote patient (ie, patient data) monitoring services (www.cchpca.org/topic/remote-patient-monitoring). Medicaid payment policies often include restrictions on the clinical indications for monitoring, the types of monitoring devices, and the health care professionals who are paid for monitoring services (eg, only home health agencies).

State regulations and payer policies for all types of digitally enhanced health services continue to evolve. It is important for physicians and other qualified health care professionals to research and understand local and regional payment policies for remote data collection and monitoring services before offering these services.

General Documentation Guidance

Documentation of all remote monitoring services should include
- Patient name and other identifying information (eg, patient identification number)
- Documented order, including clinical indications for the services provided
- Patient/caregiver agreement to receive services (Documented notification of potential financial responsibility may also be required.)
- Dates of each episode of service (eg, start and stop dates of equipment use; dates of physician, qualified health care professional [QHP], or clinical staff communication with patients and caregivers)
- Description of services provided on each date of service (eg, patient education, review of data transmission), including type of technology used
- Time, when applicable (eg, time spent in patient/caregiver communication)
- Identification and authentication by each author entering documentation into the patient's health record

Types of Remote Data Collection and/or Monitoring Services

Current Procedural Terminology (*CPT*®) describes multiple services that may include utilization of data acquired remotely by
- Patient self-collection and data transmission/submission to a physician for review and interpretation outside a face-to-face visit
- Remote physiologic monitoring with treatment management services
- Remote therapeutic monitoring of non-physiologic data (eg, level of function, adherence to treatment plan) with treatment management services

Appendix R of *CPT 2023* is a digital medicine taxonomy table for identifying and differentiating digital medicine services at a glance, including clinical data monitoring services. (The taxonomy table is not all inclusive of services that may be considered digital medicine services and does not supersede the specific coding guidance found elsewhere in *CPT*.)

Chapter 21. Remote Data Collection and Monitoring Services

Devices used for digitally storing data and/or remote physiologic or therapeutic monitoring must be medical devices as defined by the US Food and Drug Administration (FDA). Medical devices may be listed as *FDA approved* or *FDA cleared*. Storage, transfer, and access of personal health information must also comply with federal and state regulations for protection of personal health information (eg, privacy provisions of the Health Insurance Portability and Accountability Act).

Collection and Interpretation of Digitally Stored Physiologic Data

Certain codes describe specific physiologic data collection/monitoring (eg, apnea monitoring), while other codes describe more generalized services (eg, remote monitoring of physiologic parameter[s] [eg, weight, blood pressure, pulse oximetry, respiratory flow rate]). The code that most specifically describes a service should be reported.

Self-measured Blood Pressure Monitoring

#99473 Self-measured blood pressure using a device validated for clinical accuracy; patient education/training and device calibration

#99474 separate self-measurements of two readings one minute apart, twice daily over a 30-day period (minimum of 12 readings), collection of data reported by the patient and/or caregiver to the physician or other qualified health care professional, with report of average systolic and diastolic pressures and subsequent communication of a treatment plan to the patient

Self-measured blood pressure monitoring is a non–face-to-face service in which the patient or caregiver uses a home blood pressure measurement device to measure and record readings that are then provided to the ordering physician on paper or digitally (eg, email). As technology changes, these data are increasingly available for electronic transmission from the device to an application that allows the patient to directly share data with the ordering physician or other QHP.

Self-measured blood pressure monitoring is used for

- Ruling out white coat hypertension, which can prevent unnecessary treatment, adverse medication effects, and laboratory or diagnostic costs
- Identifying masked hypertension, which, if left untreated, carries a higher risk of cardiovascular disease and stroke
- Assessing control of hypertension and ensuring appropriate treatment is being ordered

Table 21-1 provides an overview of work included in each code.

Table 21-1. Self-measured Blood Pressure Monitoring by Patient	
#99473	Clinical staff or physician work • Patient education/training on self-measurement and reading collection • Home blood pressure monitoring device calibration Report once per device.
#99474	Physician work • Review report of individual and average systolic/diastolic blood pressure readings (must include ≥12 readings; patient performs/documents 2 readings 1 min apart at each measurement). • Communicate treatment plan to clinical staff or patient/caregiver. Report for a 30-d period.

Codes **99473** and **99474** are not reported for automated ambulatory blood pressure monitoring using report-generating software worn continuously for 24 hours or longer; see codes **93784–93790**.

Do not report **99473** or **99474** when reporting ambulatory blood pressure monitoring (**93784, 93786, 93788, 93790**), collection and interpretation of physiologic data (**99091**), remote physiologic monitoring and treatment management (**99453, 99454, 99457**), remote therapeutic monitoring treatment management services (**98980, 98981**), chronic care management (CCM; **99487, 99489, 99490, 99439, 99491, 99437**), or principal care management (PCM; **99424–99427**) in the same calendar month.

Example

➤ **A 16-year-old patient with moderate obesity presents with primary hypertension that is not responsive to life-style management.** The patient is struggling with dietary guidelines and exercises only during physical education. A low-dose medication is prescribed with instruction to continue the previously agreed-on diet and exercise regimen.

● indicates a new code; ▲, revised; #, re-sequenced; ✦, add-on; ★, audiovisual technology; and ◀, synchronous interactive audio.

The patient has previously been intolerant of ambulatory blood pressure monitoring but agrees to monitoring by self-measurement. The physician orders a blood pressure device validated for clinical accuracy and instructs the patient to obtain 2 readings twice daily for a 30-day period and send the results to the physician's clinical staff. The physician's documented evaluation and management (E/M) service supports moderate medical decision-making (MDM).

After the instrument is received by the patient, clinical staff calibrate the device and provide training for measurement and download and transmission of readings via the practice patient portal.

At the end of the 30-day period, the clinical staff review the patient's transmitted readings and average the systolic and diastolic pressures. The readings and calculated averages are reviewed by the physician, who communicates an ongoing treatment plan to the patient and/or caregivers.

ICD-10-CM: **I10** (hypertension) for all dates of service
CPT:
Initial date of service
   99214 (office or other outpatient E/M service with moderate MDM)
Return visit for device setup after receipt of blood pressure device
   99473 (patient education/training and device calibration)
Data analysis and patient communication after 30-day period
   99474 (collection and averaging of blood pressure readings with communication of plan of care)
   Teaching Point: At least 12 blood pressure readings must be obtained and averaged to create a treatment plan for the patient. Code **99474** includes collection, analysis, and communication of treatment plan(s) within a 30-day period.

If the patient returned for an office or other outpatient E/M service to review the readings and obtain the physician's recommended care plan, an E/M service (eg, **99214**) would be reported in lieu of **99474**.

Nonspecific Physiologic Data Collection and Interpretation

#99091   Collection and interpretation of physiologic data (eg, ECG, blood pressure, glucose monitoring) digitally stored and/or transmitted by the patient and/or caregiver to the physician or other qualified health care professional, qualified by education, training, licensure/regulation (when applicable) requiring a minimum of 30 minutes of time, each 30 days

Code **99091** *does not require active monitoring of physiologic data* or live interactive communication with the patient during the service period as is required for remote physiologic monitoring treatment management service codes **99457** and **99458** (discussed in the Remote Physiologic Monitoring Treatment Management Services section later in this chapter).

Code **99091** was assigned 1.63 relative value units (RVUs) in 2022 (facility or non-facility setting, not geographically adjusted).

Code **99091** represents a 30-day episode of care. Time spent by a physician or QHP in the following activities is included in the time supporting code **99091**:

- Access, review, and interpret data.
- Modify care plan as necessary, and communicate to patient/caregiver.
- Complete associated documentation.
- Report for minimum of 30 minutes, each 30 days.

> **If the services described by code 99091 are provided on the same day that the patient presents for an evaluation and management (E/M) service, these services should be considered part of the E/M service and not separately reported.**

Do not report **99091**
- If other, more specific *CPT* codes exist (eg, **93227**, **93272** for electrocardiographic services; **95250** for continuous glucose monitoring)
- For time spent by clinical staff
- For transfer and interpretation of data from hospital or clinical laboratory computers
- For time used to meet the criteria for care plan oversight services (**99374–99380**), personally performed CCM (**99437**, **99491**) or PCM (**99424–99427**), or remote physiologic monitoring treatment management services (**99457**, **99458**)

> *Current Procedural Terminology* **does not require use of a medical device as defined by the US Food and Drug Administration for services reported with code 99091. Live interactive contact during the reporting period is also not a required element of service for code 99091.**

● indicates a new code; ▲, revised; #, re-sequenced; ✚, add-on; ★, audiovisual technology; and ◀, synchronous interactive audio.

Example

➤ **A child with epilepsy is prescribed a wearable device that detects seizures and notifies caregivers.** The data collected by the device is transmitted to a server from which the child's physician downloads a report at the end of each 30-day period that provides the frequency of seizure detection; detailed physiologic data collected before, during, and after each seizure; and information on the patient's sleep and wake times. An additional report provides information the patient or caregiver has entered into the device diary during the reporting period. The physician spends 30 minutes or more reviewing and interpreting the data and communicating by phone with the patient or caregiver about the treatment plan. The physician reports **99091** linked to a diagnosis code for the epilepsy.

Circadian Respiratory Pattern Recording

94772   Circadian respiratory pattern recording (pediatric pneumogram), 12–24-hour continuous recording, infant

- Report code **94772** when circadian respiratory pattern recording (pediatric pneumogram), 12- to 24-hour continuous recording, is performed on an infant.
- Physicians may be required to append modifier **26** to indicate that only the professional component of this service was provided.
- Report 1 unit per recording period unless otherwise instructed by a payer.
- This code is not assigned RVUs in the Medicare Physician Fee Schedule (used by many payers). Allowable fees are determined by the payer.

Pediatric Home Apnea Monitoring Event Recording

94774   Pediatric home apnea monitoring event recording including respiratory rate, pattern and heart rate per 30-day period of time; includes monitor attachment, download of data, review, interpretation, and preparation of a report by a physician or other qualified health care professional

94775   monitor attachment only (includes hook-up, initiation of recording and disconnection)

94776   monitoring, download of information, receipt of transmission(s) and analyses by computer only

94777   review, interpretation and preparation of report only by a physician or other qualified health care professional

- Codes **94774–94777** are reported once per 30-day period.
- Codes **94775** and **94776** are reported by the home health agency because there is no physician work involved.
- Codes **94774** and **94777** are reported by the physician.
  - Code **94774** is reported by the physician when they order home monitoring, choose the monitor limits, and arrange for a home health care provider to teach the parents. It includes reviewing and interpreting data and preparation of the report.
  - Code **94777** is reported when the physician receives the downloaded information on disc or hard copy or electronically, reviews the patterns and periods of abnormal respiratory or heart rate, and summarizes, in a written report, the findings and recommendations for continuation or discontinuation of monitoring. This information is provided to the primary care physician and/or the family.
  - Codes **94774–94777** are not reported in conjunction with codes **93224–93272** (electrocardiographic monitoring). The apnea recording device cannot be reported separately. When oxygen saturation monitoring is used in addition to heart rate and respiratory monitoring, it is not reported separately.

Example

➤ **An infant born at 23 weeks' gestation, now 38 weeks old, has chronic lung disease and requires prolonged low-flow oxygen.** She continues to have occasional episodes of self-stimulated apnea lasting less than 15 seconds. She goes home with heart rate and respiratory monitoring during unattended periods and sleep. The physician orders the monitor, contacts the home health agency for its provision, and instructs the home health agency to teach the parents about cardiopulmonary resuscitation, proper attachment of the monitor leads, and resetting of the monitor. The home health agency provides the physician with the downloaded recordings. The first month's data are interpreted by the physician and a written report generated. The physician counsels the parents about the need to continue monitoring.

    Teaching Point: Report code **94774** and the appropriate *International Classification of Diseases, 10th Revision, Clinical Modification (ICD-10-CM)* code (eg, **G47.35** for congenital central alveolar hypoventilation/hypoxemia).

● indicates a new code; ▲, revised; #, re-sequenced; ✚, add-on; ★, audiovisual technology; and ◀, synchronous interactive audio.

In subsequent months, the physician receives the downloaded recordings, interprets them, and generates reports with recommendations for continued or discontinued monitoring. These services are reported with code **94777**.

Ambulatory Continuous Glucose Monitoring

95250   Ambulatory continuous glucose monitoring of interstitial tissue fluid via a subcutaneous sensor for a minimum of 72 hours; physician or other qualified health care professional (office) provided equipment, sensor placement, hook-up, calibration of monitor, patient training, removal of sensor, and printout of record

#95249   patient-provided equipment, sensor placement, hook-up, calibration of monitor, patient training, and printout of recording

95251   Ambulatory continuous glucose monitoring of interstitial tissue fluid via a subcutaneous sensor for a minimum of 72 hours; analysis, interpretation and report

- When use of an ambulatory glucose monitor is initiated and data are captured for a minimum of 72 hours, report code **95249** or **95250** on the basis of the supplier of the equipment (patient or physician office).
- Codes **95249** and **95250** do not include physician work (ie, valued for practice expense and liability only). **Table 21-2** lists the physician and clinical staff work components of codes **95249–95251**.

Table 21-2. Ambulatory Continuous Glucose Monitoring of Interstitial Tissue Fluid via a Subcutaneous Sensor (A minimum of 72 h of monitoring is required for each code.)	
95251	Physician work includes correlation of individual data points with the patient daily log and interpretation and report. Do not report more than once per month.
#95249 (patient-provided equipment only)	Clinical staff work includes sensor placement, hookup, calibration of the monitor, patient training, and printout of record. Report only once during the time a patient owns a given data receiver.
95250 (physician office–provided equipment only)	Clinical staff work includes sensor placement, hookup, calibration of the monitor, patient training, removal of the sensor, and printout of the record. Do not report more than once per month.

- Physicians report code **95249** only if the patient brings the data receiver into the physician's or other QHP's office with the entire initial data collection procedure conducted in the office.
- Report code **95249** only once for the entire duration that a patient has a receiver, even if the patient receives a new sensor and/or transmitter. If a patient receives a new or different model of receiver, code **95249** may be reported again when the entire initial data collection procedure is conducted in the office.
  - Report **95249** on the date the continuous glucose monitoring recording is printed in the office.
  - Removal of a sensor is not a required component of **95249**.
- Analysis, interpretation, and report (**95251**) may be performed with or without a face-to-face encounter on the same date of service. This service is reported only once per month.
- Code **95251** was assigned 1.02 RVUs in either a facility or non-facility setting in 2022 (not geographically adjusted).

Remote Physiologic Monitoring Services

Remote physiologic monitoring services include use of a medical device approved by the US Food and Drug Administration (FDA) to record and transmit daily recordings or programmed alerts. Codes distinguish equipment setup and patient education, device supply with transmission of data, and use of results to treat a patient under a specific treatment plan.

Do not report codes **99453**, **99454**, **99457**, and **99458** for remote physiologic monitoring services when the parameters monitored are more specifically identified by other codes.

- A physician practice may provide all components (eg, equipment supply, initial setup, calibration, training, monitoring, treatment management services) or, perhaps more frequently, only the remote physiologic monitoring treatment management component (ie, **99457** and **99458**).

Remote Monitoring Setup and Device Supply

#99453   Remote monitoring of physiologic parameter(s) (eg, weight, blood pressure, pulse oximetry, respiratory flow rate), initial; set-up and patient education on use of equipment

● indicates a new code; ▲, revised; #, re-sequenced; ✚, add-on; ★, audiovisual technology; and ◀, synchronous interactive audio.

#99454   device(s) supply with daily recording(s) or programmed alert(s) transmission, each 30 days

To report codes **99453** and **99454**, the device used must be a medical device as defined by the FDA (eg, blood glucose monitor) and the service must be ordered by a physician or QHP. *Do not report when monitoring is less than 16 days.*

> **Code 99453 describes setup and patient education provided to an individual patient. When setup and education are provided in a group setting, report an unlisted evaluation and management service (99499).**

- Codes **99453** and **99454** represent only practice expense; no physician work is valued in these codes.
- ✖ Do not report codes **99453** and **99454** in conjunction with codes for more specific physiologic parameters (eg, home apnea monitoring [**94762**]).
- ✖ Do not report **99453** and **99454** when these services are included in other *CPT* codes for the duration of time of the physiologic monitoring service (eg, **95250**, ambulatory continuous glucose monitoring of interstitial tissue fluid via a subcutaneous sensor).
- Initial setup and patient education on use of equipment (**99453**) is reported for each episode of care (begins when the remote monitoring physiologic service is initiated and ends with attainment of targeted treatment goals).

Examples

➤ **A child with epilepsy is prescribed an FDA-approved wearable device that detects seizures and notifies care-givers in addition to transmitting data to the prescribing physician.** The patient is provided with setup and education for use of the device and the program's monitoring application. The practice directly receives and monitors daily recordings and/or programmed alerts for at least a 16-day period. Education on equipment use is provided as needed. Codes **99453** and **99454** are reported.

  Teaching Point: The device must be used for monitoring for at least 16 days to report **99453** and/or **99454**. The patient and caregivers are provided separately reported treatment management services (**99457, 99458**) of at least 20 minutes in the month, as indicated.

➤ **A child with poorly controlled asthma is enrolled in a remote monitoring program.** A Bluetooth-enabled device that promotes and monitors effective inhaler use and measures forced expiratory volume in 1 second (FEV_1) and peak expiratory flow is provided to the patient by a remote monitoring technology provider. The patient's physician and/or clinical staff provide education to the patient and caregivers on device use. The physician reports code **99453**.

  Teaching Point: Because the physician practice furnishes only the initial setup and patient education, only code **99453** is reported for setup and education encounter. This service is reported only at the time of the initial 16 to 30 days of monitoring. Code **99454** would be reported by the provider of the equipment and monitoring service. See codes **99457** and **99458** for reporting 20 or more minutes of remote physiologic monitoring treatment management services during a calendar month.

Remote Physiologic Monitoring Treatment Management Services

#99457   Remote physiologic monitoring treatment management services, clinical staff/physician/other qualified health care professional time in a calendar month requiring interactive communication with the patient/caregiver during the month; first 20 minutes

#✚99458   each additional 20 minutes

Remote physiologic monitoring treatment management services include time spent in a calendar month using the results of transmitted physiologic data to treat a patient under a specific treatment plan. These services may be rendered by physicians, QHPs, and/or clinical staff working under supervision of a physician or QHP.

> **The reporting period for codes 99457 and 99458 is a calendar month. At least 20 minutes must be spent in treatment management services to report 99457.**

The time spent in activities listed in **Table 21-3** is included in the time supporting codes **99457** and **99458**.

● indicates a new code; ▲, revised; #, re-sequenced; ✚, add-on; ★, audiovisual technology; and ◀, synchronous interactive audio.

Table 21-3. Remote Physiologic Monitoring Treatment Management Services	
#99457	Physician work (performed personally or by clinical staff under physician or QHP supervision) ● Access, review, and interpret data. ● Modify treatment plan as necessary, and communicate to patient/caregiver. ● Complete associated documentation. ● Report for minimum of 20 min, each calendar month.
#✚99458	Physician work Each additional period of no less than 20 min (as previous)
Abbreviation: QHP, qualified health care professional.	

Documentation of remote physiologic monitoring treatment management must include
- An order by a physician or QHP
- *Live interactive communication* (eg, 2-way conversation via telephone or secure messaging) with the patient and/or caregiver
- Time of service of 20 or more minutes in a calendar month, including time in live interactive communication, data access, review and interpretation, and documentation

Reporting instructions
- Report code **99457** once with 1 unit of service for the initial 20 minutes of service regardless of the number of physiologic monitoring modalities performed in a given calendar month. When the time of service extends a full 20 minutes beyond the first 20 minutes, report code **99458** in addition to **99457**.

Do not report **99457** or **99458**
- ✖ For any time on a day when the physician or QHP reports an E/M service (office or other outpatient services [**99202–99205, 99211–99215**], home or residence services [**99341–99345, 99347–99350**], initial or subsequent hospital inpatient or observation services [**99221–99223, 99231–99233**], or inpatient or observation consultations [**99252–99255**]).
- ✖ For any time related to other reported services (eg, **93290**, interrogation of implantable cardiovascular physiologic monitor system).
- ✖ In conjunction with collection and interpretation of physiologic data (**99091**).
- Codes **99457** and **99458** may be reported during the same service period as CCM (**99437, 99439, 99487–99491**), PCM (**99424–99427**), transitional care management (TCM; **99495, 99496**), and behavioral health integration services (**99484, 99492–99494**). However, the time for each service must be distinct and not overlapping and must be separately documented.
- Code **99457** was assigned 0.90 RVUs in a facility setting and 1.45 in a non-facility setting in 2022. Code **99458** was assigned 0.90 RVUs in a facility setting and 1.18 in a non-facility setting. Relative value units are not geographically adjusted. At the time of this publication, 2023 RVUs were unavailable.

Example

➤ **Data are received for a child with poorly controlled asthma who is enrolled in a remote physiologic monitoring program.** Clinical staff of the ordering physician review the data and note that the patient's plan of care calls for patient contact because FEV$_1$ and/or peak expiratory flow measurements are outside a specific range. A care coordinator contacts the patient's parent to inquire about medication use and signs and symptoms. The child's physician is consulted by the care coordinator and advice or orders for a change in management are relayed to the parent. At the end of the calendar month, documentation supports 25 minutes spent in remote physiologic monitoring treatment management services with at least 1 episode of live interactive communication with the patient's caregiver. Code **99457** is reported.

Remote Therapeutic Monitoring Services

New in 2023! Code 98978 has been added for reporting device supply for remote therapeutic monitoring services for cognitive behavioral therapy.

● indicates a new code; ▲, revised; #, re-sequenced; ✚, add-on; ★, audiovisual technology; and ◄, synchronous interactive audio.

Remote therapeutic monitoring services (eg, musculoskeletal function, therapy adherence, therapy response) represent the review and monitoring of transmitted data related to signs, symptoms, and functions of a therapeutic response as opposed to physiologic data such as heart rate and rhythm. These data may represent objective device-generated integrated data or subjective inputs reported by a patient (eg, the patient's reported outcome of therapeutic exercise). These data are reflective of therapeutic responses that provide a functionally integrative representation of patient status.

Remote Therapeutic Monitoring Setup and Device Supply

Initial Setup and Patient Education

▲98975   Remote therapeutic monitoring (eg, therapy adherence, therapy response); initial set-up and patient education on use of equipment

Code **98975** is reported once per episode of care for the initial setup and patient education on use of the equipment. An *episode of care* is defined as beginning when the remote therapeutic monitoring service is initiated and ending with attainment of targeted treatment goals. **98975** is not reported for monitoring of less than 16 days.

> Codes **98975–98978** are specific to remote therapeutic monitoring services and are not used in conjunction with physiologic monitoring services (eg, **95250**, ambulatory continuous glucose monitoring).

Therapeutic Monitoring Device Supply and Transmission

▲98976   Remote therapeutic monitoring (eg, therapy adherence, therapy response); device(s) supply with scheduled (eg, daily) recording(s) and/or programmed alert(s) transmission to monitor respiratory system, each 30 days

▲98977   device(s) supply with scheduled (eg, daily) recording(s) and/or programmed alert(s) transmission to monitor musculoskeletal system, each 30 days

●98978   device(s) supply with scheduled (eg, daily) recording(s) and/or programmed alert(s) transmission to monitor cognitive behavioral therapy, each 30 days

Codes **98976–98978** are reported for 16 to 30 days of device supply (ie, do not report when device is used for <16 days of monitoring). Report these device supply codes only when equipment is supplied for use in conjunction with remote therapeutic monitoring treatment management services **98980** and **98981**. Physicians and QHPs report these codes only when supplying devices used by the patient to capture and transmit data used in remote therapeutic monitoring treatment management services. These codes may be more frequently reported by a device vendor.

Remote Therapeutic Monitoring Treatment Management Services

98980   Remote therapeutic monitoring treatment management services, physician/other qualified health care professional time in a calendar month requiring at least one interactive communication with the patient/caregiver during the calendar month; first 20 minutes

✚98981   each additional 20 minutes

Remote therapeutic monitoring treatment management service codes **98980** and **98981** are reported for a physician's or QHP's cumulative time in a calendar month spent in remote therapeutic monitoring to treat a patient under a specific treatment plan. *At least 1 interactive communication with the patient/caregiver is required* in the calendar month. Time of interactive communication with the patient/caregiver contributes to the cumulative time of remote therapeutic monitoring treatment management services.

- Code **98980** is reported once per calendar month regardless of the number of therapeutic parameters monitored.
- If the time spent in remote therapeutic monitoring treatment management services during a calendar month is less than 20 minutes, do not report **98980**.
- Report add-on code **98981** in addition to **98980** when the service time of **98980** is exceeded by at least 20 minutes. Report 1 unit of **98981** for each additional 20-minute period. Do not report **98981** for a period of less than 20 minutes.

  Do not report **98980** and **98981**

✖ In conjunction with remote monitoring of a wireless pulmonary artery pressure sensor (**93264**), collection and interpretation of physiologic data (**99091**), or remote physiologic data monitoring treatment management (**99457, 99458**)

✖ In the same calendar month as self-measured blood pressure (**99473, 99474**)

✖ For any time spent on the date of an E/M service (including home, office or other outpatient, domiciliary, rest home, or inpatient services)

● indicates a new code; ▲, revised; #, re-sequenced; ✚, add-on; ★, audiovisual technology; and ◀, synchronous interactive audio.

✖ For time counted toward separately reported CCM services (**99437, 99439, 99487–99491**), PCM services (**99424–99427**), TCM services (**99495, 99496**), or behavioral health integration services (**99484, 99492–99494**) (When provided in the same time period, each service must be separately documented and no time should be counted toward the required time for both services.)

Documentation of remote physiologic monitoring treatment management must include
- An order by a physician or QHP
- *Live interactive communication* (eg, 2-way conversation via telephone or secure messaging) with the patient and/or caregiver
- Time of service of 20 or more minutes in a calendar month

Example

➤ **An adolescent patient with moderate persistent asthma is learning to take responsibility for following a QHP's orders for use of control medication, identification and avoidance of triggers, and response to symptoms.** The QHP has prescribed remote therapeutic monitoring by using an FDA-cleared medical device that automatically transmits the patient's use of an inhaler. Initial setup of the medical device and education on its use are provided and reported with code **98975**. Code **98976** (remote therapeutic monitoring [eg, therapy adherence, therapy response]; device[s] supply with scheduled [eg, daily] recording[s] and/or programmed alert[s] transmission to monitor respiratory system, each 30 days) is reported when the patient has used the medical device for at least 16 days. (Codes **98975** and **98976** may be reported by a device vendor rather than a physician or QHP, when applicable.)

The QHP reviews the transmissions and, at least once during the calendar month, telephones the patient to discuss medication adherence. The QHP's total time spent in remote therapeutic monitoring treatment management during the calendar month is 35 minutes. Code **98980** is reported. Had time during the calendar month exceeded 39 minutes, code **98981** would have also been reported (ie, for 20 minutes beyond the first 20-minute service period).

To learn more about remote data monitoring services, see the February 2022 *Pediatrics* article, "Remote Monitoring of Patient- and Family-Generated Health Data in Pediatrics" (https://doi.org/10.1542/peds.2021-054137).

To test your knowledge of the information presented in this chapter, complete the quiz found at the end of it, after the resources. Answers to each quiz are found in **Appendix IV**.

Chapter Takeaways

This chapter discusses multiple types of remote data collection and/or monitoring services. Following are some takeaways from this chapter:
- Report the most specific *CPT* code, when applicable, for remote physiologic data monitoring services. For example, codes **95249–95251** are reported for ambulatory blood glucose monitoring, rather than **99091**, which is less specific regarding the type of physiologic data monitored.
- Documentation should include details such as the clinical indication for ordering data collection or monitoring services, dates of service, activities such as communicating findings and recommendations to the patient/caregiver, and, for time-based code selection, total time spent during the service period.

Resources

Remote Patient Monitoring

"Remote Monitoring of Patient- and Family-Generated Health Data in Pediatrics," February 2022 *Pediatrics* article (https://doi.org/10.1542/peds.2021-054137)

Digital Medical Taxonomy

Digital Medicine Taxonomy: Appendix R of *CPT 2023*

Test Your Knowledge!

1. **Which of the following services is reported with *Current Procedural Terminology* code 99091?**
   a. Physician review and interpretation of a patient's self-collected data at a face-to-face visit
   b. Clinical staff time spent monitoring remote physiologic data
   c. Physician review and interpretation of a patient's self-collected data outside a face-to-face visit
   d. Collection of patient history via patient portal before a face-to-face encounter

2. **Which of the following actions describes the work reported with code 94777?**
   a. Attachment of the monitor, download of the data, physician review and interpretation of the data, and preparation of a report
   b. Physician review of a computer analysis of the event data received over a 30-day period
   c. Physician review and interpretation of the event data collected over a 30-day period and preparation of a report
   d. Physician review and interpretation of the data collected in a calendar month and preparation of a report

3. **Which of the following codes is used to report a physician's time spent in a calendar month by using the results of transmitted physiologic data to manage a patient's treatment plan?**
   a. 99091
   b. 99457
   c. 98980
   d. b and c

4. **Which of the following data are an example of non-physiologic data that may be used in a treatment management service described by code 98980?**
   a. Results of pulse oxygen monitoring
   b. Patient-reported outcomes of therapy
   c. Daily transmissions of a patient's weight
   d. A patient's 30-day log of blood glucose readings

5. **Which of the following services may be reported on the basis of time spent by clinical staff working under supervision of a physician or qualified health care professional?**
   a. Remote physiologic monitoring treatment management services
   b. Collection and interpretation of physiologic data
   c. Pediatric home apnea monitoring
   d. Remote therapeutic monitoring treatment management services

● indicates a new code; ▲, revised; #, re-sequenced; ✚, add-on; ★, audiovisual technology; and ◄, synchronous interactive audio.

Appendixes

Additional coding resources are available at www.aap.org/cfp2023.

CPT copyright 2022 American Medical Association. All rights reserved.

I. Quick Reference to 2023 *ICD-10-CM* Pediatric Code Changes

This quick reference list does not include all changes made to *International Classification of Diseases, 10th Revision, Clinical Modification* (*ICD-10-CM*). We have made every effort to include the diagnosis code changes that most apply to pediatric practices. However, revisions and/or additional codes may have been published subsequent to the date of this printing. Refer to *Pediatric ICD-10-CM 2023* (https://shop.aap.org/pediatric-icd-10-cm-2023-8th-edition-paperback) for a complete listing of new and revised codes that apply to pediatrics, complete descriptions, and reporting instructions. Always begin in the *ICD-10-CM* alphabetical index to locate the code most specific to the condition or other reason for encounter. Codes are valid as of October 3, 2022, unless otherwise noted. (Any code updates to be implemented on April 1, 2023, will be posted at www.aap.org/cfp2023.)

Quick Reference to 2023 *ICD-10-CM* Pediatric Code Changes	
Codes followed by a dash (-) require an additional character. See *Pediatric ICD-10-CM 2023* to complete these codes.	
Activated Phosphoinositide 3-Kinase Delta Syndrome	
D81.82	Activated phosphoinositide 3-kinase delta syndrome (APDS, includes PASLI disease)
Acute or Chronic Metabolic Acidosis	
E87.20	Acidosis, unspecified
E87.21	Acute metabolic acidosis
E87.22	Chronic metabolic acidosis
E87.29	Other acidosis
Acute or Chronic Vulvovaginal Candidiasis	
B37.31	Acute candidiasis of vulva and vagina
B37.32	Chronic candidiasis of vulva and vagina
Apnea of Newborn	
P28.30	Primary sleep apnea of newborn, unspecified
P28.31	Primary central sleep apnea of newborn
P28.32	Primary obstructive sleep apnea of newborn
P28.33	Primary mixed sleep apnea of newborn
P28.39	Other primary sleep apnea of newborn
P28.40	Unspecified apnea of newborn
P28.41	Central neonatal apnea of newborn
P28.42	Obstructive apnea of newborn
P28.43	Mixed neonatal apnea of newborn
P28.49	Other apnea of newborn (includes apnea of prematurity)
Atrial Septal Defect (Congenital)	
Q21.10	Atrial septal defect, unspecified
Q21.11	Secundum atrial septal defect
Q21.12	Patent foramen ovale
Q21.13	Coronary sinus atrial septal defect
Q21.14	Superior sinus venosus atrial septal defect
Q21.15	Inferior sinus venosus atrial septal defect
Q21.16	Sinus venosus atrial septal defect, unspecified
Q21.19	Other specified atrial septal defect
Atrioventricular Septal Defect (Congenital)	
Q21.20	Atrioventricular septal defect, unspecified as to partial or complete
Q21.21	Partial atrioventricular septal defect
Q21.22	Transitional atrioventricular septal defect
Q21.23	Complete atrioventricular septal defect

Continued on next page

Appendixes

● indicates a new code; ▲, revised; #, re-sequenced; ✚, add-on; ★, audiovisual technology; and ◀, synchronous interactive audio.

Appendixes

Quick Reference to 2023 *ICD-10-CM* Pediatric Code Changes (*continued*)

Codes followed by a dash (-) require an additional character. See *Pediatric ICD-10-CM 2023* to complete these codes.

Caregiver's Noncompliance With Patient's Medical Treatment and Regimen

Z91.A10	Caregiver's noncompliance with patient's dietary regimen due to financial hardship
Z91.A18	Caregiver's noncompliance with patient's dietary regimen for other reason
Z91.A20	Caregiver's intentional underdosing of patient's medication regimen due to financial hardship
Z91.A28	Caregiver's intentional underdosing of patient's medication regimen for other reason
Z91.A3	Caregiver's unintentional underdosing of patient's medication regimen
Z91.A4	Caregiver's other noncompliance with patient's medication regimen
Z91.A5	Caregiver's noncompliance with patient's renal dialysis
Z91.A9	Caregiver's noncompliance with patient's other medical treatment and regimen

Caught, Crushed, Jammed, or Pinched In or Between Objects

W23.2XX-	Caught, crushed, jammed, or pinched in or between a moving and stationary object

Counseling

Z71.87	Encounter for pediatric-to-adult transition counseling
Z71.88	Encounter for counseling for socioeconomic factors

Disorders of Autonomic Nervous System

G90.A	Postural orthostatic tachycardia syndrome (POTS)

Hemolytic-Uremic Syndrome

D59.30	Hemolytic-uremic syndrome, unspecified
D59.31	Infection-associated hemolytic-uremic syndrome
D59.32	Hereditary hemolytic-uremic syndrome
D59.39	Other hemolytic-uremic syndrome

Heparin-Induced Thrombocytopenia (HIT)

D75.821	Non-immune heparin-induced thrombocytopenia
D75.822	Immune-mediated heparin-induced thrombocytopenia
D75.828	Other heparin-induced thrombocytopenia syndrome
D75.829	Heparin-induced thrombocytopenia, unspecified
D75.84	Other platelet-activating anti-PF4 disorders (HIT without heparin exposure)

Hepatic Encephalopathy

K76.82	Hepatic encephalopathy

Intracranial Injury With Unknown Loss of Consciousness

S06.0XA-	Concussion with loss of consciousness status unknown
S06.1XA-	Traumatic cerebral edema with loss of consciousness status unknown
S06.2XA-	Diffuse traumatic brain injury with loss of consciousness status unknown
S06.30A-	Unspecified focal traumatic brain injury with loss of consciousness status unknown
S06.31A-	Contusion and laceration of right cerebrum with loss of consciousness status unknown
S06.32A-	Contusion and laceration of left cerebrum with loss of consciousness status unknown
S06.33A-	Contusion and laceration of cerebrum, unspecified, with loss of consciousness status unknown
S06.34A-	Traumatic hemorrhage of right cerebrum with loss of consciousness status unknown
S06.35A-	Traumatic hemorrhage of left cerebrum with loss of consciousness status unknown
S06.36A-	Traumatic hemorrhage of cerebrum, unspecified, with loss of consciousness status unknown
S06.37A-	Contusion, laceration, and hemorrhage of cerebellum with loss of consciousness status unknown
S06.38A-	Contusion, laceration, and hemorrhage of brainstem with loss of consciousness status unknown
S06.4XA-	Epidural hemorrhage with loss of consciousness status unknown
S06.5XA-	Traumatic subdural hemorrhage with loss of consciousness status unknown
S06.6XA-	Traumatic subarachnoid hemorrhage with loss of consciousness status unknown
S06.81A-	Injury of right internal carotid artery, intracranial portion, NEC with loss of consciousness status unknown
S06.82A-	Injury of left internal carotid artery, intracranial portion, NEC with loss of consciousness status unknown

● indicates a new code; ▲, revised; #, re-sequenced; ✚, add-on; ★, audiovisual technology; and ◀, synchronous interactive audio.

Quick Reference to 2023 *ICD-10-CM* Pediatric Code Changes (*continued*)

Codes followed by a dash (-) require an additional character. See *Pediatric ICD-10-CM 2023* to complete these codes.

Intracranial Injury With Unknown Loss of Consciousness (*continued*)

S06.89A-	Other specified intracranial injury with loss of consciousness status unknown
S06.9XA-	Unspecified intracranial injury with loss of consciousness status unknown

Limb Girdle Muscular Dystrophies

G71.031	Autosomal dominant limb girdle muscular dystrophy
G71.032	Autosomal recessive limb girdle muscular dystrophy due to calpain-3 dysfunction
G71.033	Limb girdle muscular dystrophy due to dysferlin dysfunction
G71.0340	Limb girdle muscular dystrophy due to sarcoglycan dysfunction, unspecified
G71.0341	Limb girdle muscular dystrophy due to alpha sarcoglycan dysfunction
G71.0342	Limb girdle muscular dystrophy due to beta sarcoglycan dysfunction
G71.0349	Limb girdle muscular dystrophy due to other sarcoglycan dysfunction
G71.035	Limb girdle muscular dystrophy due to anoctamin-5 dysfunction
G71.038	Other limb girdle muscular dystrophy
G71.039	Limb girdle muscular dystrophy, unspecified

Long Term (Current) Drug Therapy

Z79.60	Long term (current) use of unspecified immunomodulators and immunosuppressants
Z79.61	Long term (current) use of immunomodulator
Z79.620	Long term (current) use of immunosuppressive biologic
Z79.621	Long term (current) use of calcineurin inhibitor
Z79.622	Long term (current) use of Janus kinase inhibitor
Z79.623	Long term (current) use of mammalian target of rapamycin (mTOR) inhibitor
Z79.624	Long term (current) use of inhibitors of nucleotide synthesis
Z79.630	Long term (current) use of alkylating agent
Z79.631	Long term (current) use of antimetabolite agent
Z79.632	Long term (current) use of antitumor antibiotic
Z79.633	Long term (current) use of mitotic inhibitor
Z79.634	Long term (current) use of topoisomerase inhibitor
Z79.64	Long term (current) use of myelosuppressive agent
Z79.69	Long term (current) use of other immunomodulators and immunosuppressants
Z79.85	Long term (current) use of injectable non-insulin antidiabetic drugs

Nontraumatic Slipped Upper Femoral Epiphysis[a]

M93.004	Unspecified slipped upper femoral epiphysis (nontraumatic), bilateral hips
M93.014	Acute slipped upper femoral epiphysis, stable (nontraumatic), bilateral hips
M93.024	Chronic slipped upper femoral epiphysis, stable (nontraumatic), bilateral hips
M93.034	Acute on chronic slipped upper femoral epiphysis, stable (nontraumatic), bilateral hips
M93.041	Acute slipped upper femoral epiphysis, unstable (nontraumatic), right hip
M93.042	Acute slipped upper femoral epiphysis, unstable (nontraumatic), left hip
M93.044	Acute slipped upper femoral epiphysis, unstable (nontraumatic), bilateral hips
M93.051	Acute on chronic slipped upper femoral epiphysis, unstable (nontraumatic), right hip
M93.052	Acute on chronic slipped upper femoral epiphysis, unstable (nontraumatic), left hip
M93.054	Acute on chronic slipped upper femoral epiphysis, unstable (nontraumatic), bilateral hips
M93.061	Acute slipped upper femoral epiphysis, unspecified stability (nontraumatic), right hip
M93.062	Acute slipped upper femoral epiphysis, unspecified stability (nontraumatic), left hip
M93.064	Acute slipped upper femoral epiphysis, unspecified stability (nontraumatic), bilateral hips
M93.071	Acute on chronic slipped upper femoral epiphysis, unspecified stability (nontraumatic), right hip
M93.072	Acute on chronic slipped upper femoral epiphysis, unspecified stability (nontraumatic), left hip
M93.074	Acute on chronic slipped upper femoral epiphysis, unspecified stability (nontraumatic), bilateral hips

Continued on next page

Appendixes

● indicates a new code; ▲, revised; #, re-sequenced; ✚, add-on; ★, audiovisual technology; and ◀, synchronous interactive audio.

Appendixes

Quick Reference to 2023 *ICD-10-CM* Pediatric Code Changes (*continued*)

Codes followed by a dash (-) require an additional character. See *Pediatric ICD-10-CM 2023* to complete these codes.

Patient's Noncompliance With Medical Treatment and Regimen

Z91.110	Patient's noncompliance with dietary regimen due to financial hardship
Z91.118	Patient's noncompliance with dietary regimen for other reason
Z91.119	Patient's noncompliance with dietary regimen due to unspecified reason
Z91.190	Patient's noncompliance with other medical treatment and regimen due to financial hardship
Z91.198	Patient's noncompliance with other medical treatment and regimen for other reason
Z91.199	Patient's noncompliance with other medical treatment and regimen due to unspecified reason

Personal History of (Corrected) Certain Conditions Arising in the Perinatal Period

Z87.61	Personal history of (corrected) necrotizing enterocolitis of newborn
Z87.68	Personal history of other (corrected) conditions arising in the perinatal period

Personal History of (Corrected) Congenital Malformations

Z87.731	Personal history of (corrected) tracheoesophageal fistula or atresia
Z87.732	Personal history of (corrected) persistent cloaca or cloacal malformations
Z87.760	Personal history of (corrected) congenital diaphragmatic hernia or other congenital diaphragm malformations
Z87.761	Personal history of (corrected) gastroschisis
Z87.762	Personal history of (corrected) prune belly malformation
Z87.763	Personal history of other (corrected) congenital abdominal wall malformations
Z87.768	Personal history of other specified (corrected) congenital malformations of integument, limbs and musculoskeletal system

Poisoning by, Adverse Effect of and Underdosing of Methamphetamines

T43.65-	Poisoning by, adverse effect of and underdosing of methamphetamines
T43.651	Poisoning by methamphetamines, accidental (unintentional)
T43.652	Poisoning by methamphetamines, intentional self-harm
T43.653	Poisoning by methamphetamines, assault
T43.654	Poisoning by methamphetamines, undetermined
T43.655	Adverse effect of methamphetamines
T43.656	Underdosing of methamphetamines

Postviral and Related Fatigue Syndromes

G93.31	Postviral fatigue syndrome
G93.32	Myalgic encephalomyelitis/chronic fatigue syndrome
G93.39	Other post infection and related fatigue syndromes

Problems Related to Housing and Economic Circumstances

Z59.82	Transportation insecurity
Z59.86	Financial insecurity
Z59.87	Material hardship

Problems Related to Sleep

Z72.823	Risk of suffocation (smothering) under another while sleeping

Reactions to Severe Stress

F43.81	Prolonged grief disorder
F43.89	Other reactions to severe stress

Rib Fracture Due to Cardiopulmonary Resuscitation

M96.A1	Fracture of sternum associated with chest compression and cardiopulmonary resuscitation
M96.A2	Fracture of one rib associated with chest compression and cardiopulmonary resuscitation
M96.A3	Multiple fractures of ribs associated with chest compression and cardiopulmonary resuscitation
M96.A4	Flail chest associated with chest compression and cardiopulmonary resuscitation
M96.A9	Other fracture associated with chest compression and cardiopulmonary resuscitation

● indicates a new code; ▲, revised; #, re-sequenced; ✚, add-on; ★, audiovisual technology; and ◀, synchronous interactive audio.

Quick Reference to 2023 *ICD-10-CM* Pediatric Code Changes (*continued*)

Codes followed by a dash (-) require an additional character. See *Pediatric ICD-10-CM 2023* to complete these codes.

Short Stature Due to Endocrine Disorder

E34.30	Short stature due to endocrine disorder, unspecified
E34.31	Constitutional short stature
E34.321	Primary insulin-like growth factor-1 (IGF-1) deficiency
E34.322	IGF-1 resistance
E34.328	Other genetic causes of short stature
E34.329	Unspecified genetic causes of short stature
E34.39	Other short stature due to endocrine disorder

Substance Use Disorder, Unspecified Pattern of Use

F10.90	Alcohol use, unspecified, uncomplicated
F10.91	Alcohol use, unspecified, in remission
F11.91	Opioid use, unspecified, in remission
F12.91	Cannabis use, unspecified, in remission
F13.91	Sedative, hypnotic or anxiolytic use, unspecified, in remission
F14.91	Cocaine use, unspecified, in remission
F15.91	Other stimulant use, unspecified, in remission
F16.91	Hallucinogen use, unspecified, in remission
F18.91	Inhalant use, unspecified, in remission
F19.91	Other psychoactive substance use, unspecified, in remission

Transfusion-Associated Dyspnea

J95.87	Transfusion-associated dyspnea (TAD)

Underimmunization Status

Z28.310[b]	Unvaccinated for COVID-19
Z28.311[b]	Partially vaccinated for COVID-19
Z28.39[b]	Other underimmunization status

Ventricular Tachycardia

I47.20	Ventricular tachycardia, unspecified
I47.21	Torsades de pointes
I47.29	Other ventricular tachycardia

Von Willebrand Disease Types

D68.00	Von Willebrand disease, unspecified
D68.01	Von Willebrand disease, type 1 (partial quantitative deficiency of Von Willebrand factor or Type 1C)
D68.020	Von Willebrand disease, type 2A
D68.021	Von Willebrand disease, type 2B
D68.022	Von Willebrand disease, type 2M
D68.023	Von Willebrand disease, type 2N
D68.029	Von Willebrand disease, type 2, unspecified
D68.03	Von Willebrand disease, type 3
D68.04	Acquired von Willebrand disease
D68.09	Other von Willebrand disease

Abbreviations: NEC, not elsewhere classified; PASLI, p110δ-activating mutation causing senescent T cells, lymphadenopathy, and immunodeficiency; PF4, platelet factor 4.

[a]Code descriptors for **M93.011–M93.013, M93.021–M93.023,** and **M93.031–M93.033** have also been revised to include "stable."
[b]Became effective April 1, 2022.

Appendixes

● indicates a new code; ▲, revised; #, re-sequenced; ✚, add-on; ★, audiovisual technology; and ◀, synchronous interactive audio.

Appendixes

II. Quick Reference to 2023 *CPT* ® Pediatric Code Changes

In this appendix, we have made every effort to include changes to procedures and services that apply to pediatric practices. However, revisions and/or additional codes may have been published subsequent to the date of this printing. This list does not include all changes made to *Current Procedural Terminology* (*CPT*) *2023*. Additionally, not all codes included in the quick reference table are further discussed in this publication (typically because of their limited use by most pediatricians). Codes not discussed elsewhere are shaded in gray. Always refer to *CPT 2023* for a complete listing of new codes, complete descriptions, and revisions. For questions or additional information on codes not discussed in this publication, please contact the American Academy of Pediatrics Coding Hotline (https://form.jotform.com/Subspecialty/aapcodinghotline). Any errata to *CPT 2023* will be posted to the American Medical Association website, www.ama-assn.org/practice-management/cpt/errata-technical-corrections. These changes take effect January 1, 2023. Do not report the changes or codes before that date.

Quick Reference to 2023 *CPT* Pediatric Code Changes	
2022	**2023**
Evaluation and Management	
99218 Initial observation care, per day, for the evaluation and management of a patient which requires these 3 key components: ● A detailed or comprehensive history; ● A detailed or comprehensive examination; and ● Medical decision making that is straightforward or of low complexity. Counseling and/or coordination of care with other physicians, other qualified health care professionals, or agencies are provided consistent with the nature of the problem(s) and the patient's and/or family's needs. Usually, the problem(s) requiring admission to outpatient hospital "observation status" are of low severity. Typically, 30 minutes are spent at the bedside and on the patient's hospital floor or unit. **99219** Initial observation care, per day, for the evaluation and management of a patient which requires these 3 key components: ● A comprehensive history; ● A comprehensive examination; and ● Medical decision making of moderate complexity. Counseling and/or coordination of care with other physicians, other qualified health care professionals, or agencies are provided consistent with the nature of the problem(s) and the patient's and/or family's needs. Usually, the problem(s) requiring admission to outpatient hospital "observation status" are of moderate severity. Typically, 50 minutes are spent at the bedside and on the patient's hospital floor or unit. **99220** Initial observation care, per day, for the evaluation and management of a patient which requires these 3 key components: ● A comprehensive history; ● A comprehensive examination; and ● Medical decision making of high complexity. Counseling and/or coordination of care with other physicians, other qualified health care professionals, or agencies are provided consistent with the nature of the problem(s) and the patient's and/or family's needs. Usually, the problem(s) requiring admission to outpatient hospital "observation status" are of high severity. Typically, 70 minutes are spent at the bedside and on the patient's hospital floor or unit.	**99218–99220** have been deleted. To report initial observation care, new or established patient, see revised codes **99221–99223**. ▲**99221** Initial hospital inpatient or observation care, per day, for the evaluation and management of a patient, which requires a medically appropriate history and/or examination and straightforward or low level medical decision making. When using total time on the date of the encounter for code selection, 40 minutes must be met or exceeded. ▲**99222** Initial hospital inpatient or observation care, per day, for the evaluation and management of a patient, which requires a medically appropriate history and/or examination and moderate level of medical decision making. When using total time on the date of the encounter for code selection, 55 minutes must be met or exceeded. ▲**99223** Initial hospital inpatient or observation care, per day, for the evaluation and management of a patient, which requires a medically appropriate history and/or examination and high level of medical decision making. When using total time on the date of the encounter for code selection, 75 minutes must be met or exceeded. (For services ≥90 minutes, use prolonged services code **99418**.) #★✚●**99418** Prolonged inpatient or observation evaluation and management service(s) time with or without direct patient contact beyond the required time of the primary service when the primary service level has been selected using total time, each 15 minutes of total time

● indicates a new code; ▲, revised; #, re-sequenced; ✚, add-on; ★, audiovisual technology; and ◀, synchronous interactive audio.

Quick Reference to 2023 *CPT* Pediatric Code Changes (*continued*)

2022	2023
Evaluation and Management (*continued*)	

2022	2023

#**99224** Subsequent observation care, per day, for the evaluation and management of a patient, which requires at least 2 of these 3 key components:
● Problem focused interval history;
● Problem focused examination;
● Medical decision making that is straightforward or of low complexity.
Counseling and/or coordination of care with other physicians, other qualified health care professionals, or agencies are provided consistent with the nature of the problem(s) and the patient's and/or family's needs.
Usually, the patient is stable, recovering, or improving. Typically, 15 minutes are spent at the bedside and on the patient's hospital floor or unit.
#**99225** Subsequent observation care, per day, for the evaluation and management of a patient, which requires at least 2 of these 3 key components:
● An expanded problem focused interval history;
● An expanded problem focused examination;
● Medical decision making of moderate complexity.
Counseling and/or coordination of care with other physicians, other qualified health care professionals, or agencies are provided consistent with the nature of the problem(s) and the patient's and/or family's needs.
Usually, the patient is responding inadequately to therapy or has developed a minor complication. Typically, 25 minutes are spent at the bedside and on the patient's hospital floor or unit.
#**99226** Subsequent observation care, per day, for the evaluation and management of a patient, which requires at least 2 of these 3 key components:
● A detailed interval history;
● A detailed examination;
● Medical decision making of high complexity.
Counseling and/or coordination of care with other physicians, other qualified health care professionals, or agencies are provided consistent with the nature of the problem(s) and the patient's and/or family's needs.
Usually, the patient is unstable or has developed a significant complication or a significant new problem. Typically, 35 minutes are spent at the bedside and on the patient's hospital floor or unit.
	99224–99226 have been deleted. To report subsequent observation care, see **99231–99233**.
	▲**99231** Subsequent hospital inpatient or observation care, per day, for the evaluation and management of a patient, which requires a medically appropriate history and/or examination and straightforward or low level of medical decision making.
	  When using total time on the date of the encounter for code selection, 25 minutes must be met or exceeded.
	▲**99232** Subsequent hospital inpatient or observation care, per day, for the evaluation and management of a patient, which requires a medically appropriate history and/or examination and moderate level of medical decision making.
	  When using total time on the date of the encounter for code selection, 35 minutes must be met or exceeded.
	▲**99233** Subsequent hospital inpatient or observation care, per day, for the evaluation and management of a patient, which requires a medically appropriate history and/or examination and high level of medical decision making.
	  When using total time on the date of the encounter for code selection, 50 minutes must be met or exceeded.
	  (For services ≥65 minutes, use prolonged services code **99418**.)
	#★✚●**99418** Prolonged inpatient or observation evaluation and management service(s) time with or without direct patient contact beyond the required time of the primary service when the primary service level has been selected using total time, each 15 minutes of total time

99221 Initial hospital care, per day, for the evaluation and management of a patient, which requires these 3 key components:
● A detailed or comprehensive history;
● A detailed or comprehensive examination; and
● Medical decision making that is straightforward or of low complexity.
Counseling and/or coordination of care with other physicians, other qualified health care professionals, or agencies are provided consistent with the nature of the problem(s) and the patient's and/or family's needs.
Usually, the problem(s) requiring admission are of low severity. Typically, 30 minutes are spent at the bedside and on the patient's hospital floor or unit.
99222 Initial hospital care, per day, for the evaluation and management of a patient, which requires these 3 key components:
● A comprehensive history;
● A comprehensive examination; and
● Medical decision making of moderate complexity.
Counseling and/or coordination of care with other physicians, other qualified health care professionals, or agencies are provided consistent with the nature of the problem(s) and the patient's and/or family's needs.
	▲**99221** Initial hospital inpatient or observation care, per day, for the evaluation and management of a patient, which requires a medically appropriate history and/or examination and straightforward or low level medical decision making.
	  When using total time on the date of the encounter for code selection, 40 minutes must be met or exceeded.
	▲**99222** Initial hospital inpatient or observation care, per day, for the evaluation and management of a patient, which requires a medically appropriate history and/or examination and moderate level of medical decision making.
	  When using total time on the date of the encounter for code selection, 55 minutes must be met or exceeded.
	▲**99223** Initial hospital inpatient or observation care, per day, for the evaluation and management of a patient, which requires a medically appropriate history and/or examination and high level of medical decision making.
	  When using total time on the date of the encounter for code selection, 75 minutes must be met or exceeded.

Continued on next page

● indicates a new code; ▲, revised; #, re-sequenced; ✚, add-on; ★, audiovisual technology; and ◄, synchronous interactive audio.

Appendixes

Appendixes

Quick Reference to 2023 *CPT* Pediatric Code Changes (*continued*)

2022	2023
Evaluation and Management (*continued*)	
Usually, the problem(s) requiring admission are of moderate severity. Typically, 50 minutes are spent at the bedside and on the patient's hospital floor or unit. **99223** Initial hospital care, per day, for the evaluation and management of a patient, which requires these 3 key components: • A comprehensive history; • A comprehensive examination; and • Medical decision making of high complexity. Counseling and/or coordination of care with other physicians, other qualified health care professionals, or agencies are provided consistent with the nature of the problem(s) and the patient's and/or family's needs. Usually, the problem(s) requiring admission are of high severity. Typically, 70 minutes are spent at the bedside and on the patient's hospital floor or unit.	(For services ≥90 minutes, use prolonged services code **99418**.) #★✚●**99418** Prolonged inpatient or observation evaluation and management service(s) time with or without direct patient contact beyond the required time of the primary service when the primary service level has been selected using total time, each 15 minutes of total time
99231 Subsequent hospital care, per day, for the evaluation and management of a patient, which requires at least 2 of these 3 key components: • A problem focused interval history; • A problem focused examination; • Medical decision making that is straightforward or of low complexity. Counseling and/or coordination of care with other physicians, other qualified health care professionals, or agencies are provided consistent with the nature of the problem(s) and the patient's and/or family's needs. Usually, the patient is stable, recovering, or improving. Typically, 15 minutes are spent at the bedside and on the patient's hospital floor or unit. **99232** Subsequent hospital care, per day, for the evaluation and management of a patient, which requires at least 2 of these 3 key components: • An expanded problem focused interval history; • An expanded problem focused examination; • Medical decision making that is straightforward or of low complexity. Counseling and/or coordination of care with other physicians, other qualified health care professionals, or agencies are provided consistent with the nature of the problem(s) and the patient's and/or family's needs. Usually, the patient is responding inadequately to therapy or has developed a minor complication. Typically, 25 minutes are spent at the bedside and on the patient's hospital floor or unit. **99233** Subsequent hospital care, per day, for the evaluation and management of a patient, which requires at least 2 of these 3 key components: • A detailed interval history; • A detailed examination; • Medical decision making of high complexity. Counseling and/or coordination of care with other physicians, other qualified health care professionals, or agencies are provided consistent with the nature of the problem(s) and the patient's and/or family's needs. Usually, the patient is unstable or has developed a significant complication or a significant new problem. Typically, 35 minutes are spent at the bedside and on the patient's hospital floor or unit.	▲**99231** Subsequent hospital inpatient or observation care, per day, for the evaluation and management of a patient, which requires a medically appropriate history and/or examination and straightforward or low level of medical decision making. When using total time on the date of the encounter for code selection, 25 minutes must be met or exceeded. ▲**99232** Subsequent hospital inpatient or observation care, per day, for the evaluation and management of a patient, which requires a medically appropriate history and/or examination and moderate level of medical decision making. When using total time on the date of the encounter for code selection, 35 minutes must be met or exceeded. ▲**99233** Subsequent hospital inpatient or observation care, per day, for the evaluation and management of a patient, which requires a medically appropriate history and/or examination and high level of medical decision making. When using total time on the date of the encounter for code selection, 50 minutes must be met or exceeded. (For services ≥65 minutes, use prolonged services code **99418**.) #★✚●**99418** Prolonged inpatient or observation evaluation and management service(s) time with or without direct patient contact beyond the required time of the primary service when the primary service level has been selected using total time, each 15 minutes of total time
99234 Observation or inpatient hospital care, for the evaluation and management of a patient including admission and discharge on the same date, which requires these 3 key components: • A detailed or comprehensive history; • A detailed or comprehensive examination; and • Medical decision making that is straightforward or of low complexity.	▲**99234** Hospital inpatient or observation care, for the evaluation and management of a patient including admission and discharge on the same date, which requires a medically appropriate history and/or examination and straightforward or low level of medical decision making.

● indicates a new code; ▲, revised; #, re-sequenced; ✚, add-on; ★, audiovisual technology; and ◄, synchronous interactive audio.

Quick Reference to 2023 *CPT* Pediatric Code Changes (*continued*)

2022	2023
Evaluation and Management (*continued*)	
Counseling and/or coordination of care with other physicians, other qualified health care professionals, or agencies are provided consistent with the nature of the problem(s) and the patient's and/or family's needs. Usually, the presenting problem(s) requiring admission are of low severity. Typically, 40 minutes are spent at the bedside and on the patient's hospital floor or unit. **99235** Observation or inpatient hospital care, for the evaluation and management of a patient including admission and discharge on the same date, which requires these 3 key components: ● A comprehensive history; ● A comprehensive examination; and ● Medical decision making of moderate complexity. Counseling and/or coordination of care with other physicians, other qualified health care professionals, or agencies are provided consistent with the nature of the problem(s) and the patient's and/or family's needs. Usually, the presenting problem(s) requiring admission are of moderate severity. Typically, 50 minutes are spent at the bedside and on the patient's hospital floor or unit. **99236** Observation or inpatient hospital care, for the evaluation and management of a patient including admission and discharge on the same date, which requires these 3 key components: ● A comprehensive history; ● A comprehensive examination; and ● Medical decision making of high complexity. Counseling and/or coordination of care with other physicians, other qualified health care professionals, or agencies are provided consistent with the nature of the problem(s) and the patient's and/or family's needs. Usually, the presenting problem(s) requiring admission are of high severity. Typically, 55 minutes are spent at the bedside and on the patient's hospital floor or unit.	When using total time on the date of the encounter for code selection, 45 minutes must be met or exceeded. ▲**99235** Hospital inpatient or observation care, for the evaluation and management of a patient including admission and discharge on the same date, which requires a medically appropriate history and/or examination and moderate level of medical decision making. When using total time on the date of the encounter for code selection, 70 minutes must be met or exceeded. ▲**99236** Hospital inpatient or observation care, for the evaluation and management of a patient including admission and discharge on the same date, which requires a medically appropriate history and/or examination and high level of medical decision making. When using total time on the date of the encounter for code selection, 85 minutes must be met or exceeded. (For services ≥100 minutes, use prolonged services code **99418**.) #★✚●**99418** Prolonged inpatient or observation evaluation and management service(s) time with or without direct patient contact beyond the required time of the primary service when the primary service level has been selected using total time, each 15 minutes of total time
99238 Hospital discharge day management; 30 minutes or less **99239** more than 30 minutes	▲**99238** Hospital inpatient or observation discharge day management; 30 minutes or less on the date of the encounter ▲**99239** more than 30 minutes on the date of the encounter
99241 Office consultation for a new or established patient, which requires these 3 key components: ● A problem focused history; ● A problem focused examination; and ● Straightforward medical decision making. Counseling and/or coordination of care with other physicians, other qualified health care professionals, or agencies are provided consistent with the nature of the problem(s) and the patient's and/or family's needs. Usually, the presenting problem(s) are self limited or minor. Typically, 15 minutes are spent face-to-face with the patient and/or family.	**99241** has been deleted. To report, use **99242**. ▲**99242** Office or other outpatient consultation for a new or established patient, which requires a medically appropriate history and/or examination and straightforward medical decision making. When using total time on the date of the encounter for code selection, 20 minutes must be met or exceeded.
99242 Office or other outpatient consultation for a new or established patient, which requires these 3 key components: ● An expanded problem focused history; ● An expanded problem focused examination; and ● Straightforward medical decision making. Counseling and/or coordination of care with other physicians, other qualified health care professionals, or agencies are provided consistent with the nature of the problem(s) and the patient's and/or family's needs.	▲**99242** Office or other outpatient consultation for a new or established patient, which requires a medically appropriate history and/or examination and straightforward medical decision making. When using total time on the date of the encounter for code selection, 20 minutes must be met or exceeded.

Appendixes

Continued on next page

● indicates a new code; ▲, revised; #, re-sequenced; ✚, add-on; ★, audiovisual technology; and ◀, synchronous interactive audio.

Appendixes

Quick Reference to 2023 *CPT* Pediatric Code Changes (*continued*)	
2022	**2023**
Evaluation and Management (*continued*)	
Usually, the presenting problem(s) are of low severity. Typically, 30 minutes are spent face-to-face with the patient and/or family. **99243** Office or other outpatient consultation for a new or established patient, which requires these 3 key components: ● A detailed history; ● A detailed examination; and ● Medical decision making of low complexity. Counseling and/or coordination of care with other physicians, other qualified health care professionals, or agencies are provided consistent with the nature of the problem(s) and the patient's and/or family's needs. Usually, the presenting problem(s) are of moderate severity. Typically, 40 minutes are spent face-to-face with the patient and/or family. **99244** Office or other outpatient consultation for a new or established patient, which requires these 3 key components: ● A comprehensive history; ● A comprehensive examination; and ● Medical decision making of moderate complexity. Counseling and/or coordination of care with other physicians, other qualified health care professionals, or agencies are provided consistent with the nature of the problem(s) and the patient's and/or family's needs. Usually, the presenting problem(s) are of moderate to high severity. Typically, 60 minutes are spent face-to-face with the patient and/or family. **99245** Office or other outpatient consultation for a new or established patient, which requires these 3 key components: ● A comprehensive history; ● A comprehensive examination; and ● Medical decision making of high complexity. Counseling and/or coordination of care with other physicians, other qualified health care professionals, or agencies are provided consistent with the nature of the problem(s) and the patient's and/or family's needs. Usually, the presenting problem(s) are of moderate to high severity. Typically, 80 minutes are spent face-to-face with the patient and/or family.	▲**99243** Office or other outpatient consultation for a new or established patient, which requires a medically appropriate history and/or examination and low level of medical decision making. When using total time on the date of the encounter for code selection, 30 minutes must be met or exceeded. ▲**99244** Office or other outpatient consultation for a new or established patient, which requires a medically appropriate history and/or examination and moderate level of medical decision making. When using total time on the date of the encounter for code selection, 40 minutes must be met or exceeded. ▲**99245** Office or other outpatient consultation for a new or established patient, which requires a medically appropriate history and/or examination and high level of medical decision making. When using total time on the date of the encounter for code selection, 55 minutes must be met or exceeded. (For services ≥70 minutes, use prolonged services code **99417**.) #★▲✚**99417** Prolonged outpatient evaluation and management service(s) time with or without direct patient contact beyond the required time of the primary service when the primary service level has been selected using total time, each 15 minutes of total time
99251 Inpatient consultation for a new or established patient, which requires these 3 key components: ● A problem focused history; ● A problem focused examination; and ● Straightforward medical decision making. Counseling and/or coordination of care with other physicians, other qualified health care professionals, or agencies are provided consistent with the nature of the problem(s) and the patient's and/or family's needs. Usually, the presenting problem(s) are self limited or minor. Typically, 20 minutes are spent at the bedside and on the patient's hospital floor or unit.	**99251** has been deleted. To report, use **99252**. ▲**99252** Inpatient or observation consultation for a new or established patient, which requires a medically appropriate history and/or examination and straightforward medical decision making. When using total time on the date of the encounter for code selection, 35 minutes must be met or exceeded.
99252 Inpatient consultation for a new or established patient, which requires these 3 key components: ● An expanded problem focused history; ● An expanded problem focused examination; and ● Straightforward medical decision making. Counseling and/or coordination of care with other physicians, other qualified health care professionals, or agencies are provided consistent with the nature of the problem(s) and the patient's and/or family's needs.	▲**99252** Inpatient or observation consultation for a new or established patient, which requires a medically appropriate history and/or examination and straightforward medical decision making. When using total time on the date of the encounter for code selection, 35 minutes must be met or exceeded.

● indicates a new code; ▲, revised; #, re-sequenced; ✚, add-on; ★, audiovisual technology; and ◀, synchronous interactive audio.

Quick Reference to 2023 *CPT* Pediatric Code Changes (*continued*)

2022	2023

Evaluation and Management (*continued*)

2022	2023
Usually, the presenting problem(s) are of low severity. Typically, 40 minutes are spent face-to-face with the patient and/or family. **99253** Inpatient consultation for a new or established patient, which requires these 3 key components: ● A detailed history; ● A detailed examination; and ● Medical decision making of low complexity. Counseling and/or coordination of care with other physicians, other qualified health care professionals, or agencies are provided consistent with the nature of the problem(s) and the patient's and/or family's needs. Usually, the presenting problem(s) are of moderate severity. Typically, 55 minutes are spent face-to-face with the patient and/or family. **99254** Inpatient consultation for a new or established patient, which requires these 3 key components: ● A comprehensive history; ● A comprehensive examination; and ● Medical decision making of moderate complexity. Counseling and/or coordination of care with other physicians, other qualified health care professionals, or agencies are provided consistent with the nature of the problem(s) and the patient's and/or family's needs. Usually, the presenting problem(s) are of moderate to high severity. Typically, 80 minutes are spent face-to-face with the patient and/or family. **99255** Inpatient consultation for a new or established patient, which requires these 3 key components: ● A comprehensive history; ● A comprehensive examination; and ● Medical decision making of high complexity. Counseling and/or coordination of care with other physicians, other qualified health care professionals, or agencies are provided consistent with the nature of the problem(s) and the patient's and/or family's needs. Usually, the presenting problem(s) are of moderate to high severity. Typically, 110 minutes are spent face-to-face with the patient and/or family.	▲**99253** Inpatient or observation consultation for a new or established patient, which requires a medically appropriate history and/or examination and low level of medical decision making. When using total time on the date of the encounter for code selection, 45 minutes must be met or exceeded. ▲**99254** Inpatient or observation consultation for a new or established patient, which requires a medically appropriate history and/or examination and moderate level of medical decision making. When using total time on the date of the encounter for code selection, 60 minutes must be met or exceeded. ▲**99255** Inpatient or observation consultation for a new or established patient, which requires a medically appropriate history and/or examination and high level of medical decision making. When using total time on the date of the encounter for code selection, 80 minutes must be met or exceeded. (For services ≥95 minutes, use prolonged services code **99418**.) #★●✛**99418** Prolonged inpatient or observation evaluation and management service(s) time with or without direct patient contact beyond the required time of the primary service when the primary service level has been selected using total time, each 15 minutes of total time
99281 Emergency department visit for the evaluation and management of a patient, which requires these 3 key components: ● A problem focused history; ● A problem focused examination; and ● Straightforward medical decision making. Counseling and/or coordination of care with other physicians, other qualified health care professionals, or agencies are provided consistent with the nature of the problem(s) and the patient's and/or family's needs. Usually, the presenting problem(s) are self limited or minor. **99282** Emergency department visit for the evaluation and management of a patient, which requires these 3 key components: ● An expanded problem focused history; ● An expanded problem focused examination; and ● Medical decision making of low complexity. Counseling and/or coordination of care with other physicians, other qualified health care professionals, or agencies are provided consistent with the nature of the problem(s) and the patient's and/or family's needs. Usually, the presenting problem(s) are of low to moderate severity.	▲**99281** Emergency department visit for the evaluation and management of a patient, that may not require the presence of a physician or other qualified health care professional ▲**99282** Emergency department visit for the evaluation and management of a patient, which requires a medically appropriate history and/or examination and straightforward medical decision making ▲**99283** Emergency department visit for the evaluation and management of a patient, which requires a medically appropriate history and/or examination and low level of medical decision making ▲**99284** Emergency department visit for the evaluation and management of a patient, which requires a medically appropriate history and/or examination and moderate level of medical decision making

Continued on next page

● indicates a new code; ▲, revised; #, re-sequenced; ✛, add-on; ★, audiovisual technology; and ◀, synchronous interactive audio.

Appendixes

Quick Reference to 2023 *CPT* Pediatric Code Changes (*continued*)	
2022	**2023**
Evaluation and Management (*continued*)	
99283 Emergency department visit for the evaluation and management of a patient, which requires these 3 key components: ● An expanded problem focused history; ● An expanded problem focused examination; and ● Medical decision making of moderate complexity. Counseling and/or coordination of care with other physicians, other qualified health care professionals, or agencies are provided consistent with the nature of the problem(s) and the patient's and/or family's needs. Usually, the presenting problem(s) are of moderate severity. **99284** Emergency department visit for the evaluation and management of a patient, which requires these 3 key components: ● A detailed history; ● A detailed examination; and ● Medical decision making of moderate complexity. Counseling and/or coordination of care with other physicians, other qualified health care professionals, or agencies are provided consistent with the nature of the problem(s) and the patient's and/or family's needs. Usually, the presenting problem(s) are of high severity, and require urgent evaluation by the physician or other qualified health care professionals, but do not pose an immediate significant threat to life or physiologic function. **99285** Emergency department visit for the evaluation and management of a patient, which requires these 3 key components: ● A comprehensive history; ● A comprehensive examination; and ● Medical decision making of high complexity. Counseling and/or coordination of care with other physicians, other qualified health care professionals, or agencies are provided consistent with the nature of the problem(s) and the patient's and/or family's needs. Usually, the presenting problem(s) are of high severity and pose an immediate significant threat to life or physiologic function.	▲**99285** Emergency department visit for the evaluation and management of a patient, which requires a medically appropriate history and/or examination and high level of medical decision making
99304 Initial nursing facility care, per day, for the evaluation and management of a patient, which requires these 3 key components: ● A detailed or comprehensive history; ● A detailed or comprehensive examination; and ● Medical decision making that is straightforward or of low complexity. Counseling and/or coordination of care with other physicians, other qualified health care professionals, or agencies are provided consistent with the nature of the problem(s) and the patient's and/or family's needs. Usually, the problem(s) requiring admission are of low severity. Typically, 25 minutes are spent at the bedside and on the patient's facility floor or unit. **99305** Initial nursing facility care, per day, for the evaluation and management of a patient, which requires these 3 key components: ● A comprehensive history; ● A comprehensive examination; and ● Medical decision making of moderate complexity. Counseling and/or coordination of care with other physicians, other qualified health care professionals, or agencies are provided consistent with the nature of the problem(s) and the patient's and/or family's needs. Usually, the problem(s) requiring admission are of moderate severity. Typically, 35 minutes are spent at the bedside and on the patient's facility floor or unit.	▲**99304** Initial nursing facility care, per day, for the evaluation and management of a patient, which requires a medically appropriate history and/or examination and straightforward or low level of medical decision making. When using total time on the date of the encounter for code selection, 25 minutes must be met or exceeded. ▲**99305** Initial nursing facility care, per day, for the evaluation and management of a patient, which requires a medically appropriate history and/or examination and moderate level of medical decision making. When using total time on the date of the encounter for code selection, 35 minutes must be met or exceeded. ▲**99306** Initial nursing facility care, per day, for the evaluation and management of a patient, which requires a medically appropriate history and/or examination and high level of medical decision making. When using total time on the date of the encounter for code selection, 45 minutes must be met or exceeded. (For services ≥60 minutes, use prolonged services code **99418**.)

● indicates a new code; ▲, revised; #, re-sequenced; ✚, add-on; ★, audiovisual technology; and ◀, synchronous interactive audio.

Quick Reference to 2023 *CPT* Pediatric Code Changes (*continued*)	
2022	**2023**
Evaluation and Management (*continued*)	
99306 Initial nursing facility care, per day, for the evaluation and management of a patient, which requires these 3 key components: ● A comprehensive history; ● A comprehensive examination; and ● Medical decision making of high complexity. Counseling and/or coordination of care with other physicians, other qualified health care professionals, or agencies are provided consistent with the nature of the problem(s) and the patient's and/or family's needs. Usually, the problem(s) requiring admission are of high severity. Typically, 45 minutes are spent at the bedside and on the patient's facility floor or unit.	#★✚●99418 Prolonged inpatient or observation evaluation and management service(s) time with or without direct patient contact beyond the required time of the primary service when the primary service level has been selected using total time, each 15 minutes of total time

99307 Subsequent nursing facility care, per day, for the evaluation and management of a patient, which requires at least 2 of these 3 key components:
● A problem focused interval history;
● A problem focused examination;
● Straightforward medical decision making.
Counseling and/or coordination of care with other physicians, other qualified health care professionals, or agencies are provided consistent with the nature of the problem(s) and the patient's and/or family's needs.
Usually, the patient is stable, recovering, or improving. Typically, 10 minutes are spent at the bedside and on the patient's facility floor or unit.
99308 Subsequent nursing facility care, per day, for the evaluation and management of a patient, which requires at least 2 of these 3 key components:
● An expanded problem focused interval history;
● An expanded problem focused examination;
● Medical decision making of low complexity.
Counseling and/or coordination of care with other physicians, other qualified health care professionals, or agencies are provided consistent with the nature of the problem(s) and the patient's and/or family's needs.
Usually, the patient is responding inadequately to therapy or has developed a minor complication. Typically, 15 minutes are spent at the bedside and on the patient's facility floor or unit.
99309 Subsequent nursing facility care, per day, for the evaluation and management of a patient, which requires at least 2 of these 3 key components:
● A detailed interval history;
● A detailed examination;
● Medical decision making of moderate complexity.
Counseling and/or coordination of care with other physicians, other qualified health care professionals, or agencies are provided consistent with the nature of the problem(s) and the patient's and/or family's needs.
Usually, the patient has developed a significant complication or a significant new problem. Typically, 25 minutes are spent at the bedside and on the patient's facility floor or unit.
99310 Subsequent nursing facility care, per day, for the evaluation and management of a patient, which requires at least 2 of these 3 key components:
● A comprehensive interval history;
● A comprehensive examination;
● Medical decision making of high complexity.
Counseling and/or coordination of care with other physicians, other qualified health care professionals, or agencies are provided consistent with the nature of the problem(s) and the patient's and/or family's needs.
	▲99307 Subsequent nursing facility care, per day, for the evaluation and management of a patient, which requires a medically appropriate history and/or examination and straightforward medical decision making.
	    When using total time on the date of the encounter for code selection, 10 minutes must be met or exceeded.
	▲99308 Subsequent nursing facility care, per day, for the evaluation and management of a patient, which requires a medically appropriate history and/or examination and low level of medical decision making.
	    When using total time on the date of the encounter for code selection, 15 minutes must be met or exceeded.
	▲99309 Subsequent nursing facility care, per day, for the evaluation and management of a patient, which requires a medically appropriate history and/or examination and moderate level of medical decision making.
	    When using total time on the date of the encounter for code selection, 30 minutes must be met or exceeded.
	▲99310 Subsequent nursing facility care, per day, for the evaluation and management of a patient, which requires a medically appropriate history and/or examination and high level of medical decision making.
	    When using total time on the date of the encounter for code selection, 45 minutes must be met or exceeded.
	    (For services ≥60 minutes, use prolonged services code **99418**.)
	#★✚●99418 Prolonged inpatient or observation evaluation and management service(s) time with or without direct patient contact beyond the required time of the primary service when the primary service level has been selected using total time, each 15 minutes of total time

Continued on next page

● indicates a new code; ▲, revised; #, re-sequenced; ✚, add-on; ★, audiovisual technology; and ◀, synchronous interactive audio.

Appendixes

Appendixes

Quick Reference to 2023 *CPT* Pediatric Code Changes (*continued*)	
2022	**2023**
Evaluation and Management (*continued*)	
The patient may be unstable or may have developed a significant new problem requiring immediate physician attention. Typically, 35 minutes are spent at the bedside and on the patient's facility floor or unit.	
99315 Nursing facility discharge day management; 30 minutes or less **99316** more than 30 minutes	▲**99315** Nursing facility discharge management; 30 minutes or less total time on the date of the encounter ▲**99316** more than 30 minutes total time on the date of the encounter
99318 Evaluation and management of a patient involving an annual nursing facility assessment, which requires these 3 key components: ● A detailed interval history; ● A comprehensive examination; and ● Medical decision making that is of low to moderate complexity. Counseling and/or coordination of care with other physicians, other qualified health care professionals, or agencies are provided consistent with the nature of the problem(s) and the patient's and/or family's needs. Usually, the patient is stable, recovering, or improving. Typically, 30 minutes are spent at the bedside and on the patient's facility floor or unit.	**99318** has been deleted. To report, see **99307–99310** (see code descriptors in previous row).

99324 Domiciliary or rest home visit for the evaluation and management of a new patient, which requires these 3 key components:
● A problem focused history;
● A problem focused examination; and
● Straightforward medical decision making.
Counseling and/or coordination of care with other physicians, other qualified health care professionals, or agencies are provided consistent with the nature of the problem(s) and the patient's and/or family's needs.
Usually, the presenting problem(s) are of low severity. Typically, 20 minutes are spent with the patient and/or family or caregiver.
99325 Domiciliary or rest home visit for the evaluation and management of a new patient, which requires these 3 key components:
● An expanded problem focused history;
● An expanded problem focused examination; and
● Medical decision making of low complexity.
Counseling and/or coordination of care with other physicians, other qualified health care professionals, or agencies are provided consistent with the nature of the problem(s) and the patient's and/or family's needs.
Usually, the presenting problem(s) are of moderate severity. Typically, 30 minutes are spent with the patient and/or family or caregiver.
99326 Domiciliary or rest home visit for the evaluation and management of a new patient, which requires these 3 key components:
● A detailed history;
● A detailed examination; and
● Medical decision making of moderate complexity.
Counseling and/or coordination of care with other physicians, other qualified health care professionals, or agencies are provided consistent with the nature of the problem(s) and the patient's and/or family's needs.
Usually, the presenting problem(s) are of moderate severity. Typically, 30 minutes are spent with the patient and/or family or caregiver.
99326 Domiciliary or rest home visit for the evaluation and management of a new patient, which requires these 3 key components:
● A detailed history;
	99324–99328 have been deleted. For domiciliary, rest home (eg, boarding home), or custodial care services, new patient, see home and residence service code **99341, 99342, 99344,** or **99345**.
	▲**99341** Home or residence visit for the evaluation and management of a new patient, which requires a medically appropriate history and/or examination and straightforward medical decision making.
	    When using total time on the date of the encounter for code selection, 15 minutes must be met or exceeded.
	▲**99342** Home or residence visit for the evaluation and management of a new patient, which requires a medically appropriate history and/or examination and low level of medical decision making.
	    When using total time on the date of the encounter for code selection, 30 minutes must be met or exceeded.
	▲**99344** Home or residence visit for the evaluation and management of a new patient, which requires a medically appropriate history and/or examination and moderate level of medical decision making.
	    When using total time on the date of the encounter for code selection, 60 minutes must be met or exceeded.
	▲**99345** Home or residence visit for the evaluation and management of a new patient, which requires a medically appropriate history and/or examination and high level of medical decision making.
	    When using total time on the date of the encounter for code selection, 75 minutes must be met or exceeded.
	    (For services ≥90 minutes, see prolonged services code **99417.**)
	#★✚▲**99417** Prolonged outpatient evaluation and management service(s) time with or without direct patient contact beyond the required time of the primary service when

● indicates a new code; ▲, revised; #, re-sequenced; ✚, add-on; ★, audiovisual technology; and ◀, synchronous interactive audio.

Appendixes

Quick Reference to 2023 *CPT* Pediatric Code Changes (*continued*)	
2022	**2023**
Evaluation and Management (*continued*)	
• A detailed examination; and • Medical decision making of moderate complexity. Counseling and/or coordination of care with other physicians, other qualified health care professionals, or agencies are provided consistent with the nature of the problem(s) and the patient's and/or family's needs. Usually, the presenting problem(s) are of moderate to high severity. Typically, 45 minutes are spent with the patient and/or family or caregiver. **99327** Domiciliary or rest home visit for the evaluation and management of a new patient, which requires these 3 key components: • A comprehensive history; • A comprehensive examination; and • Medical decision making of moderate complexity. Counseling and/or coordination of care with other physicians, other qualified health care professionals, or agencies are provided consistent with the nature of the problem(s) and the patient's and/or family's needs. Usually, the presenting problem(s) are of high severity. Typically, 60 minutes are spent with the patient and/or family or caregiver. **99328** Domiciliary or rest home visit for the evaluation and management of a new patient, which requires these 3 key components: • A comprehensive history; • A comprehensive examination; and • Medical decision making of high complexity. Counseling and/or coordination of care with other physicians, other qualified health care professionals, or agencies are provided consistent with the nature of the problem(s) and the patient's and/or family's needs. Usually, the patient is unstable or has developed a significant new problem requiring immediate physician attention. Typically, 75 minutes are spent with the patient and/or family or caregiver.	the primary service level has been selected using total time, each 15 minutes of total time

99334 Domiciliary or rest home visit for the evaluation and management of an established patient, which requires at least 2 of these 3 key components:
• A problem focused history;
• A problem focused examination; and
• Straightforward medical decision making.
Counseling and/or coordination of care with other physicians, other qualified health care professionals, or agencies are provided consistent with the nature of the problem(s) and the patient's and/or family's needs.
Usually, the presenting problem(s) are self limited or minor. Typically, 15 minutes are spent with the patient and/or family or caregiver.
99335 Domiciliary or rest home visit for the evaluation and management of an established patient, which requires at least 2 of these 3 key components:
• An expanded problem focused history;
• An expanded problem focused examination; and
• Medical decision making of low complexity.
Counseling and/or coordination of care with other physicians, other qualified health care professionals, or agencies are provided consistent with the nature of the problem(s) and the patient's and/or family's needs.
Usually, the presenting problem(s) are of low to moderate severity. Typically, 25 minutes are spent with the patient and/or family or caregiver.
99336 Domiciliary or rest home visit for the evaluation and management of an established patient, which requires at least 2 of these 3 key components:
	99334–99337 have been deleted. For domiciliary, rest home (eg, boarding home), or custodial care services, established patient, see home and residence services codes **99347–99350**.
	▲**99347** Home or residence visit for the evaluation and management of an established patient, which requires a medically appropriate history and/or examination and straightforward medical decision making.
	    When using total time on the date of the encounter for code selection, 20 minutes must be met or exceeded.
	▲**99348** Home or residence visit for the evaluation and management of an established patient, which requires a medically appropriate history and/or examination and low level of medical decision making.
	    When using total time on the date of the encounter for code selection, 30 minutes must be met or exceeded.
	▲**99349** Home or residence visit for the evaluation and management of an established patient, which requires a medically appropriate history and/or examination and moderate level of medical decision making.
	    When using total time on the date of the encounter for code selection, 40 minutes must be met or exceeded.

Continued on next page

● indicates a new code; ▲, revised; #, re-sequenced; ✚, add-on; ★, audiovisual technology; and ◄, synchronous interactive audio.

Quick Reference to 2023 *CPT* Pediatric Code Changes (*continued*)	
2022	**2023**
Evaluation and Management (*continued*)	

• A detailed history;
• A detailed examination; and
• Medical decision making of moderate complexity.
Counseling and/or coordination of care with other physicians, other qualified health care professionals, or agencies are provided consistent with the nature of the problem(s) and the patient's and/or family's needs.
Usually, the presenting problem(s) are of moderate to high severity. Typically, 40 minutes are spent with the patient and/or family or caregiver.
99337 Domiciliary or rest home visit for the evaluation and management of an established patient, which requires at least 2 of these 3 key components:
• A comprehensive history;
• A comprehensive examination; and
• Medical decision making of moderate to high complexity.
Counseling and/or coordination of care with other physicians, other qualified health care professionals, or agencies are provided consistent with the nature of the problem(s) and the patient's and/or family's needs.
Usually, the presenting problem(s) are of moderate to high severity. The patient may be unstable or may have developed a significant new problem requiring immediate physician attention. Typically, 60 minutes are spent with the patient and/or family or caregiver.
	▲**99350** Home or residence visit for the evaluation and management of an established patient, which requires a medically appropriate history and/or examination and high level of medical decision making.
	   When using total time on the date of the encounter for code selection, 60 minutes must be met or exceeded.
	   (For services ≥75 minutes, see prolonged service code **99417**.)
	#★✚▲**99417** Prolonged outpatient evaluation and management service(s) time with or without direct patient contact beyond the required time of the primary service when the primary service level has been selected using total time, each 15 minutes of total time

99339 Individual physician supervision of a patient (patient not present) in home, domiciliary or rest home (eg, assisted living facility) requiring complex and multidisciplinary care modalities involving regular physician development and/or revision of care plans, review of subsequent reports of patient status, review of related laboratory and other studies, communication (including telephone calls) for purposes of assessment or care decisions with health care professional(s), family member(s), surrogate decision maker(s) (eg, legal guardian) and/or key caregiver(s) involved in patient's care, integration of new information into the medical treatment plan and/or adjustment of medical therapy, within a calendar month; 15-29 minutes **99340** 30 minutes or more	**99339** and **99340** have been deleted. For domiciliary, rest home (eg, assisted living facility), or home care plan oversight services, see care management services codes **99491** and **99437** or principal care management codes **99424** and **99425**.

99341 Home visit for the evaluation and management of a new patient, which requires these 3 key components:
• A problem focused history;
• A problem focused examination; and
• Straightforward medical decision making.
Counseling and/or coordination of care with other physicians, other qualified health care professionals, or agencies are provided consistent with the nature of the problem(s) and the patient's and/or family's needs.
Usually, the presenting problem(s) are of low severity. Typically, 20 minutes are spent with the patient and/or family or caregiver.
99342 Home visit for the evaluation and management of a new patient, which requires these 3 key components:
• An expanded problem focused history;
• An expanded problem focused examination; and
• Medical decision making of low complexity.
Counseling and/or coordination of care with other physicians, other qualified health care professionals, or agencies are provided consistent with the nature of the problem(s) and the patient's and/or family's needs.
Usually, the presenting problem(s) are of moderate severity. Typically, 30 minutes are spent with the patient and/or family or caregiver.
	99343 has been deleted. To report, see **99341**, **99342**, **99344**, or **99345**.
	▲**99341** Home or residence visit for the evaluation and management of a new patient, which requires a medically appropriate history and/or examination and straightforward medical decision making.
	   When using total time on the date of the encounter for code selection, 15 minutes must be met or exceeded.
	▲**99342** Home or residence visit for the evaluation and management of a new patient, which requires a medically appropriate history and/or examination and low level of medical decision making.
	   When using total time on the date of the encounter for code selection, 30 minutes must be met or exceeded.
	▲**99344** Home or residence visit for the evaluation and management of a new patient, which requires a medically appropriate history and/or examination and moderate level of medical decision making.
	   When using total time on the date of the encounter for code selection, 60 minutes must be met or exceeded.

● indicates a new code; ▲, revised; #, re-sequenced; ✚, add-on; ★, audiovisual technology; and ◀, synchronous interactive audio.

Quick Reference to 2023 *CPT* Pediatric Code Changes (*continued*)

2022	2023
Evaluation and Management (*continued*)	

2022	2023
99343 Home visit for the evaluation and management of a new patient, which requires these 3 key components: ● A detailed history; ● A detailed examination; and ● Medical decision making of moderate complexity. Counseling and/or coordination of care with other physicians, other qualified health care professionals, or agencies are provided consistent with the nature of the problem(s) and the patient's and/or family's needs. Usually, the presenting problem(s) are of moderate to high severity. Typically, 45 minutes are spent face-to-face with the patient and/or family. **99344** Home visit for the evaluation and management of a new patient, which requires these 3 key components: ● A comprehensive history; ● A comprehensive examination; and ● Medical decision making of moderate complexity. Counseling and/or coordination of care with other physicians, other qualified health care professionals, or agencies are provided consistent with the nature of the problem(s) and the patient's and/or family's needs. Usually, the presenting problem(s) are of high severity. Typically, 60 minutes are spent face-to-face with the patient and/or family. **99345** Home visit for the evaluation and management of a new patient, which requires these 3 key components: ● A comprehensive history; ● A comprehensive examination; and ● Medical decision making of high complexity. Counseling and/or coordination of care with other physicians, other qualified health care professionals, or agencies are provided consistent with the nature of the problem(s) and the patient's and/or family's needs. Usually, the patient is unstable or has developed a significant new problem requiring immediate physician attention. Typically, 75 minutes are spent face-to-face with the patient and/or family.	▲**99345** Home or residence visit for the evaluation and management of a new patient, which requires a medically appropriate history and/or examination and high level of medical decision making. When using total time on the date of the encounter for code selection, 75 minutes must be met or exceeded. (For services ≥90 minutes, see prolonged services code **99417**.) #★✚▲**99417** Prolonged outpatient evaluation and management service(s) time with or without direct patient contact beyond the required time of the primary service when the primary service level has been selected using total time, each 15 minutes of total time
99347 Home visit for the evaluation and management of an established patient, which requires at least 2 of these 3 key components: ● A problem focused interval history; ● A problem focused examination; ● Straightforward medical decision making. Counseling and/or coordination of care with other physicians, other qualified health care professionals, or agencies are provided consistent with the nature of the problem(s) and the patient's and/or family's needs. Usually, the presenting problem(s) are self limited or minor. Typically, 15 minutes are spent face-to-face with the patient and/or family. **99348** Home visit for the evaluation and management of an established patient, which requires at least 2 of these 3 key components: ● An expanded problem focused history; ● An expanded problem focused examination; and ● Medical decision making of low complexity. Counseling and/or coordination of care with other physicians, other qualified health care professionals, or agencies are provided consistent with the nature of the problem(s) and the patient's and/or family's needs. Usually, the presenting problem(s) are of low to moderate severity. Typically, 25 minutes are spent face-to-face with the patient and/or family.	▲**99347** Home or residence visit for the evaluation and management of an established patient, which requires a medically appropriate history and/or examination and straightforward medical decision making. When using total time on the date of the encounter for code selection, 20 minutes must be met or exceeded. ▲**99348** Home or residence visit for the evaluation and management of an established patient, which requires a medically appropriate history and/or examination and low level of medical decision making. When using total time on the date of the encounter for code selection, 30 minutes must be met or exceeded. ▲**99349** Home or residence visit for the evaluation and management of an established patient, which requires a medically appropriate history and/or examination and moderate level of medical decision making. When using total time on the date of the encounter for code selection, 40 minutes must be met or exceeded.

Continued on next page

● indicates a new code; ▲, revised; #, re-sequenced; ✚, add-on; ★, audiovisual technology; and ◀, synchronous interactive audio.

Quick Reference to 2023 *CPT* Pediatric Code Changes (*continued*)

2022	2023
Evaluation and Management (*continued*)	
99349 Home visit for the evaluation and management of an established patient, which requires at least 2 of these 3 key components: ● A detailed history; ● A detailed examination; and ● Medical decision making of moderate complexity. Counseling and/or coordination of care with other physicians, other qualified health care professionals, or agencies are provided consistent with the nature of the problem(s) and the patient's and/or family's needs. Usually, the presenting problem(s) are moderate to high severity. Typically, 40 minutes are spent face-to-face with the patient and/or family. **99350** Home visit for the evaluation and management of an established patient, which requires at least 2 of these 3 key components: ● A comprehensive history; ● A comprehensive examination; and ● Medical decision making of moderate to high complexity. Counseling and/or coordination of care with other physicians, other qualified health care professionals, or agencies are provided consistent with the nature of the problem(s) and the patient's and/or family's needs. Usually, the presenting problem(s) are of moderate to high severity. The patient may be unstable or may have developed a significant new problem requiring immediate physician attention. Typically, 60 minutes are spent face-to-face with the patient and/or family.	▲**99350** Home or residence visit for the evaluation and management of an established patient, which requires a medically appropriate history and/or examination and high level of medical decision making. When using total time on the date of the encounter for code selection, 60 minutes must be met or exceeded. (For services ≥75 minutes, see prolonged service code **99417**.) #★✚▲**99417** Prolonged outpatient evaluation and management service(s) time with or without direct patient contact beyond the required time of the primary service when the primary service level has been selected using total time, each 15 minutes of total time
✚**99354** Prolonged evaluation and management or psychotherapy service(s) (beyond the typical service time of the primary procedure) in the office or other outpatient setting requiring direct patient contact beyond the usual service; first hour ✚**99355** each additional 30 minutes	**99354** and **99355** have been deleted. For prolonged evaluation and management services on the date of an office or other outpatient service, a home and residence service, or a cognitive assessment and care plan, use **99417** (see code descriptor in previous row).
✚**99356** Prolonged service in the inpatient or observation setting, requiring unit/floor time beyond the usual service; first hour ✚**99357** each additional 30 minutes	#★✚●**99418** Prolonged inpatient or observation evaluation and management service(s) time with or without direct patient contact beyond the required time of the primary service when the primary service level has been selected using total time, each 15 minutes of total time (Use **99418** in conjunction with **99223**, **99233**, **99236**, **99255**, **99306**, or **99310**).
#✚**99415** Prolonged clinical staff service (the service beyond the highest time in the range of total time of the service) during an evaluation and management service in the office or outpatient setting, direct patient contact with physician supervision; first hour #✚**99416** each additional 30 minutes	#✚▲**99415** Prolonged clinical staff service (the service beyond the typical service time) during an evaluation and management service in the office or outpatient setting, direct patient contact with physician supervision; first hour #✚▲**99416** each additional 30 minutes
✚**99417** Prolonged office or other outpatient evaluation and management service(s) beyond the minimum required time of the primary procedure which has been selected using total time, requiring total time with or without direct patient contact beyond the usual service, on the date of the primary service, each 15 minutes of total time (Use **99417** in conjunction with **99205** or **99215**.)	#★✚▲**99417** Prolonged outpatient evaluation and management service(s) time with or without direct patient contact beyond the required time of the primary service when the primary service level has been selected using total time, each 15 minutes of total time (Use **99417** in conjunction with **99205**, **99215**, **99245**, **99345**, **99350**, or **99483**.)

● indicates a new code; ▲, revised; #, re-sequenced; ✚, add-on; ★, audiovisual technology; and ◀, synchronous interactive audio.

Quick Reference to 2023 *CPT* Pediatric Code Changes (*continued*)

2022	2023
Evaluation and Management (*continued*)	
99446 Interprofessional telephone/Internet/electronic health record assessment and management service provided by a consultative physician, including a verbal and written report to the patient's treating/requesting physician or other qualified health care professional; 5–10 minutes of medical consultative discussion and review	▲**99446** Interprofessional telephone/Internet/electronic health record assessment and management service provided by a consultative physician or other qualified health care professional, including a verbal and written report to the patient's treating/requesting physician or other qualified health care professional; 5–10 minutes of medical consultative discussion and review
99447 11–20 minutes of medical consultative discussion and review	▲**99447** 11–20 minutes of medical consultative discussion and review
99448 21–30 minutes of medical consultative discussion and review	▲**99448** 21–30 minutes of medical consultative discussion and review
99449 31 minutes or more of medical consultative discussion and review	▲**99449** 31 minutes or more of medical consultative discussion and review
#**99451** Interprofessional telephone/Internet/electronic health record assessment and management service provided by a consultative physician, including a written report to the patient's treating/requesting physician or other qualified health care professional, 5 minutes or more of medical consultative time	#▲**99451** Interprofessional telephone/Internet/electronic health record assessment and management service provided by a consultative physician or other qualified health care professional, including a written report to the patient's treating/requesting physician or other qualified health care professional, 5 minutes or more of medical consultative time
99483 Assessment of and care planning for a patient with cognitive impairment, requiring an independent historian, in the office or other outpatient, home or domiciliary or rest home, with all of the following required elements:	▲**99483** Assessment of and care planning for a patient with cognitive impairment, requiring an independent historian, in the office or other outpatient, home or domiciliary or rest home, with all of the following required elements:
• Cognition-focused evaluation including a pertinent history and examination,	• Cognition-focused evaluation including a pertinent history and examination,
• Medical decision making of moderate or high complexity,	• Medical decision making of moderate or high complexity,
• Functional assessment (eg, basic and instrumental activities of daily living), including decision-making capacity,	• Functional assessment (eg, basic and instrumental activities of daily living), including decision-making capacity,
• Use of standardized instruments for staging of dementia (eg, functional assessment staging test [FAST], clinical dementia rating [CDR]),	• Use of standardized instruments for staging of dementia (eg, functional assessment staging test [FAST], clinical dementia rating [CDR]),
• Medication reconciliation and review for high-risk medications,	• Medication reconciliation and review for high-risk medications,
• Evaluation for neuropsychiatric and behavioral symptoms, including depression, including use of standardized screening instrument(s),	• Evaluation for neuropsychiatric and behavioral symptoms, including depression, including use of standardized screening instrument(s),
• Evaluation of safety (eg, home), including motor vehicle operation,	• Evaluation of safety (eg, home), including motor vehicle operation,
• Identification of caregiver(s), caregiver knowledge, caregiver needs, social supports, and the willingness of caregiver to take on caregiving tasks,	• Identification of caregiver(s), caregiver knowledge, caregiver needs, social supports, and the willingness of caregiver to take on caregiving tasks,
• Development, updating or revision, or review of an Advance Care Plan,	• Development, updating or revision, or review of an Advance Care Plan,
• Creation of a written care plan, including initial plans to address any neuropsychiatric symptoms, neurocognitive symptoms, functional limitations, and referral to community resources as needed (eg, rehabilitation services, adult day programs, support groups) shared with the patient and/or caregiver with initial education and support.	• Creation of a written care plan, including initial plans to address any neuropsychiatric symptoms, neurocognitive symptoms, functional limitations, and referral to community resources as needed (eg, rehabilitation services, adult day programs, support groups) shared with the patient and/or caregiver with initial education and support.
Typically, 50 minutes are spent face-to-face with the patient and/or family or caregiver.	

Continued on next page

Appendixes

● indicates a new code; ▲, revised; #, re-sequenced; ✚, add-on; ★, audiovisual technology; and ◀, synchronous interactive audio.

Appendixes

Quick Reference to 2023 *CPT* Pediatric Code Changes (*continued*)	
2022	**2023**
Evaluation and Management (*continued*)	
	Typically, 60 minutes of total time is spent on the date of the encounter. (For services ≥75 minutes, use **99417** [see code descriptor earlier in this table].)
Integumentary System	
No code	●**15778** Implantation of absorbable mesh or other prosthesis for delayed closure of defect(s) (ie, external genitalia, perineum, abdominal wall) due to soft tissue infection or trauma
15850 Removal of sutures under anesthesia (other than local), same surgeon **15851** Removal of sutures under anesthesia (other than local), other surgeon	**15850** has been deleted. To report, use **15851**. ▲**15851** Removal of sutures or staples requiring anesthesia (ie, general anesthesia, moderate sedation) #✚●**15853** Removal of sutures or staples not requiring anesthesia ✚●**15854** Removal of sutures and staples not requiring anesthesia
Cardiovascular	
None	●**33900** Percutaneous pulmonary artery revascularization by stent placement, initial; normal native connections, unilateral ●**33901** normal native connections, bilateral ●**33902** abnormal connections, unilateral ●**33903** abnormal connections, bilateral ✚●**33904** Percutaneous pulmonary artery revascularization by stent placement, each additional vessel or separate lesion, normal or abnormal connections (List separately in addition to code for primary procedure)
Digestive System: Hernioplasty, Herniorrhaphy, Herniotomy	
49560 Repair initial incisional or ventral hernia; reducible **49561** incarcerated or strangulated **49565** Repair recurrent incisional or ventral hernia; reducible **49566** incarcerated or strangulated ✚**49568** Implantation of mesh or other prosthesis for open incisional or ventral hernia repair or mesh for closure of debridement for necrotizing soft tissue infection **49570** Repair epigastric hernia (eg, preperitoneal fat); reducible (separate procedure) **49572** incarcerated or strangulated **49580** Repair umbilical hernia, younger than age 5 years; reducible **49582** incarcerated or strangulated **49585** Repair umbilical hernia, age 5 years or older; reducible **49587** incarcerated or strangulated **49590** Repair spigelian hernia **49652** Laparoscopy, surgical, repair, ventral, umbilical, spigelian or epigastric hernia (includes mesh insertion, when performed); reducible **49653** incarcerated or strangulated **49654** Laparoscopy, surgical, repair, incisional hernia (includes mesh insertion, when performed); reducible **49655** incarcerated or strangulated	**49560** and **49561** have been deleted. Report by using **49591–49596**. **49565** and **49566** and **49656** and **49657** have been deleted. Report by using **49613–49618**. **49568–49590** and **49652–49655** have been deleted. Report by using **49591–49618**. ●**49591** Repair of anterior abdominal hernia(s) (ie, epigastric, incisional, ventral, umbilical, spigelian), any approach (ie, open, laparoscopic, robotic), initial including placement of mesh or other prosthesis, when performed, total length of defect(s); less than 3 cm, reducible ●**49592** less than 3 cm, incarcerated or strangulated ●**49593** 3 cm to 10 cm, reducible ●**49594** 3 cm to 10 cm, incarcerated or strangulated ●**49595** greater than 10 cm, reducible ●**49596** greater than 10 cm, incarcerated or strangulated ●**49613** Repair of anterior abdominal hernia(s) (ie, epigastric, incisional, ventral, umbilical, spigelian), any approach (ie, open, laparoscopic, robotic), recurrent, including placement of mesh or other prosthesis, when performed, total length of defect(s); less than 3 cm, reducible

● indicates a new code; ▲, revised; #, re-sequenced; ✚, add-on; ★, audiovisual technology; and ◀, synchronous interactive audio.

Quick Reference to 2023 *CPT* Pediatric Code Changes (*continued*)

2022	2023
Digestive System: Hernioplasty, Herniorrhaphy, Herniotomy (*continued*)	
49656 Laparoscopy, surgical, repair, recurrent incisional hernia (includes mesh insertion, when performed); reducible **49657** incarcerated or strangulated	●**49614** less than 3 cm, incarcerated or strangulated ●**49615** 3 cm to 10 cm, reducible ●**49616** 3 cm to 10 cm, incarcerated or strangulated ●**49617** greater than 10 cm, reducible ●**49618** greater than 10 cm, incarcerated or strangulated ●**49621** Repair of parastomal hernia, any approach (ie, open, laparoscopic, robotic), initial or recurrent, includes placement of mesh or other prosthesis, when performed; reducible ●**49622** incarcerated or strangulated ●**49623** Removal of total or near total non-infected mesh or other prosthesis at the time of initial or recurrent anterior abdominal hernia repair or parastomal hernia repair, any approach (ie, open, laparoscopic, robotic)
Medicine: Vaccines, Toxoids	
None	#✦●**90584** Dengue vaccine, quadrivalent, live, 2 dose schedule, for subcutaneous use
Medicine: Cardiovascular	
✚**93568** Injection procedure during cardiac catheterization including imaging supervision, interpretation, and report; for pulmonary angiography	✚▲**93568** Injection procedure during cardiac catheterization including imaging supervision, interpretation, and report; for nonselective pulmonary arterial angiography ✚●**93569** Injection procedure during cardiac catheterization including imaging supervision, interpretation, and report; for selective pulmonary arterial angiography, unilateral ✚●**93573** for selective pulmonary arterial angiography, bilateral ✚●**93574** for selective pulmonary venous angiography of each distinct pulmonary vein during cardiac catheterization ✚●**93575** for selective pulmonary angiography of major aortopulmonary collateral arteries (MAPCAs) arising off the aorta or its systemic branches, during cardiac catheterization for congenital heart defects, each distinct vessel
Medicine: Behavior Management Services	
None	●**96202** Multiple-family group behavior management/modification training for parent(s)/guardian(s)/caregiver(s) of patients with a mental or physical health diagnosis, administered by physician or other qualified health care professional (without the patient present), face-to-face with multiple sets of parent(s)/guardian(s)/caregiver(s); initial 60 minutes ✚●**96203** each additional 15 minutes
Medicine: Remote Therapeutic Monitoring	
98975 Remote therapeutic monitoring (eg, respiratory system status, musculoskeletal system status, therapy adherence, therapy response); initial set-up and patient education on use of equipment **98976** device(s) supply with scheduled (eg, daily) recording(s) and/or programmed alert(s) transmission to monitor respiratory system, each 30 days	▲**98975** Remote therapeutic monitoring (eg, therapy adherence, therapy response); initial set-up and patient education on use of equipment ▲**98976** device(s) supply with scheduled (eg, daily) recording(s) and/or programmed alert(s) transmission to monitor respiratory system, each 30 days

Continued on next page

● indicates a new code; ▲, revised; #, re-sequenced; ✚, add-on; ★, audiovisual technology; and ◀, synchronous interactive audio.

Appendixes

Appendixes

Quick Reference to 2023 *CPT* Pediatric Code Changes (*continued*)	
2022	**2023**
Medicine: Remote Therapeutic Monitoring (*continued*)	
98977 device(s) supply with scheduled (eg, daily) recording(s) and/or programmed alert(s) transmission to monitor musculoskeletal system, each 30 days **0702T** Remote therapeutic monitoring of a standardized online digital cognitive behavioral therapy program ordered by a physician or other qualified health care professional; supply and technical support, per 30 days	▲**98977** device(s) supply with scheduled (eg, daily) recording(s) and/or programmed alert(s) transmission to monitor musculoskeletal system, each 30 days ●**98978** device(s) supply with scheduled (eg, daily) recording(s) and/or programmed alert(s) transmission to monitor cognitive behavioral therapy, each 30 days
0703T Remote therapeutic monitoring of a standardized online digital cognitive behavioral therapy program ordered by a physician or other qualified health care professional; management services by physician or other qualified health care professional, per calendar month	Report with **98980** or **98981** (unchanged from 2022).
Medicine: Autonomic Function Tests	
None (Prior code **0341T** was deleted January 1, 2020.)	●**95919** Quantitative pupillometry with physician or qualified health care professional interpretation and report, unilateral or bilateral
Category III	
No specific code	●**0720T** Percutaneous electrical nerve field stimulation, cranial nerves, without implantation
No specific code	●**0731T** Augmentative AI-based facial phenotype analysis with report
No specific codes	●**0733T** Remote real-time motion capture-based neurorehabilitative therapy ordered by a physician or other qualified health care professional; supply and technical support, per 30 days ●**0734T** treatment management services by a physician or other qualified health care professional, per calendar month ●✚**0770T** Virtual reality technology to assist therapy ●**0771T** Virtual reality (VR) procedural dissociation services provided by the same physician or other qualified health care professional performing the diagnostic or therapeutic service that the VR procedural dissociation supports, requiring the presence of an independent trained observer to assist in the monitoring of the patient's level of dissociation/consciousness and physiological status; initial 15 minutes of intraservice time, patient age 5 years or older ●✚**0772T** each additional 15 minutes intraservice time ●✚**0773T** Virtual reality (VR) procedural dissociation services provided by a physician or other qualified health care professional other than the physician or other qualified health care professional performing the diagnostic or therapeutic service that the VR procedural dissociation supports; initial 15 minutes of intraservice time, patient age 5 years or older ●✚**0774T** each additional 15 minutes intraservice time
Abbreviation: AI, artificial intelligence/augmented intelligence; ✎ indicates pending US Food and Drug Administration approval..	

● indicates a new code; ▲, revised; #, re-sequenced; ✚, add-on; ★, audiovisual technology; and ◀, synchronous interactive audio.

III. Vaccine Products: Commonly Administered Pediatric Vaccines

This list was current as of September 12, 2022. For updates, visit www.aap.org/cfp2023. For COVID-19 vaccines, see page 531.

CPT Product Code	Separately report the administration with *CPT* codes 90460 and 90461 or 90471–90474.	Manufacturer	Brand	No. of Vaccine Components
90702	Diphtheria and tetanus toxoids adsorbed (**DT**) when administered to <7 years, for IM use	SP	**Diphtheria and tetanus toxoids adsorbed (no trade name)**	2
90700	Diphtheria, tetanus toxoids, and acellular pertussis vaccine (**DTaP**), when administered to <7 years, for IM use	SP GSK	**Daptacel** **Infanrix**	3
90696	Diphtheria, tetanus toxoids, and acellular pertussis vaccine and inactivated poliovirus vaccine (**DTaP-IPV**), when administered to children 4–6 years of age, for IM use	GSK SP	**Kinrix** **Quadracel**	4
90697	Diphtheria, tetanus toxoids, acellular pertussis vaccine, inactivated poliovirus vaccine, Haemophilus influenza type b PRP-OMP conjugate vaccine, and hepatitis B vaccine (**DTaP-IPV-Hib-HepB**), for IM use	Merck/SP	**Vaxelis**	6
90723	Diphtheria, tetanus toxoids, acellular pertussis vaccine, Hepatitis B, and inactivated poliovirus vaccine (**DTaP-HepB-IPV**), for IM use	GSK	**Pediarix**	5
90698	Diphtheria, tetanus toxoids, acellular pertussis vaccine, Haemophilus influenza type B, and inactivated poliovirus vaccine (**DTaP-IPV/Hib**), for IM use	SP	**Pentacel**	5
90636	Hepatitis A and hepatitis B vaccine (**HepA-HepB**), adult dosage, for IM use	GSK	**Twinrix**	2
90633	Hepatitis A vaccine (**HepA**), pediatric/adolescent dosage, 2 dose, for IM use	GSK Merck	**Havrix** **Vaqta**	1
90740	Hepatitis B vaccine (**HepB**), dialysis or immunosuppressed patient dosage, 3 dose, for IM use	Merck	**Recombivax HB**	1
90743	Hepatitis B vaccine (**HepB**), adolescent, 2 dose, for IM use	Merck	**Recombivax HB**	1
90744	Hepatitis B vaccine (**HepB**), pediatric/adolescent dosage, 3 dose, for IM use	Merck GSK	**Recombivax HB** **Engerix-B**	1
90746	Hepatitis B vaccine (**HepB**), adult dosage, for IM use	Merck GSK	**Recombivax HB** **Engerix-B**	1
90747	Hepatitis B vaccine (**HepB**), dialysis or immunosuppressed patient dosage, 4 dose, for IM use	GSK	**Engerix-B**	1
90647	Hemophilus influenza B vaccine (**Hib**), PRP-OMP conjugate, 3 dose, for IM use	Merck	**PedvaxHIB**	1
90648	Hemophilus influenza B vaccine (**Hib**), PRP-T conjugate, 4 dose, for IM use	SP GSK	**ActHIB** **Hiberix**	1

Continued on next page

● indicates a new code; ▲, revised; #, re-sequenced; ✚, add-on; ★, audiovisual technology; and ◀, synchronous interactive audio.

Appendixes

Vaccine Products: Commonly Administered Pediatric Vaccines (*continued*)

CPT Product Code	Separately report the administration with *CPT* codes 90460 and 90461 or 90471–90474.	Manufacturer	Brand	No. of Vaccine Components
90651	Human Papillomavirus vaccine types 6, 11, 16, 18, 31, 33, 45, 52, 58, nonavalent (9v **HPV**), 2 or 3 dose schedule, for IM use	Merck	**Gardasil 9**	1
#90672	**Influenza** virus vaccine, quad (LAIV), live, intranasal use	AstraZeneca	**FluMist Quadrivalent**	1
#90674	**Influenza** virus vaccine, quad (ccIIV4), derived from cell cultures, subunit, preserv and antibiotic free, 0.5 mL dosage, IM	Seqirus	**Flucelvax Quadrivalent**	1
90685	**Influenza** virus vaccine, quad (IIV4), split virus, preserv free, 0.25 mL dose, for IM use	Seqirus SP	**Afluria Quadrivalent** **Fluzone Quadrivalent**	1
90686	**Influenza** virus vaccine, quad (IIV4), split virus, preserv free, 0.5 mL dose, for IM use	Seqirus SP GSK GSK	**Afluria Quadrivalent** **Fluzone Quadrivalent** **FluLaval Quadrivalent** **Fluarix Quadrivalent**	1
90687	**Influenza** virus vaccine, quad (IIV4), split virus, 0.25 mL dose, for IM use	Seqirus SP	**Afluria Quadrivalent** **Fluzone Quadrivalent**	1
90688	**Influenza** virus vaccine, quad (IIV4), split virus, 0.5 mL dose, for IM use	GSK Seqirus SP	**Fluarix Quadrivalent** **Afluria Quadrivalent** **Fluzone Quadrivalent**	1
#90756	**Influenza** virus vaccine, quad (ccIIV4), derived from cell cultures, subunit, antibiotic free, 0.5 mL dose, for IM use	Seqirus	**Flucelvax Quadrivalent**	1
90707	Measles, mumps, and rubella virus vaccine (**MMR**), live, for subcutaneous use	Merck	**M-M-R II**	3
90710	Measles, mumps, rubella, and varicella vaccine (**MMRV**), live, for subcutaneous use	Merck	**ProQuad**	4
#90620	**Meningococcal** recombinant protein and outer membrane vesicle vaccine, serogroup B (MenB-4C), 2 dose schedule, for IM use	GSK	**Bexsero**	1
#90621	**Meningococcal** recombinant lipoprotein vaccine, serogroup B (MenB-4C), 2 or 3 dose schedule, for IM use	Pfizer	**Trumenba**	1
90734	**Meningococcal** conjugate vaccine, serogroups A, C, W, and Y, quad, diphtheria toxoid carrier (MenACWY-D) or CRM197 carrier (MenACWY-CRM), for IM use	SP GSK	**Menactra** **Menveo**	1
#90619	**Meningococcal** conjugate vaccine, serogroups A, C, W, Y, quad, tetanus toxoid carrier (MenACWY-TT), for IM use	SP	**MenQuadfi**	1
90670	**Pneumococcal** conjugate vaccine, 13 valent (PCV13), for IM use	Pfizer	**Prevnar 13**	1
90732	**Pneumococcal** polysaccharide vaccine, 23 valent (PPSV23), adult or immunosuppressed patient dosage, when administered to ≥2 years, for subcutaneous or IM use	Merck	**Pneumovax 23**	1
90713	**Poliovirus** vaccine (IPV), inactivated, for subcutaneous or IM use	SP	**IPOL**	1

● indicates a new code; ▲, revised; #, re-sequenced; ✚, add-on; ★, audiovisual technology; and ◀, synchronous interactive audio.

Vaccine Products: Commonly Administered Pediatric Vaccines (*continued*)

CPT Product Code	Separately report the administration with *CPT* codes 90460 and 90461 or 90471–90474.	Manufacturer	Brand	No. of Vaccine Components
90680	**Rotavirus** vaccine, pentavalent (RV5), 3 dose schedule, live, for oral use	Merck	**RotaTeq**	1
90681	**Rotavirus** vaccine, human, attenuated (RV1), 2 dose schedule, live, for oral use	GSK	**Rotarix**	1
90611	**Smallpox and monkeypox** vaccine, attenuated vaccinia virus, live, non-replicating, preserv free, 0.5 mL dosage, suspension, for subcutaneous use	Jynneos	**Imvamune** or **Imvanex**	1
90714	Tetanus and diphtheria toxoids (**Td**) adsorbed, preserv free, when administered to ≥7 years, for IM use	MBL SP	**TDvax** **Tenivac**	2
90715	Tetanus, diphtheria toxoids and acellular pertussis vaccine (**Tdap**), when administered to ≥7 years, for IM use	SP GSK	**Adacel** **Boostrix**	3
90622	**Vaccinia (smallpox) virus** vaccine, live, lyophilized, 0.3 mL dosage, percutaneous	Sanofi Pasteur	**ACAM2000**	1
90716	**Varicella** virus vaccine (VAR), live, for subcutaneous use	Merck	**Varivax**	1
90749	Unlisted vaccine or toxoid	Please see *CPT* manual.	NA	NA

Immunization Administration (IA) Codes

IA Through 18 Years of Age With Counseling

90460	IA through 18 years of age via any route of administration, with counseling by physician or other qualified health care professional; first or only component of each vaccine or toxoid component administered (Do not report with **90471** or **90473**)
✚90461	IA through 18 years of age via any route of administration, with counseling by physician or other qualified health care professional; each additional vaccine or toxoid component administered

Immunization Administration

90471	IA, one injected vaccine (Do not report with **90460** or **90473**)
✚90472	IA, each additional injected vaccine
90473	IA by intranasal/oral route; one vaccine (Do not report with **90460** or **90471**)
✚90474	IA by intranasal/oral route; each additional vaccine

# indicates a re-sequenced code; ✚, an add-on code.

Pediatric COVID-19 Vaccine and Immunization Administration (IA) Codes

Manufacturer (Age Indication [Cap Color])[a]	*CPT* Product Code	Initial IA	Second IA	Third IA	Booster
Janssen (≥18 y)	91303	0031A	NA	NA	0034A
SARS-CoV-2 COVID-19 vaccine, DNA, spike protein, adenovirus type 26 (Ad26) vector, preserv free, 5×10¹⁰ viral particles/0.5mL dosage, for IM use					
Moderna (6 mo–5 y [blue with magenta label border])	91311	0111A	0112A	0113A	NA
SARS-CoV-2 COVID-19 vaccine, mRNA-LNP, spike protein, preserv free, 25mcg/0.25 mL dosage, for IM use					

Continued on next page

● indicates a new code; ▲, revised; #, re-sequenced; ✚, add-on; ★, audiovisual technology; and ◀, synchronous interactive audio.

Appendixes

Vaccine Products: Commonly Administered Pediatric Vaccines (*continued*)

Pediatric COVID-19 Vaccine and Immunization Administration (IA) Codes

Manufacturer (Age Indication [Cap Color])[a]	*CPT* Product Code	Initial IA	Second IA	Third IA	Booster
Moderna (6–11 y [blue with teal and purple border])	91309	0091A	0092A	0093A	NA
SARS-CoV-2 COVID-19 vaccine, mRNA-LNP, spike protein, preserv free, 50mcg/0.5 mL dosage, for IM use					
Moderna (6–11 y [dark blue with purple border])	91314	NA	NA	NA	0144A
SARS-CoV-2 COVID-19 vaccine, mRNA-LNP, spike protein, bivalent, preserv free, 25 mcg/0.25 mL dosage, for IM use					
Moderna (≥12 y [red with light blue border])	91301	0011A	0012A	0013A	NA
SARS-CoV-2 COVID-19 vaccine, mRNA-LNP, spike protein, preserv free, 100 mcg/0.5mL dosage, for IM use, Spikevax					
Moderna (≥18 y, booster [pulled from booster dose vial, blue with purple border])	91309	NA	NA	NA	0094A
SARS-CoV-2 COVID-19 vaccine, mRNA-LNP, spike protein, preserv free, 50 mcg/0.5 mL dosage, for IM use					
Moderna (≥18 y, booster [pulled from primary dose vial, red])	91306	NA	NA	NA	0064A
SARS-CoV-2 COVID-19 vaccine, mRNA-LNP, spike protein, preserv free, 50 mcg/0.25 mL dosage, for IM use					
Moderna (≥18 y [dark blue with gray border])	91313	NA	NA	NA	0134A
SARS-CoV-2 COVID-19 vaccine, mRNA-LNP, spike protein, bivalent, preserv free, 50 mcg/0.5 mL dosage, for IM use					
Novavax (≥18 y)	91304	0041A	0042A	NA	NA
SARS-CoV-2 COVID-19 vaccine, recombinant spike protein nanoparticle, saponin-based adjuvant, preserv free, 5 mcg/0.5mL dosage, for IM use					
Pfizer-BioNTech (6 mo–4 y [maroon])	91308	0081A	0082A	0083A	NA
SARS-CoV-2 COVID-19 vaccine, mRNA-LNP, spike protein, preserv free, 3 mcg/0.2 mL dosage, diluent reconstituted, tris-sucrose formulation, for IM use					
Pfizer-BioNTech (5–11 y [orange])	91307	0071A	0072A	0073A	0074A
SARS-CoV-2 COVID-19 vaccine, mRNA-LNP, spike protein, preserv free, 10 mcg/0.2 mL dosage, diluent reconstituted, tris-sucrose formulation, for IM use					

● indicates a new code; ▲, revised; #, re-sequenced; ✦, add-on; ★, audiovisual technology; and ◀, synchronous interactive audio.

Vaccine Products: Commonly Administered Pediatric Vaccines (*continued*)

Pediatric COVID-19 Vaccine and Immunization Administration (IA) Codes

Manufacturer (Age Indication [Cap Color])[a]	*CPT* Product Code	Initial IA	Second IA	Third IA	Booster
Pfizer (5–11 y [orange])	91315	NA	NA	NA	0154A
SARS-CoV-2 COVID-19 vaccine, mRNA-LNP, bivalent spike protein, preserv free, 10 mcg/0.2 mL dosage, diluent reconstituted, tris-sucrose formulation, for IM use					
Pfizer-BioNTech (≥12 y [purple])	91300	0001A	0002A	0003A	0004A
SARS-CoV-2 COVID-19 vaccine, mRNA-LNP, spike protein, preserv free, 30 mcg/0.3mL dosage, diluent reconstituted, for IM use, Comirnaty					
Pfizer-BioNTech (≥12 y [gray])	91305	0051A	0052A	0053A	0054A
SARS-CoV-2 COVID-19 vaccine, mRNA-LNP, spike protein, preserv free, 30 mcg/0.3 mL dosage, tris-sucrose formulation, for IM use, Comirnaty					
Pfizer (≥12 y [gray])	91312	NA	NA	NA	0124A
SARS-CoV-2 COVID-19 vaccine, mRNA-LNP, bivalent spike protein, preserv free, 30 mcg/0.3 mL dosage, tris-sucrose formulation, for IM use					
Sanofi-GSK (≥18 y)	91310	NA	NA	NA	0104A
SARS-CoV-2 COVID-19 vaccine, monovalent, preserv free, 5mcg/0.5 mL dosage, adjuvant AS03 emulsion, for IM use					

[a] Cap color applies only to Moderna and Pfizer-BioNTech products.

Abbreviations: *CPT, Current Procedural Terminology;* GSK, GlaxoSmithKline; IIV, inactivated influenza vaccine; IM, intramuscular; LAIV, live attenuated influenza vaccine; mRNA-LNP, messenger ribonucleic acid–lipid nanoparticle; MBL, MassBiologics; NA, not applicable; preserv, preservative; PRP, polyribosylribitol phosphate; OMP, outer membrane protein; quad, quadrivalent; SP, Sanofi Pasteur.

Appendixes

● indicates a new code; ▲, revised; #, re-sequenced; ✚, add-on; ★, audiovisual technology; and ◄, synchronous interactive audio.

IV. Test Your Knowledge! Answer Key

Chapter 1

1. *a.* *International Classification of Diseases, 10th Revision, Clinical Modification (ICD-10-CM).*

2. *b.* Always report on the basis of units included in the Healthcare Common Procedure Coding System code descriptor.

3. *d.* The code is reported for a service performed in addition to a primary service and is never reported as a stand-alone service.

4. *b.* The principal reason for the service provided on that date.

5. *c.* A diagnosis pointer in field 24E links the appropriate *ICD-10-CM* code(s) to services on each claim line.

Chapter 2

1. *b.* Procedure-to-procedure edits pair codes that should not normally be billed to the same patient by the same physician or physicians of the same specialty and same group practice on the same date.

2. *c.* This edit was deleted before its effective date.

3. *d.* Modifier **24** (unrelated evaluation and management [E/M] service by the same physician or other qualified health care professional (QHP) during a postoperative period) is appended to the E/M code to designate that the service was unrelated to the prior procedure.

4. *c.* Modifier **54** is appended to the surgery procedure code when the physician does the procedure but another physician or QHP in another group practice accepts a transfer of care and provides postoperative management.

5. *a.* True. *Current Procedural Terminology* and Healthcare Common Procedure Coding System modifiers can be appended to procedure codes in either code set when appropriate.

Chapter 3

1. *d.* All of the above. A patient's risk of increased health care use or risk adjustment is calculated by using claims data for physician services, patient demographics, health plan type, duration of coverage, and prescription drugs.

2. *a.* Learning about Healthcare Effectiveness Data and Information Set (HEDIS) measures applicable to the patient panel and proactively providing related services is a physician activity that supports HEDIS measurement.

3. *c.* The patient's experience with office staff can affect Consumer Assessment of Healthcare Providers and Systems survey results.

4. *a.* Health plans may count normal newborn care provided during the birth admission as 1 of 6 well-child visits before 15 months.

Chapter 4

1. *d.* Each relative value unit component may be independently adjusted slightly upward or downward as a function of geographic area.

2. *d.* American Academy of Pediatrics chapter pediatric councils meet with payers to discuss pediatric issues.

3. *b.* A 2-digit place of service code is entered on the claim.

4. *d.* All of the above. Conducting internal audits or reviews informs practice policy and procedures, detects missed revenue, and prevents issues with payers and outside auditors through early detection of internal errors.

5. *c.* *Assignment* refers to the patients a payer includes on your panel roster.

Chapter 5

1. *a.* The False Claims Act prohibits and establishes penalties for submitting claims for payment to Medicare or Medicaid that you know or should know are false or fraudulent.

2. *d.* Whenever a physician practice intends to enter a business arrangement that involves making referrals, legal counsel familiar with anti-kickback and physician self-referral laws should review the arrangement.

3. *b.* False. Compliance programs are required even for small practices, but they can be scalable.

4. *d.* All of the above. Compliant documentation must encompass what should be documented and safeguards from inaccuracies and potential noncompliant access to or disclosure of information.

5. *c.* Given the compressed timeline and dollars at stake, seeking legal advice is invaluable when a payer demands repayment based on atypical coding patterns.

Chapter 6

1. *d.* Critical care (hourly) is not selected on the basis of medical decision-making (MDM) or total time.

2. *c.* Emergency department services are not selected on the basis of time.

3. *d.* Time of clinical staff who obtained history and vital signs is not included in a physician's or qualified health care professional's total time on the date of the encounter.

4. *d.* b and c. Any combination of at least 2 elements of MDM that support moderate MDM is required to report a code that requires moderate MDM.

5. *a.* Presence via real-time audiovisual technology is sufficient to support presence for the key portion of an evaluation and management service provided by a resident in a rural location.

Chapter 7

1. *d.* Because the patient is seeing a physician of a different specialty (otolaryngology rather than primary care), the patient is new.

2. *b.* Review of the result of a test that was ordered between visits is included in the amount and/or complexity of data at the encounter during which the result is analyzed.

3. *b.* Follow-up evaluation and management (E/M) services initiated by the consultant or patient/family are reported as established patient visits based on the site of service (eg, established patient office visits).

4. *a.* To report services provided in an intermediate care facility for individuals with intellectual disabilities, a psychiatric residential treatment center, or a nursing facility, see codes in the Nursing Facility Services category.

5. *a.* Prolonged office E/M service (**99417**) is reported when the physician's total time on the date of the encounter exceeds the minimum time of the primary service by at least 15 minutes. Clinical staff time and time spent on other dates is not included.

Chapter 8

1. *c.* A newborn who is found to have ankyloglossia that requires release at the encounter is an example supporting an abnormal finding during a routine health examination.

2. *a.* Influenza immunization of an 18-year-old patient with physician counseling is reported with code **90460**.

3. *c.* Administration of a COVID-19 vaccine is reported with codes **0001A– 0112A**.

4. *b.* Code **99402** is appropriate for reporting 23 to 37 minutes of preventive medicine counseling to an individual patient.

5. *d.* All of the above. The problem-oriented service must be separately identifiable in the documentation and significantly beyond the work of the preventive service, and modifier **25** is appended to the code for the problem-oriented service.

Chapter 9

1. *d.* Codes **99441–99443** may be reported for the telephone evaluation and management (E/M) that is patient initiated and neither related to an E/M service within the prior 7 days nor occurring within a postoperative period.

2. *d.* All of the above. **G2012** and **G2252** are not limited to a specific asynchronous technology.

3. *b.* Online digital E/M services include the physician's or other qualified health care professional's cumulative time devoted to the patient's care over 7 days whether the time is spent addressing a single problem or multiple different problems within the 7-day period.

4. *a.* The Centers for Medicare & Medicaid Services created code **G2010** as a virtual check-in service allowing payment for evaluation of patient images and/or recorded video sent via digital technology.

5. *c.* When the reporting requirements are met, the requesting physician may report **99452** for time spent preparing for and participating in the consultative service.

Chapter 10

1. *d.* The period of service for transitional care management begins on the date of discharge and continues for the next 29 days.

2. *c.* At least 20 minutes of clinical staff time spent in chronic care management activities must be documented to support code **99490**.

3. *d.* To support principal care management, the complex chronic condition must be expected to last at least 3 months.

4. *c.* Principal care management and care plan oversight are never reported by a physician or qualified health care professional for the same patient in the same month.

5. *b.* Codes **99358** and **99359** are reported only when provided on a date other than the date of a face-to face evaluation and management service.

Chapter 11

1. *b.* These services may be covered through a plan and provider network separate from other health care services.

2. *c.* A code for dependence is reported for substance abuse with dependence.

3. *c.* Psychiatric collaborative care management **99492– 99494** are reported for activities of a behavioral health care manager working under physician supervision and in consultation with a psychiatric consultant.

4. *a.* Codes **96202** and **96203** are reported for behavior management/modification training provided to a multiple-family group of parent(s)/guardian(s)/caregiver(s).

5. *b.* False. The patient's presence is not required for the service described by code **90846**.

Appendixes

● indicates a new code; ▲, revised; #, re-sequenced; ✚, add-on; ★, audiovisual technology; and ◀, synchronous interactive audio.

Chapter 12

1 **d.** Interpretation and report is a professional component of a test.

2. **a.** Report code **36415** for all venipunctures not requiring the physician's skills to perform the procedure. See **36416** for collection of a capillary blood specimen and **36400–36410** for venipuncture requiring a physician's skill.

3. **c.** Report **87637** × 1 unit for performing the single test for SARS-CoV-2, influenza A and B viruses, and respiratory syncytial virus.

4. **d.** All of the above. Report injection of epinephrine in the office through an auto-injector with codes **J0171** and **96372** and the National Drug Code for the auto-injector.

5. **a.** Code **96127** is not valued to include physician work.

Chapter 13

1. **d.** *Scope of practice* is the term used to define the procedures, actions, and processes that are permitted for a licensed individual.

2. **b.** Qualified nonphysician healthcare professionals whose scope of practice does not include provision and independent reporting of E/M services may report assessment and management services.

3. **a.** Education and training for patient self-management are face-to-face services to an individual patient or a group of patients.

4. **c.** Modifier **33** is appropriately reported in addition to the code for medical nutrition counseling to indicate a preventive service.

5. **d.** A speech pathologist is a qualified nonphysician health care professional (QNHCP) as described in this chapter. Medical assistants are clinical staff and do not independently report services. Qualified health care professionals who may provide and independently report evaluation and management services are distinct from QNHCPs for coding purposes.

Chapter 14

1. **b.** Local or topical anesthesia is included in the global surgical package.

2. **c.** Removal of foreign bodies from skin that do not require an incision is included in the work of an evaluation and management (E/M) service and not separately reported.

3. **d.** Report **30901** when nasal packing is placed to serve a hemostatic and/or tamponade role but not when placed in the short term to administer medication. Also, report **30901** for control of hemorrhage by cautery.

4. **b.** Report **51701** for urinary catheterization to collect a clean-catch urine specimen. An E/M service and urinalysis are separately reported services.

5. **c.** Therapeutic, prophylactic, or diagnostic injections of medication other than chemotherapy are reported with code **96372**.

Chapter 15

1. **c.** Of medical decision-making, 2 of 3 elements must be met to support the code selected for an emergency department service. Time is not a factor in code selection.

2. **d.** Code **99281** does not require the presence of a physician or qualified health care professional (QHP).

3. **b.** Seventh character **D** of an *International Classification of Diseases, 10th Revision, Clinical Modification* code indicates a subsequent encounter during the healing phase of an injury.

4. **d.** All of the above. Report modifier **54** if another physician or QHP will provide care during the postoperative period. Closed treatment of nasal fracture without manipulation is included in an evaluation and management service.

5. **a.** Report **99291** × 1 unit and **99292** × 1 unit for the continuous 80-minute episode of critical care service that extended beyond midnight.

Chapter 16

1. **d.** **99463** is reported for the physician's initial admission and discharge management services when provided on the same date (regardless of the date of the newborn's birth).

2. **a.** **99465** (newborn resuscitation) is not reported in addition to **99464** (attendance at delivery).

3. **d.** The attending physician reports a category **Z38** code (liveborn infant) and **Z05.42** because the suspected infection was ruled out.

4. **c.** **99238** is reported for all discharge management services of 30 minutes or less except when admission and discharge management services are provided on the same date.

5. **a.** Subsequent visits following a consultation in the same admission are reported with codes **99231–99233**.

Chapter 17

1. **a.** When the physician has documented the total time spent on the date of the encounter, time may be used in code selection in lieu of medical decision-making (MDM).

2. **c.** Under Medicare split or shared guidelines, the individual who spent the greater portion of the combined time of service reports the service.

3. *a.* True. An outpatient evaluation and management (E/M) service provided on the same date may by separately reported, with modifier **25** appended to the outpatient code, in addition to an initial inpatient or observation E/M service.

4. *b.* When an attending physician provides both an initial face-to-face hospital service and discharge management at the same encounter, initial hospital or observation care (**99221–99223**) is reported.

5. *d.* When a physician spends 90 minutes providing initial hospital care with documentation of moderate MDM, code **99223** (≥75 minutes) is reported in conjunction with 1 unit of **99418** for the 15 minutes of prolonged service. **99418** is reported only when the primary E/M code is selected on the basis of time and is the highest code in the code category.

Chapter 18

1. *a.* Initiation of selective head or total body hypothermia (**99184**) is reported separately when provided in conjunction with neonatal critical care (**99468**, **99469**).

2. *c.* Split or shared policy applies when a physician and a qualified health care professional (QHP) of the same group practice provide critical care services.

3. *b.* Subsequent hospital inpatient or observation care (**99231–99233**) is reported for continuing care during the same admission.

4. *d.* Codes **99291** and **99292** (hourly critical care services) are reported for critical care services provided by physicians and QHPs other than the attending physician who reports daily codes.

5. *c.* Report **99479** (subsequent intensive care, infant weighing 1500–5000 grams) because subsequent intensive care is reported when the patient has previously received critical care services during the same admission.

Chapter 19

1. *c.* Append modifier **78** when a return to the operating/procedure room is necessary for a related procedure or treatment of complications during the post-operative period.

2. *d.* Both a and c. Report a reduced service or discontinued procedure when instructed by *Current Procedural Terminology* or when the procedure was significantly less than the typical service.

3. *b.* The teaching physician must be immediately available to furnish services during the entire procedure but is not required to be personally present or personally perform a procedure that is not minor, complex, or high-risk. Endoscopy requires the physician's personal presence during the procedure.

4. *b.* Code selection for left-sided heart catheterization for congenital heart defect is (**93595**) not based on the presence of normal or abnormal native connections.

5. *a.* Code **99024** is reported for manual breakdown of adhesions during the postoperative period because this work is included in the postoperative work of the procedure.

Chapter 20

1. *d.* A synchronous telemedicine service is reported with modifier **95** appended to the code for the service provided.

2. *c.* Modifier **93** signifies that a service was provided via synchronous audio-only technology.

3. *a.* The location of the physician or qualified health care professional delivering a telemedicine service is the distant site.

4. *c.* Modifier **FQ** is used only when reporting services to manage mental health or substance use disorders. Modifier **93** is reported for any service designated as eligible in *Current Procedural Terminology*.

5. *b.* False. Code selection for telemedicine services is not limited to selection based on the time spent in direct communication with the patient and/or caregiver. The requirements of the code for the service provided must be met.

Chapter 21

1. *c.* Physician review and interpretation of a patient's self-collected data outside a face-to-face visit is reported with code **99091**.

2. *c.* Code **94777** includes physician review and interpretation of the event data collected over a 30-day period and preparation of a report.

3. *b.* Code **99457** is used to report a physician's time spent in a calendar month using the results of transmitted physiologic data to manage a patient's treatment plan.

4. *b.* Patient-reported outcomes of therapy are an example of non-physiologic data that may be used in a treatment management service described by code **98980**.

5. *a.* Remote physiologic monitoring treatment management services (**99457**, **99458**) include time spent by clinical staff working under supervision by a physician or qualified health care professional.

Appendixes

Subject Index

Subject Index

Code Index

References are to pages. **Boldface** page numbers indicate the pages on which the primary code descriptions reside. *Current Procedural Terminology (CPT*) codes begin on this page; *CPT* modifiers begin on page 553; *International Classification of Diseases, 10th Revision, Clinical Modification (ICD–10–CM)* codes begin on page 553; and Healthcare Common Procedure Coding System (HCPCS) codes begin on page 556.

CPT Codes

Code Index

Summary of Changes Made to the Bright Futures/AAP Recommendations for Preventive Pediatric Health Care (Periodicity Schedule)

This schedule reflects changes approved in November 2021 and published in July 2022. For updates and a list of previous changes made, visit www.aap.org/periodicityschedule.

CHANGES MADE IN NOVEMBER 2021

HEPATITIS B VIRUS INFECTION

Assessing risk for HBV infection has been added to occur from newborn to 21 years (to account for the range in which the risk assessment can take place) to be consistent with recommendations of the USPSTF and the 2021–2024 edition of the AAP *Red Book-Report of the Committee on Infectious Diseases.*

- Footnote 31 has been added to read as follows: "Perform a risk assessment for hepatitis B virus (HBV) infection according to recommendations per the USPSTF (https://www.uspreventiveservicestaskforce.org/uspstf/recommendation/hepatitis-b-virus-infection-screening) and in the 2021–2024 edition of the AAP *Red Book: Report of the Committee on Infectious Diseases*, making every effort to preserve confidentiality of the patient."

SUDDEN CARDIAC ARREST AND SUDDEN CARDIAC DEATH

Assessing risk for sudden cardiac arrest and sudden cardiac death has been added to occur from 11 to 21 years (to account for the range in which the risk assessment can take place) to be consistent with AAP policy ("Sudden Death in the Young: Information for the Primary Care Provider").

- Footnote 33 has been added to read as follows: "Perform a risk assessment, as appropriate, per 'Sudden Death in the Young: Information for the Primary Care Provider' (https://doi.org/10.1542/peds.2021-052044)."

DEPRESSION AND SUICIDE RISK

Screening for suicide risk has been added to the existing depression screening recommendation to be consistent with the GLAD-PC and AAP policy.

- Footnote 16 has been updated to read as follows: "Screen adolescents for depression and suicide risk, making every effort to preserve confidentiality of the adolescent. See 'Guidelines for Adolescent Depression in Primary Care (GLAD-PC): Part I. Practice Preparation, Identification, Assessment, and Initial Management' (https://doi.org/10.1542/peds.2017-4081), 'Mental Health Competencies for Pediatric Practice' (https://doi.org/10.1542/peds.2019-2757), 'Suicide and Suicide Attempts in Adolescents' (https://doi.org/10.1542/peds.2016-1420), and 'The 21st Century Cures Act & Adolescent Confidentiality' (https://www.adolescenthealth.org/Advocacy/Advocacy-Activities/2019-(1)/NASPAG-SAHM-Statement.aspx)."

BEHAVIORAL/SOCIAL/EMOTIONAL

The Psychosocial/Behavioral Assessment recommendation has been updated to Behavioral/Social/Emotional Screening (annually from newborn to 21 years) to align with AAP policy, the American College of Obstetricians and Gynecologists (Women's Preventive Services Initiative) recommendations, and the American Academy of Child & Adolescent Psychiatry guidelines.

- Footnote 14 has been updated to read as follows: "Screen for behavioral and social-emotional problems per 'Promoting Optimal Development: Screening for Behavioral and Emotional Problems' (https://doi.org/10.1542/peds.2014-3716), 'Mental Health Competencies for Pediatric Practice' (https://doi.org/10.1542/peds.2019-2757), 'Clinical Practice Guideline for the Assessment and Treatment of Children and Adolescents With Anxiety Disorders' (https://pubmed.ncbi.nlm.nih.gov/32439401), and 'Screening for Anxiety in Adolescent and Adult Women: A Recommendation From the Women's Preventive Services Initiative' (https://pubmed.ncbi.nlm.nih.gov/32510990/). The screening should be family centered and may include asking about caregiver emotional and mental health concerns and social determinants of health, racism, poverty, and relational health. See 'Poverty and Child Health in the United States' (https://doi.org/10.1542/peds.2016-0339), 'The Impact of Racism on Child and Adolescent Health' (https://doi.org/10.1542/peds.2019-1765), and 'Preventing Childhood Toxic Stress: Partnering With Families and Communities to Promote Relational Health' (https://doi.org/10.1542/peds.2021-052582)."

FLUORIDE VARNISH

- Footnote 37 has been updated to read as follows: "The USPSTF recommends that primary care clinicians apply fluoride varnish to the primary teeth of all infants and children starting at the age of primary tooth eruption (https://www.uspreventiveservicestaskforce.org/uspstf/recommendation/prevention-of-dental-caries-in-children-younger-than-age-5-years-screening-and-interventions1). Once teeth are present, apply fluoride varnish to all children every 3 to 6 months in the primary care or dental office based on caries risk. Indications for fluoride use are noted in 'Fluoride Use in Caries Prevention in the Primary Care Setting' (https://doi.org/10.1542/peds.2020-034637)."

FLUORIDE SUPPLEMENTATION

- Footnote 38 has been updated to read as follows: "If primary water source is deficient in fluoride, consider oral fluoride supplementation. See 'Fluoride Use in Caries Prevention in the Primary Care Setting' (https://doi.org/10.1542/peds.2020-034637)."

CHANGES MADE IN NOVEMBER 2020

DEVELOPMENTAL

- Footnote 12 has been updated to read as follows: "Screening should occur per 'Promoting Optimal Development: Identifying Infant and Young Children With Developmental Disorders Through Developmental Surveillance and Screening' (https://doi.org/10.1542/peds.2019-3449)."

AUTISM SPECTRUM DISORDER

- Footnote 13 has been updated to read as follows: "Screening should occur per 'Identification, Evaluation, and Management of Children With Autism Spectrum Disorder' (https://doi.org/10.1542/peds.2019-3447)."

HEPATITIS C VIRUS INFECTION

- Screening for HCV infection has been added to occur at least once between the ages of 18 and 79 years (to be consistent with recommendations of the USPSTF and CDC).
- Footnote 32 has been added to read as follows: "All individuals should be screened for hepatitis C virus (HCV) infection according to the USPSTF (https://www.uspreventiveservicestaskforce.org/uspstf/recommendation/hepatitis-c-screening) and Centers for Disease Control and Prevention (CDC) recommendations (https://www.cdc.gov/mmwr/volumes/69/rr/rr6902a1.htm) at least once between the ages of 18 and 79. Those at increased risk of HCV infection, including those who are persons with past or current injection drug use, should be tested for HCV infection and reassessed annually."

HRSA
Health Resources & Services Administration

This program is supported by the Health Resources and Services Administration (HRSA) of the U.S. Department of Health and Human Services (HHS) as part of an award totaling $5,000,000 with 10 percent financed with non-governmental sources. The contents are those of the author(s) and do not necessarily represent the official views of, nor an endorsement, by HRSA, HHS, or the U.S. Government. For more information, please visit HRSA.gov.

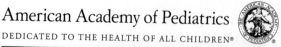
Each child and family is unique; therefore, these Recommendations for Preventive Pediatric Health Care are designed for the care of children who are receiving nurturing parenting, have no manifestations of any important health problems, and are growing and developing in a satisfactory fashion. Developmental, psychosocial, and chronic disease issues for children and adolescents may require more frequent counseling and treatment visits separate from preventive care visits. Additional visits also may become necessary if circumstances suggest concerns.

These recommendations represent a consensus by the American Academy of Pediatrics (AAP) and Bright Futures. The AAP continues to emphasize the great importance of continuity of care in comprehensive health supervision and the need to avoid fragmentation of care.

Refer to the specific guidance by age as listed in t
Bright Futures: Guidelines for Health Supervision of
of Pediatrics; 2017).

The recommendations in this statement do not ir
of medical care. Variations, taking into account in

The Bright Futures/American Academy of Pediatr
updated annually.

AGE[1]	INFANCY								EARLY CHILDHO			
	Prenatal[2]	Newborn[3]	3-5 d[4]	By 1 mo	2 mo	4 mo	6 mo	9 mo	12 mo	15 mo	18 mo	24 mo
HISTORY												
Initial/Interval	●	●	●	●	●	●	●	●	●	●	●	●
MEASUREMENTS												
Length/Height and Weight		●	●	●	●	●	●	●	●	●	●	●
Head Circumference		●	●	●	●	●	●	●	●	●	●	
Weight for Length		●	●	●	●	●	●	●	●	●	●	
Body Mass Index[5]												●
Blood Pressure[6]		★	★	★	★	★	★	★	★	★	★	★
SENSORY SCREENING												
Vision[7]		★	★	★	★	★	★	★	★	★	★	★
Hearing		●[8]	●[9] ——————→		★	★	★	★	★	★	★	★
DEVELOPMENTAL/SOCIAL/BEHAVIORAL/MENTAL HEALTH												
Maternal Depression Screening[11]				●	●	●	●					
Developmental Screening[12]								●			●	
Autism Spectrum Disorder Screening[13]											●	
Developmental Surveillance		●	●	●	●	●	●		●	●		●
Behavioral/Social/Emotional Screening[14]		●	●	●	●	●	●	●	●	●	●	●
Tobacco, Alcohol, or Drug Use Assessment[15]												
Depression and Suicide Risk Screening[16]												
PHYSICAL EXAMINATION[17]		●	●	●	●	●	●	●	●	●	●	●
PROCEDURES[18]												
Newborn Blood		●[19]	●[20] ——————→									
Newborn Bilirubin[21]		●										
Critical Congenital Heart Defect[22]		●										
Immunization[23]		●	●	●	●	●	●	●	●	●	●	●
Anemia[24]						★			●	★	★	★
Lead[25]							★	★	● or ★[26]		★	● or ★[26]
Tuberculosis[27]			★				★		★			★
Dyslipidemia[28]												★
Sexually Transmitted Infections[29]												
HIV[30]												
Hepatitis B Virus Infection[31]		★ ——————→										
Hepatitis C Virus Infection[32]												
Sudden Cardiac Arrest/Death[33]												
Cervical Dysplasia[34]												
ORAL HEALTH[35]								●[36]	●[36]	★		★	★
Fluoride Varnish[37]							←————————————————————————					
Fluoride Supplementation[38]							★	★	★		★	★
ANTICIPATORY GUIDANCE	●	●	●	●	●	●	●	●	●	●	●	●

1. If a child comes under care for the first time at any point on the schedule, or if any items are not accomplished at the suggested age, the schedule should be brought up to date at the earliest possible time.
2. A prenatal visit is recommended for parents who are at high risk, for first-time parents, and for those who request a conference. The prenatal visit should include anticipatory guidance, pertinent medical history, and a discussion of benefits of breastfeeding and planned method of feeding, per "The Prenatal Visit" (https://doi.org/10.1542/peds.2018-1218).
3. Newborns should have an evaluation after birth, and breastfeeding should be encouraged (and instruction and support should be offered).
4. Newborns should have an evaluation within 3 to 5 days of birth and within 48 to 72 hours after discharge from the hospital to include evaluation for feeding and jaundice. Breastfeeding newborns should receive formal breastfeeding evaluation, and their mothers should receive encouragement and instruction, as recommended in "Breastfeeding and the Use of Human Milk" (https://doi.org/10.1542/peds.2011-3552). Newborns discharged less than 48 hours after delivery must be examined within 48 hours of discharge, per "Hospital Stay for Healthy Term Newborn Infants" (https://doi.org/10.1542/peds.2015-0699).

5. Screen, per "Expert Committee Recommendations Rega Adolescent Overweight and Obesity: Summary Report"
6. Screening should occur per "Clinical Practice Guideline and Adolescents" (https://doi.org/10.1542/peds.2017-19 specific risk conditions should be performed at visits be
7. A visual acuity screen is recommended at ages 4 and 5 y may be used to assess risk at ages 12 and 24 months, in a Assessment in Infants, Children, and Young Adults by Pe for the Evaluation of the Visual System by Pediatricians"
8. Confirm initial screen was completed, verify results, and per "Year 2007 Position Statement: Principles and Guide (https://doi.org/10.1542/peds.2007-2333).
9. Verify results as soon as possible, and follow up, as appro

...ventive Pediatric Health Care
...an Academy of Pediatrics

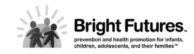

Bright Futures™
prevention and health promotion for infants, children, adolescents, and their families™

...right Futures Guidelines (Hagan JF, Shaw JS, Duncan PM, eds.
...ts, Children, and Adolescents. 4th ed. American Academy

...te an exclusive course of treatment or serve as a standard
...ual circumstances, may be appropriate.

...ecommendations for Preventive Pediatric Health Care are

Copyright © 2022 by the American Academy of Pediatrics, updated July 2022.

No part of this statement may be reproduced in any form or by any means without prior written permission from the American Academy of Pediatrics except for one copy for personal use.

| | | | MIDDLE CHILDHOOD | | | | | | ADOLESCENCE | | | | | | | | | | |
30 mo	3 y	4 y	5 y	6 y	7 y	8 y	9 y	10 y	11 y	12 y	13 y	14 y	15 y	16 y	17 y	18 y	19 y	20 y	21 y
●	●	●	●	●	●	●	●	●	●	●	●	●	●	●	●	●	●	●	●
●	●	●	●	●	●	●	●	●	●	●	●	●	●	●	●	●	●	●	●
●	●	●	●	●	●	●	●	●	●	●	●	●	●	●	●	●	●	●	●
★	●	●	●	●	●	●	●	●	●	●	●	●	●	●	●	●	●	●	●
★	●	●	●	●	★	●	★	●	★	●	★	★	●	★	★	●	●	★	★
★	★	●	●	●	★	●	★	●	←—	●10	—→	←—	●	—→		←—		●	—→
●																			
	●	●	●	●	●	●	●	●	●	●	●	●	●	●	●	●	●	●	●
●	●	●	●	●	●	●	●	●	●	●	●	●	●	●	●	●	●	●	●
									★	★	★	★	★	★	★	★	★	★	★
										●	●	●	●	●	●	●	●	●	●
●	●	●	●	●	●	●	●	●	●	●	●	●	●	●	●	●	●	●	●
★	★	★	★	★	★	★	★	★	★	★	★	★	★	★	★	★	★	★	★
	★	★	★	★															
	★	★	★	★	★	★	★	★	★	★	★	★	★	★	★	★	★	★	★
		★		★		★		←—●—→		★	★	★	★	★		←—		●	—→
									★	★	★	★	★	★	★	★	★	★	★
									★	★	★	★	←—		●	—→	★	★	★
																	—→	—→	—→
																●	—→		
									★	——————————							—→		
																			●
★	★	★	★	★															
			—→																
★	★	★	★	★	★	★	★	★	★	★	★	★	★	★	★				
●	●	●	●	●	●	●	●	●	●	●	●	●	●	●	●	●	●	●	●

...ding the Prevention, Assessment, and Treatment of Child and ...ttps://doi.org/10.1542/peds.2007-2329C).

... Screening and Management of High Blood Pressure in Children ...). Blood pressure measurement in infants and children with ...re age 3 years.

...ars, as well as in cooperative 3-year-olds. Instrument-based screening ...dition to the well visits at 3 through 5 years of age. See "Visual System ...iatricians" (https://doi.org/10.1542/peds.2015-3596) and "Procedures ...ttps://doi.org/10.1542/peds.2015-3597).

...llow up, as appropriate. Newborns should be screened, ...es for Early Hearing Detection and Intervention Programs"

...priate.

10. Screen with audiometry including 6,000 and 8,000 Hz high frequencies once between 11 and 14 years, once between 15 and 17 years, and once between 18 and 21 years. See "The Sensitivity of Adolescent Hearing Screens Significantly Improves by Adding High Frequencies" (https://www.sciencedirect.com/science/article/abs/pii/S1054139X16000483).
11. Screening should occur per "Incorporating Recognition and Management of Perinatal Depression Into Pediatric Practice" (https://doi.org/10.1542/peds.2018-3259).
12. Screening should occur per "Promoting Optimal Development: Identifying Infants and Young Children With Developmental Disorders Through Developmental Surveillance and Screening" (https://doi.org/10.1542/peds.2019-3449).
13. Screening should occur per "Identification, Evaluation, and Management of Children With Autism Spectrum Disorder" (https://doi.org/10.1542/peds.2019-3447).

(continued)

(continued)

14. Screen for behavioral and social-emotional problems per "Promoting Optimal Development: Screening for Behavioral and Emotional Problems" (https://doi.org/10.1542/peds.2014-3716), "Mental Health Competencies for Pediatric Practice" (https://doi.org/10.1542/peds.2019-2757), "Clinical Practice Guideline for the Assessment and Treatment of Children and Adolescents With Anxiety Disorders" (https://pubmed.ncbi.nlm.nih.gov/32439401), and "Screening for Anxiety in Adolescent and Adult Women: A Recommendation From the Women's Preventive Services Initiative" (https://pubmed.ncbi.nlm.nih.gov/32510990). The screening should be family centered and may include asking about caregiver emotional and mental health concerns and social determinants of health, racism, poverty, and relational health. See "Poverty and Child Health in the United States" (https://doi.org/10.1542/peds.2016-0339), "The Impact of Racism on Child and Adolescent Health" (https://doi.org/10.1542/peds.2019-1765), and "Preventing Childhood Toxic Stress: Partnering With Families and Communities to Promote Relational Health" (https://doi.org/10.1542/peds.2021-052582).

15. A recommended assessment tool is available at http://crafft.org.

16. Screen adolescents for depression and suicide risk, making every effort to preserve confidentiality of the adolescent. See "Guidelines for Adolescent Depression in Primary Care (GLAD-PC): Part I. Practice Preparation, Identification, Assessment, and Initial Management" (https://doi.org/10.1542/peds.2017-4081), "Mental Health Competencies for Pediatric Practice" (https://doi.org/10.1542/peds.2019-2757), "Suicide and Suicide Attempts in Adolescents" (https://doi.org/10.1542/peds.2016-1420), and "The 21st Century Cures Act & Adolescent Confidentiality" (https://www.adolescenthealth.org/Advocacy/Advocacy-Activities/2019-(1)/NASPAG-SAHM-Statement.aspx).

17. At each visit, age-appropriate physical examination is essential, with infant totally unclothed and older children undressed and suitably draped. See "Use of Chaperones During the Physical Examination of the Pediatric Patient" (https://doi.org/10.1542/peds.2011-0322).

18. These may be modified, depending on entry point into schedule and individual need.

19. Confirm initial screen was accomplished, verify results, and follow up, as appropriate. The Recommended Uniform Screening Panel (https://www.hrsa.gov/advisory-committees/heritable-disorders/rusp/index.html), as determined by Children The Secretary's Advisory Committee on Heritable Disorders in Newborns and Children, and state newborn screening laws/regulations (https://www.babysfirsttest.org/) establish the criteria for and coverage of newborn screening procedures and programs.

20. Verify results as soon as possible, and follow up, as appropriate.

21. Confirm initial screening was accomplished, verify results, and follow up, as appropriate. See "Hyperbilirubinemia in the Newborn Infant ≥35 Weeks' Gestation: An Update With Clarifications" (https://doi.org/10.1542/peds.2009-0329).

22. Screening for critical congenital heart disease using pulse oximetry should be performed in newborns, after 24 hours of age, before discharge from the hospital, per "Endorsement of Health and Human Services Recommendation for Pulse Oximetry Screening for Critical Congenital Heart Disease" (https://doi.org/10.1542/peds.2011-3211).

23. Schedules, per the AAP Committee on Infectious Diseases, are available at https://publications.aap.org/redbook/pages/immunization-schedules. Every visit should be an opportunity to update and complete a child's immunizations.

24. Perform risk assessment or screening, as appropriate, per recommendations in the current edition of the AAP Pediatric Nutrition: Policy of the American Academy of Pediatrics (Iron chapter).

25. For children at risk of lead exposure, see "Prevention of Childhood Lead Toxicity" (https://doi.org/10.1542/peds.2016-1493) and "Low Level Lead Exposure Harms Children: A Renewed Call for Primary Prevention" (https://www.cdc.gov/nceh/lead/docs/final_document_030712.pdf).

26. Perform risk assessments or screenings as appropriate, based on universal screening requirements for patients with Medicaid or in high prevalence areas.

27. Tuberculosis testing per recommendations of the AAP Committee on Infectious Diseases, published in the current edition of the AAP Red Book: Report of the Committee on Infectious Diseases. Testing should be performed on recognition of high-risk factors.

28. See "Integrated Guidelines for Cardiovascular Health and Risk Reduction in Children and Adolescents" (http://www.nhlbi.nih.gov/guidelines/cvd_ped/index.htm).

29. Adolescents should be screened for sexually transmitted infections (STIs) per recommendations in the current edition of the AAP Red Book: Report of the Committee on Infectious Diseases.

30. Adolescents should be screened for HIV according to the US Preventive Services Task Force (USPSTF) recommendations (https://www.uspreventiveservicestaskforce.org/uspstf/recommendation/human-immunodeficiency-virus-hiv-infection-screening) once between the ages of 15 and 18, making every effort to preserve confidentiality of the adolescent. Those at increased risk of HIV infection, including those who are sexually active, participate in injection drug use, or are being tested for other STIs, should be tested for HIV and reassessed annually.

31. Perform a risk assessment for hepatitis B virus (HBV) infection according to recommendations per the USPSTF (https://www.uspreventiveservicestaskforce.org/uspstf/recommendation/hepatitis-b-virus-infection-screening) and in the 2021–2024 edition of the AAP Red Book: Report of the Committee on Infectious Diseases, making every effort to preserve confidentiality of the patient.

32. All individuals should be screened for hepatitis C virus (HCV) infection according to the USPSTF (https://www.uspreventiveservicestaskforce.org/uspstf/recommendation/hepatitis-c-screening) and Centers for Disease Control and Prevention (CDC) recommendations (https://www.cdc.gov/mmwr/volumes/69/rr/rr6902a1.htm) at least once between the ages of 18 and 79. Those at increased risk of HCV infection, including those who are persons with past or current injection drug use, should be tested for HCV infection and reassessed annually.

33. Perform a risk assessment, as appropriate, per "Sudden Death in the Young: Information for the Primary Care Provider" (https://doi.org/10.1542/peds.2021-052044).

34. See USPSTF recommendations (https://www.uspreventiveservicestaskforce.org/uspstf/recommendation/cervical-cancer-screening). Indications for pelvic examinations prior to age 21 are noted in "Gynecologic Examination for Adolescents in the Pediatric Office Setting" (https://doi.org/10.1542/peds.2010-1564).

35. Assess whether the child has a dental home. If no dental home is identified, perform a risk assessment (https://www.aap.org/en/patient-care/oral-health/oral-health-practice-tools/) and refer to a dental home. Recommend brushing with fluoride toothpaste in the proper dosage for age. See "Maintaining and Improving the Oral Health of Young Children" (https://doi.org/10.1542/peds.2014-2984).

36. Perform a risk assessment (https://www.aap.org/en/patient-care/oral-health/oral-health-practice-tools/). See "Maintaining and Improving the Oral Health of Young Children" (https://doi.org/10.1542/peds.2014-2984).

37. The USPSTF recommends that primary care clinicians apply fluoride varnish to the primary teeth of all infants and children starting at the age of primary tooth eruption (https://www.uspreventiveservicestaskforce.org/uspstf/recommendation/prevention-of-dental-caries-in-children-younger-than-age-5-years-screening-and-interventions1). Once teeth are present, apply fluoride varnish to all children every 3 to 6 months in the primary care or dental office based on caries risk. Indications for fluoride use are noted in "Fluoride Use in Caries Prevention in the Primary Care Setting" (https://doi.org/10.1542/peds.2020-034637).

38. If primary water source is deficient in fluoride, consider oral fluoride supplementation. See "Fluoride Use in Caries Prevention in the Primary Care Setting" (https://doi.org/10.1542/peds.2020-034637).